Brain circuits and functions of the mind

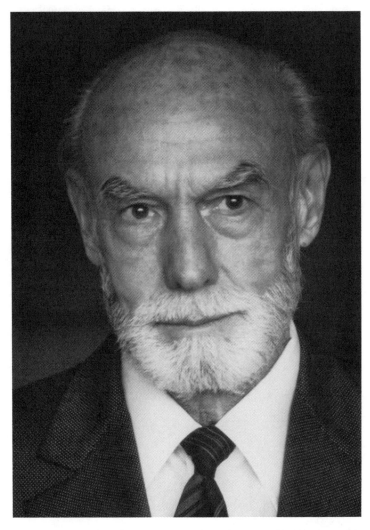

Roger Sperry at 68. Photograph taken by Lois E. MacBird for an article announcing Sperry's Nobel Prize in Caltech's *Engineering and Science*, November, 1981.

Brain circuits and functions of the mind

Essays in honor of Roger W. Sperry

Colwyn Trevarthen, Editor

University of Edinburgh

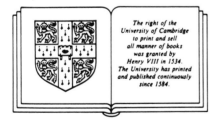

The right of the
University of Cambridge
to print and sell
all manner of books
was granted by
Henry VIII in 1534.
The University has printed
and published continuously
since 1584.

Cambridge University Press

Cambridge

New York   *Port Chester*

Melbourne   *Sydney*

Published by the Press Syndicate of the University of Cambridge
The Pitt Building, Trumpington Street, Cambridge CB2 1RP
40 West 20th Street, New York, NY 10022, USA
10 Stamford Road, Oakleigh, Melbourne 3166, Australia

First published 1990

Printed in the United States of America

Library of Congress Cataloging-in-Publication Data
Brain circuits and functions of the mind.

Includes bibliographies and index.
1. Neural circuitry.   2. Neurophysiology.
3. Neuropsychology.   4. Cerebral dominance.   5. Sperry,
Roger Wolcott, 1913–   .   I. Sperry, Roger Wolcott,
1913–   .   II. Trevarthen, Colwyn B. [DNLM: 1. Brain
—physiology.   2. Neurobiology.   3. Psychophysiology.
WL 103 B8135]
QP363.3.B72   1989   591.1′88   89-9852
ISBN 0-521-26102-3
ISBN 0-521-37874-5 (pbk.)

British Library Cataloguing in Publication Data
Brain circuits and functions of the mind: essays in
    honor of Roger W. Sperry.
    1. Man. Brain
    I. Trevarthen, Colwyn B.   II. Sperry, Roger W.
    612′.82

    ISBN 0-521-26102-3 (hard covers)
    ISBN 0-521-37874-5 (paperback)

Contents

Contributors   x

Foreword: Coordination of movement as a
  key to higher brain function: Roger W.
  Sperry's contributions from 1939 to 1952
    Edward V. Evarts   xiii

Editor's preface: Roger W. Sperry's lifework
  and our tribute
    Colwyn Trevarthen   xxvii

**Part I: Specification of behavioral nerve net-
  works in invertebrates   1**

1 **Ontogenesis of neuronal nets:** The che-
  moaffinity theory, 1963–1983
  Rita Levi-Montalcini   3
Introduction and historical survey of early
  findings   3
The "rebellious graduate student" and the
  evidence for chemical specificity   5
Behavioral and histological basis of the
  chemoaffinity theory   6
Recollections from a remote past   8
Chemoaffinity and the nerve-growth factor
  studies at a crossroad   9
The in-vivo neurotropic effects of
  NGF   9
The in-vitro neurotropic effects of
  NGF   10
Local control of neurite growth by
  NGF   12
Chemoaffinity and neurotropism: The same

or two different properties of nerve
  fibers?   14
The road ahead   15
References   16

2 **The chemoaffinity hypothesis:** An appre-
  ciation of Roger W. Sperry's contribu-
  tions to developmental biology
  *R. Kevin Hunt and
    W. Maxwell Cowan*   19
Introduction   19
Antecedents   24
The development of the chemoaffinity
  hypothesis   39
Chemoaffinity and developmental
  biology   62
Postscript   68
References   70

3 **Retinotectal connections made through
  ectopic optic nerves**
  Emerson Hibbard   75
Introduction   75
Eye rudiments grafted to hindbrain or
  spinal regions of amphibian embryos   76
Eye rudiments grafted to forebrain or mid-
  brain regions of amphibian embryos   76
Eye rudiments grafted to genetically eye-
  less embryos   77
Optic nerve experimentally deflected to ab-
  normal entry sites   78
Hypertrophy in regenerating optic cells
  that fail to make endings   79
Conclusions   82

Acknowledgments   83
References   83

4   **Neural reconnection between the eye and the brain in goldfish**
Myong G. Yoon   86
Topographic pattern of the visual projection   86
Sperry's theory of neuronal specificity   87
Retinotectal size-disparity experiments   87
"Systems-matching" hypothesis versus "topographic-regulation" hypothesis   88
Tectal reimplantation after rotation or inversion   89
Reciprocal transplantation between the tectum and the forebrain   92
Retention of topographic addresses and topographic polarity by reciprocally translocated and rotated tectal reimplants   93
Regulative modification of topographic addresses in accord with the original topographic polarity   96
Acknowledgments   99
References   99

5   **The case for chemoaffinity in the retinotectal system:** Recent studies
Ronald L. Meyer   101
Introduction   101
Macrotopography in the visual projection   103
Stability of tectal markers   110
Polarity in tectal markers   111
Plasticity   111
Chemoaffinity models allowing for plasticity   115
Future of chemoaffinity   120
References   121

Part II: Split-brain studies of perception, motor coordination, and learning in cats and monkeys, and comparisons to humans   125

6   **The role of the corpus callosum in the representation of the visual field in cortical areas**
Giovanni Berlucchi and Antonella Antonini   129

Callosal connections and the representation of the vertical meridian of the visual field   129
Experiments with "split-chiasm" cats and the representation of the periphery by callosal connections   131
Callosal connections and visual maps in the superior colliculus   133
Visual Maps and callosal connections in the monkey   133
The corpus callosum and binocular interaction   134
Is the callosal pathway involved in inhibitory interactions between cells in the two hemispheres?   135
Plasticity in the development of the callosal system   136
Conclusions   136
References   137

7   **Studies of visual perception and orienting in cats with fore- and midbrain commissure section**
John S. Robinson and Theodore J. Voneida   140
Introduction   140
Our earlier studies of cognitive processing in the split-brain animal   140
Recent studies of changes in orienting and attending behavior resulting from commissurotomy   142
General discussion   152
Forebrain commissures and midbrain decussations: Differing effects of midline section   153
Conclusions   154
Acknowledgments   155
References   155

8   **Brain pathways in the visual guidance of movement and the behavioral functions of the cerebellum**
Mitchell E. Glickstein   157
Preliminaries   157
Introduction   157
Preferential and forced eye–hand coordination in split-brain monkeys   158
Finger use in split-brain monkeys   160
Visual-motor connections and conditioning   161

Contents

Visual input to the pontine nuclei and
cerebellum 161
Pontine receptive fields, laterality, and the
visual guidance of movement 161
The cerebellum and bimanual
control 163
The cerebellum and motor learning 163
Conclusions 165
Acknowledgments 165
References 165

9 Intermanual transfer, interhemispheric
interaction, and handedness in man and
monkeys
Bruno Preilowski 168
Coordination of the two hands in split-
brain patients 169
Intermanual transfer in monkeys and
handedness 173
Conclusions as to the role of the corpus
callosum in motor coordination of the
hands 178
Acknowledgments 179
References 179

10 Hemispheric specialization in monkeys
Charles R. Hamilton 181
Statement of the problem 181
Evidence for hemispheric specialization in
animals 182
Our experiments with monkeys 184
The overall picture 192
References 193

11 A corticolimbic memory path revealed
through its disconnection
Mortimer Mishkin and
Raymond R. Phillips 196
Experiment I: Memory failure after
crossed corticolimbic lesions, without
commissurotomy 197
Experiment II: Opening up a crossed
corticolimbic pathway by sparing
area TEa 201
Experiment III: Memory failure after
crossed corticolimbic lesions,
but only if combined with
anterior commissurotomy 204
Comment 208
Acknowledgments 209
References 209

Part III: Cerebral hemispheres and human
consciousness 211

12 Partial hemispheric independence with
the neocommissures intact
Joseph E. Bogen 215
Some extracallosal unifying
mechanisms 217
Some examples of nonverbal cross-
cueing (and of its failure) in the
human with complete cerebral
commissurotomy 218
Other sources of "mental duality" 220
A quantitative anatomy argument for significant hemispheric independence with
neocommissures intact 221
Experimental evidence for significant hemispheric independence with respect to
learning 221
Results with cortical spreading depression
(CSD), including a digression on methodological critiques 223
Hemispheric independence in the intact
human 225
Conclusion 227
References 228

13 Regulation and generation of perception
in the asymmetric brain
Jerre Levy 231
Some historical considerations 232
Brain-damaged and split-brain patients: An
inconsistency? 234
Behavior, perception, and hemispheric reg-
ulation in split-brain patients 234
Activation and specialization of the hemi-
spheres in normal people 240
Conclusion 245
Acknowledgments 246
References 246

14 The neurobiological basis of
hemisphericity
Harold W. Gordon 249
Prologue 249
Introduction 249
Concepts and confusions concerning hemi-
spheric functions 250
Neurobiological bases of cognitive function
and individual differences 251
The cognitive laterality battery 252

Hemispheric asymmetry and
psychopathology 254
Hormone concentrations and cognitive
function 256
Diurnial or sleep–wake variation in hemi-
spheric functional balance 258
Cognitive asymmetries and specific disabili-
ties or special talents 259
Epilogue 262
References 263

15 **Long-term semantic memory in the two
cerebral hemispheres**
Dahlia W. Zaidel 266
Introduction 266
What is the nature of long-term semantic
memory? 266
Long-term semantic memory in commissu-
rotomy patients 269
Performance of patients with unilateral
lesions 274
Semantic relationships among concepts
stored in LTM: Normal subjects 277
Concluding remarks 278
Acknowledgments 279
References 279

16 **Hughlings Jackson on the recognition of
places, persons, and objects**
*Oliver L. Zangwill and
Maria A. Wyke* 281
Introduction 281
Jackson on recognition of places 282
Case studies, since Jackson, of loss of tem-
poral memory associated with spatial dis-
orientation for place 283
Comparative incidence of right- and left-
hemisphere lesions in loss of topographi-
cal memory 284
Jackson on the recognition of persons 284
Laterality of hemisphere lesion and
prosopagnosia 285
Visual agnosia and the recognition of
objects 286
Lissauer on "mind blindness," and two
contrasting cases of visual
agnosia 287
Visual object agnosia and unilateral
lesions 288
Conclusions 289
References 291

17 **Lessons from cerebral commissurotomy:
Auditory attention, haptic memory, and
visual images in verbal associative-
learning**
*Brenda Milner, Laughlin Taylor, and
Marilyn Jones-Gotman* 293
Dichotic-listening tests of hemispheric
differences 293
Delayed matching-to-sample tests of haptic
shape perception: Right-hemisphere su-
periority; memory loss 294
Image-mediated verbal learning after cere-
bral commissurotomy 297
Acknowledgments 302
References 302

18 **The saga of right-hemisphere reading**
Eran Zaidel 304
Prologue: At Caltech 304
The classical tradition 305
The dramatic conflict 306
Interlude: A change of scene; at
UCLA 311
Working through 311
Resolution: A second look at right-
hemisphere reading in aphasics 314
Conclusion: A happy ending? 316
Epilogue 317
References 317

19 **The role of the right cerebral hemisphere
in evaluating configurations**
*Lawrence I. Benowitz, Seth Finkelstein,
David N. K. Levine, and
Kenneth Moya* 320
Introduction 320
Nonverbal communication in patients with
right-hemisphere lesions 321
Emotional behavior, emotional state, and
self-evaluation 324
Thought and language 325
Conclusions 330
Acknowledgments 331
References 331

20 **Growth and education in the hemispheres**
Colwyn Trevarthen 334
Transmission of culture by brain growth: A
new approach 335
Cortical growth in utero 336
Three steps by which cells become con-

nected in the central nervous
system 337
The neurobiology and genetic significance
of motives 339
Intrinsic regulation of brain growth
and the social transmission of
knowledge 340
Cultural intelligence in infants and
toddlers 341
Lateral asymmetries in early expressive
communication and in perception of
expressions 343
Genetic disorders of brain growth that
block development of symbolic
intelligence 347
"Inner expression" is made coherent by
asymmetric cerebral motives for communication from the start 349
Brain growth after birth: New
evidence 351
Evidence from psychological developments
to adolescence 353
Conclusions 356
References 357

21 **Hemispheric specialization in the aged
brain**
Robert D. Nebes 364
How cognitive processes change in old
age 364

Perceptual asymmetries in the elderly 365
Age and lateral asymmetry of memory
abilities 367
Selective spatial disability in the elderly –
An artifact? 368
Conclusion 369
References 370

22 **Forebrain commissurotomy and conscious
awareness**
Roger W. Sperry 371
Split-brain man 373
Functional asymmetry 375
Minor-hemisphere consciousness 377
Incompleteness of psychological
division 379
Implications for consciousness in the nor-
mal intact brain 381
Formula for psychophysical
interaction 383
Acknowledgments 386
References 386

Appendix A: Publications of Roger W.
Sperry 389

Appendix B: Students and collaborators of
Roger W. Sperry 396

Index 399

Contributors

Antonella Antonini
Istituto di Fisiologia Umana
Università di Verona
Strada Le Grazie
37134 Verona, Italy

Larry I. Benowitz
Department of Psychiatry
Harvard Medical School
Mailman Research Center 315
McLean Hospital
Belmont, Massachusetts 02178

Giovanni Berlucchi
Istituto di Fisiologia Umana
Università di Verona
Strada Le Grazie
37134 Verona, Italy

Joseph E. Bogen
Department of Neurological Surgery
School of Medicine
University of Southern California
1645 Poppy Peak Drive
Pasadena, California 91105

W. Maxwell Cowan
Howard Hughes Medical Institute
6701 Rockledge Drive
Bethesda, Maryland 20817

Edward V. Evarts
(d. July 2, 1985)

Formerly of the Laboratory of
    Neurophysiology
National Institutes of Mental Health
Bethesda, Maryland 20205

Seth Finkelstein
Department of Neurology
Harvard Medical School
Mailman Research Center 315
McLean Hospital
Belmont, Massachusetts 02178

Mitchell E. Glickstein
Department of Anatomy
University College
Gower Street
London, England

Harold W. Gordon
Western Psychiatric Institute and Clinic
University of Pittsburgh
3811 O'Hara Street
Pittsburgh, Pennsylvania 15261

Charles R. Hamilton
Division of Biology
California Institute of Technology
Pasadena, California 91125

Emerson Hibbard
Department of Biology
Pennsylvania State University
University Park, Pennsylvania 16802

R. Kevin Hunt
Department of Neuroscience
Children's Hospital Medical Center
300 Longwood Avenue
Boston, Massachusetts 02115

Marilyn Jones-Gotman
McGill University
Montreal, Quebec, Canada

Rita Levi-Montalcini
Institute of Cell Biology
Via Romagnosi 18A
C. N. R.
00196 Rome, Italy

David N. K. Levine
Department of Neurology
Harvard Medical School
Mailman Research Center 315
McLean Hospital
Belmont, Massachusetts 02178

Jerre Levy
Department of Behavioral Sciences
University of Chicago
Green Hall
5848 S. University Avenue
Chicago, Illinois 60637

Ronald L. Meyer
Developmental Biology Center and
Department of Developmental and Cell
   Biology
University of California, Irvine
Irvine, California 92717

Brenda Milner
McGill University
Montreal, Quebec, Canada

Mortimer Mishkin
Laboratory of Neuropsychology
National Institutes of Mental Health
9000 Rockville Pike
Bethesda, Maryland 20205

Kenneth Moya
Department of Psychiatry
Harvard Medical School
Mailman Research Center 315

McLean Hospital
Belmont, Massachusetts 02178

Robert D. Nebes
Geriatric Psychiatry Program
Western Psychiatric Institute and Clinic
University of Pittsburgh
3811 O'Hara Street
Pittsburgh, Pennsylvania 15261

Raymond R. Phillips
Laboratory of Neuropsychology
National Institutes of Mental Health
9000 Rockville Pike
Bethesda, Maryland 20205

Bruno Preilowski
Department of Psychology
University of Tübingen
Field Station Weissenau
Rasthalde 3
D-7980 Ravensburgh/Weissenau
Federal Republic of Germany

John S. Robinson
Formerly of the Department of Psychiatry
Brain-Behavior Research Center
University of California
Eldridge, California 95431

Roger W. Sperry
Division of Biology
California Institute of Technology
Pasadena, California 91125

Laughlin Taylor
McGill University
Montreal, Quebec, Canada

Colwyn Trevarthen
Department of Psychology
University of Edinburgh
7 George Square
Edinburgh EH8 9JZ, Scotland

Theodore J. Voneida
Department of Neurobiology
Northeastern Ohio Universities College of
   Medicine
P.O. Box 95
Rootstown, Ohio 44272

Maria A. Wyke
Institute of Psychiatry
London, England

Myong G. Yoon
Department of Psychology
Life Sciences Centre
Dalhousie University
Halifax, Nova Scotia, Canada B3H 4J1

Dahlia W. Zaidel
Department of Psychology

University of California, Los Angeles
Los Angeles, California 90024

Eran Zaidel
Department of Psychology
University of California, Los Angeles
Los Angeles, California 90024

Oliver L. Zangwill
(d. October 12, 1987)
Formerly of Kings College
Cambridge University
Cambridge, England

Foreword: Coordination of movement as a key to higher brain function: Roger W. Sperry's contributions from 1939 to 1952

Edward V. Evarts
(d. July 2, 1985)
Formerly of the Laboratory of Neurophysiology
National Institutes of Mental Health

Roger Sperry's career has had many phases: he has been a student of English literature, a physiological and a cognitive psychologist, a zoologist, an anatomist, and a philosopher, and has studied with individuals as diverse as Stetson at Oberlin, Weiss at Chicago, and Lashley at Harvard. I have been given the privilege (and at the same time the challenge) of writing an overview of Sperry's research, expressing my own ideas as to his achievements. As I began my writing, however, I soon realized that his contributions are too numerous and too varied for me to cover: he has made important discoveries in developmental neurobiology, in brain mechanisms for control of movement, and in the cognitive psychology of hemispheric specialization. Sperry's contributions in the second of these areas (control of movement) are the ones to which I have elected to devote this essay, since it is this area of Sperry's work that has had the most direct influence on my own thinking and scientific career.

Sperry's interest in movement and visuomotor coordination began very early, for he was associated with Stetson at Oberlin and his later work on developmental neurobiology and nerve regeneration involved observations of motor behavior. His first studies in Weiss's laboratory dealing with motor behavior (Sperry 1939, 1940) concerned the functional results of muscle transposition in the hind limb of the rat. This work was followed by observations on the functional effect of crossing the peroneal and tibial nerves in the rat (Sperry 1941). When he began these experiments, the weight of previous experimental evidence favored the view that complete or nearly complete functional adaptation could occur following nerve crossing or muscle transposition. Sperry's work showed that in the rat, however, reversal of flexor and extensor movements persisted indefinitely after transposition of the dorsiflexor and plantar extensor muscles. Sperry noted that under circumstances in which dorsiflexion was called for, the transplanted dorsiflexor muscle contracted, producing extension, and vice versa. A corresponding result was obtained (Sperry 1941) when the peroneal and tibial nerves were crossed. No sign of reeducative correction of function of the crossed peroneal and tibial nerves ever appeared.

One of Sperry's next contributions in this area dealt with the consequences of crossing nerves and muscles in the forelimb of the rat. Sperry (1942a) noted that in human patients, reeducation was reported to occur more readily after transposition of arm muscles than after transposition of leg muscles. Sperry's experiments on the forelimb of the rat, however, yielded results that were in essential agreement with his earlier findings on the hindlimb. Thus, both for nerve crosses and for muscle transpositions, the motor neurons to the test muscles continued permanently to discharge in their original innate action phase without adjustment to the reversed anatomical arrangement. The single exception to this lack of adaptation involved what Sperry referred to as a "trick" adjustment that was accomplished by the action of the intact musculature of the shoulder and a mechanical locking of the elbow joint rather than by corrective adjustment of the action of the muscles. The result obtained with transposition of muscles and crossing of nerves was then extended to sensory nerves (Sperry 1943a). In this study, sensory nerves were crossed and it was found that in spite of prolonged training under various conditions, the maladaptive spinal reflexes remained in every case without any evidence of a reorganization of central connections.

Contrasting features of adaptation in mammalian and amphibian species

The work of Sperry on consequences of transposition of muscles and crossing of nerves of the rat is of particular importance in relation to work by Weiss and others on amphibians, and in contrasting results in mammals and amphibians, Sperry (1945b) points out that the complete functional restoration that can occur in amphibians is not achieved through practice, adaptation, and experience, but is determined by growth-regulating factors. Thus, Sperry stated (1945b, p. 358) that

> apparently the same factors which are responsible in ontogeny for the development of normally adaptive anatomical and physiological neuron relationships between center and periphery remain influential in adult nerve regeneration. This particular type of adaptation is correlated with the lasting embryonic lability of amphibian tissues, and apparently does not occur in the mammalian organism except in early embryonic stages (Weiss 1935, 1936; Sperry 1941).
>
> After disarrangements in amphibians which cannot be entirely remedied by such growth-organizing factors and which therefore necessitate reeducative correction, as after reorientation and transplantation of muscles, limbs, and eyes, then a maladaptive effect inevitably ensues which remains uncorrected.

It is especially valuable to read Sperry's conclusions and speculations in his review (1945b) on the problem of central nervous reorganization, since he gives such a clear statement of his thinking about higher nervous function and the role that the cerebral cortex may have in adaptation. Thus, he wrote that

> on the motor side, the evidence suggests a limit in the minimum size of the functional units which are subject to dissociation and recombination by learning. Corollary to the conclusion that learning depends upon reorganization in the higher centers is the further deduction that reeducative dissociation and reintegration of motor patterns must therefore be restricted by the degree of refinement in the relations between the higher centers and the spinal motor system. One would consequently expect to see an increase in capacity for effecting detailed motor reorganization by reeducation in passing from the lower vertebrates through the mammals to man, correlated with the appearance and increasing elaboration of the corticospinal system. A marked increase of this kind is indicated by the data available. The urodele amphibian, for example, does not correct or even inhibit the normal action of the entire limb after transplantation has made the normal limb coordination detrimental to the animal (Weiss 1937). In the lower vertebrates it appears to be only generalized movements and orientations of the whole organism that can be recombined by learning. Even the rat is apparently not able to correct or even inhibit separately the movements of one limb joint after muscle and nerve crosses, indicating that the minimum functional units subject to dissociation and recombination by learning are considerably larger in the rat than in man and involve possibly movements of the limb as a whole. In man, not only the action of a single limb joint but even that of individual muscles about a joint can be dissociated and readapted to some extent (Sperry 1945b, p. 359).

As we recall this early phase of Sperry's work, it may be of interest to attempt to identify links between his early ideas on motor reorganization and coordination following nerve crosses and muscle transposition and his later experiments on the callosum and chiasm. It seems to me that in the passage just quoted, one can see that Sperry was thinking of the significance of differences between adaptation processes in lower and higher forms and that this in turn was forming the basis for his subsequent work on the cerebral cortex and the corticocortical connections within and between the hemispheres. But, before discussing Sperry's work on the cerebral cortex, it will be valuable to consider another line of work with lower vertebrates that he began at almost the same time as his work on nerve crossing and muscle transposition in the rat.

In 1942, Sperry (1942b) published a report describing the effects on visuomotor coordination in the newt of eyeball rotations of 180° accompanied by optic-nerve section carried out so as to favor random reassortment of the regenerating fibers. When recovery of reactions to visual stimuli occurred, the motor responses corresponded to the rotated position of the retina and involved erroneous spatial localization and other abnormalities of visual coordination dependent on the reversed visual field. These reversed reactions persisted without modification by experience despite their maladaptive character.

In undertaking this work, the underlying issue that Sperry addressed was similiar to the one that had been addressed in the studies on nerve crossing and muscle transposition in the rat. Thus, in introducing his report on visuomotor coordination in the newt after regeneration of the optic nerve, Sperry (1943c) began by pointing out that Stone and Zaur (1940) had shown that normal vision with accurate spatial localization of small moving objects was exhibited by amphibians following regeneration of a severed optic nerve. At the time that Sperry began his work involving optic-nerve section, the question remained as to whether the normality of the restored vision in the amphibian was due to a selective synaptic termination of the regenerating optic-nerve fibers in the same central loci to which they were originally directed or, alternatively, to a functional reorganization after indiscriminate regrowth of the optic-nerve fibers. In his observations on the newt after regeneration of the optic nerve, Sperry clearly showed that visually guided behavior following restoration of vision after

optic-nerve section and eye rotation conformed in all cases to the orientation of the retina. Visually guided behavior was normal in the 12 animals in which the eyeball had been left in a normal position and was systematically inverted and reversed when the retina had been rotated by 180°. This finding led Sperry to conclude that

> regenerating optic nerve fibers arising from different retinal loci must be distinguished from each other in the centers according to the relative location of their ganglion cell bodies in the retinal field, probably by differential physico-chemical properties imposed on them by a polarized differentiation of the retina in development. The experiments thus extend the demonstration of peripheral nerve specificity in amphibians (Weiss 1942) to include the fibers of the optic tract (Sperry 1943c, p. 53).

Sperry extended this study by an analysis of the retinal projection to the optic lobe in anurans, combining studies on optic-nerve regeneration with central lesions in parts of the optic lobe that mediated vision for particular subsectors of the visual field. Sperry reasoned that since there is an orderly projection of the retina on the optic lobe, localized lesions within a particular part of the optic lobe should produce blind spots in a particular part of the visual field. These blind spots could be detected by noting the sectors of the visual field in which a lure could be held without eliciting a motor response on the part of the animal and then showing that the blind spot was indeed localized by shifting the lure into a region to which the animal responded promptly. Sperry (1944) found that the types of scotomata produced by optic-lobe lesions following optic-nerve regeneration conformed consistently to those that had resulted in animals without the optic-nerve section and regeneration. This meant, of course, that a given segment of retina projected to precisely the same part of the optic lobe before and after regeneration of a cut optic nerve. This finding clinched the argument that there was specificity of loci both in the central target territory of the regenerating optic-nerve fibers and in the array of optic-nerve fibers themselves.

Additional work on the specificity of optic-nerve regeneration was carried out by Sperry in an experiment involving crossing of the optic nerves and contralateral transplantation of the eye. The results of these experiments were consistent with those of the earlier work, and demonstrated that the functional relations between retina and brain visual centers are strictly and systematically predetermined by growth-regulating factors irrespective of functional adaptation (Sperry 1945a).

At the time that Sperry published his work on specificity of regenerating optic-nerve fibers and lack of plasticity in visual motor patterns in amphibians, he was a member of the staff of the Yerkes Laboratories of Primate Biology, where he had moved in 1943. At that time, Yerkes Laboratories were jointly operated by Harvard University and Yale University, and the director of the laboratories was Karl S. Lashley. Sperry had moved from the University of Chicago to the Biology Department of Harvard University when he received his PhD from the University of Chicago in 1941, and had then moved to the Yerkes Laboratories when Lashley assumed the position of director and moved there from his position in the Psychology Department at Harvard University at Cambridge in 1943. As already noted in the quotations from Sperry's review article (1945b) on reorganization following nerve crossing and muscle transposition, Sperry felt that there was greater potential for reorganization on the basis of experience at higher levels of the nervous system. He believed that while adaptation due to learning was virtually absent in lower forms, it was, to a certain degree at least, present in higher forms, especially in primates. Thus, while Sperry was carrying out his experiments on the specificity of optic-nerve regeneration in amphibians, he was at the same time carrying out analogous experiments on primates at the Yerkes Laboratories of Primate Biology.

In reporting the failure of any reorganization following nerve crossing or muscle transposition in the rat, Sperry (1945b) noted that a number of reports from the clinical literature had suggested that movement reorganization following such procedures became increasingly possible as experiments were conducted in higher forms, and this in turn led Sperry to be increasingly interested in the higher levels of the nervous system and especially in the cerebral cortex. In his work on monkeys, Sperry's object was to discover whether or not there might be any major differences in capacity for readaptation between the rat and the monkey and to find out whether the results in the monkey would not approach closely those reported for man. It was hoped that such a comparison of the monkey and the rat might yield some clues to fundamental differences in organization of the central nervous system of these two forms that might explain in part the superior adaptability of the primates.

In his experiments on the effects of crossing nerves to antagonistic limb muscles in the monkey, Sperry (1947a) dissected free the nerve branches to the primary flexor and extensor muscles of the elbow and cross-united the nerves so that the nerves were forced to regenerate into muscles antagonistic to those that they had formerly supplied. Sperry noted that nerves of the arm rather than of the leg were chosen because, in human subjects at least, it appeared that motor readjustment might occur more readily in the arm. Following nerve regeneration and reestablishment of connections with muscle, all animals showed reversed movements. As a result, the animals avoided use of the impaired arm. Reversed movements in the monkeys, however, were much less conspicuous than they had been in the rat after similar nerve-crossing operations. Again, unlike the rat, there gradually appeared positive readaptation. The readaptation was usually preceded by a period of inhibition, when the occurrence of a reversed movement led to the cessation of movement. In summarizing these results, Sperry notes that the superior readaptive capacity of the monkey was readily apparent:

> the monkey is quick to halt reversed movements, as well as to find new ways of accomplishing various acts without using the abnormally innervated muscles. Positive correction in the contraction phase of the test muscles was also eventually achieved. The active coordination

of the cross innervated muscles became smooth and automatic in the course of two years in some reactions which received constant daily practice in regular cage activities. The rat, on the other hand, was found to repeat the reversed movements indefinitely without correction and even without inhibition of the reversed action.

Regarding the problem of the neurologic basis of the monkey's superiority, there are a number of known factors that appear significant. First, there are the obvious advancements in the structure of the primate nervous system and its associated end organs, of which the following may be listed as particularly pertinent: (a) the more highly developed sensorimotor cortex; (b) the more elaborate connection systems between the spinal limb centers and the higher levels of the brain, especially the corticospinal tracts and the dorsal funiculi and medial lemniscus system; (c) the increased ratio of sensory to motor fibers in the limb nerves; (d) the increase in number and differentiation of sensory nerve terminations in the skin, tendons, muscles and joints; and (e) the mechanical arrangement of the muscles and skeleton of the primate limb so as to permit a much greater range of variation in limb movements than is possible in the rat.

To these anatomic differences may be added a number of functional differences which showed up in the course of the experiments. First, the monkey appears to have a greater capacity for detecting the presence of abnormal movements and for sensing in some degree the location and nature of the motor difficulty. Whereas the rat may continue indefinitely to repeat without modification a movement in reverse and seems meanwhile to remain oblivious of the reversed action, the monkey indicates by its behavior a more direct awareness of when and where an error has been made. The beginning of a single movement in reverse is often sufficient in the monkey to disrupt the activity going on at the moment. Sometimes it appears that the monkey stops and concentrates its attention on the member that is at fault. This is particularly true when the limb is being used in a "voluntary" manner, as in reaching for or handling something.

This difference in capacity for perceiving the presence and location of adverse reactions is correlated with a second factor, namely, a difference in the way the animals naturally use their limbs. The rat is not adapted, like the monkey, for finely controlled, deliberate, delicate movements of individual limbs or separate segments of the limbs, as in manipulation. It is in movement of this sort that learning appears to occur most readily. Both the aforementioned factors are therefore probably important in the monkey's superiority: the ability to make discriminate voluntary movements of individual limbs and parts of the limb, and also the perceptual capacity to attend to such specific movements, to guide them and to note their effects.

There is a third possible factor, not unrelated to the two already indicated, which may also account in part of the monkey's quicker detection and inhibition of reversed movements, namely, a greater dependence of the motor control of limb movement on sensory cues, especially those originating within the limb itself. In the rat the adverse sensory effects resulting from movement of one joint in reverse is not sufficient, as in the monkey, to disrupt the motor sequence. The aforementioned three factors together make the reversed action of cross innervated muscles inconspicuous in the monkey as compared with the rat.

Another factor of significance is the greater diversity of limb movement present normally in the monkey. The rat tends to use a limb as a whole in a stereotyped manner, with relatively few variations of the coordination pattern. In the monkey, however, the various limb segments may act differentially, being flexed, extended or rotated in various combinations, with a large variety of possible permutations of the coordination pattern. Because dissociation in the action of cross innervated muscles is a prerequisite of readaptation, the monkey, with a high degree of such functional dissociation already present normally, has a great advantage over the rat, in which the limb muscles are more rigidly bound together in restricted functional associations.

The ability to activate the test muscles in many different combinations with other limb muscles opens the possibility for their activation in the new proper combination to suit the crossed innervation. It is necessary in learning a new motor skill to achieve the new coordination a first time, whether by directed effort or by accidental blunder. Once made, the new coordination can be reinforced by further repetition and practice. In the rat the proper coordination was apparently never achieved, even a single time. The limb always worked in the old patterns, without any trial variations. It remained questionable whether the motor system of the rodent is so organized as ever to permit the required reassociation of muscle function. The ability of the monkey to make diversified trial coordinations would seem to be an extremely important item.

Another factor favoring motor reeducation in the monkey is the fact that learning plays a much greater role in the original ontogenetic acquisition of motor coordinations. The monkey to start with is, therefore, already more experienced than the rat in learning new arm coordinations. Furthermore, it is to be expected that coordinations established largely by learning in the first place will be more easily reorganized by the learning process than those built into the system by processes of growth and maturation (Sperry 1947a, pp. 470–2).

This section from Sperry's comments on the significance of the adaptation following nerve crossing in monkeys is quoted at such length because it seems to me to be one of the most insightful statements that has ever appeared concerning the functional significance

of afferent input and of the cerebral cortex in the primate for control of the limb movement. Sperry also proposed that the fundamental difference in the adaptation in rat and monkey might depend on the fact that greater learning was possible in the monkey.

Within this same paper (Sperry 1947a) on the effects of nerve crosses in the monkey, Sperry described the effects of lesions of various parts of the cerebral cortex on adaptations that had occurred following nerve crosses. Unfortunately, the number of monkeys studied and the regions of cortex that were extirpated did not provide sufficient data to allow any firm conclusions as to those parts of the cerebral cortex that were critical. It would have been most interesting if selective lesions had been carried out in cortical areas now referred to as "premotor cortex." Recent observations (Wise 1984) suggest that premotor cortex is especially important for adaptability, flexibility, and coordination of the sort that would be important in the adaptation following nerve crosses. It would be most interesting to have data on the consequences of premotor cortex lesions for adaptations of the type that Sperry found to occur following nerve process in the Macaque.

At the same time that Sperry was studying the effects of nerve crosses on the upper limb of the monkey, he carried out a new type of experiment in the amphibian, studying the nature of functional recovery following regeneration of the oculomotor nerve that had been divided in amphibians. These new experiments on the oculomotor system provided still more evidence that the readjustment process in the amphibian is dependent upon an embryonic plasticity and reversibility of neuron specification rather than central readjustment due to learning. Thus, there was little evidence for a central reorganization of the type that occurred in the primate, but instead there was evidence for a fundamentally different process: the capacity of amphibia to exhibit adaptations following a variety of nerve crosses depended upon the capacity of motor neurons to shift their myotypic specificity in the adult. In contrast, Sperry noted that

in mammals the specificity in the motor neurons of the limb as well as of the oculomotor system presumably becomes irreversibly determined very early in development.

There may be a tendency in the course of evolution for the specification of the nerve centers and the adjustment of their connections to become more and more dependent on peripheral regulation wherever possible. If so, this would account further for the difference between amphibians and mammals and between the limb and oculomotor centers in respect to recovery following nerve regeneration (Sperry 1947c, p. 313).

Sperry pursued the issue of patterning of synaptic associations in regeneration of fiber tracts by studying the effects of brain transsections in adult water newts. In these experiments, all the descending central fiber tracts that link the primary visual centers with medulla and spinal cord were severed and then, once regeneration had been demonstrated, experiments were carried out to determine whether the adjustment of the central connections might be dependent upon functional types of adaptation such as learning or whether it was regulated by factors intrinsic to the regeneration process itself (Sperry 1948). In general, it was found that regeneration took place and the lost functions were restored in an orderly and systematic manner.

Having demonstrated that the severed descending tracts from visual systems to spinal cord could regenerate in otherwise intact animals, Sperry studied the visuomotor coordination in animals in which hemisection of descending tracts was combined with eye rotation. In these instances, the animals showed maladaptive responses to eye rotation following regeneration of descending tracts just as would have been the case for eye rotation in otherwise intact animals. Likewise, the effects of optic-lobe lesions in animals with hemisection of the descending tracts were similar to those of optic-lobe lesions in intact animals.

These experiments added another stage to the demonstration of neuronal specification, showing that this specification extended from the retina through the optic lobe and into descending tract systems innervating the spinal cord. Sperry concluded that

> differential biochemical affinities exist between the higher and lower level neurons and that the selective patterning of synaptic connections is regulated by these affinities in accordance with a modernized chemotactic interpretation of the developmental organization of neuronal interconnections (Sperry 1948, p. 65).

In 1946, Sperry moved from the Yerkes Laboratories of Primate Biology in Orange Park, Florida (where he was associated with Harvard University), back to the University of Chicago, where he joined the Department of Anatomy and continued work on factors determining the specification of terminations of optic-nerve fibers within the tectum. While in the Department of Anatomy, however, Sperry maintained a keen interest in physiological psychology, an interest that may have been strengthened while he was at the Yerkes Laboratories of Primate Biology, where he was associated with Donald Hebb, Austin Riesen, Karl Lashley, and a number of other physiological psychologists. Indeed, one of the best summaries of his work on developmental neurobiology (Sperry 1951) appeared in a *Handbook of Experimental Psychology* edited by S. S. Stevens. Figure F.1 from Sperry's article in this handbook diagrams his experiment involving excision of the optic chiasm and crossuniting the optic nerves.

This figure showing optic chiasm surgery is reproduced here because just at the time that this article was appearing in 1951, Sperry was about to suggest to Ronald Myers, then a combined MD/PhD student at the University of Chicago, that it might be worthwhile to combine lesions of the optic chiasm with lesions of the corpus callosum in an experiment aimed at examining the role of the corpus callosum in transfer of information between the cerebral hemispheres. In discussing the start of Sperry's work on the corpus callosum, I would like to "flash back" to the Yerkes Laboratories in 1945, and to Sperry's studies on the role of corticocortical connections, studies that are of special historical interest because they provide

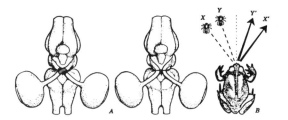

Figure F.1. Contralateral transfer of retinal projection on the brain. (**A**) By excising the optic chiasma and cross-uniting the four optic-nerve stumps as diagrammed, the central projection of the two retinas can be interchanged. (**B**) After optic-nerve regeneration, the animals respond as if everything viewed through either eye were being seen through the opposite eye. For example, when a lure is presented at *X* or at *Y*, the animal strikes at *X'* or at *Y'*, respectively. (From Sperry 1951.)

a link between Sperry's work on coordination after nerve crossing and muscle transposition with his work on the role of the great commissures.

One of Sperry's first studies on the role of corticocortical connections dealt with the issue of horizontal intracortical fibers in the cerebral control of limb movement (Sperry 1945c, 1947b). In seeking to address this general issue, Sperry selected the arm area of the cerebral motor cortex because of its importance in refined manipulatative voluntary movements of the hand and digits. Sperry wrote:

> In coordinated arm movements, the action at each joint of the limb must be regulated with reference to the action at all the other joints, and also the movement of the arm as a whole must be directed with respect to the posture and action at joints in the rest of the body. Cerebral regulation of arm movement would seem accordingly to require an integrated interaction or interplay of some kind among the various electrostimulable foci in the cortex for movement of these separate parts. It was proposed to find out what functional effect would follow the separation of these cortical foci from one another in the foregoing manner by a series of multiple intersecting incisions (Sperry 1947b, p. 275).

In the experiments stimulated by these ideas, Macaque monkeys received multiple intersecting knife cuts through the thickness of the cerebral cortex, these knife cuts being carefully carried out beneath the surface of the pia as to leave the blood supply intact. It was found that when the incisions were confined to the exposed cortex and extended only as deep as the upper part of layer VI, the effects on motor coordination were negligible.

The negative result that Sperry obtained in these experiments was *not* interpreted to mean that horizontal intracortical fibers have no function at all. His result was merely described as negative and he was cautious not to overinterpret it. As a matter of fact, it is interesting to note that he emphasized that his negative result applied to "intracortical, as distinguished from intercortical, integration" (Sperry 1947b, p. 275). Sperry was referring to the corpus callosum and other great commissures when he spoke in this quoted passage of *inter*cortical integration and one may assume that as he was writing this essentially negative result on the effects of subpial cross-cutting of cerebral cortex, he was wondering what might have been the effect of sectioning the corpus callosum.

During the years when Sperry was at Orange Park (1943–6), his own negative experiments on intracortical horizontal connections were discussed with Lashley and others in connection with the negative experiments of other investigators (e.g., Akelaitis 1941) on the lack of effects of interruption of the corpus callosum in neurological patients. I, myself, was a member of the staff at the Yerkes Laboratories in Orange Park a few years after Sperry left to go to Chicago, and during the years after his negative experiments on subpial sectioning but before his experiments on the corpus callosum, there were often lunchtime discussions of the negative outcomes and speculations as to what the experiments might mean. Lashley himself had actually carried out some preliminary (negative, of course) experiments involving section of the corpus callosum (see textbooks on physiological psychology by Morgan [1943] and Morgan and Stellar [1950], where a personal communication from Lashley is given). The same sorts of discussions that I had with Lashley may have gone on when Sperry was on the staff, and, thus, when Sperry left Orange Park and went to Chicago, he carried with him knowledge of the apparently negative results of corpus callosum section in man and subhuman animals and, in addition, was equipped with a wealth of experience as to the effects of nerve interruptions, including interruption of the optic chiasm. It was with this background that Sperry suggested to Ronald Myers in early 1952 that it might be worthwhile to examine the role of the corpus callosum in transfer of information between the hemispheres by combining an interruption of the corpus callosum with an interruption of the optic chiasm.

In connection with preparing this paper concerning Sperry's work, I phoned Ronald Myers to get his recollections of the events surrounding the experiment on the effects of combined interruption of the optic chiasm and corpus callosum in the cat, and, in what follows, I will use a number of the details that Myers provided. Myers started college at the University of Chicago in 1947 and then, in 1950, got a summer job with Roger Sperry in the Department of Anatomy; he actually began in Sperry's lab as a worker to make money rather than as a graduate student. He then stopped work to begin his first year in medical school in 1950, but when he entered the joint MD/PhD program and could begin his graduate research, he returned to Sperry's laboratory, where the scientific collaboration between Sperry and Myers began. The first project that Myers worked on involved an examination of the hypothesis that direct-current fields in the visual system were significant in pattern recognition and discrimination. This work involved setting up techniques for testing visual discrimination in cats, following which there were implantations of insulators or short-circuiting devices. These experiments were negative, but they were important in providing the techniques that were subsequently used in the experiments on the corpus callosum.

Early in 1952, Sperry made the crucial suggestion to Myers that it would be a good idea to examine the role of the corpus callosum in transfer between the hemispheres. When I talked to Myers on the phone, we discussed the possible origins of Sperry's idea for this experiment, and Myers had the following suggestions: (1) The roles of intra- and interhemi-

spheric connections were extensively discussed at Orange Park. When Myers mentioned this to me, I, of course, agreed, since my own initial research at Orange Park (suggested by Lashley) was concerned with the role of intrahemispheric corticocortical connections. Thus, one source of Sperry's suggestion was the general interest in significance of corticocortical connections as this had been expressed at Orange Park. (2) Sperry had become interested in the role of commissural connections in connection with his work involving optic chiasm section and interocular transfer of learning in fish. (3) Myers pointed out to me that Lashley himself had at one time done experiments involving section of the corpus callosum, and although these experiments were not published, it appears that the results of the experiments did find their way (via a personal communication) into a text of psychology by Clifford Morgan (1943). Thus, there are a number of indications that Sperry had been thinking about the great cerebral commissure for a number of years prior to going to Chicago in 1946.

In our phone conversation, Myers recalled the excitement with which the results of the initial experiments were awaited: both he and Sperry were well aware of the negative results of Akelaitis, and did not really know what to expect. As described in the initial report (Myers and Sperry 1953), however, the results were unequivocal. The combined callosum/chiasm section prevented interhemispheric transfer of a visual habit.

The concept of corollary discharge

Starting with observations on the effect of eye rotation associated with section of the optic nerve, Sperry (1943b) had demonstrated that such inversions of the normal connection of the visual system resulted in persistent abnormal movements on the part of the animal. Initially, Sperry used these behavioral aberrations as a basis for inferring the pattern of synaptic termination of regenerating optic-nerve fibers and then, in 1950, he published a paper using these abnormal movements as a basis for a theory that has had a great impact on ideas as to central programming of movement. His theory was suggested by the abnormalities of the spontaneous optokinetic response produced by visual inversion in fishes and amphibians. Sperry (1950) noted that following eye rotation in fishes and amphibians, circling persists indefinitely with no reeducation. In experiments done in 1942 and 1943, Sperry had shown that the same type of spontaneous optokinetic response produced by visual inversion could be produced by contralateral transplantation of the eyeball with inversion on only one axis and also by cross connection of the optic nerves to the wrong sides of the brain. Sperry introduced his 1950 paper by noting that

> the importance of the central mechanisms underlying these phenomena for the normal visual perception of space and motion prompted an attempt to find out something about the neural apparatus involved, using the forced circling of eye rotation as an indicator. The investigation was started with teleost fishes in which the circling phenomenon is particularly pronounced. In addition to various advantages which the fishes offer with respect to surgery, maintenance, and observation, the brain is comparatively simple and is much less susceptible to diaschisis than is that of the higher vertebrates (Sperry 1950, p. 482).

Having produced the continuous circling in fish by eye rotation, Sperry proceeded to extirpate various parts of the nervous system to determine the structures that were essential for the circling behavior. The cerebellum, forebrain, and inferior lobe could be extirpated without eliminating the circling. To his surprise, Sperry found that even labyrinthectomy could be carried out without eliminating circling.

In discussing the mechanisms underlying circling, Sperry raised two possibilities. The first explanation was the simpler, but it was one that Sperry rejected:

> An interpretation . . . could be conceived as follows: With the eye rotated, any movement that is visually initiated or guided, like that involved in centering the gaze on a peripheral object, would only

exaggerate, instead of resolving, the stimulating situation which induced it. This in turn would reinforce in cyclic fashion more of the same (erroneous) response. This interpretation has an advantage in that it can be expressed in purely reflex terms without requiring the assumption of an illusory spinning sensation in the animal.

It is difficult, however, to believe that the smooth, continuous forced circling which is made consistently in the same direction and which simulates exactly the circling produced by actual rotation of the visual field could be merely a repeatedly frustrated attempt to orient with reference to some visual object or a succession of such objects. Such an interpretation meets with further difficulties when applied to the urodele amphibians like *Triturus*. These animals make localizing and orientating movements of the head in any direction across the visual field. The spinning reactions of inverted vision, on the other hand, occur only toward one side, the direction of which correlates consistently with that of the circling produced by actual rotation of the visual scene. It is not unreasonable to assume, therefore, that an illusory spinning of the visual field, such as accompanies visual inversion in man, is present also in the lower vertebrates and that this is primarily responsible for the forced circling.

Assuming the whirling sensation to be present, it clearly could not result from the retinal stimulation in and of itself. Retinal inversion can exist only with reference to extra-retinal surroundings. It is the inversion with reference to the body and its movement (as registered in the nerve centers) that is crucial. Exactly the same pattern of excitations entering the brain from the retina may, in one instance, arouse the spinning reaction and in another, not, depending entirely upon the direction of the animal's movement accompanying the retinal influx. This is illustrated in Figure [F.]2. It applies to the whirling sensation in man as well as to the overt spinning of the fish. Thus, the

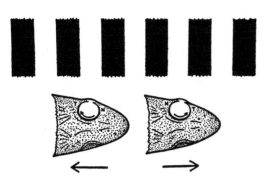

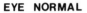

EYE NORMAL   EYE INVERTED

Figure F.2. The normal fish swimming backward is subjected to the same retinal stimulus as the fish with rotated eye moving forward. The same retinal influx that does not cause spinning in the former case does in the latter because of the direction of movement with which it is combined. *N* and *T* mark nasal and temporal poles of the eye. (From Sperry 1950.)

direction of the movement of the perceiving animal is one of the critical factors that condition the central effects of the retinal stimulus (Sperry 1950, pp. 486–8).

Having rejected the idea that the continuous circling behavior was a purely optic phenomenon resulting from the fact that the animal's responses tended to exaggerate rather than eliminate the retinal error, Sperry went on to propose his famous theory of corollary discharge:

> Another possibility must be considered, namely, that the kinetic component may arise centrally as part of the excitation pattern of the overt movement. Thus, any excitation pattern that normally results in a movement that will cause a displacement of the visual image on the retina may have a corollary discharge into the visual centers to compensate for the retinal displacement. This implies an anticipatory adjustment in the visual centers specific for each movement with regard to its direction and speed. A central adjustor factor of this kind would aid in maintaining stability of the visual field under normal conditions during the onset of sudden eye, head and body movement. With the retinal field rotated 180 degrees, any such anticipatory adjustment would be in di-

ametric disharmony with the retinal input, and would therefore cause accentuation rather than cancellation of the illusory outside movement.

The postulation of such a central kinetic factor would help account also for certain other phenomena in movement perception such as the illusory displacement of the visual field in man when the eyeball is moved passively as when tapped with the finger tips and the lack of such displacement when the same movement of the eye in space is brought about through an active response. It would provide a neural basis for what Helmholtz called the sensation of the "intensity of the effort of will." The need for some kind of central mechanism to eliminate blurring of vision between fixations in eye movement has long been recognized (Sperry 1950, p. 488).

Here, then, was Sperry's postulate as to the existence of corollary discharge, a concept that has had such a major impact on subsequent ideas as to central programming of movement. Recent reviews have shown how this concept has now become enmeshed in almost all thinking as to central organization of movement. Extensive references to Sperry's impact are seen in a recent paper (McCloskey 1981). An earlier review is seen in a paper by Evarts (1971). One person who was especially influenced by Sperry's concept was Hans-Lukas Teuber:

> as von Holst and Mittelstaedt, and quite independently, Professor Sperry, have pointed out, an organism which moves has to take its own movements into account. While looking into the world, he must be able to distinguish those movements of the environment that are environmentally produced from those movements that are consequences of the organism's own action (Teuber 1966, p. 579).

Before leaving this issue of corollary discharge and the impact of Sperry's ideas in the area of motor control, it would be worthwhile to point out that following Sperry's postulation of corollary discharges from motor into sensory centers, there have, in fact, been numerous microelectrode recordings in behaving primates that have demonstrated the existence of such corollary discharge. These have been made for visual centers such as the superior colliculus (Wurtz and Goldberg 1972) as well as for somatosensory centers (Fromm and Evarts 1982). Thus, Sperry's ideas as put forward in his 1950 paper have stimulated studies of neuronal activity in behaving animals that have indeed demonstrated the occurrence of discharges occurring in sensory areas in association with volitional active movement.

Neurology and the mind–brain problem

It is apparent in Sperry's early writings that he was indeed interested in the relevance of the studies he carried out in lower animals for higher brain function. Thus, in discussing the spontaneous optokinetic response following visual-field rotation in fishes and amphibians, Sperry considered the illusory movements of the visual field that result from visual inversions in man and considered the possibility of neural mechanisms that might give rise to corresponding cerebral events. Thus, Sperry was most interested in the relations between brain and conscious experience. From the standpoint of these relations, one of his especially important papers, published in 1952, just as the 1950 paper on corollary discharge, has had an immense impact on the ideas of those investigators studying brain mechanisms of movement. The impact was especially great because Sperry suggested a new and different approach to the mind-brain problem. Sperry wrote that

> An analysis of our current thinking will show that it tends to suffer generally from a failure to view mental activities in their proper relation, or even in any relation, to motor behavior. The remedy lies in further insight into the relationship between the sensori-associative functions of the brain on the one hand and its motor activity on the other. In order to achieve this insight, our present one-sided preoccupation with the sensory avenues to the study of mental processes will need to be supplemented by increased attention to

the motor patterns, and especially to what can be inferred from these regarding the nature of the associative and sensory functions. In the machine, the output is usually more revealing of the internal organization than is the input. Similarly in the case of our thinking apparatus an examination of its terminal operations and finished products may be more enlightening than any amount of analysis of the transport of raw materials into it (Sperry 1952, p. 296).

In initiating my review of some of Sperry's contributions to brain research, I pointed out that I intended to focus on that area of his work that was especially concerned with motor coordination and central control of movement and the paper that is the source of the just-quoted passage had an especially great impact on the thinking of investigators interested in the interface between motor behavior and higher brain function. Sperry's 1952 paper is of a special importance because it links the brain mechanisms underlying control of movement with the brain mechanisms underlying conscious experience and thought. From the standpoint of investigations that may be carried out in subhuman animals, this linkage is extremely important. Thus, if one accepts the notion that those parts of the brain especially concerned with control of movement may in fact be the very same areas serving to prepare the central nervous system for generation of behavior, then it becomes possible to plan experiments in which one uses microelectrodes to pick up activity of cells in motor and premotor structures with the idea that unobserved preparatory and planning processes in the animal may be reflected in these motor and premotor structures. My own early work was in both biology and psychology, and, like Sperry, I was associated with Karl Lashley at the Yerkes Laboratories of Primate Biology in Orange Park, Florida. Partly as a result of my Orange Park years, I always followed Sperry's work closely, and as I began to develop techniques for recording activity of nerve cells in intact behaving animals, Sperry's ideas had a great impact on the way in which my own work developed.

At the time that I began studying activity

of cells in awake behaving animals, the major approach of behaviorally oriented neurophysiologists was to study sensory systems, and to seek behavioral correlates of altered input/output relations by looking at various relays within the sensory systems. As it turned out, however, those studies that sought to observe changes in the visual pathways in association with altered responsiveness to visual inputs generally failed to observe the correlates until the loci of recordings reached those structures that were somewhat more motor than sensory in their function. This is seen clearly in the case of the early studies of Wurtz, who began with investigations of neuronal activity in the waking primate in the primary visual cortex, where it turned out that the responsiveness of neurons depended almost entirely upon the stimuli that were falling on the retina and not upon the way in which the animal was prepared to utilize the information generated by retinal signals. Within structures that are related to control of movement, however, there was a marked difference. Thus, it has been abundantly demonstrated that the "set," expectancy, preparatory state, and a variety of other central events are associated with marked changes both in the resting levels of neuronal activity and in the patterns of neuronal response in regions that we refer to as "premotor" in their function. Sperry's idea that thought should be conceived of in relation to brain mechanisms underlying control of movement led to a shift in the customary perspective with which scientists viewed the interrelation of cerebral and motor processes. Thus, Sperry wrote that

> instead of regarding motor activity as being subsidiary, that is, something to carry out, serve, and satisfy the demands of the higher centers, we reverse this tendency and look upon the mental activity as only a means to an end, where the end is better regulation of overt response. Cerebration, essentially, serves to bring into motor behavior additional refinement, increased direction toward distant, future goals, and greater over-all adaptiveness and survival value. The evolutionary increase in man's capacity for

perception, feeling, ideation, imagination, and the like, may be regarded, not so much as an end in itself, as something that has enabled us to behave, to act, more wisely and efficiently (Sperry 1952, p. 299).

Concluding comments

This citation from Sperry's paper on neurology and the mind-brain problem will end my consideration of his individual works. I have omitted considering the work on the great commissure because other contributors will deal fully with the enormous impact of the work that he started on the corpus callosum. What I have tried to do in my review is to show how his work on developmental neurobiology and motor coordination has led to so much of present-day behavioral neurobiology. I can only marvel at the numerous different areas that Sperry was able to contribute to simultaneously! What astonishes me especially in reviewing Sperry's publications in the years 1939–52 is that there were such immense contributions prior to the work on the corpus callosum. And, finally, I cannot close without adding a personal note expressing the extent to which I am indebted to him for the conversations that we have had over the years and for the very great influence that his ideas have had in directing my own research.

References

Akelaitis, A. J. 1941. Studies on the corpus callosum. II. The higher visual functions in each homonymous field following complete section of the corpus callosum. *Arch. Neurol. Psychiat.* 45: 788–96.

Evarts, E. V. 1971. Feedback and corollary discharge: A merging of the concepts. *In* E. V. Evarts, E. Bizzi, R. E. Burke, M. DeLong and W. T. Thach, Jr. (eds.) *Central Control of Movement*. The MIT Press, Cambridge, pp. 86–112.

Fromm, C., and E. V. Evarts. 1982. Pyramidal tract neurons in somatosensory cortex: Central and peripheral inputs during voluntary movement. *Brain Res.* 238: 186–91.

McCloskey, D. I. 1981. Corollary discharges: Motor commands and perception. *In* V. B. Brooks (ed.) *Handbook of Physiology. Vol. II. Motor Control, Part 2*. American Physiological Society, Bethesda (MD), pp. 1415–47.

Morgan, C. T. 1943. *Physiological Psychology*. McGraw-Hill, New York.

Morgan, C. T., and E. Stellar. 1950. *Physiological Psychology*, 2nd ed. McGraw-Hill, New York.

Myers, R. E., and R. W. Sperry. 1953. Interocular transfer of a visual form discrimination habit in cats after section of the optic chiasma and corpus callosum. *Anat. Rec.* 115: 351–2.

Sperry, R. W. 1939. The functional results of muscle transposition in the hind limb of the Albino rat. *Anat. Rec.* 75 (Suppl.): 51 (abstract).

–1940. The functional results of muscle transposition in the hind limb of the rat. *J. Comp. Neurol.* 73: 379–404.

–1941. The effect of crossing nerves to antagonistic muscles in the hind limb of the rat. *J. Comp. Neurol.* 75: 1–19.

–1942a. Transplantation of motor nerves and muscles in the forelimb of the rat. *J. Comp. Neurol.* 76: 283–321.

–1942b. Reestablishment of visuomotor coordinations by optic nerve regeneration. *Anat. Rec.* 84: 470 (abstract).

–1943a. Functional results of crossing sensory nerves in the rat. *J. Comp. Neurol.* 78: 59–90.

–1943b. Effect of 180 degree rotation of the retinal field on visuomotor coordination. *J. Exp. Zool.* 92: 263–79.

–1943c. Visuomotor coordination in the newt (*Triturus viridescens*) after regeneration of the optic nerve. *J. Comp. Neurol.* 79: 33–55.

–1944. Optic nerve regeneration with return of vision in anurans. *J. Neurophysiol.* 7: 57–69.

–1945a. Restoration of vision after crossing of optic nerves and after contralateral transplantation of eye. *J. Neurophysiol.* 8: 15–28.

–1945b. The problem of central nervous reorganization after nerve regeneration and muscle transposition. *Quart. Rev. Biol.* 20: 311–69.

–1945c. Horizontal intracortical organization in the cerebral control of limb movement. *Proc. Soc. Exp. Biol. Med.* 60: 78–9.

–1947a. Effect of crossing nerves to antagonistic limb muscles in the monkey. *Arch. Neurol. Psychiat.* 58: 452–73.

–1947b. Cerebral regulation of motor coordination in monkeys following multiple transection of sensorimotor cortex. *J. Neurophysiol.* 10: 275–94.

–1947c. Nature of functional recovery following regeneration of the oculomotor nerve in amphibians. *Anat. Rec.* 97: 293–316.

–1948. Orderly patterning of synaptic associations in regeneration of intracentral fiber tracts mediating visuomotor coordination. *Anat. Rec.* 102: 63–75.

–1950. Neural basis of the spontaneous optokinetic response produced by visual inversion. *J. Comp. Physiol. Psychol.* 43: 482–9.

–1951. Mechanisms of neural maturation. *In* S. S. Stevens (ed.) *Handbook of Experimental Psychology*. Wiley, New York, pp. 236–80.

–1952. Neurology and the mind-brain problem. *Am. Scientist* 40: 291–312.

Stone, L. S., and I. Zaur. 1940. Reimplantation and transplantation of adult eyes in the salamander (*Triturus viridescens*) with return of vision. *J. Exp. Zool.* 85: 243–69.

Teuber, H. -L. 1966. Summation: Convergences, divergences, lacunae. *In* J. C. Eccles (ed.) *Brain and Conscious Experience*. Springer-Verlag, New York, pp. 575–83.

Weiss, P. 1935. Homologous (resonance-like) function in supernumerary fingers in a human case. *Proc. Soc. Exp. Biol. Med.* 33: 426–30.

–1936. Selectivity controlling the centralperipheral relations in the nervous system. *Biol. Rev.* 11: 494–531.

–1937. Further experimental investigations on the phenomenon of homologous response in transplanted amphibian limbs. IV. Reverse locomotion after the interchange of right and left limbs. *J. Comp. Neurol.* 67: 269–315.

–1942. Lid-closure reflex from eyes transplanted to atypical locations in *Triturus torosus*. *J. Comp. Neurol.* 77: 131–69.

Wise, S. P. 1984. The nonprimary motor cortex and its role in the cerebral control of movement. *In* G. Edelman, W. M. Cowan, and E. Gall (eds.) *The Dynamic Aspects of Cortical Function*. Wiley, New York.

Wurtz, R. H., and M. E. Goldberg. 1972. Activity of superior colliculus in behaving monkey. III. Cells discharging before eye movements. *J. Neurophysiol.* 35: 575–86.

Editor's preface: Roger W. Sperry's lifework and our tribute

Colwyn Trevarthen
Department of Psychology
University of Edinburgh

This book celebrates the work of a man who has combined remarkable talents for discovery in both biological and psychological sciences – a man whose visionary insights into the development and functioning of the brain have given us a new understanding of human nature.

Born in Hartford, Connecticut, on August 20, 1913, Roger Wolcott Sperry graduated from Oberlin College in 1935 with a degree in English Literature, after which his life took a decisive turn to science. MA research in experimental psychology at Oberlin under the guidance of polymath R. H. Stetson opened the prospect of a life career exploring the intriguing processes of brain and mind. Though Stetson specialized in motor phonetics and the analysis of rhythm, his wide scholarship encouraged an interest in philosophy and the humanities as well as in empirical research. Sperry's first publication, in 1939, on coordination of muscle-action currents in human arm movements, gave prophetic statement to his own holistic vision of psychoneural research, as in the following. This extract also demonstrates a precision with words that has never left him:

> An objective psychologist, hoping to get at the physiological side of behavior, is apt to plunge immediately into neurology trying to correlate brain activity with modes of experience. The result in many cases only accentuates the gap between the total experience as studied by the psychologist and neural activity as analyzed by the neurologist. But the experience of the organism is integrated, organized, and has its meaning in terms of coordinated movement (Sperry 1939, p. 295).*

From that first exercise in behavioral physiology, advance was bold and swift. Doctoral research at Chicago with the top developmental neurobiologist of the period, Paul A. Weiss, taught Sperry the use of surgical techniques with the stereomicroscope, which he applied and developed in much of his later work. Weiss had demonstrated that movement patterns of amphibia were self-created in the embryo, and were apparently independent of specific nerve connections. By transplanting limb-buds and rerouting motor nerves, Weiss had found that salamanders could reconstruct excellent sequential control of limb muscles, fitting not the locomotor usefulness of the movements, but the embryonic origins of the different muscles – and regardless of the resultant derangements in their neural connections. These findings appeared to call for a fundamental reformulation of the prevailing textbook switchboard-connection theories of central nervous integration. Sperry felt Weiss's results in amphibians might be explained by a more highly specific form of control in the growth of nerve circuits than any existing theory had supposed.

In his doctoral research, Sperry examined related questions in rats, testing fiber connection versus impulse specificity (erregungspeci-

*Appendix A presents a full list of Roger Sperry's publications in chronological order.

ficität) theory by transplanting the insertions of extensor and flexor muscles of the limbs and cutting and interchanging their nerve supply. In 1941, he reported that this mammalian motor system, contrary to the then-prevalent doctrine, was hard-wired and highly resistant to reeducation. Except for some editing out of false moves of the forelimbs, the wrongly connected nerves or muscles continued indefinitely, unlike those in Weiss's amphibia, to produce maladaptive reversed limb movements. Edward Evart's foreword to this volume explains the significance of this early study.

It was striking that limb movements in the same animal species widely chosen by psychologists for experiments on learning could be so rigidly programmed. The observation led Sperry, in 1945, to review the use of corrective nerve and muscle surgery for motor losses in humans (Sperry 1945). He convinced surgeons that motor-nerve transplants were being carried out too freely, under the erroneous belief that the human brain could easily learn infinite new uses for motor nerves after they had been surgically connected to foreign muscles.

From 1941 to 1946, Sperry worked in Karl Lashley's lab, first as a Fellow of the National Research Council at the Harvard Biological Laboratories and then as a Fellow of Harvard University at the Yerkes Laboratories of Primate Biology in Orange Park, Florida. With Lashley, he published one paper on the effects of thalamic lesions in rats on olfactory learning, gaining firsthand acquaintance with Lashley's techniques. By then, however, his main interest had become focused on the laws that fitted nerves into functional networks in development. He confirmed an amazing finding of Robert Matthey in Switzerland and Leon Stone at Yale that after a newt's eye had been dissected from the head and replaced, the optic nerve could regrow connections to the brain and normal vision would return.

Analyzing the behavior of such animals more closely, Sperry showed further that when a transplanted eye had been rotated 180°, the newt's movements to catch food after recovery of vision were entirely misdirected, precisely as predicted by the theory that cells at each retinal point had reconnected themselves to the same

place in the brain as before surgery. All visual reactions became reversed like those of a person who has just put on inverting ocular prisms. Adaptive visuomotor coordination was never regained. This proved that the regenerating fibers beyond the scrambled tangle at the rejoined optic nerve had somehow unsorted themselves and grown back into the brain in a precise order, guided by some pathfinding principle in which learning played no part. This now classic finding contradicted the nerve-growth doctrine of the 1930s, in which the growth and termination of developing nerves was inferred to be essentially diffuse and nonselective, with earlier views of chemotropic and bioelectric guidance seemingly disproven.

Sperry's demonstration that the adaptive wiring of brain connections for behavior can be achieved in the growth process itself did much to resolve ongoing nature/nurture disputes of the 1930s and 1940s, at the center of which ethologists were pitting instincts and inheritance against the behaviorist's "prenatal conditioning." These early projects of Sperry exhibit qualities that were to secure him a lasting place in the history of brain research. The surgical, histological, and behavioral techniques were of the highest degree of skill and elegance and the reports are models of clear, concise reasoning and lively expression. Rita Levi-Montalcini, in Chapter 1, gives us an intimate glimpse of Sperry at the time when his neurospecificity studies were making him famous.

After returning to Chicago in 1946 as Assistant Professor of Anatomy, Sperry extended his nerve-growth experiments in amphibia to the cutaneous, vestibular, and other sensory and motor systems. From 1948, he also spent winter months at the Lerner Marine Laboratory at Bimini, British West Indies, working on small tropical fish collected from the nearby tide pools and reefs. His experiments showed that regeneration of the nerves going from eye to brain and from the brain to the muscles of eyes and fins (both of which make intricate movements in these marine species) obeyed the law of innate specification of connections. With Norma Deupree, a fellow biologist whom he married in December 1949, he carried out an important study at Bimini demonstrating that motor nerves prefer to regenerate connections to their own muscles; connections to wrong muscles were weaker. This suggested that the salamanders Weiss had studied were atypical and, years later, Richard Mark (1974) showed this to be the case.

In 1950, Sperry reported that fish and amphibians with vision surgically inverted consistently displayed another peculiar type of behavior. Quiet if not caused to swim, they proceeded to move in accelerating circles as soon as they stirred. This circling behavior was cured only by removal of the midbrain, where the optic nerves terminate. It was not affected after removal of the labyrinths or severance of the oculomotor muscles. Sperry concluded that the midbrain was the site of a predictive adjustment of visual perception from inside the brain, triggered by the motor impulse to turn and anticipating the sensory displacement caused by the movement. The retinal information regarding placement of the external world relative to the animal's head was reversed along the front/back axis as a consequence of the surgery. Instead of serving to stabilize the perceived world during movement, it had the reverse effect, signaling that the world was drifting away. As a result, the locomotor system worked harder to catch up, thereby worsening the illusory drift – like a kitten chasing its tail. Sperry proposed that there was an internal brain signal, which he named a "corollary discharge from efference." Such a "central kinetic factor," he pointed out, would help explain both perception of self-movement and the constancy of the visually perceived surroundings during movement. The discovery of this fundamental cognitive principle that coordinated perception with movement was also made simultaneously and independently by Erik von Holst and Horst Mittelstaedt, in Germany, in the optomotor reflexes of the praying mantis. They called it the reafference principle and explained it, under the name of efference-copy, by the same mechanism as proposed by Sperry.

Building on ideas learned at Oberlin, Sperry theorized that perception is basically a preparation to respond. In an essay entitled "Neurology and the Mind–Brain Problem," written in the Adirondack mountains on a forced year's leave from research to recover from tuberculosis, he argued in 1952 that deductions about the central unknowns of consciousness are better inferred from the patterns of motor output rather than those of sensory input, as is customary. He also questioned integrationist and anticonnectionist views of the Gestaltists and his teacher Lashley, indicating that mind–brain theories were better based on patterns of response than on postulated "field processes" or "mass action" in the sensory cortex. He showed prophetic insight into questions now being tackled by systems engineers and cognitive scientists who are trying to model intelligence with computational machines, and into questions that relate natural (or "ecological") categories of perceptual processing to the problems of coordination that the brain has to solve in order to make movements that use terrain or objects efficiently.

Wolfgang Kohler, Karl Lashley, and others were theorizing in the 1950s that form recognition was the result of "field" effects generated from transitory electrical or magnetic fields arising between active and inactive grey matter or of interference configurations generated by waves of activity spreading in random cortical fiber feltworks. To test such ideas, Sperry made minute criss-cross cuts under microscopic control throughout the visual cortex, riddled it with tantalum wires to short-circuit any electrical fields, and implanted leaves of mica to interrupt local transverse current. Such use of the stereomicroscope for mammalian brain surgery was a Sperry innovation, as well as the improvization of his own custom-made surgical instruments. To assess the behavioral effects of these cross-cut/implant operations, he and his students at Chicago, most notably Nancy Miner (who also worked on the formation of somatosensory nerve connections in frogs) and Ronald Myers, subjected the cats to extreme tests of perceptual ability to discriminate basic features of visual forms. They found virtually no losses in vision and concluded that form perception must depend on passage of information into and out of the small circumscribed cortical blocks or vertical columns, presumably interconnected by neuronal linkages lying below the cortical grey matter. The training and testing in these and other experiments in Sperry's lab were carried out in compact two-choice training boxes that fit easily on a small table and allowed a maximum of trials with a minimum of time, space, and effort. The apparatus was an original design of Sperry's based on principles of the Lashley jumping stand that had proven so successful for rats.

Ronald Myers, taking a PhD under Sperry at Chicago, along with his MD, elected for his doctoral thesis to work on problems of the corpus callosum, the function of which by then had become a major enigma and the proposed next project on Sperry's research agenda. Myers applied the stereomicroscope to work out a delicate operation to cut the crossover of visual nerves (*optic chiasm*) under the cat's brain, so each eye would lead to only one cerebral hemisphere. In 1953, he and Sperry reported not only transfer of visual pattern memory between the hemispheres in chiasm-sectioned cats, but also that this transfer was abolished when the fiber bridge between the hemispheres, the *corpus callosum,* was cut. Thus was created what Sperry in later years labeled the "split-brain" and with which his name is associated in the minds of psychology students everywhere. The results proved that the functions of the corpus callosum, which previously had escaped detection, include the transmission of perceptual learning from one to the other hemisphere. Edward Evarts reports on Ron Myers' recollection of the origins of the split-brain research, which go back to Sperry's years with Lashley.

Sperry became Section Chief at the National Institute for Neurological Diseases and Blindness under Seymour Kety in 1952. Meantime, he also remained Associate Professor of Psychology at Chicago while awaiting completion of a new building at Bethesda. Then, in 1954, Sperry moved to the Hixon Chair of Psychobiology at the California Institute of Technology, Pasadena. Viktor Hamburger, on the occasion of the presentation to Sperry of the Ralph W. Gerard Prize of the Society for Neuroscience in 1979, recalled how the offer of a chair in Psychobiology at Caltech arose from Sperry's impressive presentation of his chemoaffinity concepts of brain development to a Symposium of the Growth Society in 1950 (Sperry 1951; Hamburger 1979).

At Caltech, extensions of the split-brain studies revealed that monkeys as well as cats show independent learning, perception, and memory in the two brain halves after transection of the optic chiasm and forebrain commissures. With Myers and other graduate students and postdoctoral workers, including John Stamm and Alan Schrier, work continued unabated through the fifties on the divided awareness and learning of split-brain cats, confirming the role of the commissural fibers in memory formation and exploring routes by which vision or touch accesses voluntary limb movements (Sperry 1961). The technique was extended to monkeys with contributions into the sixties and beyond from Gil French, Mitch Glickstein, Colwyn Trevarthen, Chuck Hamilton, Betty Vermeire, Joe Bossom, John Steiner, Michael Gazzaniga, Evelyn Lee-Teng, Rochelle Gavalas, and the list goes on (see Appendix B); Ted Voneida, Jack Robinson, Doug Webster, James Carl, Giovanni Berlucchi, and others continued work with cats.

With the cerebral hemispheres surgically disconnected, monkeys were able to learn simultaneously two mutually contradictory visual discrimination habits in the right and left half-brains, showing the split-brain monkey must therefore possess double and separate realms of consciousness. In the cat, each disconnected hemisphere directed movements of the whole body, but with monkeys, hand movements on the side of the seeing hemisphere were, at least in the immediate postsurgical period, less willing to respond and, if forced into action, were clumsy, as if the monkeys became partially blind each time this hand was used. Crossed pathways linking each half of the cortex to the opposite hand were clearly superior for guiding fine exploratory movements of the fingers. John Downer, in London, had found the same effects in his split-brain monkeys, and in the 1970s, the physiological and anatomical basis for it was clarified by beautiful studies of Jacoba Brinkman and Hans Kuypers in Holland. Related split-brain projects were used to reveal shifts of attention between the two separated halves of the cortex and the effects on perception of preparatory sets to move in particular ways. The results gave a fresh view of the global design of the mammalian brain for awareness, learning, and voluntary action (Sperry 1967).

Many surgical experiments utilized the

unique advantages of having two brains governing one body. The minimum piece of cortex needed to retain tactile or visual learning was determined by progressively ablating cortex from the "experimental" hemisphere until functional losses occurred. The other half-brain was left intact so that near-normal behavior might continue outside the training situation (Sperry 1961). Other studies analyzed differences in transfer through various commissural segments and recent findings demonstrate the presence of basic hemispheric differences in rhesus monkeys (see Chapter 10). Sperry continued through the 1960s to perform the majority of the split-brain surgeries required by the laboratory, ably assisted by Lois MacBird. Some students preferred to do their own surgery, and all who worked on split-brain projects were encouraged to learn the surgery before leaving. When a flare-up of Sperry's TB in 1958 interrupted his scheduled surgeries, Harbans Arora filled in for a year and a half, supplying the laboratory requests for split-brain subjects.

Between 1950 and the mid-1970s, Sperry continued to direct, in parallel, research on the formation of nerve circuits in lower vertebrates – goldfish, cichlid fish, salamanders, and frogs. Collaborators in this work were Harbans Arora, Ivan-Jean Weiler, Domenica Attardi, John Ronald Cronly-Dillon, Norma Deupree, Richard Mark, Ronald Meyer, Emerson Hibbard, Margaret Scott, and Myong Yoon. Some twenty articles were published, explaining, defending, and extending Sperry's theory that the innate basis for cerebral functions is determined genetically through highly refined physiochemical coding of cellular pathways and connections. Although new methods for following nerve growth have since revealed competitive epigenetic processes involved in sorting out functional connections, every attempt so far to overthrow the chemospecificity theory by experiment has been forced to invoke some such similar basic selective principle. Sperry had certainly won his battle against the theories of the 1930s, which had universally assumed there was no way that complex, precisely organized nerve networks for behavior could be adaptively prewired for function by the growth process itself.

In 1965, he wrote:

It now appears that the complicated nerve fiber circuits of the brain grow, assemble and organize themselves through the use of intricate chemical codes under genetic control. . . .

In regard to the inheritance of a given behavior pattern, it is no longer so much a question of whether the machinery of growth is capable of installing it, as to whether the survival rate may be better if the behavior is kept flexible by having it learned in each generation and thus adaptable to external conditions and adjustable to changes (Sperry 1965a).

In this context, Sperry also stressed the strong possibility that learning itself is the consequence of submicroscopic modifications within already existing cerebral connections, the anatomical design of which is prewired according to minutely specified genetic instructions. These innate factors predetermined adaptive goals, categories of experience, and intricately coordinated forms of action. His 1955 publication on the conditioned reflex was the first to attribute the new neural connections linking conditioned stimulus and response, not to lasting engram changes, but to a transient facilitatory set. The real new engram connections he allocated to a different "perceptual expectancy" system, presumed to be not much simpler nor more readily localizeable than with other forms of learning.

Sperry's tendency to encourage students and other associates to follow their own ideas for research resulted often in projects outside the foregoing trends. In particular, aspects of learning and memory in newly hatched chicks were explored by a sizeable group in the laboratory, including Drs. Arthur Cherkin and Evelyn Lee-Teng, Geoffrey Magnus and Larry Benowitz, and Karen Gaston and Karen Greif. Occasionally, projects were conducted with rats but in a special room in the basement instead of in the main top-floor laboratory because of Sperry's allergy to rats acquired in the early days in Lashley's lab at Harvard.

In 1960, Joseph Bogen, a Los Angeles neurosurgeon, announced to Sperry that he had a patient with severe intractable epilepsy, who might be helped by cerebral commissurotomy. Dr. Bogen had earlier done research at Caltech in Van Harreveld's group down the passage from Sperry's lab and thus was well acquainted with the Caltech split-brain findings and also with the earlier 1940s' reports by Akelaitis on the effects of commissurotomy in human epileptics – reports that had prompted Sperry's split-brain work in the beginning. Bogen's patient was having progressively frequent and severe life-threatening seizures as a result of head injuries sustained as a paratrooper. Following further consultations and a thorough consideration of many pros and cons, Bogen's chief, Philip Vogel, performed, in 1962, with Bogen's assistance, a total neocortical commissurotomy on this patient (Bogen and Vogel 1963).

Soon thereafter, Sperry and Bogen, with a new graduate student, Michael Gazzaniga, brought in to help with the testing and transportation, began systematic analyses in the Caltech lab of the effects of the commissurotomy on perception, speech, and motor control. Instead of relying on standard neurological procedures, original testing methods were devised based on principles learned from split-brain animals. That year, the first report of their test results, along with clinical observations made by Bogen, appeared in the *Proceedings of the National Academy of Sciences USA,* describing the resultant left-right division of consciousness in a human being (Gazzaniga, Bogen, and Sperry 1962). In the same year, Norman Geschwind and Edith Kaplan, in Boston, described split-brain phenomena in a human patient with lesion pathology, also basing their explanation on the animal split-brain work of the previous decade (Geschwind and Kaplan 1962).

During the next three years, several days a week for one to two hours and often on weekends after testing sessions, Sperry and Gazzaniga reviewed the test data obtained to date and planned the next steps in coming tests, and Gazzaniga shuttled across town to keep Bogen informed and to get his input. It was immediately clear in the new patient of Vogel and Bogen that awareness of objects seen by both halves of the brain (in left and right halves of the visual field) or felt in the left or right hand was rich and intelligent, but that, just as in the earlier animal studies, the left and right mental realms were as separate as if they were in separate heads. Only when the subject shifted his visual fixation or passed the stimulus object from one hand to the other did the one hemisphere know what the other was perceiving. Conclusions reached previously in animals, only after difficult surgery and many weeks or months of laborious training, could be obtained in only a few minutes in this patient by simply having him describe verbally what he had or had not experienced.

The one extraordinary defect, quite unlike anything seen in animals, was that the subject was unable to verbally describe experiences of the left half of the visual field or of the left hand. Though both hemispheres were conscious, only the left could speak or write. A more startling result, however, for any neuropsychologist aware of the classical loss of language produced by a lesion restricted to the left cerebral cortex, was that the right hemisphere, though predictably speechless, could nevertheless, comprehend speech fairly well. It picked up information quickly from utterances made by the left half-brain, it could read common words flashed to the left visual field, and it could follow verbal instructions. It was, however, conspicuously weak at calculating and in both comprehending and thinking with verbal propositions. Jerre Levy and Eran Zaidel (Chapters 13 and 17, respectively) discuss the meaning this finding has for central regulatory processes of consciousness and for localization of language in the brain.

Sperry's interest after 1967 turned increasingly to the more elusive, less readily testable mental faculties of the nonspeaking right hemisphere, referred to then as the "minor" (supposedly mentally retarded) hemisphere. In a 1968 doctoral study, Levy succeeded in showing that imagination of spatial relations and transformations in space were more highly developed on the right side of the brain. Her test conditions clearly ruled out mere praxic assymmetry in favor of true cognitive processing. This led to the idea that the human brain housed two different, complementary kinds of cognitive strategy – two kinds of consciousness. The finding was reported that same year by Levy and Sperry to the National Academy of Sciences and was quickly followed the next year by a series of three papers on "the other side of the brain" by Bogen, supported by his extensive clinical tests with the patients.

Thereafter, a growing team of researchers, working under Sperry's direction on the small population of the Vogel/Bogen commissurotomy patients, helped to explore what proved to be an extraordinary state of divided asymmetric mental activity. Studies by Bob Nebes, Harold Gordon, Joe Bogen, Jerre Levy, Colwyn Trevarthen, Bruno Preilowski, Laura Franco, Eran Zaidel, Dahlia Zaidel, Leah Ellenberg, and others (see Appendix B) yielded further evidence that the verbal left hemisphere kind of consciousness was offset in the right hemisphere by a different set of mental processes, superior to the left at comprehending visuospatial constructions.

Taken together, the implications of these and later findings on left–right cognitive differences reach into all areas of human mental life and have excited public and scholarly interest like no other topic in brain science in recent times. In brief, it was found that the surgically separated left hemisphere is in immediate command of fluent speech and able to generate and retain phonological images of speech sounds. It is capable of serial logical propositions such as are expressed in spoken gestural or written language, and it powerfully encodes and is adept at the kind of combinatorial and systematic logic required for some kinds of formal mathematical or musical thought. The right hemisphere, in contrast, has superior mastery of the immediate experience of forms in visual, auditory, and haptic domains. It can remember these experiences better, can distinguish and remember faces better, has richer reactions to colors, and to affective tone of the voice and its musical quality. It perceives more easily the abstract resemblances of forms in topological but not Euclidean geometry. These differences are summarized in Sperry's Nobel Address (Sperry 1982). Recent tests with commissurotomy patients support findings with brain-damaged and normal subjects showing the right half of the brain to have greater involvement in emotional communication and the mediation of direct social interactions (see Chapter 18).

This research has stimulated a great flowering of laterality studies in patients with lateralized brain injury and in normal subjects for perceptual, cognitive, and motoric asymmetries. Acceptance of the hypothesis that the hemispheres are innately wired for different psychological processes (genetic variations in handedness or lateralization of language being but two manifestations of a complex hereditary regulation of human mental life) has caused reappraisal of the reasons for variety in different people's educational performance and intellectual aptitudes. Obviously, the aims of educators and employers would benefit by responding to any such natural mental variation.

Reflection on the manifestations of conscious awareness in the surgically divided brain led Sperry, in 1965, to publish the first of a remarkable series of philosophical papers. Under the title "Mind, Brain and Humanist Values," he proposed a new mentalistic monist theory of mind that breaks with established behaviorist traditions in giving subjective experience a prime controlling role in brain function and behavior.

> Mental forces direct and govern the inner impulse traffic, including its electrochemical and biophysical aspects. . . . In the brain model proposed here, the causal potency of an idea, or an ideal, becomes just as real as that of a molecule, a cell, or a nerve impulse. Ideas cause ideas and help evolve new ideas. They interact with each other and with other mental forces. . . . The present scheme would put mind back into the brain of objective science and in a position of top command (Sperry 1965b, p. 82).

Though greeted with some skepticism initially, this mentalist view of consciousness based on emergence and downward causation was destined within 10 years to replace behaviorism as the dominant foundational philosophy of behavioral science.

Consciousness is conceived as an entirely natural process, emerging from activity in cerebral networks, different from, but also inseparable from, the neural activity generating it. Its control over neuronal activity is gained by virtue of its higher "functionalist" and "downward-control" properties. He portrays consciousness as a special instance of a general principle, "macrodeterminism," in which the higher, more evolved forces throughout nature exert control over their lower components. "In emergence of new entities, the parts are captured, contained, and controlled by the higher, previously nonexistent properties of the new whole." Conversely, he recognizes that the highest of human motives are constrained by inherent cerebral design. He contends that this view, integrating macro- with microdeterminism and the causal reality of mental states is a more valid foundation for all science, not just psychology, with "endless humanistic implications for philosophy, religion and human values," providing science and all of us with a new outlook on existence (Sperry 1983, 1988).

Notwithstanding his participation, in the mid-1960s, in a Vatican Conference, and his election to the Pontifical Academy of Sciences, Sperry is a thoroughgoing sceptic about God-given values, if these are in conflict with "this-world" values based in the truths of (reformed nonreductionist) science. His early renunciation of the traditional science-values dichotomy evoked some hostile criticism initially, but, after the mid-1970s, gained wide acceptance in what is now seen as a new era in value philosophy. He believes the new world view of science offers the best guide to human values, social policy, and a future in harmony with nature's limited resources, about which he has great concern. His conception of the new mentalist paradigm in psychology and of the important reconciliations it brings for some of the long-standing "tensions" between scientific and religious belief is presented in his most recent publication (Sperry 1988). This philosophy also has, he argues, promising potential as an ideological base for a world system of justice, one that will encourage nations with their necessarily different cultural, political, and religious systems to find common cause and mutual respect.

Sperry has always advocated objective scientific enquiry as the brain's most reliable basis for arriving at belief and now argues that the same applies to value judgments. His "emergent interactionist" approach engenders a new scientific respect for the human spirit and for all evolving nature in which he sees it impossible to separate the creative forces from creation itself. His ideas meet resistance from established materialist doctrines on the one side and dualist systems of belief on the other, but they have also attracted increasing interest and

admiration from thinkers not accustomed to taking advice from brain science. Sperry's arguments in these areas derive unique force from the fact that their originator has a lifetime of experience exploring the brain and how it and its behavioral outputs are formed. His rich and original thinking about human consciousness and the importance of values and emotion are given lucid expression in his book with Eccles, Prigogine, and others entitled *Nobel Prize Conversations* (1985).

Roger Sperry has received many high honors, particularly for his neurospecificity and split-brain discoveries, including:

The Oberlin College Distinguished Alumni Citation (1954)

The Howard Crosby Warren Medal of the Society of Experimental Psychologists (1969)

The Distinguished Scientific Contribution Award of the American Psychological Association (1971)

The California Scientist of the Year Award (1972)

Corecipient of the William Thomas Wakeman Research Award of the National Paraplegia Foundation (1972)

The Passano Foundation Award (1973)

The Claude Bernard Science Journalism Award (1975)

The Karl Lashley Award of the American Philosophical Society (1976)

The Albert Lasker Basic Medical Research Award (1979)

The Wolf Prize in Medicine (1979)

The Ralph W. Gerard Prize of the Society for Neuroscience (1979)

The Nobel Prize in Physiology/Medicine for 1981, shared in half with Torsten Wiesel and David Hubel

He is a member of the National Academy of Sciences of the United States, the American Academy of Arts and Sciences, the Pontifical Academy of Sciences, the American Philosophical Society, Foreign Members of the Royal Society of the United Kingdom, the American Psychological Association, the Society for Neuroscience, and other learned societies. He received honorary DSc degrees from Cambridge and Rockefeller universities, the University of Chicago, and Kenyon and

Oberlin colleges before being forced to forego participation in ceremonies by a progressive neuromotor impairment from primary lateral sclerosis.

Sperry, the dedicated researcher, is a taciturn, socially reticent person with a rich private life, who shuns formalities and loves to vacation in remote, wild places. With the company and help of his wife Norma and children Tad and Jan, he has enjoyed remarkable success hunting giant fossil dinosaur bones and record-breaking ammonites in the deserts and canyons of the southwestern states, or catching big fish off the shores of Baja California. Indeed, when the announcement of his Nobel Prize came, he and Norma were camping alone on a beach in Baja about 18 miles below La Paz with their dog Chadwick. They had been left stranded by a hurricane and were out of touch for days with Caltech, all roads back being impassable by ordinary vehicles; meantime, they continued to snorkel, fish, and explore the regional islands in their Zodiac inflatable. Sperry is no mean artist, as scientific illustrations in this book taken from his large collection show. His home is scattered with his own sculptures, ceramic and other pieces, including busts of his family and life drawings concocted in what he refers to as "antibrainstrain evenings."

We know Sperry best as an inspiring teacher, uncannily perceptive of his associates' personal qualities and aspirations, and a quietly devastating communicator with a precise, ironic sense of humor.

This book is a tribute by one-time students to their teacher, and by research colleagues, to a paragon of scientific skill. We have all learned by sharing Sperry's untiring interest in the brain and its workings. His powerful, challenging, uncompromising theories and meticulous techniques, applied always with pragmatic "problem oriented" or "What difference does it make?" priorities, and with methodologies adaptable to contingencies of the hunt, have inspired us and led us to fruitful questions of our own that we have spent years exploring. As a psychobiologist, he has strategically combined insights from a cluster of related fields in efforts to advance understanding of some of the brain's deepest questions. Most of us have ben-

efited from discussions in his office, in which a directness and clarity of logic may have left us shaken, perhaps, but in possession of a new and better idea of what we were trying to prove. Trying to win an argument with Sperry is an exhausting, but highly profitable, business. There are many references to this feature of his tutelage in our individual statements. Above all, we, his students, have joined in the excitement of teamwork at a frontier of psychobiology way out in front of the world. The laboratory in the monastic peace of Caltech has been a wonderful place to work. Even when we felt left alone and temporarily uninspired (for Sperry almost never imposed himself and could at times withdraw austerely), the current of decades of careful, inner-directed, and greatly interested effort carried us onward.

Roger, please understand that we have each undertaken to give our own story, attempting to fit it in, as we see it, to your endeavor. Of course, none of us is competent over the whole spectrum and we have our own preoccupations. We know you will be disappointed that none of us has ventured far toward appraisal of your most recent philosophical writings, and we decided not to bring anyone in from outside to do this. You have made large steps through difficult places and we, naturally enough, wish to look hard at the ground at our feet before we contemplate setting off in those directions. We hope you will see that a fair part of your philosophy has rubbed off on us, nevertheless.

It is an unfortunate necessity that the contributors to this book are only a part of the group that has worked in Sperry's academy, supported by the remarkable institution of Caltech. Some major contributors to many of his scientific enterprises are absent, regretfully. I single out a few of these. First of all is Ronald Myers, who carried out brilliant first steps in the development of the split-brain technique, both the surgery and the behavioral testing. Then there is Harbans Arora, who assimilated Roger's skill in microsurgery with fish and amphibia, carrying out important experiments on regrowth of visual and motor connections in cichlids, and then extended his talents to help with split-brain monkey surgery.

Nica Attardi made some marvelous retinal ablations and histological analyses in goldfish to test the chemoaffinity theory. In the early 1960s, Michael Gazzaniga assisted in the initial testing of the human commissurotomy patients with Sperry and Bogen, and then became strongly devoted to the human studies that advanced faster and more easily than did the animal work and with greater general impact. During the same years, Richard Mark was conducting experiments on bimanual targeting in split-brain monkeys and innovated strategic analyses of motor innervation in salamanders, which gave substance to the concept of competitive innervation of neuromuscular connections, and led to new ideas about how learning could be related to neuroembryology. These and many other contributors to the steady flow of research over a third of a century are listed in Appendix B.

Of those who gave technical and administrative help in the Psychobiology lab at Caltech, first in Kerckhoff and then in the Alles and Church buildings, special mention should be made of Lois MacBird, who, from the 1950s to 1983, kept things, and us, in order. Lois gave efficient help with an amazing range of practical tasks, including surgery and animal and human testing, recording and filming commissurotomy patients, and keeping records. Her love for the animals joined with that of Nancy Miner and Eef Goedemans led to a common observation that the animals received better treatment in this lab than the human workers. We are glad that Lois's excellent photographic skills are represented here in Sperry's portrait. After 1967, for nine years, Dahlia Zaidel assisted Sperry with his experiments in the commissurotomy patients, both simian and human, reaching a stage of expertise near the end where she was devising and conducting tests on her own. In Chapter 15, the latest direction of this work is reported. From 1965 to 1985, Eef Goedemans gave expert care to the animals, their testing, and technical assistance.

With great sadness, we note the deaths of two of our contributors. Edward Evarts died on July 2, 1985, shortly after completing his generous and scholarly foreword, which reviews Sperry's early work on the neural mechanism of motor control. Ed was an old friend of Sperry's, following him to the Yerkes Laboratory of Primate Biology at Orange Park in 1949 and joining him at the National Institute of Health when, in 1953, Ed became Chief of the Physiology Section at the Laboratory for Clinical Science of the National Institute of Mental Health, and, in 1971, Chief of the Laboratory of Neurophysiology. Ed Evarts' illustrious career was centered on cortical motor control. He appreciated that early scientific work with Stetson gave Sperry a clear view of the significance of motor processes. It is easy to overlook the importance to cognition generally of factors ennabling preparedness for movement, and to forget that perception serves primarily to initiate, guide, and give value and purpose to coordinated movements.

Oliver Zangwill, Emeritus Professor of Experimental Psychology of Cambridge University and Fellow of Kings College, was weakened by the effects of a stroke when he undertook to write an historical essay on Hughlings Jackson's clinical observations that gave prophetic insights into the functions of the hemispheres. Generously assisted by Maria Wyke, he wrote recollections of a great epoch in neuropsychology that only an "old timer" could give us. Oliver was himself a pioneer in neuropsychology, who, in the 1940s, helped gain recognition for the special functions of the right hemisphere. He examined commissurotomy patients at Caltech with Roger about 1970 and he wrote an important essay based on this experience, discussing the problem of consciousness and its divisibility (Zangwill 1974). Oliver Zangwill died in Cambridge on October 12, 1987.

With delight and pride, we note that Rita Levi-Montalcini received a Nobel Prize in Psysiology/Medicine in 1986. She and Stanley Cohen, research colleagues of Viktor Hamburger, were honored "for their twin contributions to the understanding of substances that influence cell growth." The importance of Nerve-Growth Factor, and its relevance to Sperry's work on neuronal specificity, is made clear in Chapter 1.

Collecting these essays from busy people has not been without its problems. Some were more prompt in their responses than others, and quicker to react to editorial comments. At times, the editor was himself preoccupied with other matters. All contributors joined in enthusiastically and expressed their pleasure at having an opportunity to indicate their affection, gratitude, and admiration to Roger Sperry. This made the editor's responsibility an enjoyable one. It is a pleasure to have our book completed in his 75th year. We wish Roger and Norma the very best.

Acknowledgments

In the early planning of this volume, Lois MacBird helped in remembering and locating people. Chuck Hamilton, Jerre Levy, and Ron Meyer assisted with the initial editing; the quality of the chapters owes much to their comments and advice. Paula Mathieson gave invaluable, expert attention to the arduous task of obtaining permissions, and she prepared the list of Roger's publications. Ulla Hipkin, Rhona Fraser, and Cindy White dealt efficiently and cheerfully with typing of considerable parts of the manuscript. Finally, Susan Milmoe and Ian Jeffers of Cambridge University Press have been unfailingly helpful and encouraging.

The Editor wishes to report that many chapters for this book were written in 1983 and revised, ready for publication, in 1984. He thanks the authors for their patience.

References

Bogen, J. E., and P. J. Vogel. 1963. Treatment of generalized seizures by cerebral commissurotomy. *Surg. For.* 14: 431–33.

Gazzaniga, M. S., J. E. Bogen, and R. W. Sperry. 1962. Some functional effects of sectioning the cerebral commissures in man. *Proc. Natl. Acad. Sci. USA* 48: 1765–9.

Geschwind, N., and E. Kaplan. 1962. A human cerebral deconnection syndrome. *Neurol.* 12: 675–85.

Hamburger, V. 1979. Roger Sperry. *Neurosci. Newslett.* 10: 5–6.

Mark, R. F. 1974. *Memory and Nerve-Cell Connections.* Oxford University Press, London.

Nobel Prize Conversations. 1985. *Nobel Prize Conversations with Sir John Eccles, Roger Sperry, Ilya Prigogine and Brian Josephson,* at the Dallas Isthmus Institute (with a commentary by Norman Cousins). Saybrook, Dallas.

Sperry, R. W. 1939. Action current study in movement coordination. *J. Gen. Psychol.* 20: 295–313.

–1945. The problem of central nervous reorganization after nerve regeneration and muscle transposition. *Quart. Rev. Biol.* 20: 311–69.

–1951. Regulative factors in the orderly growth of neural circuits. *Growth Symp.* 10: 63–87.

–1961. Cerebral organization and behavior. *Science* 133: 1749–57.

–1965a. Embryogenesis of behavioral nerve nets. *In* R. L. Dehaan and H. Ursprung (eds.) *Organogenesis.* Holt, Rinehart and Winston, New York, pp. 161–85.

–1965b. Mind, brain, and humanist values. *In* J. R. Platt (ed.) *New Views of the Nature of Man.* University of Chicago Press, Chicago, pp. 71–92.

–1967. Split-brain approach to learning problems. *In* G. C. Quarton, T. Melnechuk, and F. O. Schmitt (eds.) *The Neurosciences: A Study Program.* Rockefeller University Press, New York, pp. 714–22.

–1982. Some effects of disconnecting the cerebral hemispheres. *Science* 217(4566): 1223–6.

–1983. *Science and Moral Priority.* Columbia University Press, New York. 1985 edition, Greenwood/Praeger, Westport (CT).

–1988. Psychology's mentalist paradigm and the religion/science tension. *Am. Psychol.* 43: 607–13.

Zangwill, O. L. 1974. Consciousness and the cerebral hemispheres. *In* S. J. Dimond and J. G. Beaumont (eds.) *Hemisphere Function in the Human Brain.* Paul Elek, London.

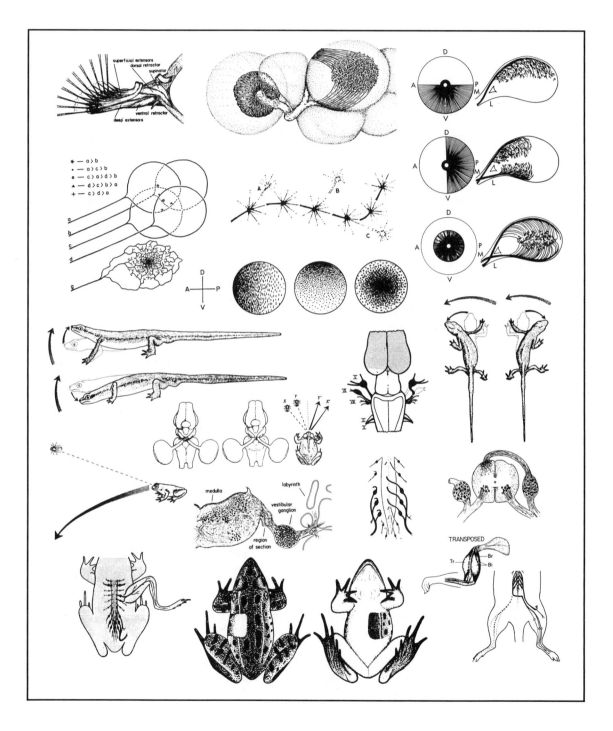

When Roger Sperry was in his twenties, he formulated a conception of brain morphogenesis and the formation of nerve circuits that directly challenged the thinking of his day. In the footsteps of the great Santiago Ramon y Cajal, he saw nerve cells seeking to link up according to a chemical coding of their surfaces and responding in a similar way to coded surfaces belonging to other cells in the interneuronal matrix. Sperry thought this would be the best explanation for innate behaviors, and he doubted that the orderly and intricate patterns familiar to neuroanatomists or the behaviors that psychologists study could come about in any other way. He saw learning filling out and refining lines of transmission in the neurone network that had been given most of its connections according to a gene-regulated chemoaffinity code. This was quite a claim in the 1940s. Through the years, Sperry has had to defend his theory against attempts to reduce the genetic contribution, and evidence that early phases of nerve growth on regeneration are uniselective and diffuse. The chapters in this part discuss the current state of this rich field of neurobiological research that Sperry's early experiments helped to establish. They demonstrate that the chemoaffinity theory is very much alive and well, nearly fifty years after its first formulation.

Rita Levi-Montalcini was one of the discoverers of a chemical substance that undoubtedly does influence survival and growth of nerve fibers. Her chapter (Chapter 1) gives a glimpse of Sperry as he was when she met him in 1950, at a meeting organized by Viktor Hamburger. The Nerve-Growth Factor leads to the discovery of surface features that may answer the riddle of the molecular basis of chemoaffinity.

R. Kevin Hunt and W. Maxwell Cowan (Chapter 2) present a remarkable historical analysis of neuroembryological research, showing how Sperry's experiments applied and extended classic principles of organismic differentiation and morphogenesis brilliantly to elucidate pattern formation in connections of sensory, central, and motor nerves.

Emerson Hibbard (Chapter 3) describes experiments that elegantly show selective pathfinding in growing nerves when these have been made to enter the body at a site far from the normal one.

Myong G. Yoon (Chapter 4) has made quite amazing operations on his goldfish, putting the workhorse of this field, the retinotectal system, through every kind of surgical rearrangement to test the selectivity and plasticity of the regrowing optic nerves.

Finally, Ronald L. Meyer (Chapter 5) presents us with a thorough review and theoretical discussion of this same goldfish retinotectal system, examining the various hypotheses by which mapping, ordering, and flexible adjustment of terminals can be explained. The data give strong support to the chemoaffinity theory. These scholarly analyses enable us to see Sperry's work in the context of the present-day understanding of problems he set out to clarify at the start of his scientific career.

1 Ontogenesis of neuronal nets: The chemoaffinity theory, 1963–1983

Rita Levi-Montalcini
Institute of Cell Biology

Introduction and historical survey of early findings

The "instructive" stimulus has gone the way of the philosopher's stone, an agent dimly akin to it in certain ways. Embryonic development at the level of molecular differentiation must therefore be an unfolding of preexisting capabilities, an acting-out of genetically encoded instructions; the inductive stimulus is the agent that selects or activates one set of instructions rather than another (Medawar 1967, p. 107).

This statement, formulated by Medawar in his usual remarkably incisive way, illustrates the sharp turn that took place in the sixties in basic concepts of developmental biology, mainly in consequence of the tremendous advances realized in the field of immunology under the leadership of scientists such as Medawar, Burnett, and Yerne.

The acceptance of the selective versus the instructive theory of developmental processes, based on theoretical considerations and experimental evidence obtained in immunology, occurred in such a smooth and silent way as to pass almost unnoticed by the majority of biologists. About the same period, though through an entirely different approach, a young psychologist, Roger Sperry, operated single-handedly the same revolution in the still-unnamed field of neurosciences. In this field, which at that time consisted of three different and distinct areas of research known as neuroanatomy, neurophysiology, and behavior, such a revolution could not, however, go unnoticed since it touched upon a problem of vital importance for investigators engaged in studies at these three different levels. All of them, even if in possession of different tools and scientific backgrounds, were attempting to find an answer to a long-standing and unsolved question that had preoccupied students of the nervous system even before it became the object of direct experimental analysis. To what extent are the structure, functional interconnections, and activity of the nervous system, as evaluated from the behavior of the whole organism, dependent upon the genetic program, and to what extent are they the result of experience, trial and error? The importance of the problem and the reason why it was so hotly disputed are obvious, if one considers the close linkage between this question and the task of assessing the role played by hereditary and environmental factors in higher brain functions such as intelligence, talent, and behavior. A definition of the respective roles of these factors is of vital concern not just to the student of the nervous system, but to the whole of mankind.

Toward the end of the past century, the founding fathers in the fields of neuroanatomy and neurophysiology, S. Ramon y Cajal and C. S. Sherrington, had provided decisive evidence for the key role played by hereditary factors, the genetic basis of heredity being at that time unknown, in the building of the nervous system. But their concept that the function of the nervous system depends upon a preestablished program underwent a full 180° reversion in the first four decades of this century.

Largely responsible for imposing this new trend in thought were two leading figures in the fields of psychology and developmental neurology: K. S. Lashley, the psychologist, and P. Weiss, the experimental neuroembryologist. Through entirely different methodological approaches and experimental designs, Lashley and Weiss had provided what seemed foolproof evidence against the hypothesis that selectivity in nerve connections regulated by inheritance is basic for the function of the nervous system. In view of the great influence exerted by these men, it is worth mentioning their experimental approach and findings.

In an attempt to find out whether and to what extent learning capacities are localized by fixed anatomical arrangements in given brain centers, Lashley submitted maze-learning rats, prior to the test, to extensive cortical lesions, which resulted in the disconnection of different cortical areas and destruction of most of them. The finding that the maze-solving ability did not decrease as a result of lesions in a specific location, but only as a consequence of increasing the extent of the lesion, was taken by Lashley as evidence for the importance of global rather than localized cortical brain function. "The learning process and the retention of habit," he states, "are not dependent upon any finely localized structural change within the cerebral cortex. The results (of these experiments) are incompatible with theories of learning by changes in synaptic structures, or with any theories which assume that particular neural integrations are dependent upon definite anatomical paths specialized for them. . . . The mechanisms of integration are to be sought in dynamic relations among the parts of the nervous system rather than in details of structural differentiation" (Lashley 1929, p. 176). As the leading psychologist in the twenties and following two decades, Lashley played a decisive role in channeling brain research in this direction, and, perhaps also because his theories agreed well with the prevailing philosophical trend, he exerted a considerable appeal on his contemporaries in psychology. The brain, according to Lashley, would have been endowed with an almost unlimited adaptation capacity, and cor-

tical areas, as well as other sectors of the brain, would be functionally interchangeable. "In retrospect," as commented upon by Kandel and Spencer, "Lashley's rejection of a cellular-connection approach was premature. Not only were the experiments in fact too crude to be meaningful, but also the lack of aseptic procedures in performing these experiments may well have resulted in widespread infections which would have obscured differences attributable to locus-specific damage" (Kandel and Spencer 1968, p. 67).

The trend against heritable specificity in neuronal circuits and synaptic connections received at the same time strong support from experiments that were not aimed at finding the basic mechanism underlying higher brain functions, but rather at establishing the ontogeny of behavior at the much lower level of complexity that governs reflex activity and spontaneous motion.

In the twenties, Weiss reported that supernumerary limbs transplanted in close proximity to the anterior or posterior limbs of amphibian tadpoles exhibited, upon reaching adult stage, the same motility as the adjacent host limb: they underwent flexion or extension every time and synchronously with the motion of the proper limb, in spontaneous as well as reflex activity. This phenomenon, designated by Weiss as "homologous or myotypic response" (Weiss 1928, 1931, 1936), occurred also when the transplanted leg, explanted from donors of different species, was larger in size than that of the host, as in the case of a graft of the limb-bud of *Amblystoma punctatum* in a tadpole of *Mexicanum*. Even more impressive, according to Weiss, was the finding that the synchrony in motion occurred also when the transplanted limb was taken from the opposite side of the body and was, therefore, a mirror image of that of the recipient tadpole. In these cases, the simultaneous contraction of the host and of the donor legs resulted in a scissor movement of the limbs that counteracted each other with obvious disadvantage to the animal. The same phenomenon took place when individual muscles rather than the whole limb were transplanted in proximity to the homologous muscle. These findings, based on extensive though not all too rigorous experimental evidence, led Weiss to submit the "resonance principle" (Weiss 1931), which states that the peripheral end organs, in this case the motor end plates of the host's and donor's muscles, pick up only those nerve signals to which they are attuned by their biochemical constitution, and this would differ from one muscle to another. Each muscle, through the agency of its end plates, establishes a selective relationship with motor-nerve cells, issuing nerve messages that differ in range and other parameters from the impulses dispatched by other nerve cells. "The conclusion was being drawn," as commented later by Sperry, "that selective communication in the nervous system must be based not on selectivity among synaptic connections, as the classical textbook doctrine would have it, but rather upon some kind of qualitative selectivity among the signals carried by different fiber types: that is, some kind of impulse specificity. . . . In the resonance principle, the old telephone switchboard analogy was replaced by a radio broadcasting concept of communication. The anatomical connections were inferred to be diffuse and nonselective" (Sperry 1965, p. 163).

Although the resonance principle had to be abandoned on the basis of electrophysiological studies by Wiersma, who produced evidence against it (Wiersma 1931), still the doctrine of impulse specificity seemed in the late thirties as the most plausible explanation of the phenomenon of the homologous response. Likewise, the ability of the central nervous system to adapt to any change imposed by the experimenter in the peripheral nerve-to-muscle connections, with no apparent disarrangement of function, was considered as in favor of the hypothesis that selective neuronal connections are not essential for building the normal orderly function of the nervous system (Weiss 1955).

The "rebellious graduate student" and the evidence for chemical specificity

It was against this historical background that Sperry's revolution took place. "Reversing the major trend of current thinking," as phrased recently by Viktor Hamburger, one of Sperry's admirers and a leading authority in the field of neuroembryology, "he [Sperry] postulated that synaptic connections are highly selective and that the precision of neuronal circuitry can be accounted for only by chemical affinities between nerve terminals and their target cells" (Hamburger 1981, p. 154). Sperry, as Hamburger reminds us, was Weiss's graduate student and it was under his guidance that he obtained his PhD degree in 1941. He then spent six postdoctoral years with K. Lashley. "During this period," writes Hamburger, "he managed to disprove Lashley's notion of equipotentiality of cortical structures. I know of nobody else who has disposed of cherished ideas of both his doctoral and postdoctoral sponsor, both at that time the acknowledged leaders in their fields" (Hamburger 1979, p. 5).

The studies that were to result in the formulation of the chemoaffinity theory took their start from a series of rigorously planned and systematically performed experiments, undertaken while Sperry was still Weiss's graduate student. In order to find out whether functional adjustment would occur in rather simple experimental situations, Sperry switched nerve connections between antagonistic muscles, which command a reverse movement in the rat's ankle. According to the prevailing notion that "behavior, function, practice, experience, learning and conditioning mold and shape the fiber pathways in a functionally adaptive communication system" (Sperry 1965, p. 161), one would have expected that the operated animals would have learned to adapt to the novel situation and suffer no functional maladaptation. This expectation, however, did not materialize. In no instance, not even after extensive practicing, did the animal learn to correct the reversal of motor coordination consequent to the substitution of flexor with extensor muscles (Sperry 1941, 1943a). Experiments with sensory rather than motor nerves gave an even more impressive demonstration of the lack of any functional adjustment to the abnormal nerve connections with their end organs. Dramatic evidence of this failure to adjust to new situations was obtained by Sperry in experiments of disconnection of sensory nerves from the left paw of adult rats and connection of the same nerves with the homologous cutaneous field of the right side. Noxious stimuli such as an electric shock applied to the left paw, evoked pain reaction from the uninjured right paw, which was lifted and licked in an attempt to mitigate the pain, whereas the left leg was pressed even harder on the electrode (Sperry 1943a). On the basis of these and other experimental findings to be considered in the following section, Sperry formulated his principle of neuronal specificity, which states that connections between nerve centers in the cerebrospinal axis, and between neuronal elements and target organs and tissues at the periphery, occur through the agency of nerve circuits rigidly specified according to a genetic program, and are not dependent upon function and learning (Sperry 1951, 1955a, 1955b, 1958). This principle, which to the 1983 neurobiologist appears obvious in the light of evidence accumulated from other sectors of biological sciences, and most of all from genetics, was not at all self-evident in the early forties when the anticonnectivity trend had the support of leading scientists of the time. Sperry's early experiments led the way to the classical and celebrated studies on retinotectal connections, which were to become his favorite object of investigation, pursued at first at the behavioral level and then at the histological and electrophysiological levels and subsequently studied by an increasing number of other investigators.

Behavioral and histological basis of the chemoaffinity theory

In searching for a system particularly favorable for a behavioral analysis, Sperry chose the visual system of lower vertebrates: fishes and amphibians. This most fortunate choice was prompted by reports from other laboratories (Matthey 1925; Stone 1944) on the remarkable regenerative properties of sectioned optic nerves in these species and on the restoration of normal visual function in animals submitted to transection of this nerve-fiber system. An additional advantage considered by Sperry is to be found in the highly developed visual function in both species; motion of objects elicits in amphibians the optokinetic reflex, which serves remarkably well as an index of the restoration (Sperry 1943b).

The first objective of these studies, which Sperry began at the Chicago Laboratory, was to ascertain whether the recovery of function was due to the reestablishment of connection of the transected optic nerves with matching nerve cells in the optic tecta (the visual brain center in these vertebrates) or whether the regenerating nerve fibers connected first at random, with rearrangement of correct synaptic connections taking place later, to bring about the return of normal function. In order to answer this question, Sperry combined the transection of optic nerves in newts and in adult frogs with the surgical rotation of the eye bulbs by 180° on their optic stalks. Upon recovery, the animals were submitted to the visual test and found to behave on the basis of an inverted reception of visual stimuli: small objects moving in the visual field elicited an inverted optokinetic reflex. The maladaptive visuomotor response persisted indefinitely, and did not undergo correction after repeated trials and experience. Recovery of the normal optokinetic reflex took place, however, immediately after the eye bulb was returned, through a new surgical intervention, to its normal position, even if the second operation was performed as late as four and one-half years after the first inversion (Sperry 1951, 1955b, 1958). Misdirection of response to a visual lure occurred also upon transection of the two optic nerves, transplantation of the eyes to the controlateral orbit, and connection of each of the two proximal nerve stumps with the distal one of the opposite nerve. The results of these experiments provided unequivocal evidence against the hypothesis that vision undergoes restoration in these lower vertebrates through functional readjustment consequent to experience and learning, and offered strong arguments in favor of the hypothesis that return of vision (normal or altered) was due to reestablishment of preexisting connections between optic-nerve fibers and matching neurons in the tecta. As phrased by Sperry, "Under the conditions of the experiments, the orderly patterning of the central hook-ups could not be ascribed to any kind of functional adaptation. Animals do not learn to see things up-side-down and backwards. In fact it was

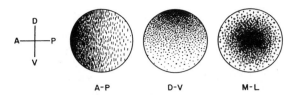

Figure 1.1. Diagrams illustrating how each retinal locus might acquire its unique properties through polarized differentiation of the retinal field in development: A-P, anteroposterior; D-V, dorsoventral; M-L, mediolateral gradient. A combination of the three gradients would impress a unique specificity on each retinal ganglion cell. (After Sperry 1951, with permission.)

possible to show that these animals were at a greater disadvantage with inverted vision than with no vision at all" (Sperry 1951, p. 67).

To account for this orderly restoration of vision, whether normal or inverted, Sperry submitted the hypothesis that the retinal differentiation must occur along two mediodorsal and anteroposterior gradients (to these two, he later added a third rostrocaudal axis.) The embryogenic constitution of each retinal locus (Figure 1.1) would stamp the optic fibers with a unique combination of labels. "Our general conclusion," stated the young Roger Sperry at the 1951 Growth Symposium, in bold and defiant opposition to his master and sponsor, Paul Weiss, "was that the optic fibers do not obey the rule of random termination but instead form their terminals both in regeneration and in development in a highly selective and discriminative manner in accordance with specific affinities and incompatibilities between the ingrowing fibers and the central neuron. A fiber from any given retinal point apparently is predisposed to terminate on the cells of a particular area of the optic lobe" (Sperry 1951, p. 69).

Sperry's hypothesis, which at that time was formulated on the basis of an extraordinary intuition rather than any experimental evidence, received very strong support eleven years later from histological studies he performed with Attardi. Only three decades later, however, was unequivocable proof provided for a topographic gradient of molecules in the retina, as is reported in the last section of this chapter (see p. 16).

The elegant Attardi–Sperry experiments were enthusiastically received when the two articles appeared in 1963 (Attardi and Sperry 1963; Sperry 1963), as indicated by extensive quotation of these papers in the literature. Here I shall briefly summarize the results and procedures that are illustrated in detail in the originals. The experiments consisted of the combination in adult goldfishes of surgical section of optic nerves and destruction of half-retinas. A few weeks later, when behavioral tests gave evidence for the restoration of the visual function, the animals were sacrificed and the connections between the regenerated optic fibers and neurons in the optic tecta were examined in histological sections, processed according to a specific staining technique that allows recognition of regenerated axons. The regenerating optic fibers bypassed the area of the tecta vacant of fibers as a result of the destruction of half-retina and established synaptic contact with neurons in the same quadrants of the optic tecta that had provided their terminal station prior to their transection. Regenerating axons selected, apparently at a distance, the pathway that would bring them to the correct sector of the optic tectal lobes. "The outgrowing fibers," commented Sperry two years later, "are guided by a kind of probing chemical touch that leads them along exact pathways in the enormously intricate guidance program that involves millions and perhaps billions of different chemically distinct brain cells [Figure 1.2]. By selective chemical preferences, the respective nerve fibers are guided correctly to their separate channels at each of the numerous forks of decision points which they encounter as they travel to what is essentially a multiple Y-maze of possible channels" (Sperry 1965, p. 170).

In Sperry's (1963) article, the term "chemoaffinity," used many times in previous original and review articles, appears in the title as if to stress the importance of these histological studies in providing the long-sought evidence that growing and regenerating nerve fibers are guided by selective

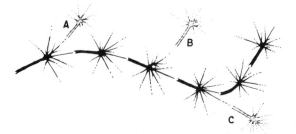

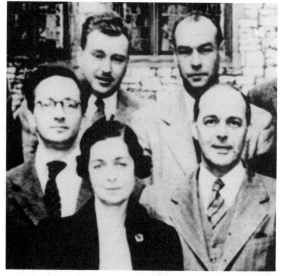

Figure 1.2. Schematic representation of sequential steps in chemotactic guidance of a growing nerve fiber. Multiple filopodia constantly reach out in front of the advancing fiber tip, testing the environment in all directions. The critical factors determining which filopodia will form the strongest attachments, and thereby direct the route of growth, are apparently chemical. Numerous alternative paths, like those represented at A, B, and C, are open, mechanically feasible, and may even be established temporarily, but fail to survive because of differential selective adhesion. (After Sperry 1965, with permission.)

Figure 1.3. Some participants of the Conference on Genetic Neurology, University of Chicago, March 1944. Top row: J. Piatt and R. Sperry; bottom row: H. Hyden, R. Levi-Montalcini, and P. Weiss.

chemical affinity between matching neurons and other neuronal or nonneuronal systems. It seems therefore justified to consider the year 1963 as that of the birth of this theory, which was to open a new, most fertile field in neurobiology. Other contributors to this volume will comment on the most extensive literature on this topic and on the present status of the problem. I shall instead consider, in the following section, studies on the ontogenesis of neuronal nets pursued at the same time as those of Sperry and co-workers, but with entirely different techniques and goals. Their bearing on some aspects of the problem investigated by Sperry justifies an excursion to this related area of neurobiological studies.

Recollections from a remote past

It was a cold early Spring day in 1949 when I first met Sperry at a conference organized by Paul Weiss on Genetic Neurology at the University of Chicago (Figure 1.3).

At this first encounter, I was impressed by some resemblance of Roger with Gary Cooper, the famous hero of the movies of those years. During the entire conference, he was most of the time silent, as if lost in thoughts unrelated to the topic presented by the speak-

ers. "Gary Cooper is dreaming of his Far West prairies and of the taming of wild horses," I whispered to my neighbor, who happened to be a young Italian. Sperry was to move to the Far West in the early fifties, to become, three decades later, even better known than Gary Cooper, though for different achievements. At the conference, we exchanged only a few words since Roger was not inclined to engage in long talks, and he inspected with some curiosity the frail person that I was. He listened, however, with attention to the report of the phenomenon that I had just discovered, consisting in the orderly migration of thousands of nerve cells in an incipient stage of differentiation in the thoracic spinal cord of chick embryos (Levi-Montalcini 1950). In subsequent years, I followed his work with great interest and growing admiration. I doubt if he took too much interest in my studies on the effects of mouse sarcomas transplanted into the body wall of chick embryos, or in the conclusion that the growth-promoting effects elicited by these tumors on sensory and sympathetic cells of the embryos bearing the transplants were due to a humoral factor released by the neoplastic cells (Levi-Montalcini 1952). Neither Roger nor I would have predicted that the Nerve-Growth Factor (as this humoral agent was to become known) would provide a new lead for the study of the chemical nature of factors leading to the formation of neuronal circuits. Indeed, at that time, his own and my field of interest seemed to share little in common.

Chemoaffinity and the Nerve-Growth Factor at a crossroad

The study of the retino-tectal system "opened the gates," as stated by Sperry, "for similar interpretation on many other borderline observations where chemotropic explanations of nerve growth had long appeared possible but had been withheld or were considered suspect because of the dominant long-term bias against anything suggestive of chemotaxis, chemotropism or neurotropism" (Sperry 1965, p. 170). In considering some of these findings, Sperry comments, "The orderly cell migration described in the beautiful studies of Levi-Montalcini (Levi-Montalcini 1964) come immediately to mind in this regard" (Sperry 1965, p. 170). If these studies had already provided evidence in favor of neurotropism, it remained for the interaction between the Nerve-Growth Factor (NGF) and the target cells to offer a most valuable model with which to investigate the molecular basis of nerve guidance under rigorous controlled conditions. A first hint that the still-unidentified growth factor released from some mouse sarcomas was endowed with neurotropic activity was indicated by the penetration into the small and large veins of embryos bearing transplants of these tumors of sympathetic fiber bundles. Likewise, the massive invasion of excretory organs such as the mesonephroi (organs that are not innervated by sympathetic fibers in untreated embryos) suggested that the humoral agent released by the tumors had the property of channeling the nerves inside the efferent section of the vascular system and the mesonephroi, structures that serve the function of clearing the embryonic tissues of waste products. NGF released in excessive quantities from neoplastic

nerve cells in embryos bearing grafts of these tumors is carried away through these systems (Levi-Montalcini 1952, 1966). It was, however, only when the NGF protein molecule became available in a purified form and in rather large amounts from the mouse salivary glands (Cohen 1960) that the hypothesis of a NGF neurotropic effect received definite support, as will be reported in the following.

The in-vivo neurotropic effects of NGF

In one of his excellent essays on the early history of neuroembryology, entitled "S. Ramon y Cajal, R. G. Harrison and the Beginnings of Neuroembryology," Viktor Hamburger (1980) pays homage to the "extraordinary conceptual insight and observational power which characterizes his [Cajal's] genius." He was referring to Cajal's ideas about guidance of nerve-fiber growth. But, as stated by Hamburger, "Ingenious as it was, the neurotropism theory has not fared well. It is true that not very extensive efforts have been made to test it and that practically all experiments, both in vivo and in vitro to that effect have given negative results. . . . But the negative results of Weiss and others are not a final verdict either. When such efforts are unsuccessful, one can always raise the question of whether the experimental design was sufficiently subtle. Anyway, neurotropism has been pronounced dead as recently as 1976" (by Weiss 1976). "As it happened," continued Hamburger, "the deceased was resurrected in the same book by R. Levi-Montalcini" (Hamburger 1980, p. 609). Hamburger then describes the results of the experiments that I reported in that volume (Levi-Montalcini 1976) and in a subsequent more extensive article with some of my associates (Menesini-Chen, Chen, and Levi-Montalcini 1978). In view of the relevance of these findings to the problem under consideration, I shall briefly mention the experimental approach and the results.

Minute amounts in the order of a few micrograms of a highly purified solution of NGF were injected daily with a mouth micropipette into neonatal rats in proximity of the two loci coerulei of the brainstem medulla. The treatment did not result in any adverse effect. Seven to ten days later, the animals were sacrificed. The cerebrospinal axis and the adjacent sympathetic and sensory ganglia as well as the surrounding soft tissues were dissected out and processed for histofluorescence studies, sectioned serially, and examined with an optic microscope equipped with a UV light source. Control littermates injected in the same way with the vehicle solution and another group of age-matched neonatal rats injected systemically with the NGF were prepared by the same procedure. The study of a large number of rodents injected intracerebrally with NGF revealed the presence, in the dorsolateral funiculi of the spinal cord and in the ventrolateral cordons of the brain stem, of intensely fluorescent fiber bundles. The sympathetic nature of these fibers was ascertained by tracing their origin to the adjacent, markedly enlarged paravertebral sympathetic ganglia (Figures 1.4 and 1.5). Neither in vehicle-injected nor in systemically NGF-injected neonatal rats was this fluorescent fiber system present in the cerebrospinal axis and EM studies revealed that the fiber bundles in the NGF-intracerebrally injected neonatal rats consisted of very thin axons, most likely collaterals of stem axons, channeled inside the neural tube as a consequence of the local high-NGF concentration.

It is important to call attention to the fact that, in order to gain access inside the spinal cord and brainstem, sympathetic nerve fibers departed to a marked extent from their normal route, which is directed peripherally rather than centripetally, and toward different organs and tissues. Discontinuation of NGF intracerebral injections resulted in the progressive reabsorption and total disappearance of these ectopic adrenergic fiber systems, thus providing additional evidence for their total dependence upon local administration of NGF. Since NGF was injected into the medulla of neonatal rats, its only possible access to the sympathetic ganglia (which underwent remarkable volume increase) was by diffusion along the neural tube and along the dorsal roots into the adjacent sympathetic chain ganglia. The same dorsal roots, infused with NGF, made multiple channels available to the aberrant adrenergic fibers, enabling them to gain entrance to the spinal cord and the medulla (Menesini-Chen et al. 1978; Levi-Montalcini, Menesini-Chen, and Chen 1978).

These findings gave the first proof, as mentioned by Hamburger, of a neurotropic nerve-guidance effect elicited by this protein molecule in vivo. Evidence for a neurotropic effect of NGF in vitro will be considered in the following section.

The in-vitro neurotropic effects of NGF

Experiments performed in the early seventies (Charlwood, Lamont, and Banks 1972), employing a method devised two decades earlier, gave suggestive evidence for an orientating or chemotactic effect elicited by capillary tubes filled with an aqueous solution of salivary NGF on sensory fibers emerging from embryonic ganglia cultured in vitro (Levi-Montalcini, Meyer, and Hamburger 1954). These findings, however, as acknowledged by the authors, were inconclusive. They could not be taken as unambiguous evidence for chemotaxis. "It is possible," they stated, "that the side of each ganglion facing away from the source of NGF is completely screened from the influence of the source by the bulk of the ganglion" (Charlwood et al. 1972, p. 106). Subsequent studies from other laboratories brought additional support (Chamley, Goller, and Burnstock 1973; Ebendal and Jacobson 1977). However, not one of the experimental systems devised by the last investigators afforded rigorous and unequivocable evidence that NGF could guide nerve growth in vitro. This was to come from two more recent different experimental approaches, directed to establish (a) whether an NGF neurotropic effect was dissociated and independent from its well-known neurotrophic effect, and (b) whether NGF actually guided axonal elongation or simply enhanced the survival of axons that happen, by random growth, to be located near the NGF source.

The first question was answered by inspecting the growth pattern of axons from dissociated embryonic nerve cells in vitro in presence of an NGF source. The results seemed to provide evidence for dissociation of the neurotropic and neurotrophic effects of NGF (Letourneau 1978). However, evidence for an

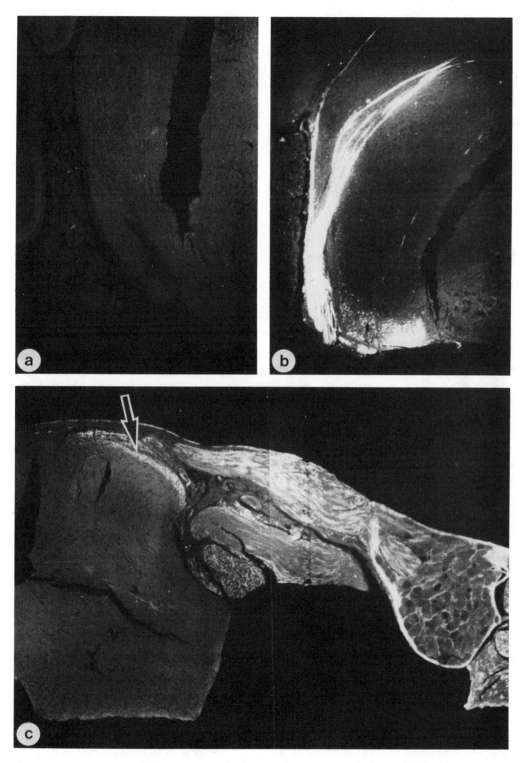

Figure 1.4. Transverse sections through the middle level of the medulla oblongata of (A) a control and (B) a littermate experimental rat. The latter was treated daily for a 10-day period with intracerebral NGF injections. (C) Transverse section through thoracic level of the spinal cord, dorsal root, and sensory ganglion of an NGF-intracerebrally injected 10-day-old rat. Adrenergic nerve fibers emerging from adjacent sympathetic ganglion (not shown in figure) gain access into the spinal cord (arrow) by enganging into an abnormal path through the ganglion and sensory dorsal root. (After Levi-Montalcini et al. 1978.)

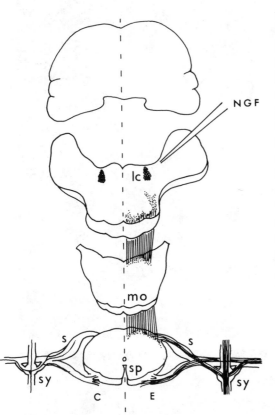

Figure 1.5. Diagrammatic representation of sympathetic fiber bundles that enter into the spinal cord and medulla oblongata from adjacent sympathetic ganglia in NGF-intracerebrally injected neonatal rats. Left half: control (C). Right half: experimental (E) case. NGF, site of injection of NGF into the floor of the fourth ventricle; lc, locus coeruleus; mo, medulla oblongata; sp, spinal cord; s, sensory ganglia; and sy, sympathetic ganglia. Sympathetic fibers run across the sensory ganglion and enter into the neural tube with the dorsal roots. (After Levi-Montalcini 1976.)

NGF directional effect on sensory axons was apparent only in 60% of the inspected nerve fibers, so the problem of whether NGF is endowed with a neurotropic effect could not be considered as definitely settled on the basis of these findings. Unequivocable evidence for a chemotactic effect was obtained one year later in a different in-vitro system. In view of the most impressive demonstration of this effect obtained by Gundersen and Barrett (1979), it is worth reporting in some detail their experimental design and the results.

Spinal root ganglia dissected out from 7–12-day chick embryos were incubated in a nu-trient medium supplemented with 5–10 biological units (BU) of NGF, a procedure that results in the production of a dense fibrillar halo that spreads around the explant within the first 24 hours of culture. At the end of the first day of culture, the cover slip with the ganglion was placed in an observation chamber and viewed with an inverted phase-contrast microscope. A micropipette filled with 1–50 BU of NGF and a tip diameter of 2–4 μm was positioned about 25 μm from the growth cone of an axon at about 45° from the fiber's longitudinal axis. Sequential micrographs of the motion of the growth cone exposed to NGF flowing out at a slow and constant rate from the pipette tip through a perfusion device show that the axons turn and grow toward the NGF source within 21 minutes (Figure 1.6). Upon successive displacement and repositioning of the micropipette, the axons adjusted their orientation according to the new position of the NGF source. They did not turn toward pipettes filled with other media or a low-NGF-concentration solution.

Subsequent, more detailed, and extensive studies by the same authors (Gundersen and Barrett 1980) were aimed at ascertaining whether the NGF property to impart directional cues to growing or regenerating nerve fibers of receptive neurons was due to growth changes consequent to an increased adhesion of the fiber to the substratum produced by NGF. The results did not favor this hypothesis. Attempts to identify the molecular mechanism underlying the NGF chemotactic effect consider the possibility that it results from an increase in the intracellular level of cAMP (cyclic adenosine 3′,5′ monophosphate) and calcium. This problem is under active investigation in this and other laboratories (Griffin and Letourneau 1980; Pfenninger and Johnson 1981).

Local control of neurite growth by NGF

Another feature of the NGF effects on axonal growth from its target cells was uncovered with a different in-vitro system. The growing axons and the cell bodies were separately submitted to the action of NGF in an apparatus comprising three chambers (Campenot 1977). Briefly, small cell clusters dissociated from the superior cervical ganglion of newborn rats were

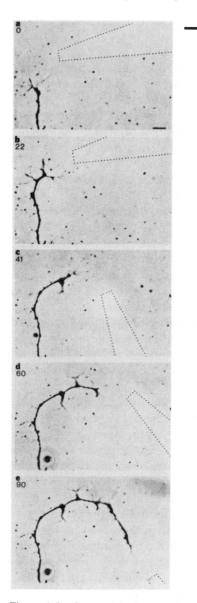

Scale Bar = 10 μm

Figure 1.6. Sequential photographs of a dorsal-root growth cone bathed in NGF (1 BU/ml) and exposed to an NGF gradient created by outflow from a micropipette containing NGF at 50 BU/ml. Numbers indicate time (in minutes) after the onset of perfusion by micropipette, and dotted lines outline the micropipette in its successive placements. The growth rate for this axon was 72 μm/hour. After 90 minutes, the axon had grown 108 μm and had turned almost 160° relative to its original direction of growth. Scale bar equals 10 μm. (After Gundersen and Barrett 1979, with permission; copyright 1979 by the American Association for the Advancement of Science.)

cultured in the central compartment of the system in a medium enriched with NGF. A barrier virtually impermeable to fluid, provided by teflon dividers sealed to the coverslip with silicone grease, separated the central chamber from the two lateral chambers. In one of them, but not in the other, NGF was added to the nutrient medium. Neurites regularly penetrated the barrier and extended into the side compartment containing an NGF-enriched medium, but did not bypass the barrier nor undergo elongation in the chamber devoid of NGF. Removal of NGF in the side compartment, where axons had already entered, resulted in their withdrawal and/or degeneration, whereas their cell bodies survived in excellent condition in the central NGF-rich chamber.

The conclusion was reached that "growth and probably survival of neurites depends upon NGF present in their local environment, regardless of the Nerve-Growth Factor concentration, to which other portions of the neuron are exposed" (Campenot 1977, p. 4516). In two subsequent, more extensive investigations (Campenot 1982a, 1982b), the experimental design was further perfected and the concept of local control of neurite growth was elaborated in great detail. The main result of these most accurate studies is that the NGF concentration in the local environment of the neurite exerts an important control over its growth, and lends support to the hypothesis that tissue NGF levels in different organs and tissues regulate their sympathetic innervation in vivo.

Campenot subsequently calls attention to the difference between the chemotactic or neurotropic effect demonstrated in vitro, mainly by the results reported by Gundersen and Barrett (1979, 1980), and the "local control effect" brought to light by his own investigations. In commenting on the previous in-vivo experiments that showed that sympathetic nerve fibers gain access inside the cerebrospinal axis upon NGF injections into the medulla oblongata of neonatal rats (Levi-Montalcini 1976; Menesini-Chen et al. 1978), Campenot states that these experiments "can be interpreted in the same manner as the experiments with compartmentalized cultures, i.e., the sympathetic fibers entered the central nervous system . . . when the ordinarily NGF-deficient central nervous system was provided with NGF. . . . These experiments neither demonstrate nor rule out that growth cones show chemotactic behavior, thereby elongating preferentially along a gradient of increasing NGF. A simple trophic requirement of direct exposure of the growth cone to extracellular NGF would be sufficient to confine neurite elongation in regions containing NGF" (Campenot 1982a, p. 2). However, this hypothesis takes no account of the main findings of the in-vivo experiments that have no counterpart in Campenot's in-vitro system. In order to gain access inside the neural tube, sympathetic nerve fibers (or their collaterals branching out from the stem axons) reversed their normal peripherally directed course and engaged into a new path, never followed before, that took them from the ganglia in a centripetal direction, to penetrate inside the central nervous system. The concept of local control of NGF elongation and branching is based on the assumption that a fluctuating NGF level regulates these processes, but it cannot explain the most atypical redirected elongation pattern exhibited by adrenergic fibers in the in-vivo experiments.

Equally difficult to accept, and indeed surprising, is the following statement by the same author: "I know of no convincing demonstration of the phenomenon (the NGF neurotropic effect) in sympathetic neurons" (Campenot 1982a, p. 2). Leaving aside the extensively documented evidence that NGF affects in a similar, if not identical, way sensory and sympathetic neurons (for an extensive documentation of the similarity of NGF effects on sensory and sympathetic neurons, see review articles by Levi-Montalcini, 1966, and Levi-Montalcini and Angeletti, 1968), and that the in-vivo experiments proved the NGF neurotropic effect, it is a universally accepted principle that a given biological effect uncovered in a model system need not be validated by submission to a test in all other like systems. According to Campenot, one could object also to the formulation of the chemoaffinity theory by Sperry, which was based only on his studies on the retinotectal connection in lower vertebrates. The significance of Sperry's theory rests in fact on the extrapolation that the same principle is valid also for other, as yet not investi-

gated, wiring systems in lower and higher vertebrates.

Chemoaffinity and neurotropism: The same or two different properties of nerve fibers?

The first time that the concept of chemoaffinity was enunciated in nonambiguous terms was in a lecture that Sperry delivered at a Growth Symposium and that was published in 1951 (Sperry 1951). This concept was further elaborated in the following years. At the first International Neurochemical Symposium held in Oxford in 1954, Sperry stated, "The kind of chemoaffinity required for the selective linkage of sensory and central neurons is not unlike that observed among other biological phenomena, a number of examples of which are well known in the laboratory" (Sperry 1955a, p. 79), and he quotes the specific affinity of a single species of motile sperm only for unfertilized eggs of its kind, the bacteriophage attachment to only bacteria of a particular strain, the property of dissociated cells of a sponge to recombine selectively with their own kind, and concludes, "The selective chemoaffinities involved in synaptic formation in the nervous system are special only in their extreme refinement. They go beyond the order of species, tissues, and even of organ specificity, almost in some instances, to that of the individual cell" (*ibid.*, p. 79). At present, as stated by Viktor Hamburger, "the chemoaffinity hypothesis can be considered as consisting of three basic components: chemical identity of like neurons belonging to the same strain, such as a motor pool, selective matching affinity of growth cones with chemical cues in their local micro environment which they encounter along their pathway, and selective affinity of nerve terminals and their targets in synapse formation" (Hamburger 1981, p. 154).

The concept of neurotropism was formulated by Ramon y Cajal in the last decade of the past century (Ramon y Cajal 1888). It remained, however, for the Nerve-Growth Factor to provide definite evidence in favor of the hypothesis that growing and regenerating nerve fibers are receptive to the chemotactic cues provided by this protein molecule. In commenting on the effects, reported in previous pages, of intracerebral NGF injections in neonatal rats, in reference to this chemotactic response, Griffin and Letourneau wrote, "A dramatic *in-vivo* finding is that the injection of nerve growth factor (NGF) into the brain of young rats induces abnormal growth of axons from peripheral sympathetic neurons into the spinal cord and up to the site of NGF injection" (Griffin and Letourneau 1980, p. 156). The rigorous *in-vitro* experimental approach by Gundersen and Barrett provided, as already mentioned, a most impressive proof of this neurotropic effect.

It is, however, all too apparent that the concept of neurotropism differs in many important respects from that of chemoaffinity; it deals, in fact, with the role played by diffusible factors, possibly released by end organs and tissues, in imparting directional instruction to growing or regenerating nerve fibers, and makes no mention of a genetically programmed blueprint for the building of neuronal circuits and formation of selective synaptic connections between axons and matching neuronal or non-neuronal cell populations. Neurotropism, in other words, stresses the role of the microenvironment rather than that of the genetic program imprinted in each component of neuronal circuits. In elaborating on these complementary rather than identical factors in the formation of neuronal nets, we stated in a previous article:

> The recognition of such a role (neurotropic NGF role) played by diffusible factors in directing nerve fibers toward their matching end organs and tissues does not contradict the firmly established and today generally accepted concept that neuronal nets are genetically determined and not modifiable by extrinsic environmental factors. It acknowledges, however, a restricted degree of freedom to the growing fibers into the general frame of these preestablished programs. The axonal tip of the fibers moves along gradients of diffusion of trophic and tropic factors released by end organs, according to a time schedule which is very similar if not identical in all developing organisms. Neurotropism would assist rather than determine the course of nerve fibers toward their correct destination. The effects

produced by intracerebral NGF injections in neonatal rodents should be regarded as a grossly magnified and almost charicatural representation, but not misrepresentation of what happens in normal neurogenesis, where developmental processes unfold in temporal and topographic sequences which are the same for all systems and mask with their precision the underlying intrinsic (genetic) and extrinsic (environmental) factors which interact at each step in the building of the final product, maybe the whole organism or the formation of neuronal circuits (Menesini-Chen et al. 1978, p. 80).

Both concepts of chemoaffinity and of neurotropism emphasize the role of chemical factors as diffusible or structural components of cell membrane in the building of neuronal nets. NGF "instructs" genetically selected populations of neurites, guiding them toward their correct matching cells. This protein molecule, and other like factors, produced by target cells might, as submitted by Purves, "be considered mediators of chemoaffinity in a broad sense" (Purves 1981, p. 239).

The road ahead

"But the final step, from position specificity to chemoaffinity, remains to be taken. So far, chemoaffinity is an abstract concept devoid of substantial content. . . . It is a challenge to the molecular neuroembryologist to give it a concrete meaning" (Hamburger 1975, p. 172).

These two past decades have not seen the solution of the problem outlined by Sperry (1965) of identifying the chemical nature of the factors responsible for imparting specificity to the partners that interconnect in the formation of nerve nets. This problem was and still is beyond the resolution power of conventional biochemical techniques, but it can now be approached, as prefigured by Hamburger (1975) with newly developed, more powerful tools.

Before mentioning a most promising line of investigation along these lines, it is worth recalling the value of relating concepts in the two once-segregated fields of inquiry, one dealing with the problem of identifying the nature of the chemical factors that confer like or complementary connotations to the partners of neuronal circuits and the other investigating the spectrum of action of NGF in the differentiation of its target nerve cells. At present, the retinotectal fiber connections still represent the best, if not the only, preparation with which to test the chemoaffinity theory (see, however, Purves and Lichtman 1983). A similar leading role pertains to NGF. In fact, this protein molecule represents the only NGF that has been identified in an unequivocable way and submitted to extensive structural, ultrastructural, and biochemical studies. At the time of this writing, advances are taking place at an unprecedented pace in both areas of investigation, thanks to the development of new methodological approaches and the availability of tools and techniques borrowed from molecular biology and immunology. Some of these advances bring the two fields into closer relation. The now routinely used technique of producing monoclonal antibodies to different antigens, according to the most ingenious method devised by Kohler and Milstein (1975), has already found invaluable application in all sectors of biology. It is possible that no sector of neuroscience will profit more from the exploitation of this technique than those dealing respectively with differentiation of different nerve-cell populations and of the building of wiring circuits among them. New avenues opened by the advent of recombinant DNA technology and of monoclonal antibodies are most competently discussed in three recent articles (Sutcliffe et al. 1983; Chaudhari and Hahn 1983; McKay 1983).

In conclusion, it is of particular interest in reference to the problem first prospected by Sperry more than three decades ago on the role of chemospecificity in the building of neuronal circuits to see how his hypothesis that the retinal ganglion cells undergo chemical specification according to two ortogonal molecular gradients (Figure 1.1) has received a most gratifying confirmation from recent studies that made use of this monoclonal antibody technique. By this method, Trisler, Schneider, and Nirenberg (1981) identified a monoclonal antibody that recognizes an antigen that is thirty-five times more concentrated in the dorsal than in the ventral portions of the chick retina. Im-

munofluorescence studies, reported in the same article, support the hypothesis that the antigen molecules are distributed in the retina on the basis of cell position rather than cell type. Perhaps these most important findings should be viewed as only a first step along the line indicated by Sperry when he stated, "The nature of the biochemistry of the specificity factors that underlie the demonstrated selectivity in nerve growth . . . remains, of course, an open field untouched as yet, with relatively little in the way of evidence to curb creative speculation" (Sperry 1965, p. 172). Nevertheless, they prove that the Chemoaffinity Theory is now amenable to rigorous verification.

References

Attardi, D. G., and R. W. Sperry. 1963. Preferential selection of central pathways by regenerating optic fibers. *Exp. Neurol.* 7: 46–64.

Campenot, R. B. 1977. Local control of neurite development by nerve growth factor. *Proc. Natl. Acad. Sci. USA* 74: 4516–19.

–1982a. Development of sympathetic neurons in compartmentalized cultures. I. Local control of neurite growth by nerve growth factor. *Dev. Biol.* 93: 1–12.

–1982b. Development of sympathetic neurons in compartmentalized cultures. II. Local control of neurite survival by nerve growth factor. *Dev. Biol.* 93: 13–21.

Chamley, J. H., I. Goller, and J. Burnstock. 1973. Selective growth of sympathetic fibers to explants of normally densely innervated autonomic effector organs in tissue culture. *Dev. Biol.* 31: 362–79.

Charlwood, K. A., D. M. Lamont, and B. E. C. Banks. 1972. Apparent orientating effects produced by nerve growth factor. *In* E. Zaimis (ed.) *Nerve Growth Factor and its Antiserum.* Athlone Press, London, pp. 102–7.

Chaudhari, N., and W. E. Hahn. 1983. Genetic expression in the developing brain. *Science* 220: 924–8.

Cohen, S. 1960. Purification of a nerve growth promoting protein from the mouse salivary gland and its neurocytoxic antiserum. *Proc. Natl. Acad. Sci. USA* 42: 302–11.

Ebendal, T., and C. O. Jacobson. 1977. Tissue explants affecting extension and orientation of axons in cultured chick embryo ganglia. *Exp. Cell Res.* 105: 379–87.

Griffin, C. G., and P. C. Letourneau. 1980. Rapid retraction of neurites by sensory neurons in response to increased concentrations of nerve growth factor. *J. Cell Biol.* 86: 156–61.

Gundersen, R. W., and J. N. Barrett. 1979. Neuronal chemotaxis. Chick dorsal-root axons turn toward high concentration of nerve growth factor. *Science* 206: 1079–80.

–1980. Characterization of the turning response of dorsal root neurites toward nerve growth factor. *J. Cell Biol.* 87: 546–54.

Hamburger, V. 1975. Changing concepts in developmental neurobiology. *Persp. Biol. and Med.* 12: 162–78.

–1979. Roger Sperry. *Neurosci. Newslett.* 10: 5–6.

–1980. S. Ramon Cajal, R. G. Harrison, and the beginnings of neuroembryology. *Perso. Biol. and Med.* 23: 600–16.

–1981. Historical landmarks in neurogenesis. *Trends in Neurosci.* 4: 1951–5.

Kandel, E. R., and W. A. Spencer. 1968. Cellular neurophysiological approaches in the study of learning. *Physiol. Rev.* 48: 60–134.

Kohler, G., and C. Milstein. 1975. Continuous cultures of fused cells secreting antibody of predefined specificity. *Nature (London)* 256: 495–7.

Lashley, K. S. 1929. *Brain Mechanism and Intelligence: A Quantitative Study of Injuries to the Brain.* University of Chicago Press, Chicago.

Letourneau, P. C. 1978. Chemotactic response of nerve fiber elongation to nerve growth factor. *Dev. Biol.* 66: 183–96.

Levi-Montalcini, R. 1950. The origin and development of the visceral system in the spinal cord of the chick embryo. *J. Morphol.* 86: 253–84.

–1952. Effects of mouse tumor transplantation on the nervous system. *Ann. N.Y. Acad. Sci.* 55: 330–43.

–1964. Events in the developing nervous system. *In* D. P. Purpura and J. P. Schade (eds.) *Progress in Brain Research, Growth and Maturation of the Brain,* Vol. 4. Elsevier, Amsterdam, pp. 1–26.

–1966. The nerve growth factor: Its mode of action on sensory and sympathetic nerve cells. *Harvey Lectures* 60: 217–59.

–1976. The nerve growth factor: Its role in growth differentiation and function of the sympathetic adrenergic neuron. *In* M. A. Corner and D. F. Swaab (eds.) *Progress in Brain Research: Perspectives in Brain Research,* Vol. 45. Elsevier, Amsterdam, pp. 235–46.

Levi-Montalcini, R., and P. U. Angeletti. 1968. Nerve growth factor. *Physiol. Rev.* 48: 534–69.

Levi-Montalcini, R., M. G. Menesini-Chen, and J. S. Chen. 1978. Neurotropic effects of the nerve growth factor in chick embryos and in neonatal rodents. *Zoon* 6: 201–12.

Levi-Montalcini, R., H. Meyer, and V. Hamburger. 1954. In-vitro experiments on the effects of mouse sarcoma on the sensory and sympathetic ganglia of the chick embryo. *Cancer Res.* 14: 49–57.

Matthey, R. 1925. Récupération de la vue aprés résection des nerfs optiques chez le Triton. *Cont. Rend. Soc. Biol.* 93: 904–6.

McKay, R. D. G. 1983. Molecular approaches to the nervous system. *Ann. Rev. Neurosci.* 6: 527–46.

Medawar, P. B. 1967. *The Art of the Soluble.* Methuen, London.

Menesini-Chen, M. G., J. S. Chen, and R. Levi-Montalcini. 1978. Sympathetic nerve fiber in growth in the central nervous system of neonatal rodents upon intracerebral NGF injection. *Arch. Ital. Biol.* 116: 53–84.

Pfenninger, K. H., and M. P. Johnson. 1981. Nerve growth factor stimulates phospholipid methylation in growing neurites. *Proc. Natl. Acad. Sci. USA* 78: 7797–800.

Purves, D. 1981. Selective formation of synapses in the peripheral nervous system and the chemoaffinity hypothesis of neural specificity. *In* M. Cowan (ed.) *Studies in Developmental Neurobiology (Essays in Honor of Viktor Hamburger).* Oxford University Press, New York and Oxford, pp. 231–42.

Purves, D., and J. W. Lichtman. 1983. Specific connections between nerve cells. *Ann. Rev. Physiol.* 45: 553–65.

Ramon y Cajal, S. R. 1888. *Estructura de la Retina de las Aves.* Thorpe and Glick (trans.) Thomas, Springfield (IL), 1972.

Sperry, R. W. 1941. The effect of crossing nerves to antagonistic muscles in the hind limb of the rat. *J. Comp. Neurol.* 75: 1–19.

–1943a. Functional results of crossing sensory nerves in the rat. *J. Comp. Neurol.* 78: 59–90.

–1943b. Effect of 180 degree rotation of the retinal field on visuomotor coordination. *J. Exp. Zool.* 92: 263–79.

–1951. Regulative factors in the orderly growth of neural circuits. *Growth Symp.* 10: 63–87.

–1955a Problems in the biochemical specification of neurons. *In* H. Waelsch (ed.) *Biochemistry of the Developing Nervous System. Proceedings of the First International Neurochemical Symposium.* Academic Press, New York, pp. 74–84.

–1955b. Functional regeneration in the optic system. *In* W. F. Windle (ed.) *Regeneration in the Central Nervous System.* Thomas, Springfield (IL), pp. 66–76.

–1958. Physiological plasticity and brain circuit theory. *In* H. F. Harlow and C. N. Woolsey (eds.) *Biological and Biochemical Bases of Behavior.* University of Wisconsin Press, Madison, pp. 401–21.

–1963. Chemoaffinity in the orderly growth of nerve fiber patterns and connections. *Proc. Natl. Acad. Sci. USA* 50: 703–10.

–1965. Embryogenesis of behavioral nerve nets. *In* R. L. DeHaan and H. Ursprung (eds.) *Organogenesis,* Vol. 6. Holt, Rinehart and Winston, New York, pp. 161–85.

Sutcliffe, J., R. J. Milner, T. M. Shinnick, and F. E. Bloom. 1983. Identifying the protein products of brain-specific genes with antibodies to chemically synthesized peptides. *Cell* 33: 671–82.

Stone, L. S. 1944. Functional polarization in retinal development and its reestablishment in regenerating retinae of rotated grafted eyes. *Proc. Soc. Exp. Biol. Med.* 57: 13–14.

Trisler, G. D., M. D. Schneider, and M. Nirenberg.

1981. A topographic gradient of molecules in retina can be used to identify neuron position. *Proc. Natl. Acad. Sci. USA* 78: 2145–9.

Weiss, P. A. 1928. Erregungspecifität und erregungsresonanz. *Ergeb. Biol.* 3: 1–151.

–1931. Das Resonanzprinzip des Nerventätigkeit Wien. *Klin. Wochenschr.* 39: 1–17.

–1936. Selectivity controlling the central-peripheral relations in the nervous system. *Biol. Rev.* 11: 494–531.

–1955. Nervous system (neurogenesis). *In* B. H. Willier, P. A. Weiss, and V. Hamburger (eds.) *Analysis of Development.* Saunders, Philadelphia, pp. 346–401.

–1976. Neurobiology in statu nascendi. *In* M. A. Corner and D. F. Swaab (eds.) *Progress in Brain Research: Perspectives in Brain Research,* Vol. 45. Elsevier, Amsterdam, pp. 7–38.

Wiersma, C. A. G. 1931. An experiment on the "resonance theory" of muscular activity. *Arch. Néerl. Physiol.* 16: 337–45.

The chemoaffinity hypothesis: An appreciation of Roger W. Sperry's contributions to developmental biology

R. Kevin Hunt
Department of Neuroscience
Children's Hospital Medical Center
and

W. Maxwell Cowan
Howard Hughes Medical Institute

Introduction

In citing his seminal work on hemispheric localization and its implications for consciousness and mentation, the Nobel Prize Committee appropriately recognized what will undoubtedly remain as Roger Sperry's major contribution to neuroscience. But it would be unfortunate if this recognition were to obscure, in any degree, the importance of his fundamental contributions to developmental biology in general, and to neuroembryology in particular. For just as his studies of the corpus callosum were to transform our understanding of higher brain function, his ingenious experiments on the regeneration of nerve connections and the bold conceptual advance provided by his chemoaffinity hypothesis completely revolutionized neuroembryology, and secured a place for him alongside such distinguished figures as S. Ramon y Cajal, J. N. Langley, Hans Spemann, Johannes Holtfreter, and Ross Harrison (see Hamburger 1981). In this chapter, we briefly reexamine Sperry's developmental studies over the quarter century from 1940 to 1965 and attempt to place his work and ideas within the appropriate historical context in order to make clear the magnitude of his contribution.

THE CHEMOAFFINITY HYPOTHESIS AND ITS EXPERIMENTAL FOUNDATION

The significance of new conceptual developments in science can generally be assessed by the difficulty one encounters when trying to recapture the thought patterns, ideas, and even the language that were in vogue before the new concepts came to be accepted. And when the conceptual advance was of the magnitude of Roger Sperry's and was supported by a painstaking body of work over 25 years or more, it is difficult to summarize in a few pages the key elements that led to the advance or to adequately describe the confusion and misconceptions that his work laid to rest.

Any attempt to evaluate Sperry's contribution to developmental neurobiology, and to trace its embryological antecedents, must be informed by an appreciation not only of the experimental strategies he adopted and the ideas that those strategies gave rise to, but also of the historical background against which his work was carried out. Sperry's own review of 1965 gives us some glimpse of the problem of the "embryogenesis of behavioral nerve nets" as it was viewed in the 1930s:

> The old problem of how all the information required to build a complete organism can be compacted and funneled through the microscopic dimensions of the zygote – and the problem involved in the reading out of all this genetic information, step by step, in development – is encountered in probably its ultimate and most challenging form in the developmental organization of the brain and nervous system.... Here, in addition to the many problems of morphogenesis and cytodifferentiation common to other organs and organ systems, formidable

enough in themselves, is the problem of the wiring of this whole system for behavior.

For a long time it was believed that the developing embryo avoided the whole problem by letting the growth process spin out a random, diffuse, unstructured, essentially equipotential transmission network; a blank slate as it were, leaving behavior, function, practice, experience, learning, and conditioning to mold and shape the fiber pathways into a functionally adaptive communication system. The old saying prevailed: "Function precedes form in the development of the nervous system" (Sperry 1965, p. 161).

Moving to the present, he goes on to say in the same essay:

> Today, by contrast, . . . some researchers are taking an almost diametrically opposite stand – to emphasize that the great bulk of behavioral circuitry of the nervous system, especially in infrahuman vertebrates, is built in. That is, the behavioral networks are organized in advance of their use, by growth and differentiation primarily, with relatively little dependence on function for their orderly patterning. The center of the problem has thus shifted from the province of psychology to that of developmental biology. . . . A key concept in the more recent, more genetically oriented outlook on these matters, is that of the chemical differentiation or qualitative specificity of individual nerve cells and fibers and its influence on the formation of fiber pathways and connections . . . the extent to which the cytochemical specificity of the individual nerve cells and fibers determines the kinds of structural linkages that neurons form.

The work that led to this new perspective was largely due to Sperry himself, and began with a critical analysis of the earlier "functionalist" position and the first clear formulation of its central ideas: the interchangeability of young nerves, the nonselectivity of central and peripheral innervation, and the modification by function and experience of maladaptive connections. Then, having defined the issues, Sperry set about to systematically test each point in a sustained series of experiments that were at once elegant in their simplicity and formidable in their rigor.

Although the experiments were to progress through a variety of neural systems – from the motor innervation of the limbs through the somatosensory and vestibular systems to the projection of the retina upon the optic tectum, and were to be carried out on a variety of animals, in newts, frogs, several different teleosts, and even mammals – the general strategy was parsimonius and organized around two dominant themes. The first strategy was to surgically force upon the animal a set of behaviorally maladaptive nerve connections and then test its ability, through function and experience, to either correct the connections so formed or to replace them with functionally adaptive circuits. The second strategy was to challenge growing axons with an expanded range of potential targets, to provide them with an opportunity to innervate both appropriate and inappropriate cells or tissues, and then to assess the degree to which the axons connect selectively with particular targets while rejecting others. We shall later consider in some detail many of the studies in which these two strategies were employed, but it is appropriate here to mention a few of the most striking experiments to give something of the flavor of his work and style.

As a graduate student under Paul Weiss at the University of Chicago, Sperry began his experimental work in 1938 with a series of studies on the innervation of the limbs in young rats (see the foreword). In the first experiments, he surgically transposed the flexor and extensor muscles of the foot to see if, in time, the animals could "learn" to make the correct foot movements as the "functionalist" view would predict (Sperry 1940). In a second study, he first cross-united the peroneal and tibial nerves in one group of rats, and, in a second group of animals, he crossed the nerve branches to two specific antagonist muscles, the gastrocnemius and the anterior tibial, and at the same time removed all the other muscles that act upon the ankle joint (Sperry 1941). In yet a third study, the analysis was extended to antagonistic muscles in the forelimb (Sperry 1942). In each case, the movements of the relevant foot during normal walking, and after reflex or electrical stimulation of the appropriate nerves, were carefully monitored, often for several months. In all these studies, the critical findings were the same: the movements elicited were always maladaptive, the animal flexing its foot when extension was called for and vice versa, and the rats showed "no adjustments, either immediate by means of automatic reflex regulation or gradual, by means of a learning or conditioning process" (Sperry 1940, p. 399). The consistency of the findings permitted only one conclusion: motoneurons are not interchangeable, and even prolonged function is powerless to correct behaviorally maladaptive neuromuscular connections.

Shortly after these studies, Sperry began to exploit the ability of amphibians to regenerate central neural connections. He began by confirming that in newts, whose optic nerves were transected and allowed to regenerate, visual function could be completely restored, as judged by visually guided strike responses to lures placed at various positions in the field of view of the affected eye. In other cases, the eye was rotated 180° *in situ* at the time of nerve transection; in these animals, recovery of function was accompanied by consistently misdirected visual responses: whenever a lure was placed in the visual field of the rotated eye, the animals would always turn toward a position 180° away from the lure (see Figure 2.1). As Sperry reported:

> They displayed definite photokinetic reactions to rotation of the visual field, but the responses were made in the reverse direction. When the drum was revolved counterclockwise about the animals, they slowly turned their heads to the right in the direction opposite to that in which the visual field was moving. . . . When a small moving lure was held above the animals, they turned their heads downward; when it was held in front of them, they turned around and looked behind them; and when it was held behind them and slightly to one side, they started forward. . . . Spa-

tial localization of small objects was thus consistently erroneous in direct correlation with retinal rotation (Sperry 1943b, p. 39).

Similar misdirected visuomotor reflexes were later demonstrated in frogs with 180°-rotated eyes; these results were particularly dramatic since frogs normally respond to lure stimuli with sharply directed prey-catching strikes, Figure 2.1B:

> When a fly was held in front of the animals within easy jumping distance, they wheeled rapidly to the rear instead of striking forward. Contrariwise, when the lure was held in back of them and a little to the side they struck forward into space. When the animals came to rest in such a position that the lure could be presented well below eye level, they tilted the head upward and snapped at the air above. When the lure was held above the head and a little caudal to the eye the animals struck downward in front of them and got a mouthful of mud and moss. When the lure was presented successively in front of the animals they kept shifting around in circles as if the lure had appeared behind them each time instead of in front (Sperry 1944, p. 64).

In a companion series of studies, Sperry (1945a) tested visual behavior in newts and frogs after surgical cross-union of the left and right optic nerves, or after contralateral transplantation of one eye. Following optic-nerve regeneration and recovery of vision, the animals with contralaterally transplanted eyes reproducibly misdirected their responses in either the horizontal or the vertical dimension of visual space, depending on whether the left-to-right transplantation had inverted the eye anteroposteriorly or dorsoventrally. In the animals whose left and right optic nerves had been cross-united, there was a similar one-axis reversal of visuomotor reflexes: the animals predictably responded to a visual stimulus as if it had been presented in the visual field of the other eye. In every case, the animal retained its exact pattern of maladaptive visuomotor localization, over many months of visual test-

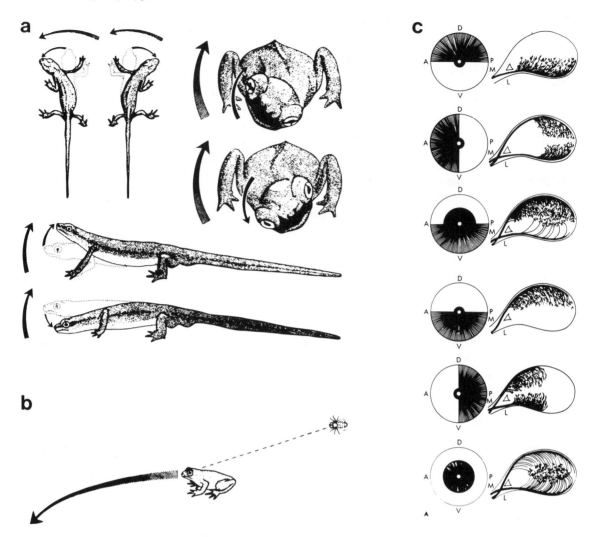

Figure 2.1. **(A)** Normal and 180°-misdirected visuomotor "following" reactions in newts that had recovered visual function after optic-nerve transection (Sperry 1946). Each pair of newts illustrates the reactions to a particular lure position, and contrasts normal responses seen after simple transection of the optic nerve (and its regeneration) with misdirected responses of newts whose eyes had been rotated through 180° at the time of the nerve transection. (*Top left*) When a lure was placed in front of the newt and to the animal's left, the newt with normally oriented eyes slowly turned its head toward the left, indicating that the regenerated optic-nerve fibers again mediated accurate visuomotor localization. By contrast, the newt with rotated eyes responded to the same stimulus by turning its head to the *right*, away from the stimulus. The same pair of newts are shown responding to other lure positions (*top right* and *bottom*). In each case, when the eyes had been left in their normal anatomical orientation, the regenerated optic fibers mediated normal visuomotor localization, whereas the reactions of the newts whose eyes had been rotated were always directed 180° away from the lure. (From Sperry 1951a.) **(B)** 180°-misdirected visuomotor "striking" reaction to a lure placed in the visual field of an adult frog that had recovered visual function following optic-nerve transection and 180°-rotation of the eye (Sperry 1944). Here a lure behind and above the frog has evoked a strike directed below and in front of the animal. (From Sperry 1951a.) **(C)** Summary of the histological findings of Attardi and Sperry (1963) following the surgical excision of specific portions of the retina and transection of the remaining optic-nerve fibers in adult goldfish. Regenerating optic-nerve fibers from the surviving partial retinae had apparently reinnervated only their correct parts of the tectum and had regrown selectively through their

ing, with no signs of improved visuomotor performance:

> The majority of cases were retained longer than two months after recovery of vision; four were kept longer than four months; and one as long as five and one half months. The reversed optikenetic reactions, spontaneous circus movements, and erroneous spatial localization of small objects were all present up to the time of sacrifice. There was no oppositive correction in any case of any of the reversed reactions (Sperry 1945a, p. 18).

From a consideration of these behavioral data, and from observations on the disordered arrangement of the nerve fibers at the site of the lesion, and on the localized scotomas (blind spots) that occurred after restricted tectal lesions, Sperry (1943a, 1943b, 1944, 1945a) concluded that during regeneration, the axons of retinal ganglion cells must grow back to their original projection sites and that even prolonged function is unable to modify maladaptive visual connections.

In the late 1940s and early 1950s, Sperry carried out an important series of studies on cutaneous innervation with his student Nancy Miner. In one set of experiments (Sperry and Miner 1949), surgical cross-union of the cranial nerves that mediate cutaneous sensation of the face resulted in misdirected motor reflexes in response to discrete tactile stimulation. In another group of experiments (Miner and Sperry 1950; Miner 1956), an extra hindlimb bud was grafted onto the trunk of a number of tadpoles. Although the supernumerary limbs were limited in their mobility, after metamorphosis, pinching of the limbs evoked a specific withdrawal of the frog's normal hind limb. At Sperry's suggestion, Miner (1956) also rotated the trunk skin of tadpoles through 180°, so that the white belly skin was transposed to the back and the spotted back skin was moved to the belly (see Figure 2.12A). After metamorphosis, stroking the belly skin on the frog's back evoked specific limb-wipes to the belly (the original position of the skin), whereas tickling the transplanted back skin on the frog's belly consistently evoked wipes to the back. Again, the pattern of maladaptive reflexes failed to improve over many months of testing. As we shall see later, these experiments were important in the development of the notion that neuron specificity can be induced by association with a peripheral sensory receptor, but for the moment, it will suffice to make the point that they served to bring the somatosensory system into line with Sperry's emerging connectionist view:

> The results appear to eliminate mechanical guidance and functional adaptation as the factors responsible for the neural organization mediating cutaneous local sign in amphibians. They indicate the existence of a refined constitutional specificity among the cutaneous nerve fibers and in the integumentum itself. The patterning of synapses between sensory and central neurons is tentatively explained in terms of our chemoaffinity theory of synapse formation (Sperry and Miner 1949, p. 422).

And so the work progressed, applying the same critical test experiments to a wide range of systems, including the vestibular system

---

normal pathways to the tectal lobe. Six variations of the experiment are depicted, each showing the retinal ablation to the left and a tracing of the contralateral optic tectum (dorsal view) to the right to show the typical pattern of silver-stained axons and terminals from the optic-nerve fibers that had regenerated from the residual and regenerated fibers. Fibers from the dorsal retina innervated only the lateral half of the tectum, where the dorsal retina normally projects in intact goldfish. The medial half of the textum, previously innervated by the (now excised) ventral half of the retina, had been "bypassed" by the regenerating dorsal fibers. Moreover, all of the regenerated dorsal optic-nerve fibers had reached the tectum via their normal pathway – the lateral brachium of the tract; the medial brachium of the tract, normally filled by optic fibers from ventral retina, was missing. The remaining rows show other retinal ablations and regenerated optic-fiber patterns. In each case, the regenerated fibers from the partial retina had "bypassed" large areas of vacant tectum and confined their terminal arbors to the part of the tectum they normally innervate. (After Sperry 1965.)

(Sperry 1945b), the regenerating spinal cord and brainstem of goldfish (Sperry 1948b), and the innervation of the tail-fin and eye muscles of *Astronotus* fish (Sperry and Dupree 1956; Arora and Sperry 1957; Sperry and Arora 1965). Then in the early 1960s, he returned to the visual system and, taking advantage of the distinctive staining of regenerating axons, carried out a now classical series of experiments on the regeneration of optic-nerve fibers in the goldfish. With Arora, he cross-sutured the medial and lateral brachia of the optic tract and observed that although the regenerating optic fibers entered the tectum through an abnormal route, they coursed abruptly across the tectal surface, bypassing the inappropriate half of the tectal lobe, and only terminated when they had grown into their appropriate target zone (Arora and Sperry 1962; Sperry 1965). With Attardi, he selectively ablated various parts of the retina, leaving, in different animals, only the central retina, the anterior or posterior retina, or the dorsal or ventral half-retina. Silver-stained preparations, made a few weeks after the optic nerve was crushed, showed that the regenerating axons from the surviving portion of the retina selectively terminated in their original target zone, again often bypassing large areas of noninnervated tectum (Figure 2.1C). Moreover, not only were the termination zones remarkably specific, but the main fiber bundles appeared to have "homed in" rather directly on their target region, often coursing along "shortcuts" at right angles to the normal direction of fiber growth (Attardi and Sperry 1963; Sperry 1963). Accordingly, the chemoaffinity model was extended to include selective growth to the target as well as matching of the fibers with the target cells themselves:

> Our thesis that specific chemical affinities govern neuronal synapsis . . . may be extended on the basis of the present findings to include the patterning of central fiber pathways. Not only the details of synaptic association within terminal centers, but also the routes by which the fibers reach their synaptic zones would seem to be subject to regulation during growth by differential chemical affinities (Attardi and Sperry 1963, p. 62).

We also find that fibers from neighboring points in the retina tend to segregate at the first opportunity within the nerve scar and may remain thus segregated through the chiasma and all the way to the tectum. It is apparent from the results that not only the synaptic terminals, but also in these fishes, the route by which the growing optic fibers reach those terminals, is selectively determined, presumably on the basis of similar or identical chemoaffinity factors (Sperry 1963, p. 706).

Thus it was that the working framework of developmental neurobiology changed from one of functional selection among equipotential neural nets to one of chemically labeled nerve cells and prefunctional "hard-wiring" of neural connections by selective growth and recognition of chemically matched cells. Later in this chapter, we will return to these experiments as we trace the evolution of the concepts of chemoaffinity and neuronal specificity. Yet the initial conceptual leap, from upside-down visual striking to notions of fieldlike differentiation and chemical matching between two neuronal arrays, must be appreciated not only for its boldness, but also for its ability to draw together a number of embryologic ideas, whose origins we now consider.

Antecedents

RAMON Y CAJAL, HIS, AND NEUROSCIENCE AS A CELLULAR DISCIPLINE

The emergence of neuroscience as a cellular discipline occurred after an unusually long gestation. It was more than fifty years after the formulation of the cell theory that Wilhelm His (1886) first proposed what is now known as the *neuron doctrine*. According to this, individual neurons are the fundamental cellular units of the nervous system, each neuron being anatomically discrete, embryologically distinctive, and, in a sense, functionally independent. It followed from this that the axon is to be regarded as a protoplasmic extension of the neuron, "an outgrowth from a single cell which is its genetic, trophic and functional center." At about the same time, and quite independently, Santiago Ramon y Cajal (1890; 1905; 1908) recognized the specialized structures at the ends of growing axons, which he called "growth cones" (Figure 2.2A). Writing some time later (1909), he was to go well beyond his initial simple description when he referred to the growth cones as:

> a sort of club or battering ram, endowed with exquisite chemical sensitivity, with rapid ameboid movements, and with impulsive force by which it is able to proceed forward and overcome obstacles met in the way, forcing cellular interstices, until it arrives at its destination (Ramon y Cajal 1917, p. 599).

From his careful study of Golgi-impregnated sections of embryonic neural tissue, he was convinced that the axons of young neuroblasts were highly selective in their direction of outgrowth, and that they "sensed" their way through the complex landscape of the embryonic nervous system before selectively associating with their preferred target cells in the nervous system itself or in the periphery. Drawing upon earlier notions of "tropism" from experimental physiology and embryology (Roux 1888; Bohn 1897), Ramon y Cajal proposed a theory of chemotropism to explain the selective outgrowth of axons and the specificity of the connections they formed:

> How does the mechanical development of nerve fibers occur, and wherein lies that

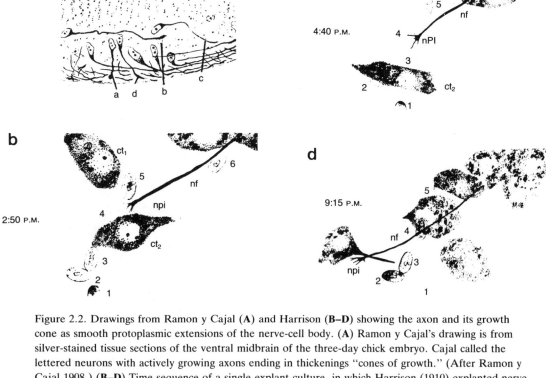

Figure 2.2. Drawings from Ramon y Cajal (**A**) and Harrison (**B–D**) showing the axon and its growth cone as smooth protoplasmic extensions of the nerve-cell body. (**A**) Ramon y Cajal's drawing is from silver-stained tissue sections of the ventral midbrain of the three-day chick embryo. Cajal called the lettered neurons with actively growing axons ending in thickenings "cones of growth." (After Ramon y Cajal 1908.) (**B–D**) Time sequence of a single explant culture, in which Harrison (1910) explanted nerve cells onto clotted lymph and challenged them to grow out axons *in vitro*. Harrison's (1910, p. 816) original legend read: "Three views of a growing nerve fiber, observed alive in a clotted lymph preparation. 1, 2, 3, 4, 5, red blood corpuscles in fixed position; *ct₁* and *ct₂*, single cells which were seen to wander across the field: *nf*, nerve fiber; *npl*, growing end of motile protoplasm. (**B**) As seen at 2:50 p.m., two days after isolation of the embryonic tissue. (**C**) As seen at 4:40 p.m., the same day. Note change in form and position of the loose cells. (**D**) As seen at 9:15 p.m., the same day. Movement of cells has covered over the proximal part of the fiber."

marvelous power which enables nerve fibers from very distant cells to make contact directly with certain other nerve cells or the mesoderm or ectoderm without going astray or taking a roundabout course?

Without wanting to deny the importance of . . . mechanical influence, especially in the growth of the nerve fibers from the retina to the brain and vice versa, I believe that one could also think of processes like the phenomenon called Pfeffer's chemotaxis, whose influences on the leukocytes was established by Massary and Bordet. . . .

If a chemotaxic sensitivity of the neuroblasts is assumed, then it must be supposed that these cells are capable of amoeboid movement and are responsive to certain substances secreted by cells of the epithelium or mesoderm. *The processes of the neuroblasts become oriented by chemical stimulation, and move toward the secreted products of certain cells* (Ramon y Cajal 1894, p. 146, emphasis added).

In the 1890s, again apparently independently, J. N. Langley advanced rather strong evidence that regenerating preganglionic fibers to the superior cervical ganglion can selectively reestablish connections with the correct classes of postsynaptic cells in the ganglion. Langley's observations on the return of specific sympathetic functions and the inescapable evidence that many, if not all, of the preganglionic fibers had selectively reinnervated the class of ganglion cells they had previously contacted, led him to essentially the same conclusion as Ramon y Cajal:

The regenerated fibres do not grow out past the superior cervical ganglion, but end in the ganglion itself. Further, the fibres from each spinal nerve end in connection with their proper nerve cells. Thus the fibres of the 1st thoracic nerve again become connected with nerve cells supplying the nictitating membrane and pupil and leave entirely on one side the nerve cells supplying the blood vessels and the muscles of the hairs. The fibres of the 4th thoracic nerve pick out the nerve cells supplying the blood vessels and the hairs, and pass by the nerve cells supplying the pupil. . . . The only feasible explanation appears to me to be that the sympathetic fibres grow out along the peripheral piece of nerve . . . spreading amongst the cells of the ganglion, and that *there is some special chemical relation between each class of nerve fibre and each class of nerve cell,* which induces each fibre to grow towards a cell of its own class and there to form its terminal branches. *At bottom then the phenomenon would be a chemotactic one* (Langley 1895, pp. 283–4, emphasis added).

It is worth noting in the light of later work (see Sperry 1963) that both Ramon y Cajal and Langley recognized that during development or regeneration, erroneous axonal connections could be formed and that, at later stages, many of these were probably eliminated.

Ramon y Cajal later wrote:

There is no doubt that, at first, many imperfect connections are formed. . . . But these incongruences are progressively corrected, up to a certain point, by two parallel methods of rectification. One of these occurs in the periphery, and is the atrophy through disuse of superfluous and parasitic ramifications, in combination with the growth of sprouts. The other occurs in the ganglia and spinal centres; by this there would be a selection, due to the atrophy of certain collaterals and the progressive disappearance of disconnected and useless neurones, of the sensory-motor fibres capable of being useful (Ramon y Cajal 1928, p. 279).

Meanwhile Langley observed:

. . . in certain conditions pre-ganglionic nerve fibres are able to form endings in connection with nerve cells not belonging to their own class. . . . It will be noticed that the abnormalities of innervation were greater in the cases in which the regeneration was recent than in those in which it was of long standing. And this suggests that the abnormal connections which are first formed gradually atrophy . . . (Langley 1897, pp. 227, 230).

In retrospect, it is remarkable that such clearcut observations and such well-formulated hypotheses should have been ignored for so long and that for almost three decades, the view that prevailed was that neural connectivity is to all intents and purposes random and that in some way function selects the appropriate circuitry out of equipotential neural networks (Weiss 1941b; 1941c.) However, when we recall that Ramon y Cajal (1954) considered it necessary in his last major work to reaffirm the even more basic concept – that neurons are anatomically discrete entities and that axons are protoplasmic extensions of neuronal somata – it is perhaps not so surprising that the more complex issue should have become mired in confusion and misunderstanding. And it is perhaps appropriate that both sets of issues should later be clarified by a single individual, Ross G. Harrison.

In 1906, Harrison reported the results of a series of extirpation studies in amphibian embryos that once and for all laid to rest the curious, but long-held, notion that axons are formed by the concerted action of a long chain of supporting (Schwann) cells. In the critical experiments, Harrison showed that removal of the neural crest led to the normal outgrowth of motor axons from the spinal cord in the complete absence of Schwann cells, and that after the reciprocal ablation (i.e., removing the neural tube, while leaving the neural crest intact), produced sensory fibers and Schwann cells in the periphery, but no motor nerves. The definitive test, namely, inducing axonal outgrowth from nerve cells into an essentially cell-free medium, came shortly thereafter. In an abstract published in 1907, and a longer paper published in 1910, Harrison described the successful development of the technique of tissue culture and its application to the problem of axonal outgrowth. The rationale for this new approach, and the limitations of the earlier *in-vivo* extirpation data, were clearly stated:

> . . . in all of the first experiments the nerve fibers had developed in surroundings composed of living organized tissues, and that the possibility of the latter contributing organized material to the nerve element stood in the way of rigorous proof of the view that the nerve fiber was entirely the product of the nerve center. The really crucial experiment remained to be performed, and that was to test the power of the nerve centers to form nerve fibers within some foreign medium which could not by any possibility be suspected of contributing organized protoplasma to them (Harrison 1910, p. 790).

Explanting fragments of embryonic nervous tissue onto a solid clot formed by frog lymph, he observed in hanging-drop cultures, the outgrowth of neurites from cells in the tissue fragments, and was thus able to confirm in the most direct possible way Ramon y Cajal's earlier speculations about the dynamic role of the growth cone, and to establish for the first time the importance of a solid substratum for growing neural processes, Figures 2.2B–D). As he said:

> These observations show beyond question that the nerve fiber develops by the outflowing of protoplasm from the central cells. This protoplasm retains its amoeboid activity at its distal end, the result being that it is drawn out into a long thread which becomes the axis cylinder. No other cells or living structures take part in this process. . . . While at present it seems certain that the mere outgrowth of the fibers is largely independent of external stimuli, it is, of course, probable that in the body of the embryo there are many influences which guide the moving end and bring about contact with the proper end structure (Harrison 1907, p. 118).

PRIMARY INDUCTION AND THE
ROLE OF THE "ORGANIZER"

If the nature of axonal outgrowth was revealed by these imaginative experiments, the antecedent question about the origin of the neural plate and the associated neural crest was to be clarified some years later by Harrison's compatriot, Warren H. Lewis, and by his close friend, German embryologist Hans Spemann. Using the techniques of tissue extirpation and heterotopic transplantation, Spemann (1901; rev. 1938) and Lewis (1904; 1906; 1907a; 1907b) established that for each organ, one can define a group of embryonic cells that, although morphologically indistinguishable from the surrounding embryonic tissues, later forms that organ. Complete extirpation of the relevant group of cells led to absence of the corresponding organ, whereas heterotopic transplantation of the same population of cells to a foreign site in a host embryo could result in the formation of a complete and apparently normal supernumerary organ, whose development proceeded on a normal schedule and often resulted in an organ of normal size and form, with no missing or extra parts. Lewis (1904; 1907a; 1907b), for example, defined the rudimentary eye field, as including the optic vesicle, the associated optic stalk, and its forebrain attachment site, at a stage when the vesicle itself was recognizable only as a slight outpocketing of the neural tube. Moreover, when a portion of the eye-field, so defined, was left in the host embryo (as a result of a partial ablation), it usually had the potential to reconstitute a complete (albeit miniature) eyeball – indicating, as Spemann expressed it, that "the presumptive optic vesicles and optic stalks together with the presumptive material for the chiasma are more or less equipotential" (Spemann 1938, p. 53). Interspecies grafting (first introduced by Bohn, 1897), provided direct confirmation that it was indeed the heterotopically transplanted tissue that gave rise to the supernumerary organ (Harrison 1935).

Similar grafting strategies helped to identify instances in which cell groups acquire specific tissue fates by interacting with other embryonic cells in their neighborhood. Perhaps the best studied example of this was the development of the lens in which inductive interactions, between the optic vesicle and the overlying head ectoderm, evoke a specific tissue commitment from the latter, to form the lens of the eye (Lewis 1904; Spemann 1938). Spemann (1938) had shown that after ablation of the eye-field in newt or frog embryos, a lens did not form on the operated side. In a complementary series of experiments, Lewis (1903;

1907a) grafted optic vesicles from embryos of *Rana sylvatica* into contact with body ectoderm in *Rana palustris* or body ectoderm from *Rana palustris* in place of the normal ectoderm overlying the optic vesicle in *Rana sylvatica*. From these experiments, he concluded that

> (1) The lens is absolutely dependent for its origin on the influence of the optic vesicle on the ectoderm. (2) There is no predetermined area of ectoderm which must be stimulated in order that a lens may arise; the ectoderm is probably equipotential as regards its lens-forming power; more than this even, the ectoderm of R. sylvatica is equipotential with that of R. palustris in this regard (Lewis 1903, p. 2; and see Figure 2.3A).

In yet another series of grafting experiments in frog embryos, Lewis (1907c) reported that transplantation of the dorsal lip of the blastopore could give rise to a supernumerary neural tube, notochord, and surrounding mesoderm in the host embryo. At the time, he favored the view that the transplanted tissue gave rise to most of the supernumerary structures as the result of self-differentiation, but when this preparation was later taken up by Spemann and his students, it became clear that the tissue of the dorsal lip was acting as an inductive focus capable of redirecting the developmental fate of the ectoderm of the host embryo.

In an important paper on the transplantation of small pieces of neural plate and epidermis published in 1918, Spemann reported in passing that transplants, which included the dorsal lip of the blastopore, could form an entire secondary neuraxis, much as Lewis (1907c) had previously found. By 1921, Spemann had adopted the method of interspecies grafting as a means of distinguishing graft and host contributions in experiments of this kind, and this led three years later to his classical study with Hilde Mangold (Spemann and Mangold 1924) involving grafts of dorsal-lip tissue from the near-white embryos of *Triton cristatus* into the darkly pigmented embryos of *T. taeniatus*. In these cases, "the unpigmented *cristatus* cells can be clearly distinguished, over long periods of time, from

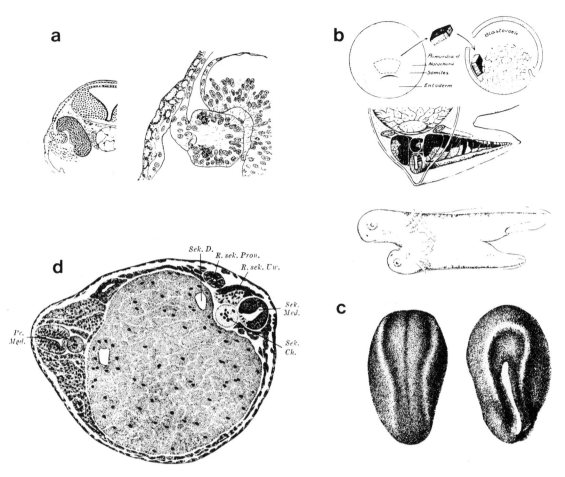

Figure 2.3. Summary of key experiments on embryonic induction, by Lewis (1903, 1904, 1907a–c), on the eye lens of Ranid embryos (**A**), and by Spemann and Mangold (1924) on the primary organizer of Urodele embryos (**B–D**). (**A**) Lewis demonstrated that nonfacial ectoderm from a host species can be induced to form a lens placode by a grafted optic cup from a donor species. Here an optic vesicle has been grafted to a heterotopic position posterior to the ear vesicle and, three days later, histologic sections were prepared through the region of the transplant. These low- and high-power tracings show the relations of the heterotopic eye cup formed by the transplant and the *Rana sylvatica* lens formed from, and as yet attached to, the nonfacial ectoderm of the host embryo. (After Lewis 1904.) (**B**) Operative schematic, together with sketches of the principal findings, for the organizer experiment of Spemann and Mangold (1924). The dorsal lip of the blastopore, from a donor embryo of the near-white species *Triton cristatus* has been transplanted into a host embryo of the darkly pigmented *T. taeniatus*. Such transplants were observed to induce a secondary neuraxis, often leading to a frankly double embryo. The dark-cell/white-cell species difference allowed the contributions of graft and host tissue to the secondary embryo to be determined and, as shown in the cross section, most of the neural material in the secondary embryo derived from induced host tissue. (**C**) These drawings show a normal early neurula stage embryo of *T. taeniatus* on the left and a *T. taeniatus* host embryo, of the same stage, which had earlier received a blastopore-lip graft from a white *T. cristatus* donor. (**D** This section is taken from a more mature embryo following a similar *cristatus*-into-*taeniatus* transplant of the blastopore lip. Spemann (1938, p. 146) notes that "The notochord of the secondary embryo (Sek. Ch) has been formed from the implant (*cristatus*), the medullary tube (Sek. Med.) and somites (R. sek. Uw.) partly from the implant, partly from the host." (After Spemann 1938.)

the pigmented *taeniatus* . . . cells, and the part supplied by the transplanted dorsal lip tissue can thus be sharply delimited from the regions induced by it" (Spemann and Mangold 1924, p. 169). Marked grafts of this kind provided strong evidence, Figure 2.3B, that much of the secondary embryo was formed from host material. As they stated:

> The structure of the secondary embryonic primordium is quite complete . . . all organ primordia, such as the neural tube with otocysts, notochord, somites, pronephros and perhaps also intestine, can be present and relatively well developed.
>
> Part of this secondary embryonic primordium always derives from the implant, which can be sharply distinguished from its surroundings by virtue of its different histological characteristics. The size and position of this component are very variable, depending, undoubtedly, on the size and point of origin of the implant. Host tissue prevails in the neural tube; *cristatus* cells are either absent . . . or they form only a narrow strip. . . . In contrast, implant tissue predominates in the notochord; in fact, the notochord consisted completely of cristatus cells in all cases except one . . . where small groups of host cells are interspersed. . . . The somites assume an intermediate position: they can be composed completely of *cristatus* cells . . . or completely of host cells . . . or they can be chimeric, i.e., composed of both (Spemann and Mangold 1924, pp. 172–3).
>
> The causal relationships in the origin of the secondary embryonic anlage are still completely in the dark. The only point that is certain is that somehow an induction by the implant occurs. . . . It is very probable that the inducing action of the implant already begins very early and that it consists at first in inducing its new environment to participate actively in the invagination. . . . The inducing action of the implant could have run its course with this instigation of invagination; everything else could be merely the

consequence of this secondary gastrulation. . . . But there is another possibility, namely that the implant continues to exert determinative influences on its surroundings. For instance, the long, narrow strip of *cristatus* cells in the neural plate could have caused the adjacent cells, which otherwise would have become epidermis, to differentiate likewise into neural plate . . . (Spemann and Mangold 1924, p. 174).

In recognition of the fact that the dorsal lip of the blastopore somehow orchestrates an entire set of covert, but patterned, determination steps that define the long axis of the embryo and a number of its future organ fields, Spemann called it the *organizer,* a term that will always be associated with his name, and for his discovery of the phenomenon of primary induction, he received the Nobel Prize in 1935.

PATTERN DETERMINATION IN
EMBRYONIC ORGAN FIELDS

The concept of fields and gradients in embryonic development is an old one, which antedates by several years Spemann's discovery of the organizer and Harrison's characterization of the fieldlike differentiation of individual organ rudiments. The studies of Boveri (1901; 1902; 1910) on nuclear versus cytoclasmic control of differentiation, although best remembered for their contribution to the chromosomal theory of inheritance, served to focus attention on the graded organization of egg cytoplasm and its potential role in evoking spatially ordered differentiation among equivalent nuclei. The field concept thus arose as a conceptual treatment of individuation in the embryo and an attempt to define territories and domains of cells and to account for the progressive restriction of "potencies" within individual populations of cells, while their ultimate fate was to become integrated with other groups of cells to form coherent organs. Although a generation or more of distinguished scientists were to address this issue (Child 1915, 1941; Gurwitsch 1922; Weiss 1926; Huxley and de Beer 1934; Waddington, 1934, 1940), the work of Ross Harrison and his students merits special attention since it established the framework against which Sperry's later studies are to be viewed.

In 1915, Harrison began a lengthy series of studies on relations of symmetry in the developing forelimb of the salamander embryo. Defining the limb field by extirpation and heterotopic transplantation, Harrison (1918, 1921) reworked Driesch's (1894) concept of self-differentiating "equipotential systems" and devised a series of experimental tests for regional determination within the limb field (Figure 2.4). When any half of the surgically defined limb field was ablated, the residual half often developed into a whole, perfectly formed, limb – even though the outgrowth of the limb was usually delayed and though it frequently remained half-normal size until a rather advanced stage of larval maturation. When two noncomplementary halves of this surgically defined limb field – one grafted from a donor embryo and the other from the host's limb field – were surgically grafted together, the two pieces melded together and often formed a single harmonious limb of normal size that developed along a normal schedule of outgrowth and maturation. In other experiments, Harrison (1918) fused two whole limb fields together and observed that, while the initial outgrowth was enlarged and only adjusted its size over several days or weeks, this preparation was also able to integrate the two organ plans into a single harmonious structure.

> On the whole, these experiments show that, while quantitatively the limb-forming tissue is unequally distributed in the four quadrants of the area usually extirpated, there is no qualitative difference in the potencies of the cells of the four quadrants. . . . While the ectodermal covering is indifferent, the mesoderm of the limb bud constitutes a specific self-differentiating system, which . . . in itself is an equipotential system . . . (Harrison 1918, p. 459).

Finally, in perhaps his best remembered experiments on the limb, Harrison (1921) went on to examine the effects of disorienting the limb field relative to the embryo's body plan by surgically rotating limb fields through 180° *in situ,* and grafting left limbs onto the right

side of the body at a site that does not normally form limbs. In these experiments, he established that the limb fields of early embryos can adapt to an up–down misalignment and go on to form a right-side-up forelimb, whereas at later stages, the limb field never adapts and always forms a limb whose orientation and handedness match the original disposition of the graft in the donor animal. Equally important was his finding that regional determination is progressive, and based on the sequential polarization of the field with respect first to its anteroposterior and then its dorsoventral axis; this was based on the finding of an intermediate stage in which the limb field could adapt to up–down (dorsal-to-ventral) inversion, but not an anteroposterior misalignment. At this stage:

> . . . the asymmetry of the limb is determined by two factors, the polarization of the anteroposterior axis of the limb bud and the orientation of the limb bud with respect to the dorsoventral polarization of its organic environment (Harrison 1921, p. 110).

In subsequent studies by Harrison (1921, 1933, 1936, 1945) and a succession of students (Nicholas 1924, 1955; Stultz 1936; Swett 1937; Stone 1944, 1960, 1966; Yntema 1955), the principle of progressive regional determination in organ fields was extended to include the amphibian hindlimb, ear, and eye. Included among the many observations on this topic were the findings that (1) many of the grafted limbs and ears could form twinned organs, whose rules of mirror symmetry were well-defined. (2) Rotated organs possess a second means of correcting their postural disharmony with the host body plan – a poorly understood process by which they physically "derotate" *in situ* a few degrees a day over many weeks (while maintaining an internally perfect form), and ultimately come to lie in normal orientation on the body. (3) At early stages of development, when, for example, a rotated limb can adapt to a new orientation *in situ* or on the flank, there is already sufficient information in the field to direct the outgrowth of a perfectly formed limb whose orientation matches the original disposition of the field in the donor embryo. And (4) simple alterations in the graft-

a

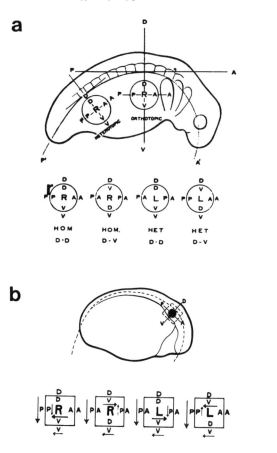

b

c

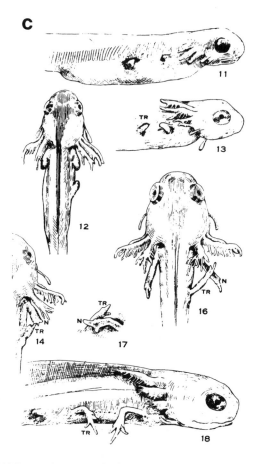

Figure 2.4. Summary of some of Harrison's (1918, 1921, 1936) experiments on fieldlike differentiation of the forelimb (**A**) and ear (**B**) in the salamander, *Ambystoma maculatum (A. punctatum)*, with drawings of the sequential stages in the outgrowth of a left-handed forelimb on the right side of the body (**C**). (**A**) This drawing of a tail-bud larva shows the normal (orthotopic) position occupied by the limb field as a circle with its relations to the major anteroposterior (A-P) and dorsoventral (D-V) axes of the embryo. Also drawn as a second circle marked "heterotopic" are the position and axial relations of a grafted limb-rudiment taken from a donor larva and placed at a position on the host flank that does not normally form limbs. Harrison (1921) performed both orthotopic and heterotopic transplants and a variety of surgically induced misalignments in which the grafted limb field was inverted or rotated with respect to the major axes of the host's body. Four such variations are shown below the embryo silhouette. Grafts from the same side of the body – Harrison called them "homopleural" – could be normally oriented (*far left*) or rotated so as to invert both the A-P and D-V axes (*near left*). Grafts from the opposite side of the body – Harrison called them "heteropleural" – can be inverted in either the A-P axis alone (*near right*) or the D-V axis alone (*far right*). (**B**) A "neural-tube" stage larva showing the normal position and axial relations of the ear field and, below the embryo silhouette, the four variations of surgical alignment as applied to the ear by Harrison (1936). (After Harrison 1945.) (**C**) Harrison's drawings show the sequential outgrowth of a *left*- handed but right-side-up limb, at a heterotopic flank position on the *right* side of a host larva, following surgical implantation of a *right* donor limb-field in 180°- rotated orientation. The growth of the transplant (TR) occurred at about the same rate as the host's normal forelimb (N). The numbers (11–18) from Harrison's original figure, depict the transplanted limb at successive intervals from 5–16 days postoperation. (11) Lateral view, five days after operation; (12, 13) dorsal and lateral views of the same individual at eight days after operation; (14, 15) dorsal and lateral views of the same embryo at twelve days after operation; (16, 17) dorsal and lateral views of the same specimen at sixteen days after operation. A second case is shown (18), drawn from a

ing protocols – for example, leaving a portion of host limb or ear in the site of a graft or including an annulus of surrounding nonlimb or ear material in a rotated graft – could evoke the expression of instructions already present in an early limb or ear field.

Harrison's "systems" characterization of pattern determination in embryonic organ fields established that a set of instructions is present in the organ field at an early stage, and yet individual regions within the field become only gradually committed to forming specific parts of the organ pattern. In this, and in formulating the idea that local cell fate can be specified in accordance with cell position along an anteroposterior and dorsoventral axis, Harrison provided two essential elements in Sperry's later chemoaffinity hypothesis, as well as a set of explicit predictions as to how position-determining features may be established in the retina and optic lobe.

TISSUE AFFINITIES IN EMBRYONIC CELLS

The most direct evidence for selective affinities among embryonic cells derived not from Harrison, but rather from Johannes Holtfreter, one of Spemann's most distinguished students. Holtfreter had devoted most of his research effort in the 1920s and 1930s to elucidating the chemical basis of embryonic induction and had produced much of the evidence for various nonspecific inductions that eventually brought the search for chemical inducers to a disappointing halt. In 1939, Holtfreter turned his attention to morphogenetic cell movements in gastrulating embryos and began to examine the ways in which cells from the different primary germ layers – endoderm, ectoderm, and mesoderm – behave when confronting one another *in vitro*.

The concept of tropisms between cells was not a new one. Roux (1888, 1894, 1895) had observed that embryonic frog cells isolated in an artificial medium would either associate in groups and form spherical aggregates or, alternatively, would migrate away and isolate themselves. Roux was of the opinion that mutual attraction or repulsion rather than chance movements brought the cells together or drove them apart, and spoke of "positive and negative cytotropisms," which he thought to be operating through cell-specific chemical stimulants that diffused into the environment and set up concentration gradients (Holtfreter 1939, p. 190). Similarly, Bohn (1897), while studying fused partial embryos from different species of amphibians and using the pigment differences in the chimeras to follow cell fates, concluded that "cells arising from the same germ layer unite to form continuous sheets, while cells from different germ layers tend instead to separate from each other" (Bohn 1897, p. 586). And Wilson had reported in 1907 that dissociated sponge cells could, under certain circumstances, reaggregate and reconstitute a whole organism with normal tissue relations. Unfortunately, the impact of these findings seems to have been blunted somewhat by the larger concerns of the papers in which they appeared, and it was not for some years that they entered the mainstream of embryological thinking, in large part due to Holtfreter's work.

Holtfreter (1939) began by examining the behavior of isolated fragments of newt gastrulae *in vitro*. Then, by combining pairs of fragments from similar or dissimilar embryonic tissues and carefully mapping the tissue patterns formed after dissociation and reaggregation of the cells, he was able to show, among many other things, that single fragments of an

---

specimen preserved until twenty-eight days after operation, where the transplanted limb is now quite mature. In both cases, but especially in the more mature case (18), the grafted limb grew out with left-handed symmetry – its A-P axis reversed relative to the host limb, but its dorsoventral axis in normal relation to the host body. These, among many results, led Harrison (1921) to conclude that the fieldlike differentiation of the limb reaches a stage of commitment or *determination* in two axial steps, with the A-P axis becoming insensitive to body cues from the host before the D-V axis. The two cases whose drawings are shown had been operated upon at the intermediate stage when the A-P axis is now unresponsive to the host, but the D-V axis is still able to adapt to cues defining the host body plan. (After Harrison 1945.)

embryo are able not only to self-differentiate, but, in many cases, to self-assemble into more mature tissue patterns. Figure 2.5A, for example, illustrates the sequential morphology of head neural-plate fragments, which maintained a segregation of presumptive epidermis and brain as the fragment rounded up, and went on to form discrete tissue assemblies recognizable as eye, forebrain, skin, and olfactory pit. When two or more dissimilar fragments, such as endoderm and ectoderm, were artifically recombined *in vitro,* one tissue was observed to gradually envelope the other. As the component tissues matured, giving rise to differentiated cell types such as skin and cartilage, one cell type was segregated into a solid tissue mass in the center of the aggregate and the other formed a discrete outer shell around it. For a particular pair of starting tissues, one member tended to move to an internal position and form the core, while the other member nearly always formed the outer shell. More complex recombinations, involving three or more tissue fragments, also showed stereotypic patterns of association and segregation: some combinations formed concentric layers, with tissue A external to tissue B, which in turn was external to tissue C; in yet other combinations, one tissue would envelop the second, while the third might be excluded from the structure altogether. Holtfreter (1939) coined the term *Gewebaffinitat* (tissue affinity) to explain the resulting tissue patterns. As he concluded:

> It seems advantageous . . . to introduce a more fitting term for the forces that are instrumental in these processes of attraction and repulsion. Henceforth we shall apply the term *affinity,* which . . . may be either positive or negative, it may be graded in its intensity, and may approach the point of neutrality. These gradations may change during development, increasing or decreasing between two cell generations, or they may repeat themselves in cycles (Holtfreter 1939, p. 198).

More importantly, Holtfreter viewed these affinities as properties of the surfaces of the cells and conceived of their operation as being critically dependent upon direct cell-to-cell contact.

In our isolation and combination experiments, carried out on embryonic amphibian material, the question of a chemotropic distant effect between cells has not even been touched upon. All the phenomena here described occurred while the various kinds of cells and tissues were in direct mutual contact. What was actually observed was an orderly union as well as nonunions and self-isolations. The events proceeded in an age- and tissue-specific manner, removed from the embryo as a whole, in a purely protective, indifferent medium, without the participation of a physically structured substrate. . . . These stimulatory affinities share with the hypothetical cytotropism the capacity to bring about gradations of attraction and repulsion between cells, which lead to directional changes in their form and position. . . . As a means of the self-sorting of embryonic regions these phenomena are of great significance. They lead to the anatomical segregation of physiologically different organ primordia and to their recombination with other parts of the embryo. They provide a unified explanation for local migration and constriction movements in whole cell complexes, starting with those in gastrulation and being continued during organogenesis (Holtfreter 1939, p. 224).

In subsequent studies, Holtfreter (1943a, 1943b, 1944) extended these observations to a consideration of changes in individual cell shape and adhesiveness, examined a wide range of embryonic stages, and dramatically demonstrated the formation of distinct tissue layers from dissociated cell suspensions derived from two and three embryonic tissues. Remarkably, the tendencies of particular tissue pairs, or threesomes, to become spatially segregated (e.g., the tendency of neural plate fragments to segregate internal to presumptive epidermis) could be recapitulated by dissociated cells. Indeed, the active sorting of neural plate and epidermal cells, from a randomly intermingled mixed cell suspension, has become one of the classic images of experimental embryology (Figures 2.5B–2.5D).

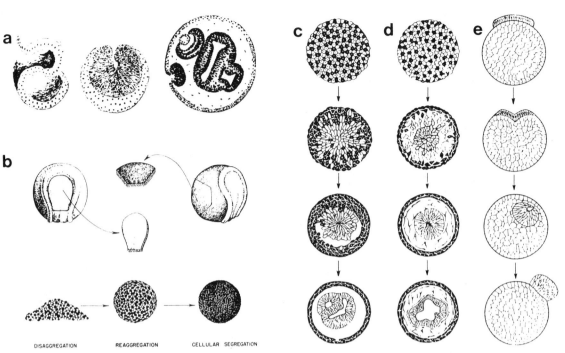

Figure 2.5. Holtfreter's analysis of tissue affinities of amphibian embryonic cells, including (**A**) the self-organization of tissues from simple explants cultured *in vitro,* and (**B**) the preparation of mixed cell aggregates from dissociated cell suspensions from two or more tissues, followed by (**C**) the sorting out of cell components to form segregated tissues within the aggregate. (**A**) On the *left* is shown a fresh explant, upon excision from a newt neurula, containing a portion of head neural plate together with a larger piece of adjacent prospective epidermis. A day later *(center* panel), the two tissues had tightly united, and the prospective epidermis had begun to envelope the neural anlage. The neural-plate tissue had sunk in to form a groove and the beginnings of a tubelike structure. Several days later (on the *right*), the explant had differentiated into brain, including an eye and nasal pit, surrounded by an epidermal capsule. (After Holtfreter 1939.) (**B**) The preparation and analysis of mixed cell aggregates began by excising two embryonic tissues – neural plate (white cells) and prospective epidermis (black cells) in these drawings – and dissociating them in alkali solution. After the cells had been "thoroughly intermingled" *(bottom left),* they were allowed to reaggregate in normal saline *(bottom center).* Within hours, the initial steps in cellular segregation were evident in the disappearance of one type of cell from the surface of the aggregate *(bottom right).* (**C**) Such aggregates were then prepared for histologic inspection at various times after the reaggregation step and used to reconstruct a temporal sequence of sorting out (vertical column). Over time, the neural-plate cells were observed to withdraw from the surface of the aggregate, to coalesce in a central core, and to differentiate into neural structures; concurrently, the prospective epidermal cells (black) were observed to withdraw from the core of the aggregate, to form an outer rind around the core of neural cells, and, finally, to differentiate into an epidermal capsule. (**D**) In a slightly more complex variant of the experiment, reaggregates were made after mixing cell suspensions from three embryonic tissue sources – neural plate, prospective epidermis, and neural fold. Again a reproducible pattern of cellular segregation was observed, with the neural-fold cells taking up the space between the outer rind of epidermal cells and the inner core of neural cells. (**E**) In still another variant, explants of two tissues were combined – a piece of neural plate (grey) was placed atop a solid mass of ventral endoderm. The neural fragment was observed to fold inward and form a tubelike structure, at first moving into the mass of endoderm as if to form a central core. Within a day, however, although the two tissues remained segregated, the neural tissue had been extruded from the core of the endodermal material. The reproducibility of segregated patterns, the tendency of certain tissues to envelop some tissues and extrude others, and the dynamic changes in the behavior of tissues when the explants and cell suspensions were taken from embryos of advancing age led Holtfreter to postulate a dynamic system of positive and negative tissue affinities as a driving force behind the morphogenetic movements that shape embryonic organs and tissue patterns. (**B–E**, after Townes and Holtfreter 1955.)

Holtfreter's ideas were later taken up and refined by Paul Weiss and his students. In 1947, Weiss and Albert Tyler independently proposed that many adult and embryonic cell types possess unique cell surface molecules, similar in their actions to antibodies and their related antigens, which mediate a lock-and-key type of affinity between one cell and another. Later, Moscona, after demonstrating the sorting out of specific cell types from differentiated tissue and organs (Moscona and Moscona 1952), was to establish the existence of cell surface factors that directly and selectively promote adhesive association of particular cell types with other cells of the same class (Moscona 1957, 1962). Townes and Holtfreter (1955) were to analyze the behavior of a wide variety of embryonic tissues in mixed cell aggregates, fixing the aggregates at various stages of maturity, and carefully charting the sorting out of homologous cells into the core-and-shell configurations that Holtfreter had earlier described. And novel quantitative treatments were to be introduced by Trinkaus and Groves (1955), by Steinberg (1958, 1962), and by Curtis (1967).

Holtfreter was not slow to recognize the implications of his findings for neural development:

> The concept of cytotropism has found favorable support especially among neurologists since it seemed to provide an explanation for the directed growth of nerves if it is assumed that attracting stimuli emanate from the future effector organ. Some investigators (Kappers, Child and others) considered a difference in electrical potential to be important while others (Ramon y Cajal, Tello) assumed that specific chemical substances may act as stimulators. Indeed, several authors interpreted the behavior of outgrowing axons toward other cells in the explant in terms of chemotropism (Holtfreter 1938, p. 223).

But, even as he provided the working material for chemoaffinity in neural development, Holtfreter (1939) bowed to the dominant view of Weiss that nerve growth is nonspecific and controlled by simple mechanical factors, and toward the end of his 1939 paper wrote:

The interpretation of these findings has been rejected by Weiss (1934) on the strength of his counterarguments. . . . On the basis of further extensive tests in plasma cultures in which neural tissue was confronted with other kinds of tissue, or with extracts of crushed tissues or chimeric agents applied to one side, he concluded that the outgrowing nerve fiber does not respond to chemotactic stimulation, and that the direction of its growth is determined primarily, if not exclusively, by mechanical factors.

What is important here is to point out that on the basis of these investigations of Weiss, which thus far have remained unchallenged, *cytotropism has not been experimentally demonstrated for animal tissues* (Holtfreter 1939, p. 223; emphasis added).

THE RISE OF THE FUNCTIONALIST VIEW OF NEURAL DEVELOPMENT

The view of neural development that rose to prominence in the 1930s was an amalgam of several functionalist ideas that had existed since the midnineteenth century. The first of these ideas viewed the adult nervous system as a diffuse network of connections in which the orderly processing of information was directed by the coded properties of neural signals that were thought to encode information about their site of origin, the sensory modality they subserved, and the behavioral action patterns that they initiated. Such signals were assumed to evoke responses in the network only in the behaviorally appropriate neurons whose "resonance" properties were activated by the specific "frequencies" of the encoded message (Herring 1913; Bok 1917; Head 1920; Weiss 1924). This idea seems to have stemmed from the notion that vertebrate behavior is much too complex to be explained on the basis of simple connectivity and reflex actions. As Herrick expressed it:

No complication of separate and insulated reflex arcs, each of which is conceived as giving a one-to-one relation between stimulus and response, and no interconnection of such arcs by elaborate switchboard devices can conceivably yield the type of behavior which we actually find in higher vertebrates. . . . The mechanisms of traditional reflexology seem hopelessly inadequate (Herrick 1930, p. 645).

The resurgence of this idea in the 1930s was catalyzed by a number of contemporary trends including the rise of Gestalt psychology, the growing emphasis of the role of environmental factors in determining animal behavior among ethologists of the period, the electrical field theory of cortical function with its emphasis on diffuse connectivity and on the absence of localized function, and a large body of clinical evidence claiming virtually complete functional recovery after nerve injuries (Head 1920; Lashley 1929, 1942; Weiss 1936; Goldstein 1939; Gerard 1941; reviewed by Sperry 1945b, 1951b, 1955, 1958).

The second idea was that although the adult brain contains anatomically well-defined pathways and connections, these neural circuits are forged by function and experience out of an initially equipotential neural network in the embryo. It was thought that the pathways that mediate useful adaptive behavior were in some way favored by the functional compatibility of the participating neurons and were reinforced by the animal's experience, whereas other connections whose activation led to maladaptive behavior were gradually eliminated. Kappers (1971) had proposed a theory of neurobiotaxis, which, although largely discredited as a general theory of axon guidance, had contributed at least one persisting idea. This held that enduring synaptic associations were favored between neurons with similar patterns of electrical discharge, and the general idea drew strength from Coghill's (1929, 1930) studies on behavioral development in Urodeles. Coghill proposed that the sharp, "individuated" behaviors and orderly behavior patterns seen in mature animals were sculpted by experience out of the crude thrashing behavior observed in early larvae. A number of earlier observations and ideas were recast in a functionalist perspective. These included the idea first propounded by Roux (1881) that development consists of two phases, a prefunctional phase of growth and

tissue assembly, and a later period of functional refinement. Evidence for the elimination of many early formed axonal branches (Speidel 1933) and for the peripheral control of cell numbers in the spinal cord and ganglia (Shorrey 1909; Detwiler 1920; Hamburger 1934) during this second "functional" phase of development, a wide range of observations on cultured neurons (Harrison 1910; Lewis and Lewis 1912; Lewis 1922; Levi 1934), and even Ramon y Cajal's (1928) notion of "disuse atrophy," were all recast as vehicles for eliminating functionally maladaptive pathways and connections (Weiss 1941b, 1941c).

But perhaps the most important idea that contributed to the functionalist view was the notion that axon growth is largely a nonselective process controlled, in the main, by mechanical factors. That mechanical factors are important in neural outgrowth was hardly in question (one can find strong evidence in support of this in the writings of His [1886], Ramon y Cajal [1905, 1908, 1928] and perhaps most eloquently in Harrison's paper of 1910):

> The configuration of the various organs of the embryo affords certain paths of predilection, such as small channels or grooves, in which nerve fibers are found to grow. These factors, together with the predetermination of the initial directions of outgrowth within the cell . . . itself, will account for the main features in the topography of the peripheral nervous system (Harrison 1910, p. 843).

What was at issue was the question whether such nonspecific guiding mechanisms led to the formation of *nonspecific patterns* of connections. In the 1930s, this notion was taken up and strongly advocated by Paul Weiss. And it was he, more than any other single figure, who was to force functionalist ideas into the center of neuroembryological thinking and discussion.

In the early 1920s, Weiss had made the remarkable observation that if a supernumerary limb is grafted close enough to a host salamander's own limb so as to receive some of its nerve supply from the brachial segments of the spinal cord, it could move in unison with the host's own limb. Weiss (1924) initially explained this so-called *homologous response* by proposing that each muscle possessed a specific *resonance* that enabled it to "decode" and respond selectively to neural impulses that were behaviorally appropriate for that muscle and that muscle alone. Later, when it was evident from electrophysiologic studies (Wiersma 1931) that muscles always contracted whenever action potentials passed down their motor nerves, Weiss directed attention to the relevant motoneurons. He now suggested that although motoneurons innervate embryonic muscles nonselectively, each muscle stamps upon its innervating nerve a unique resonance property by a process of end-organ induction, which he called "modulation" or "myotypic specification," and that, thereafter, activation of the spinal motor pools was decoded selectively by those motoneurons with the proper resonant frequencies. In 1936, Weiss claimed to observe homologous responses in the muscles of a limb grafted *backwards* onto a host salamander, despite the fact that the resulting movements were "at cross purposes" with those of the animal's normally oriented leg; moreover, this homologous response was said to have persisted throughout the life of the animal. This required some modification of the original functionalist view, since it suggested that the modulation of motor-neuron resonance by individual muscle fibers was not organized on the basis of behavioral utility to the animal as a whole (Weiss 1936, 1941b). Weiss went on to perform an exhaustive series of follow-up experiments that involved forcibly restricting the innervation of supernumerary limbs, cross-uniting the axons of motoneurons to antagonistic muscles, eliminating or disarranging sensory nerves, and transplanting individual muscles in frog larvae (Weiss 1932, 1935, 1936, 1937a–d, 1941a, 1941b). The cardinal weakness in Weiss's evidence was, as we shall see, the assumption that his surgical derangements had in fact precluded selective peripheral innervation of muscles by the normal motor pools (Grimm 1971). Nevertheless, the data seemed to Weiss to reaffirm the general principle of the homologous response, so that, in 1941, he could state that

> At present, the view best in agreement with the facts, although not entirely free

from difficulties, is the following. . . . Each muscle exerts, by virtue of its individual protoplasmic specificity, a correspondingly specific influence upon its motor nerve fibers. As a result, the nerves acquire specific differentials which match and centrally represent the variety of muscles. The biceps muscle, for instance, would gradually transform any nerve fibers connecting with it into strictly biceps-specific fibers. . . . This hypothetical process of appropriation of the motoneurons by their muscles has been called *"modulation"* (P. Weiss 1936). . . . According to this view, a nerve fiber which has been severed from its erstwhile connections and switched to another muscle, would lose its former specificity and acquire the new one. However, it seems that nerve fibers, as they grow older, lose their plasticity and become irreversibly ingrained. . . . A *young* nerve, which after connecting with a biceps muscle had become biceps-specific, can still be transposed to a triceps muscle and assume triceps-specificity, thus changing its central tune. However, after having been under prolonged influence of its original biceps contact, transfer to the triceps has no longer any retuning effect, and the nerve responds centrally as if the muscle at the end were still a biceps (Weiss 1941b, pp. 524–5).

From the most radical surgical derangements, he went on to find evidence that seemed to preclude the formation of selective connections and stressed the interchangeability of neurons:

> A brief list may indicate the range of nonselectivity. First, with regard to regeneration: Motor fibers can connect with sensory organs . . . a dorsal root (Weiss 1935) or a sensory nerve (Weiss 1934) forced upon a muscle can mediate its contraction. Any motor nerve will connect with any muscle. It even connects with spinal cord when inserted into it (Weiss 1932). In deplantation experiments . . . innervation of limb and trunk muscles was obtained from . . . spinal cord, medulla

oblongata, midbrain and forebrain...
(Weiss 1941b, p. 184).

Thus, it came about that in little more than a decade, the rather strong evidence adduced by Ramon y Cajal, Langley, and others was thrust aside, and, at the same time, their clearly formulated hypotheses of chemotropism, directed axon growth, and chemospecific association of pre- and postsynaptic cells were either neglected or intentionally ignored. And, in their place, a loose fabric of functionalist ideas came to the fore: the notion that the adult nervous system is more like a radio and less like a telephone switchboard; that, during development, the connections are assembled more or less haphazardly; that axonal outgrowth is governed by the crudest of mechanical guides; that function and experience help to reinforce and select behaviorally adaptive circuits from the initially diffuse neural network; that individual neurons, regardless of their class, are largely interchangeable – at least until a very late stage of maturation; that the "resonance properties" of neurons enable them to respond selectively to behaviorally specific impulse traffic although the neural networks themselves are anatomically diffuse; and that end-organ contacts, established at random in the embryonic periphery, serve to induce these resonance properties and so begin the cascade of resonance tuning and functional selection of neurons that in the last analysis determine the functional capacities of the brain and spinal cord.

The development of the chemoaffinity hypothesis

EVIDENCE THAT MOTONEURONS ARE NOT INTERCHANGEABLE

The development of the chemoaffinity hypothesis was a gradual process, involving a succession of ingenious experiments and bold leaps, but restrained throughout by Sperry's deference to his mentor, Paul Weiss, and hampered by continual redefinition and repeated recasting of the functionalist view, by Weiss and others during the late 1930s and 1941. As Sperry himself saw it in his retrospective review of 1965:

...with the advent of the chemoaffinity interpretation, the campaign for impulse specificity was promptly abandoned. By 1947, even the strongest opponents of chemical selectivity...had come well around toward a reversal of their earlier position of the 1930's (Weiss 1947). This turnabout of opinion did not come easily after the heavy investment of the preceding two decades against both chemical selectivity on the one hand and fiber connection specificity on the other. It was accomplished in the literature more by verbal subtleties....

For example, "chemotaxis" and "chemotropism" were first attacked on an antiselectivity basis, but when this no longer seemed wise, the terms were carefully defined (Weiss and Taylor 1944) to include the concept of attraction from a distance, and from then on the attack was shifted to the implied distance effects. Instead of chemotaxis and chemotropism, terms like "selective contact guidance" and "preferential contact affinities"... are used (Weiss 1947). After the renunciation of Cajal's concept of "selective attraction" it is allowed that there may be selective "proximity" effects in addition to those of direct "contact" (Weiss 1947). "Selective fasciculation" was used initially to describe the tendency of any fiber to follow along those particular preceding fibers that had happened blindly to succeed in achieving a terminal connection, whereas now it is coming to be used more and more to mean the selective segregation in growth of similar fiber types as conceived earlier by Cajal....

Specificity in fiber connections was denied for many years as a basis for selective communication in nerve circuits. When the ground started to become shaky on this point, the attack . . . was shifted to decry the notion of absolute invariance in the development of anatomical relations, something that never was much questioned and is largely irrelevant to the issue. The term "resonance" originally used to suggest that muscles respond selectively to specific impulse frequencies

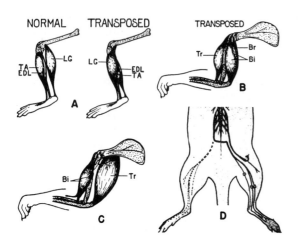

Figure 2.6. Summary of nerve-end-organ disarrangements in rats that resulted in sensory and motor dysfunctions that remained uncorrected by experience. (**A**) Transposition of opposing flexor and extensor muscles of hind limb (Sperry 1940, 1941). (**B**) Same in forelimb (Sperry 1942). (**C**) Reinnervation of triceps extensor muscle by antagonist nerve from biceps flexor muscle. (**D**) Contralateral crossed-innervation of right foot by nerves from left foot (Sperry 1943c). (Figures from Sperry 1958.)

... (Weiss 1928, 1931) has survived to the present, but only by undergoing repeated metamorphoses ... (pp. 165–6).

At the same time, it must be admitted that Sperry's own thinking underwent a steady gradual evolution beginning with his studies on the innervation of the rat hindlimb.

The experimental design of these experiments is schematized in Figure 2.6. It was the first of the two experimental paradigms that Sperry was to apply to one system after another in a repeated series of tests: surgically force a set of behaviorally maladaptive connections upon the animal and then, over a period of time, assess the animal's ability to adapt to the experimental situation (see the foreword). Sperry's conclusions from this initial series of experiments were clear cut:

No adaptive functional adjustment of the nervous system took place in these rats after the connections from the spinal centers to antagonistic limb muscles had been exchanged. The crossing of the peroneal and tibial nerves and the crossing of the pure muscular branches of these nerves

resulted in an awkward and thoroughly abnormal foot movement in the former case and in a complete reversal of foot movement in the latter, neither of which was ever corrected by automatic reflex regulation or by a gradual learning or conditioning process.... The organization of the intrinsic motor patterns themselves must depend primarily on central rather than peripheral factors.

Permanent retention of the original incidence of discharge of the motor nerve fibers after their regeneration into foreign antagonistic muscles also demonstrates that nerve cells in juvenile and adult stages of the rat are no longer in a sufficiently labile condition to be respecified by foreign muscles (Sperry 1942).

The concept of myotypic respecification was to reappear in Sperry's later work on the neuromuscular systems of fish (Sperry 1950b; Sperry and Dupree 1956; Arora and Sperry 1957) before giving way to the idea of selective reinnervation of individual muscles by their original motoneurons (Sperry and Arora 1965; Mark 1965). But, in the early 1940s, it appears to have served as the basis for an uneasy peace between Sperry and his mentor. By emphasizing that the motoneurons themselves could not be interchanged, the critical point was made that neither muscle-decoding properties nor experience acting to correct the miswired neuromuscular connections could be invoked *in the periphery* to explain coordinated movements. At the same time, Sperry was willing to interpret his findings in functionalist terms as late as 1950, as when discussing the first of his experimental studies on motor regeneration in fish, he wrote:

How ... neuronal specificity influences the discharge pattern in the spinal centers remains speculative. Physiological sensitization of the motor cells to particular modes of central excitation has been suggested as one possibility. The central connections are assumed, in this case, to be sufficiently diffuse and non-selective so that all motoneurons within a unilateral limb center are bombarded by all modes of central excitation.

Another possibility which is in accord with a chemoaffinity concept of synaptic patterning assumes that the specificity of motoneurons determines the kinds of synaptic endings which can be formed upon the motor cells. The establishment of synaptic associations is supposed to depend upon selective affinities between the motor and association neurons (Sperry 1941, 1950a). Respecification of a regenerated motoneuron by a foreign muscle is assumed to cause a breakdown of the original synaptic endings and the formation of new ones from a different set of internuncials (Sperry 1950b, p. 285).

This cautious interpretation not only reflects a deep respect for Weiss's views, but Sperry's judicious evaluation of the limitations of his own data. His detailed experiments on the reinnervation of mammalian muscles (Sperry 1940, 1941, 1942, 1945b), in which he found that the induced maladaptive behavior was never corrected, offered few insights into the mechanisms controlling nerve-muscle specificity in normal development, and this was true also of his experiments involving the cross-innervation of muscles in fish in which he obtained a recovery of normal motor function. Whether it was for this reason or because historically the visual system had provided none of the underpinnings of the functionalist position, in the early 1940s, Sperry turned his attention to the problem of the regeneration of connections in the teleost and amphibian visual systems.

THE SPECIFICITY OF REGENERATING OPTIC-NERVE FIBERS

Sperry's (1943a) initial experiment on the newt visual system involved rotating the eyeball through 180° (without disturbing the optic nerve) and subsequently testing optokinetic reflexes and prey localization. The demonstration of 180°-misdirected reflexes provided strong evidence that visually guided behavior was not dependent upon functional decoding of "visual impulses," and the persistence of the maladaptive behavior throughout the life of the animals made it clear that visual connections cannot be either shaped or corrected by experience.

But the amphibian visual system offered even more. In 1926, Matthey (1926a–c) had shown that in adult Urodeles, transplanted eyes were able to regenerate their optic nerves, and furthermore, that the recovered newts were able to navigate normally about their terrarium and to localize small objects in their visual fields. Matthey's papers also contained the intriguing observation that when examined historically, many of the regenerated nerves showed considerable disorder and quite atypical intermingling of the optic-nerve fibers. One of Harrison's students, Leon Stone, and his coworkers had also transplanted eyes in larval and adult salamanders and newts and confirmed the recovery of visual function, not only after simple regeneration of the optic nerve, but, in some adult cases, even after the degeneration and subsequent regeneration of the retina itself (Stone and Ussher 1927; Beers 1929; Stone, Zaur, and Farthing 1934). But perhaps the most interesting finding in the literature available to Sperry was the casual observation by Stone's group that, among the cases showing normal optokinetic and lure reactions, there were several animals in which the grafted eyes were anatomically misaligned by 90° or even 180°, and several others in which subsequent histological examination seemed to indicate that the optic fibers had regrown to inappropriate brain centers. If correct, the observations "suggested that some sort of functional adaptation might be involved" (Sperry 1951a, p. 242).

Sperry was quick to recognize the importance of this finding and to seize on the opportunity that regeneration of the newt optic nerve presented. In 1943, he undertook a detailed investigation of visual responses in a series of seventy adult newts whose optic nerves had been crushed or cut, including fifty-eight in which one eyeball had been intentionally rotated through 180° and the nerve stumps deliberately twisted and tangled at the time of operation. As noted earlier, the patterns of 180° misdirection of visuomotor behavior in these animals were stereotyped, persistent, and striking, even though in a minority of the animals with rotated eyes, degeneration of the retina had delayed the reappearance of visual responses by more than fifty days. The optic nerves were examined histologically in representative cases (Figure 2.7).

In the ten cases in which the nerves had regenerated . . . from the point where they were cut, the point of severance was clearly marked by an extreme entangling of the fibers which took a very crooked and devious course through this region. . . . After crossing the gap to the proximal stump, the regenerating axons are apparently guided along the parallel framework left by the degenerating nerves. The appearance of the regenerated fibers beyond the scar region through the chiasma along the central tracts to the optic tectum was not noticeably different from that of normal animals (Sperry 1943b, p. 43).

But, by contrast, in the cases in which the retina had degenerated and regenerated,

. . . no distinct scar region was present at the point where the nerve had been severed . . . considerable intermixing and

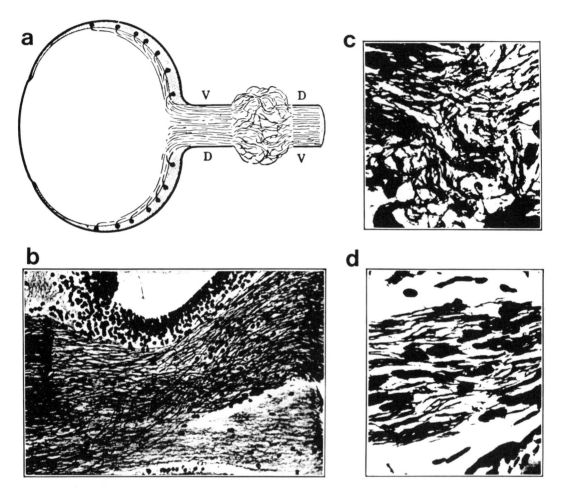

Figure 2.7. Histologic checks on the fiber patterns in regenerated optic nerves, accompanying Sperry's (1943, 1945a) studies on misdirected visuomotor reflexes in newts and frogs after optic-nerve transection and 180°-rotation or contralateral transplantation of the eye. "Despite extreme intermixing of the regenerating fibers in the scar region and despite rotation or inversion of the opposing nerve stumps as diagrammed in (**A**), the fibers reestablish their functional associations in the brain in an orderly manner. The photomicrographs show the interwoven, nonparallel course of the regenerated optic fibers in animals that had shown orderly functional recovery. (**B**) Optic-nerve regeneration scar in a newt. (**C**) Regenerated optic chiasma in a frog, following contralateral transplantation of the eye. (**D**) Regenerated optic nerve of a newt, following retinal degeneration and regeneration." (Figure and original legend from Sperry 1951a, p. 247.)

crossing of the fibers was apparent throughout the course of the nerve from retina to chiasm. . . . The contortion and intermixing of fibers was more extensive in these cases than in the regions proximal and distal to the scar in the other animals, due probably to the disintegration of the old nerve framework . . . (giving) . . . further evidence that the course of individual axons . . . [was] not predetermined by old pathways (Sperry 1943b, p. 44).

Just as the behavioral findings offered compelling evidence against the prevailing functionalist view, the finding that the regenerating optic fibers had become disordered in their initial regrowth greatly strengthened Sperry's position. Surely, an active and highly selective mechanism must be called into play when the fibers reach the visual centers in order to reestablish something akin to their original synaptic relations in the optic lobe. As we shall see, the finding of nerve entanglements and the later disentanglement of the regenerated fibers distal to the scar is one of many passing observations in Sperry's (1943b) paper (together with the first statements about the fieldlike differentiation of the retina, selective fasciculation, and collateral withdrawal) that would be developed in more detail in subsequent studies (Sperry 1945a, 1950a, 1951a, 1951b, 1963). But the 1943 paper remains remarkable mainly for its clear articulation of the hypothesis of chemical specification of retinal ganglion cells and their optic fibers:

> . . . the ganglion cells of the retina including their optic fiber axons *must differ intrinsically from one another according to their location in the retinal field. . . . The results require that ganglion cells of each quadrant of the retina have intrinsic physico-chemical qualities distinguishing them from the ganglion cells of the other retinal quadrants.* Ganglion cells located in different regions of any one quadrant must likewise have distinctive physico-chemical properties. . . . The original polarity of the retina is evidently restored after degeneration and regeneration in these adult Urodeles, probably through organizing influences spreading from the ciliary margin of the retina and perhaps also from

other structures in the eyeball which resist degeneration (Sperry 1943b, pp. 45–6, emphasis added).

CHEMICAL SPECIFICATION OF THE TECTUM
FOR TOPOGRAPHIC CONNECTIONS

In discussing his newt experiments, Sperry (1943b) left open the nature and expression of these optic-fiber specificities, advancing his favored view as but one possibility among many:

> Another possible interpretation . . . [is] . . . that these neuron specificities act primarily on the growth process in regeneration and in embryonic development to influence the formation of central synaptic connections. The specification of nerve fibers by their end-organs is considered to be an important factor in regulating the establishment of proper anatomical associations between peripheral and central neurons. Accordingly, in the case of the present experiment, the optic fiber specificity induced by differentiation of the retina may permit the various kinds of regenerating fibers to form specific central connections owing to differential affinities and incompatibilities between the ingrowing axons and the central neurons (Sperry 1943b, p. 47).

Sperry was also well aware of the implications of *retinal* specificity for neuronal differentiation in the *visual centers:*

> The foregoing interpretation assumes, of course, a differentiation of the neurons of the optic tectum, not merely in respect to their functional relations with lower centers, but also in physico-chemical properties that are capable of influencing growth processes previous to and irrespective of the adaptability of the functional results. According to the hypothesis of end-organ induction of central connection specifically, it is presumed that the central neurons become specified originally through a series of successive induction steps (Sperry 1943b, p. 50).

It is evident that his views about the development of the central target structures were still vaguely rooted in the notion of end-organ specification (Weiss 1936, 1941b) and were clearly hindered by the limited data available on the anatomical arrangement of retinal fibers in the amphibian optic lobe (Stroer 1939). It was to this issue that his next work was directed.

His important paper, published in 1944, is often remembered mainly for its telegraphic descriptions of inverted visuomotor strike responses in several species of anurans subjected to adult or larval eye rotation (see Figure 2.1), but its real and most lasting contribution derives from the lesion studies it reported. For these, Sperry ablated specific quadrants of the optic lobe and found that, in each case, this resulted in an immediate localized scotoma in the visual field of the contralateral eye, thus proving, in what was at the time the most direct possible way, that the retina projects in a *topographically* ordered manner across the surface of the optic tectum.

> When tested within an hour of operation the five animals with the anterior part of the lobe intact made no response when the lure was shown in the back part of the visual field but struck vigorously and accurately when it was shown in front. The five animals in which the ventral part of the lobe remained intact made no response when the lure was presented anywhere in the visual field above them but turned or struck forward readily when it was presented below eye level. When the lure was presented behind the five cases in which the posterior part of the lobe was intact, they turned quickly so as to face the lure in preparation to strike just as do normal animals but, when they had thus turned and the lure was directly in front of them, they made no further response until it was again moved to the back part of the visual field. By repeating the performance these animals could be made to turn around in circles without ever striking at the lure . . . (Sperry 1944, p. 65).

It was a simple step from this to predict what the nature of the retinal projection upon the tectum would be in frogs whose optic nerves had recently regenerated:

> The types of scotoma produced in . . . cases with regenerated optic nerves conformed consistently with those which had resulted in the foregoing group of normal animals. . . . Two additional cases . . . from the experimental group which had recovered reversed vision were also tested. A lesion in the anterior part of the optic lobe in one of them abolished responses to the lure presented behind the animal. When the lure was held in front, this animal responded by turning around to the rear in characteristically reversed manner. In the other case a medial tectal lesion abolished responses to the lure when it was held below eye level but did not eliminate the reversed reactions to the lure when it was presented well above eye level . . . *it may be concluded that the ingrowing optic fibers reestablish functional associations in the same topographical areas of the optic lobe in which they originally terminated and that no major reorganization of secondary synaptic relations is involved in the recovery of function* (Sperry 1944, p. 66, emphasis added).

Armed with this evidence for a topographically ordered projection between the eye and brain of normal frogs, and for the quadrant-specific reconnection by regenerating optic fibers in the optic lobe, Sperry (1944) proposed the next element of his chemoaffinity hypothesis, namely, a matching specificity of the neurons in the target area that did not involve an appeal to end-organ induction, modulation, or other such notions.

> The orderly topographical arrangement of functional relations found in the optic lobe after optic nerve regeneration is difficult to explain without assuming that *the secondary neurons of the optic tectum are also biochemically dissimilar,* possessing differential affinities for fibers arising from different retinal quadrants . . . it is conceivable that a basic embryonic specification arises through central self-differentiation of the central nuclear mass itself. Under such conditions the conjecture that specification of tectal neurons may be induced via the more early dif-

ferentiating motor and adjustor systems becomes unnecessary (Sperry 1944, pp. 67–8).

If Holtfreter had provided, as it were, the raw materials for chemoaffinities between embryonic cells, it remained to explain how a pattern of physicochemical specificities might arise during the development of sheets of neurons such as those in the retina and tectum. An important first step toward answering this was Sperry's simplifying assumption that the chemical diversity of the fibers in the optic nerve must in some way reflect the position of their cell bodies in the layer of retinal ganglion cells.

> It is easiest to conceive of this retinal cell differentiation as being orderly and continuous so that the difference between cells located far apart across the retina is greater than that between cells which are nearer together. *The development of such a condition is readily interpreted embryologically in terms of a polarized, field differentiation of the optic cup.* The retinal field would thus become, in respect to cellular differentiation of the ganglion layer a true "field" in the physical sense of the term (Sperry 1943b, pp. 45–6).

Drawing upon the embryological studies of Harrison (1921), which pointed to a progressive determination of pattern in embryonic fields, Sperry then made the first of several explicit predictions about the embryonic origins of chemospecificity in the amphibian retina:

> Presumably if rotation of the retinal field or its anlage were carried out at a sufficiently early stage of development, the polarity of retinal differentiation would be regulated so that normal vision would be restored (Sperry 1943b, p. 46).

The further development of this idea to include a fieldlike differentiation along two orthogonal retinal or tectal axes seems to have been arrived at intuitively, as Sperry suggests in his 1951 review:

> The qualitative specificity must parallel the topography of the retinal field. This means a true "field" distribution of qualitative properties among the retinal ganglion cells from which the optic fibers originate and among the tectal neurons on which they terminate. It means, furthermore, that the retina must be differentiated with respect to at least two axes of the eyeball in order that each locus may have biochemical properties different from those of all other loci (Sperry 1951a, p. 258).

Again, as we have seen, there was good historical precedent for this notion in the work of Harrison (1921, 1936) on the development of limb and ear primordia, and, beginning in 1945, Sperry was to adopt Harrison's experimental strategy for his exhaustive series of studies on eye rotations and left/right eye transplants.

> The interest in contralateral eye transplantation for the present experiment lies in the fact that the eyeball cannot be shifted from the orbit on one side of the head across to the other without reversing it on one of its axes. If the transplanted eye be correctly oriented on its optic axis, then it may also be correctly oriented on either, but not both, the dorsoventral or the nasotemporal axis. If one of these is correct, the other will be inverted.... Hence if recovery were to conform with the previous results, it follows that the appearance of the visual field should be spatially inverted on one cross dimension (Sperry 1945a, pp. 19–20).

As noted earlier, the animals with left-to-right eye transplants did indeed confirm his prediction – the animals accurately localized the lure in one dimension of visual space, but misdirected their response in the other, in accordance with the surgical misalignment of either the anteroposterior (nasotemporal) or the dorsoventral axis of the eye (Figure 2.8A). A similar one-dimensional reversal of visuomotor reflexes occurred in animals in which the left and right optic nerves had been surgically cross-united and allowed to regenerate into the ipsilateral optic lobe (Figure 2.8B).

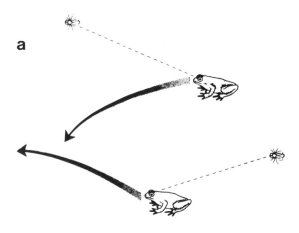

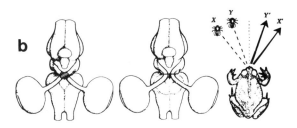

Figure 2.8. Persistent errors in visuomotor localization in frogs, following optic-nerve regeneration from contralaterally transplanted eyes or after surgical cross-union of the left and right optic nerves (Sperry 1945a). (**A**) When the eye had been implanted with its dorsoventral axis upside down (*top*), the frog was observed to strike correctly with reference to the nasotemporal (anteroposterior) dimension of the visual field, but inversely with reference to the dorsoventral dimension. When the eye had been implanted with its anteroposterior axis reversed, the strikes were misdirected in the nasotemporal dimension. (After Sperry 1951a.) (**B**) Surgical cross-union of the left and right optic nerves is diagrammed to the left; the pattern of visual strikes observed following optic-nerve regeneration is schematized to the right. In the author's words: "After optic-nerve regeneration the animals respond as if everything viewed through either eye were being seen through the opposite eye. For example, when a lure is presented at X or at Y, the animal strikes at X' or Y' respectively." (Figure and legend from Sperry 1951a, p. 246.)

Localization of small objects in space as tested with a housefly impaled on a fine wire was quite accurate when the lure was presented . . . exactly in the midsagittal plane. At all other positions, however,

the lure was erroneously localized at a corresponding point on the opposite side of the mid-plane. These errors of localization were quite precise. When the lure was held close to the midsagittal plane in front of the animals, they struck close to the lure but on the opposite side of the midline. When the lure was held at increasing distances away from the midplane, the errors were correspondingly greater to the opposite side (Sperry 1945a, p. 18)

With this evidence for one-axis reversed vision, Sperry (1945a) made an equally bold prediction about the visual behavior to be expected from embryonically rotated eyes:

> To attain a complete differential specificity of all retinal loci the retinal field must undergo differentiation on at least two separate axes. Possibly as in the developing limb bud (Harrison 1921), the anteroposterior and dorsoventral axes are determined separately in the order given. If so, one would expect that contralateral eye transplantation carried out at increasingly early embryonic stages would begin at a certain point to yield normal vision after dorsoventral inversion while continuing to yield inverted vision after nasotemporal inversion (Sperry 1945a, p. 27).

A few years later, Sperry (1951b) set out this prediction even more clearly, and formalized his proposal in terms of quantitative differences along two or more qualitatively distinct gradients, as schematized in Figure 2.9.

> We suggested that this optic fiber specificity might be brought about through a polarized field-like differentiation of the retina in development with the specificity of the ganglion cells being extended into the optic fibers throughout their length. It was also suggested that normal vision might prevail if the retina or its anlage were rotated prior to the stage at which its polarity had become irreversibly fixed.
>
> It was necessary to conclude further that the retinal differentiation must occur on at least 2 axes. A dorsoventral differ-

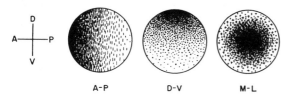

Figure 2.9. "Diagrams illustrating how each retinal lucus might acquire its unique properties through polarized differentiation of the retinal field in development. Differentiation on the anteroposterior (A-P), or nasotemporal, axis alone would not be sufficient as all points along lines perpendicular to the A-P axis would remain equivalent. The addition of a dorsoventral (D-V) gradient, qualitatively distinct from the former, however, would endow each retinal point with its distinct local properties. A separate mediolateral (M-L) or radial differentiation, by itself, or in combination with either the A-P or the D-V gradient would not be adequate, but superimposed upon the combination of the first two, might increase the degree of differentiation." (Figure and original legend from Sperry 1951b, p. 69.)

entiation alone, for example, would not be sufficient because the anterior and posterior retinal quandrants would be indistinguishable. An anteroposterior differentiation superimposed upon the dorsoventral, however, would stamp the fibers from each retinal locus with a unique combination of qualities. . . . One is reminded of Harrison's (1921) studies showing the establishment of an anteroposterior and a dorsoventral axis in the differentiation of the early limb bud. It was suggested that contralateral transplantation of the eye or its anlage during the critical developmental stages might similarly reveal a separate determination of two such axes in retinal differentiation (Sperry 1951b, p. 68).

His prediction that normal vision would follow early eye rotation in embryos was confirmed in salamanders by Stone (1944, 1960, 1966; see also Hunt and Piatt 1974) and later in *Xenopus* by Jacobson (1968); and the prediction that one-axis reversals would be found in contralaterally transplanted embryonic eyes was soon to be confirmed in two species of newt by Szekely (1954, 1966) and some years later in *Xenopus* by Hunt and Jacobson (1972a, 1972b). But more germane to the development of Sperry's ideas was the

extension of the chemoaffinity hypothesis to include an explicit proposal as to how the retinal specificities that mediate the proposed affinities might arise during embryonic development. The ganglion cell layer was conceived of as behaving like a classic embryonic field undergoing progressive differentiation first in its anteroposterior and then in its dorsoventral dimension, and in the process acquiring a pattern of chemical differences that are graded and smoothly ordered across the entire retinal cell sheet.

ON THE CHEMOAFFINITIES THAT
GOVERN THE EFFERENT PATHWAYS
OF THE OPTIC TECTUM

In 1948, Sperry published two studies that broadened the base for his ideas on the chemical specification of neurons in the visual pathway. The first described the orderly return of visuomotor responses, as well as the recovery and persistence of 180°-misdirected vision from rotated eyes, following optic-nerve regeneration in several species of teleost fish (Sperry 1948a). Although this study provided no new conceptual insights, it was typical of Sperry to seek a broad comparative approach for his ideas, and, at the same time, it paved the way for his analysis of the optic lobe, not only as the recipient of an ordered retinal input, but also as the source of inputs to the brainstem and spinal cord, that mediate visuomotor behavior (Sperry 1948b). The key experiments in this second study involved transecting the brainstem either unilaterally or bilaterally, just caudal to the midbrain, in normal adult newts and in cases in which both eyes had been rotated 180° without disruption of the optic nerves. Following regeneration of the tectal efferent pathways, the first group of animals showed normal visuomotor responses, whereas the second group showed a restoration of 180°-misdirected vision (Sperry 1948b). In the latter group, the eyes were subsequently "reset" by surgical derotation back into their normal anatomical orientation in the orbit. Immediately after recovery from the anesthetic, the newts showed normal visuomotor reflexes indistinguishable from those in unoperated animals. The animals were then subjected to yet another operation: localized ablations were made in the medial quadrant of the optic lobe, and the animals were retested shortly following the lesion.

> The effects of these lesions were found to be similar to those obtained in normal cases, namely, an elimination of all responses to the lure when it was presented anywhere in the dorsal part of the visual field plus retention of normal reactions to the lure when it was presented in the ventral portions of the visual field. Had there been a functional adjustment in the optic lobe to suit random connections in the lower centers, the above operation should have impaired vision in the ventral as well as in the dorsal quadrants. Apparently, however, the afferent system had retained its original organization and the efferent relations had been adjusted accordingly (Sperry 1948b, p. 71).

Sperry's interpretation of these complex experiments again began by emphasizing the absence of functional adjustment, but proceeded directly to extend the chemoaffinity theory beyond the input to the optic lobe to include the synaptic relations of its efferents to the brainstem and spinal cord:

> That learning or any adaptation through functional adjustment might be responsible has been ruled out by the fact that the central associations were restored in the same systematic manner even though the eyes had been previously rotated 180° making the functional results of recovery highly maladaptive.
>
> The results are explicable on the assumption that *the regenerating fibers differ in character in accordance with their different afferent associations* and that this constitutional specificity was able to influence in a selective manner the type of functional associations which were formed in the efferent centers. *It must be concluded that the lower-level neurons likewise differ qualitatively among themselves,* for, if they were all alike, there would have been no basis on which the regenerating fibers could have established associations selectively. Presumably the formation of synaptic connections in the

spinal and medullary centers is regulated by differential affinities between various types of regenerating fibers and the different kinds of lower-level neurons (Sperry 1948b, pp. 72–3, emphasis added).

Thus, the chemoaffinity hypothesis was broadened to include the sensory-motor circuits of the brain and spinal cord, and so became a general theory to account for the formation of connections within the central nervous system. In its most general form, the hypothesis suggests that all neuronal populations are subject to a patterned chemical differentiation, and that chemical compatibilities mediate the development of highly selective connections between each group of neurons in a polyneuronal circuit.

STUDIES ON THE VESTIBULAR AND SOMATOSENSORY SYSTEMS

Although Sperry's studies on the vestibular and somatosensory systems are less well known than his studies of the visual system and historically occupy a less central position in the development of the chemoaffinity hypothesis, in fact, they contributed significantly to the generalization of the theory in at least four respects. First, by applying the same experimental paradigms to the vestibular nerve and to the sensory nerves of the limbs and trunk, Sperry obtained a wealth of new data that established beyond doubt that the recovery of function following regeneration of these nerves was based on the selective reconnection within the brain and spinal cord of the regenerating axons, and that function and experience play little or no role in forging these connections. Second, they incorporate into the chemoaffinity hypothesis the interesting notion that neuronal specificities can be induced in sensory neurons by the end organs innervated by their outgrowing axons. (We later consider this issue in greater detail, but here it may be remarked that this notion is reminiscent of Weiss's concept of "modulation" or "myotypic specification".) Third, the vestibular and somatosensory experiments provided the first evidence for a refined differentiation of the nonneural periphery – of sensory receptors both by *class* and by *position,* and for the notion of "cutaneous local sign," which provide the cornerstone of Sperry's least well-appreciated, but arguably his most significant, contribution to general embryology. Finally, these studies provided the first clear statement that the chemoaffinities that govern synaptic connections are based not only upon the position of the relevant neurons in embryonic fields, but also upon their distinctive cellular phenotype, including their functional specializations, end-organ relations, and the sensory modalities they subserve.

The vestibular system. The vestibular system offered a number of attractions. Not the least of these was the fact that the VIIIth nerve was readily accessible to surgical intervention, and rather simple behavioral tests could be devised to evaluate vestibular function following interruption of the nerve and its subsequent regeneration.

Moreover, as Sperry wrote in 1951:

From the nature of vestibular reflexes it is evident that the fibers that supply the crista of any one semicircular canal must have different reflex relations in the hindbrain from the fibers supplying the crista of either of the other canals. Similarly the fibers to each of the approximately seven separate end organs of the amphibian labyrinth must have their own special linkages. . . . At the same time . . . fibers supplying different parts of a single end organ, such as those to the utricular macula, must have differential central associations to match their functional diversity (Sperry 1951a, p. 248).

He accordingly transected the VIIIth nerve bilaterally in adult *Hyla squirrela,* along with the root fibers of cranial nerve VII, and teased the residual fibers in the VIIIth nerve stump to introduce disorder in the initial pattern of fiber outgrowth (Sperry 1945c). The profound disturbance of equilibrium caused by the surgery was never corrected in control cases in which VIIIth nerve regeneration was prevented. In the experimental cases, however, there was an orderly restoration of vestibular reflexes to tilting and angular acceleration of the animal

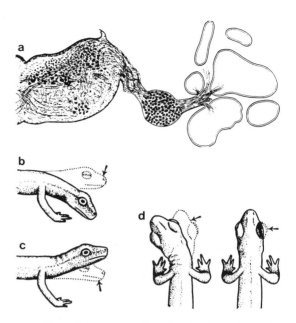

Figure 2.10. Restoration of vestibular and somatomotor reflexes in frogs and newts following transection and regeneration of identified cranial nerves. (A) Following transection of vestibular nerve roots bilaterally in *Hyla* frogs, the root fibers were able to regenerate into their medullary nuclei as indicated by this "diagrammatic section through regenerated vestibular nerve root at its entrance into the medulla. Fibers connected to the various sensory endings in the semicircular canals, the utriculus, the sacculus, and the lagena become intertangled at the point of nerve section, but they nevertheless reestablish central reflex relations in a systematic pattern." (Figure and original legend from Sperry 1951a, p. 249.) (B–D) Sperry and Miner (1949) transected the trigeminal nerve root and assayed sensorimotor withdrawal reflexes following centripetal regeneration of the Vth nerve. Sharply defined head-withdrawal reflexes were restored, which accurately localized a punctate stimulus on the face and evoked head withdrawal away from the stimulus. In addition (D, *right*), the corneal reflex was also restored such that punctate stimulation of the cornea evoked withdrawal of the eye into its eye socket followed by closure of the eyelids. (From Sperry 1951a.)

in the three primary planes of the body (Figure 2.10A). Again there was no evidence of learning in the process, and the recovered reflexes survived later decerebration. In separate studies on tadpoles (Sperry, 1945b, 1946), the optic nerves were completely excised at the time the VIIIth nerves were cut. These tadpoles also showed recovery of vestibular function, including vestibularly induced compensatory eye movements, despite the fact that in the absence of optic nerves, such vestibuloocular reflexes were of no adaptive value to the animal.

The vestibular studies thus provided, in a second sensory system, an observation similar to the orderly return of visuomotor localization following regeneration of the optic nerve (Sperry 1943b, 1944). Although the strategies used to exclude function stopped short of applying Sperry's second paradigm of surgically forcing a set of maladaptive connections upon the animal (in the sense that rotation of the vestibular periphery, analogous to eye rotation, was not performed), careful histologic examination of the VIIIth nerve scars showed chaotic intermingling of the regenerated fibers reminiscent of the scarred regions in regenerated optic nerves (Figure 2.10A).

Viewed as a whole, the findings led to the important inference that chemoaffinity must apply not only to neurons of different *"field" positions* within a sensory array, but also to neurons *of different functional classes:*

> Evidently, the different neuron types among the heterogeneous collection of divided sensory root fibers were able to reestablish functional relations with the secondary central cells in a discriminating manner. Judging from the number of different kinds of sensory end organs supplied by nerves VII and VIII, one would estimate that at least eleven distinct classes of fibers regenerated from the point of transection with ample opportunity for a chaotic interspersion into abnormal pathways (Sperry 1951a, p. 250).

In some respects, the inferences drawn from the return of vestibular function closely paralleled those drawn from the visual system studies, but they also led to several new conclusions. As Sperry expressed it in the 1951 growth symposium:

> The results indicate that the sensory fibers innervating the various end organs of the labyrinth *differ from one another in quality*. For example, those fibers connected with the crista of the horizontal semicircular canal differ from those connected with the crista of the anterior or posterior vertical canals and these differ in turn from those supplying the macula of the utriculus, etc.

> The end organs themselves must undergo a correlated differentiation. In the case of the macula of the utriculus the functional relationships suggest a biaxial polarized specification similar to that of the retina such that fibers to any given point in the macula may be stamped with unique properties distinguishing them from all other macular fibers. The central neurons of the vestibular nuclei must also be qualitatively specified, for if they were all alike and indistinguishable there would be no basis on which the ingrowing vestibular fibers could form their proper differential reflex relations.

> Considering the manner in which the labyrinth differentiates (Harrison 1936) and the way in which the innervation of its sense organs is developed . . . it seems probable that here, as in the optic fibers, *central synapsis is governed from the periphery with the end organs leading the way in differentiation and inducing specificity in their nerve fibers*. In the labyrinth, however, bodies of the nerve cells are not embedded within the end organ tissue, as they are in the retina, but lie in the ganglion at some distance with only their fiber tips in contact. We are therefore obliged to assume in this case that terminal fiber connections are sufficient for the induction of specificity in the peripheral nerve cells.

> This idea that an end organ may impose specific chemical changes in its nerve fibers, and that this in some way determines its functional relations with the centers – something which we have now come to regard as a general principle in neurogenesis – was suggested by Weiss . . . in 1936 under the term "modulation" to account for the "homologous" or "myotypic" function of supernumerary limbs (Sperry 1951b, pp. 72–3).

Integumental specification and somatosensory connections. From 1947 through 1951, Sperry and his student Nancy Miner performed a variety of surgical rearrangements on the somatosensory system of tadpoles and frogs (Sperry and Miner 1949; Miner and Sperry 1950; Sperry 1951a, 1951b; Miner, 1951a, 1951b, 1956). The experiments are among the most ingenious that Sperry performed and, at the same time, among the most difficult to interpret. Historically, they drew heavily on his sustained interest in the problem of cutaneous innervation and seems to have begun with his early fascination with the problem of sensory local sign.

> A patient on the examining table with eyes closed is capable of localizing with considerable accuracy a pin prick applied anywhere on the body surface. . . . Similarly the dog or cat turn directly to the point where a flea is biting and even the frog displays pretty fair localization of cutaneous stimuli. There is something about impulses entering the brain from different points on the body surface that registers the cutaneous locus from which they arise and we refer to this as the "local sign" quality of cutaneous sensibility . . . for accurate localization, it is necessary that the central synaptic associations of the cutaneous fibers be neatly adjusted during development to suit the pattern of peripheral innervation (Sperry 1951b, p. 75).

He had first addressed this issue in his dissertation studies on motor innervation in the rat hindlimb (Sperry 1943c) when he examined the capacity of young rats to localize cutaneous stimuli following surgical rerouting of nerves from the left to the right hind foot (Figure 2.6D). Although the operations were performed as early as the fourteenth day postnatally, the painful stimuli were never consistently localized and the resulting maladaptive behavior was never corrected: when the right foot was stimulated, the animal would raise and lick its left foot, while bearing down on the offending stimulus with the right foot. From this, Sperry (1943c) was led to infer that sensory nerves are not interchangeable and that, in some sense, cutaneous "local sign" must be, as we would now say, hardwired early during development.

The analysis was later extended to the sensory nerves of amphibians in two unpub-

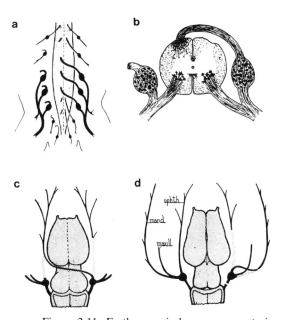

Figure 2.11. Further surgical rearrangements imposed on the somatosensory system of the frog by Sperry (1951) and by Sperry and Miner (1949). (A–B) After surgical excision of the dorsal roots from the left hindlimb in tadpoles, the contralateral roots (from the right leg) were transected and cross-united to the left dorsal horn of the spinal cord. When stimulated at specific positions on the right leg, after metamorphosis, the frogs showed the appropriate place-specific withdrawal reflex – except that instead of withdrawing the stimulated right limb, the anesthetic left limb was withdrawn. (After Sperry 1951b.) (C–D) Sperry and Miner's (1949) study featured a number of ingenious surgical rearrangements on the identified branches of the trigeminal nerve V. In (C), the right ophthalmic nerve root has been cross-united to the left ophthalmic nerve. The left root has been completely resected so as to thwart regeneration of trigeminal axons from the left ganglion back into its own terminal field. In (D), the proximal stump of the right ophthalmic nerve has been surgically cross-united to the distal segment of the mandibular nerve on the same side. The mandibular root has also been completely excised to prevent reinnervation of the mandibular nerve field by mandibular fibers. In both instances, peripheral regeneration of the sensory nerves led to sensory mislocalization and the maladaptive reflexes were never corrected by practice. (After Sperry 1951a.)

lished experiments (Sperry 1951a, 1951b), one of which is illustrated in Figures 2.11A and 2.11B. The experiments were designed to examine the effects of surgically rearranging the connections of cutaneous nerves to the trunk in frog tadpoles, so that upon metamorphosis, sensory stimuli from one side of the body would be carried to the opposite (wrong) side of the spinal cord. As in his previous experiments on rats, he found the responses to cutaneous stimulation to be persistently maladaptive and the animal's behavior was never corrected by practice:

> We have been able to eliminate functional adaptation as the responsible factor by experiments like the following: when skin flaps, with original innervation retained, are transposed in frog tadpoles across the midline of the back, from the left to the right side, the frogs, after metamorphosis, wipe erroneously with the left leg at the former site of the skin flap when it is stimulated on the right side. After contralateral cross connections of the sensory nerve roots of the hindlimb in frog tadpoles, the metamorphosed frogs make characteristic, but useless and maladaptive responses of the left limb when the right foot is stimulated ... (Sperry 1951b, p. 76).

In 1949, with Miner, he reported a detailed series of experiments on sensorimotor reflexes following surgical rearrangement of the trigeminal nerve, Figures 2.10B to 2.10D. In the first experiment, the central root of the trigeminal nerve was transected in a group of newts at various larval and postmetamorphic stages. To disrupt all topographic order within the root, the nerve roots were teased apart during the intracranial transections. Despite this, when sensitivity was restored, there was full recovery of the normal place-specific withdrawal reflexes.

> Different reactions could be elicited from different cutaneous points as follows: (a) depression of the head from the dorsal tip of the snout, (b) elevation of the head from the ventral tip of the chin, (c) lateral withdrawal of the head from the edge of the jaw anterior to the eye, (d) combined lateral and downward withdrawal from a point intermediate between those of a and c, (e) withdrawal of the eye from the cornea and surrounding skin.
> The recovered responses were quite

normal in character.... The recovered reflexes survived decerebration and were abolished in three cases so tested by resection of the regenerated fifth root (Sperry and Miner 1949, pp. 406–7).

The same experiment was carried out with limited success in frogs (*Rana catesbiana*) and in the best cases (in which the root transection was carried out at tadpole stages) there was an orderly return of function. Histologic examination of the regenerated nerves confirmed that, as in the optic and vestibular nerve studies, during regeneration there was a "haphazard intermixing" of the nerve fibers in the scar, and it followed that the recovery of place-specific reflexes could not be ascribed to "any combination of mechanical and timing factors" (Sperry and Miner 1949, p. 410).

In other newts and tadpoles, a variety of more complex rearrangements were forced upon the different branches of the trigeminal nerve including cross-union of the left and right ophthalmic nerves, inserting the cut distal end of the mandibular nerve into the proximal stump of the ophthalmic, and cross-uniting the trigeminal and facial nerves. The rationale of these experiments was quite explicit as stated for the first group:

> If the central organization of the localizing reflexes were predetermined by developmental forces, the wiping responses, after metamorphosis, ought to be directed at the wrong side of the snout upon stimulation of the left ophthalmic area. If, on the contrary, the central organization were acquired through function, the frogs might soon come to direct their wiping responses correctly toward the point stimulated (Sperry and Miner 1949, p. 417).

In fact, the behavioral patterns observed were consistent and strictly in accordance with the structuralist prediction:

> ... tactile stimuli applied to the left ophthalmic area elicited wiping responses of the contralateral limb directed toward the right ophthalmic area. Also the right eye was retracted instead of the left. When a small piece of filter paper dampened in dilute acetic acid was placed on

the left side of the snout, the frogs repeatedly wiped at the wrong side failing to remove the paper (Sperry and Miner 1949, p. 417).

Similarly, after successful mandibular/ophthalmic cross-unions, head withdrawal reflexes were irreversibly misdirected: stimulating the jaw from below caused normal elevation on the unoperated side, but depression response into the stimulus on the operated side – as if the stimulus had originated from the region normally supplied by the ophthalmic nerve. And, significantly, no improvement occurred in these maladaptive responses during the four months or more that the animals were studied. However, when the trigeminal nerve was cross-united with the central stump of the facial (with the facial ganglion removed), *normal* sensorimotor reflexes were observed. In about two months, the corneal "eye-withdrawal" reflex had returned, and most cases showed place-specific head withdrawal to stimulation of the face.

> Histological examination . . . confirmed that the fact that the root fibers of V had regenerated into the brain via the seventh root pathway as intended . . . so we may assume that the ingrowing fibers managed to reach trigeminal neuropil (Sperry and Miner 1949, pp. 413–14).

Sperry and Miner were quick to perceive the larger implications of their findings:

> To explain the orderly formation of reflex relations in the trigeminal sensory nuclei under the conditions of the foregoing experiments it is necessary to conclude that the sensory neurons supplying different cutaneous areas differ in character. The sensory root fibers associated with different cutaneous loci must somehow be distinguished from one another in the centers. . . .
> Furthermore the nature of the localizing responses requires that the sensory neuron specificity correspond with the topography of the trigeminal cutaneous field. . . . For example, neurons innervating loci far distant from one another must be less similar in their bio-

chemical constitution than those supplying adjacent areas. . . . It would seem impossible that this could be attained in the absence of a corresponding qualitative differentiation of the skin itself.
> . . . Taken together the findings suggest that the development of cutaneous local sign depends upon a highly refined field-like differentiation of the entire integument plus a parallel differentiation of the primary sensory neurons. The specification of the sensory fibers, perhaps imposed in part by induction from the cutaneous field, would make possible an orderly, selective formation of reflex relations in the centers on a chemical affinity basis. This interpretation implies a correlated specificity among the second order neurons, which, in turn, must be distinguishable according to their various efferent relations in order that the invading root fibers may form the appropriate linkages (Sperry and Miner 1949, p. 419).

Although their experiments did not address the question of modality specificity, it is clear that they were not unaware of the problem:

> The present experiments furnish no information regarding the additional dimension of differentiation among the trigeminal neurons required for the various sense modalities like pain, touch, and temperature. Presumably the local sign specificity would have to be superimposed upon this modal differentiation (Sperry and Miner 1949, p. 421).

In her doctoral dissertation Miner (1951a, 1951b, 1956) applied the "choice" and "cross-union" paradigms to the dorsal root ganglion cells of the trunk region in frog tadpoles. Her first experiment was to remove ganglia 8–10 unilaterally in *Rana clamitans* tadpoles at foot-paddle stages. These ganglia normally supply the hindlimb; yet, after metamorphosis, most of the frogs showed well-localized foot-withdrawal reflexes upon stimulation of the experimental limb – including thirteen cases in which histology later confirmed that ganglia 8–10 were absent on the operated side. Miner's

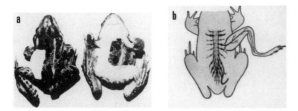

Figure 2.12. (**A**) These two photographs show, in dorsal and ventral views, a postmetamorphic frog whose trunk skin had been excised and rotated through 180° at earlier tadpole stages. The grafted skin had "self-differentiated," leaving the frog with green back skin on its left belly and white belly skin on its left back. Sensory stimuli applied to the grafted skin after metamorphosis evoked place-specific wiping reflexes directed not at the stimulus, but at the original position of the stimulated skin. (After Miner 1956.) (**B**) In a second preparation, shown schematically, Miner (1956) grafted a supernumerary limb-bud onto a host tadpole at a dorsolateral trunk position in between the tadpole's own forelimb and hindlimb bud. After metamorphic transformation, stimuli to specific positions on the supernumerary limb evoked position-specific withdrawal reflexes of the ipsilateral hindlimb. Histologic checks confirmed that the extra limb had been innervated by the adjacent thoracic ganglia. (After Sperry 1951b.)

(1956) remaining two experimental variations are shown in Figure 2.12. When an extra limbbud was grafted to the dorsal thoracic region of a midlarval *Rana pipiens* tadpole, a full but immobile supernumerary leg developed between the frog's own fore- and hindlimb (Figure 2.12B). Punctate or dilute-acid stimulation of the immobile leg evoked place-specific limbwithdrawal reflexes of the frog's own ipsilateral fore- or hindlimb. Yet of the three experiments Miner (1956) carried out, perhaps the most striking involved excising the trunk skin on one side of *R. pipiens* tadpoles and replacing it in 180°-rotated orientation. In the successful cases, which were tested after metamorphosis, the skin had self-differentiated so that the graft had developed typical spotted green (back) skin on the belly and white (belly) skin on the back (Figure 2.12A). And stimulation of the grafted back skin on the belly evoked hindlimb wipes to the back, whereas stimulation of the belly skin on the back evoked misdirected wipes of the forelimb toward the belly. Thus, not only were the wipes directed at the original position of the skin, but the choice of limb was appro-

priate for the misidentified target – belly wipes being normally mediated by the forelimb and back wipes by the hindlimb. Occasional "normal" wipes were also seen, but these could be eliminated by surgically cutting around the perimeter of the graft so as to interrupt branches of axons from the surrounding unrotated skin.

Since in all three groups of experiments, the patterns of misdirected reflexes remained more or less unchanged over many months of testing, Miner (1956) reaffirmed the view that "function" cannot by itself shape the relevant neural circuitry and concluded:

> It has seemed necessary to infer that cutaneous fibers supplying different local areas in the skin differ chemically from one another, and it has been suggested that the central reflex patterning is achieved through a selective synaptic termination of the root fibers that is regulated by specific chemical affinities between the sensory fibers and the central neurons (Miner 1956, p. 161).

Like the earlier vestibular studies, the work on cutaneous nerves also advanced the notion that chemoaffinity labels might arise, not only by self-differentiation within fieldlike neural anlagen, but also by *end-organ induction*. The notion that the peripheral structures differentiate first and somehow "lead the way" in shaping the differentiation of the related neural centers was not new to Sperry (see, for example, Detwiler 1920, 1936), and selective induction was generally accepted as a central concept in any theory of differentiation (Spemann rev. 1938). Sperry and Miner's observations on "integumental specification" of local sign in sensory axons afforded an attractive bridge between the emerging chemoaffinity hypothesis and Weiss's idea of modulation – a kind of "cutaneotypic" variation on Weiss's notion of the myotypic specification of motoneurons. But the alternative explanation involving an independent and parallel differentiation of the sensory neurons and the targets in both center and periphery, followed by the selective innervation by both branches of the sensory axon, was also considered.

Finally, and perhaps most importantly, the work on the somatosensory system, together with the earlier vestibular studies, established a clear imperative for the progressive fieldlike differentiation of the nonneural periphery of the embryo, and so paved the way for a general theory for the spatial control of differentiation, and for marking cell positions in the embryo with appropriate chemical labels.

> Such evidence as we now have . . . seems sufficient to warrant the conclusion that almost the entire nervous system is subject to a refined differentiation . . . which in many regions approaches the level of the individual nerve cell. The bulk of the somatic and visceral periphery likewise must undergo a similar subtle specification insofar as differential motor or sensory functions prevail. This would include, in addition to . . . [the retina, skin, muscles, and vestibular end organs] . . . already mentioned and other specialized sensory and motor organs, such structures as the fascias and other subcutaneous connective tissues, the ligaments, tendons, joint surfaces, the periosteum of the bones, and the parts of the various viscera.

RETURN TO THE VISUAL SYSTEM AND THE EMERGENCE OF A DYNAMIC THEORY OF NERVE GROWTH

Sperry returned to the visual system in the early 1960s when he carried out a series of histological studies with Harbans Arora and Dominica Attardi on optic-nerve regeneration in adult fish. The studies were broadly conceived and addressed a number of issues, including the restoration of color vision and other functional properties, after optic-nerve transection (Arora and Sperry 1963). In his discussion of these experiments, he extended his notions of chemoaffinity in the retina and tectum to encompass the idea that chemical labels denoting *cell class* must be superimposed upon the labels that define *cell position*. According to this view, ganglion cell axons not only identify tectal cells at the appropriate loci, but, by some chemical matching mechanism, must also recognize the appropriate classes of tectal relay cells to mediate "on" and "off" responses and color vision. But perhaps these studies are best

remembered for the experiments with partial lesions of the retina that provided the first direct evidence that regenerating optic fibers can bypass inappropriate regions of the tectum and selectively reinnervate their normal target zones (Attardi and Sperry 1963), and for those in which optic fibers were forced into inappropriate pathways to the tectum yet nevertheless succeeded in growing back to their normal target regions (Arora and Sperry 1962; Arora 1963; Sperry 1965). But, conceptually, the most profound impact of these studies was the broadening of the chemoaffinity hypothesis itself to include the chemical guidance of axonal growth.

As we have seen, the notion that chemoaffinities might mediate the selection of pathways by growing axons and the selective fasciculation of axons with similar chemical identities was not entirely new. Indeed, it was quite explicit in Ramon y Cajal's lively description of the growth cone and his concept of chemotropism. And Sperry himself had initially considered, but then rejected, the possibility of chemospecific bundling of optic axons in his paper on the return of vision in rotated newt eyes.

> Another possibility is that fibers from the same region of the retina tend to adhere to each other during regeneration because of preferential surface affinities (selective fasciculation) so that the whole optic tract is normally oriented with an orderly arrangement as it approaches the visual centers. However, the interweaving and crossing of fibers, not only in the scar region, but also throughout the course of the nerve in those cases in which retinal degeneration occurred does not support this assumption (Sperry 1943b, pp. 47–8).

And his histological examination of the region of the nerve scar when a frog eye was transplanted to the contralateral side had also led him to think that axonal guidance was essentially a mechanical process:

> Although the peripheral and central nerve stumps necessarily met each other in an inverted position there was no indication in the scar region of an orderly inversion

of the fiber pattern to correct this. . . . On the whole the fiber pattern in the chiasma offered no support for assuming that the turning of fibers to one side or the other was determined by other than mechanical factors . . . the optic fibers did not regenerate in straight parallel lines maintaining their original interneural pattern but instead showed considerable interweaving and rearrangement (Sperry 1945a, p. 26).

But a few years later, in a remarkable passage from his 1951 lecture to the Growth Society, he was to openly entertain a role for chemical guidance when he stated:

It remains possible, although the old idea has been under fire in recent times, that the chemical effects of neuronal differentiation may be influential in determining not only terminal linkages but also the course of the growing nerve fibers and thereby the configuration of connecting pathways. We would visualize the growing fiber tips as responding, not so much to chemicals diffusing in the tissue fluids, as to the local, stabilized chemical properties of the differentiating cells and intercellular ground substance which the tips encounter in their advancement. . . . It is not difficult to conceive of chemical guidance based on the selective reinforcement and resorption of the exploratory filaments and incipient branches of the advancing fibers. . . . There is also suggestion that the neuronal differentiation results in variant fiber growth potentials such that the elongating processes of different types of neurons may respond diversely, each in a characteristic manner, to the same chemical substrate (Sperry, 1951b, p. 84)

This theme was taken up anew by Attardi and Sperry (1963) in their work on cichlid fish (*Astronotus ocellatus*) and goldfish (*Crassus auratus*). Using the Bodian silver stain to visualize retinal axons in the optic tract and their terminals in the synaptic layers of the tectum, they first described the normal anatomy of the teleost visual pathway, including the divergence of the fibers from the dorsal and ventral retina into separate brachia of the optic tract:

Before entering the midbrain tectum the primary optic tract divides into two main bundles, the medial and lateral optic tracts. These course along the medial and lateral circumference of the optic lobe, respectively, giving off fibers all along the periphery. . . . The medial tract . . . consists of fibers arising in the ventral part of the retina . . . [which] . . . spread fanlike into the dorsal portion of the tectum from its medial border. Conversely, the fibers of the lateral tract arise in the dorsal retina and spread from the ventral border of the lobe into its ventral and lateral areas (Attardi and Sperry 1963, p. 49).

Taking advantage of the differential coloration of normal and regenerating fibers, they then proceeded to describe the time course of reinnervation of the tectum after intraorbital transection of the optic nerve.

At 3 to 4 days after nerve section, the whole distal segment of the optic nerve and the two [brachia] . . . appear to have degenerated.

At 4 to 7 days . . . the optic fibers have started to regenerate and have become mixed and entangled in a dense and swollen neuromatous growth. . . .

At 10 to 12 days . . . the regenerated fibers start to reinnervate the optic lobe. Small groups of fibers exit from each bundle at different points along the circumference of the lobe and enter . . . the underlying plexiform layer particularly in the border regions.

At 14–18 days when visual function is being restored, the plexiform layer formed by the regenerated fibers is visible in all areas of the optic tectum (Attardi and Sperry 1963, pp. 53–4).

This, in turn, set the stage for the various experimental manipulations in which specific portions of the retina were surgically excised prior to nerve transection (Figure 2.1C). When the anterior half of the retina was excised, the regenerated fibers from the remaining posterior retina were seen to reestablish the normal pattern of medial and lateral bundles, but to confine their terminals to the rostral half of the tectal lobe where they normally terminate. When the posterior retina was ablated, the two bundles of regenerated fibers coursed along the medial and lateral borders of the lobe to their normal innervation zone in the posterior half of the tectum while giving off no branches to the anterior half of the tectum (Figure 2.1D). After two kinds of peripheral retinal ablations, the central retinal fibers were similarly found to regenerate selectively to their normal terminal zones in the center of the tectum. But the most telling experiments were those in which either the ventral or the dorsal half of the retina was excised. The results of these experiments are shown in Figure 2.1C and Figure 2.13A, and in the words of the authors:

> When the dorsal half of the retina was removed and the optic nerve of the same side severed, the remaining fibers originating in the ventral half of the retina regenerated and were found to enter the medial bundle. The route of the lateral bundle was left empty. . . . The parallel and plexiform layers were restored in the dorsal tectum only. Conversely, when the ventral half of the retina was removed, nearly all of the regenerated fibers were found to enter the lateral bundle, and only the ventral half of the cortex was reinnervated (Attardi and Sperry 1963, pp. 55–7).

These results provide direct microscopical confirmation of earlier deductions that the regenerating optic axons reconnect selectively in matching loci of the tectal field to restore an orderly topographic projection of the retina upon the tectum. *In addition the findings disclose for the first time an unexpectedly high degree of specificity in the choice of central pathways taken by the fibers en route to their terminal stations.* The results would appear to dispell any remaining doubts that the growing optic fibers are destination bound (Attardi and Sperry 1963, p. 61, emphasis added).

In a companion series of studies, Arora and Sperry (1962) surgically cross-united the medial and lateral brachia of the optic tract in *Astronotus ocellatus,* in an attempt to determine "whether the nerve bundles, if deliberately directed into the wrong channels, would grow into the foreign tracts and perhaps establish connections in foreign regions of the tectum" (Arora and Sperry 1962, p. 389). Yet after the recovery of visual function some 30–40 days later, the fish were found to be able to *correctly* localize moving objects in the visual fields of the operated eyes. And Bodian preparations of the brains (Figure 2.13B) revealed that "each fiber bundle, instead of growing ahead into its foreign channel, crossed back toward its original pathway and entered its own sector of the tectum" (Arora and Sperry 1962, p. 389).

Arora (1963) repeated in a more refined way the "bundle transplant" experiments, teasing away the posterior fascicle from the lateral bundle at the tectal border, and forcibly inserting it into the medial border of the ipsilateral optic lobe. Again the regenerated fibers were found to grow to the correct posterolateral region of the ipsilateral lobe, and to co-innervate that region with the corresponding fibers from the undisturbed eye. Commenting on the corrective course taken by these experimentally misrouted fibers, Sperry emphasized the idea of destination-bound growth:

> It is a common and repeated observation that fibers growing through the parallel (fiber) layer (of the tectal lobe) by-pass those regions of the tectum inappropriate for an orderly mapping of the retinotectal projections under conditions where the mechanical opportunities are equal for different fiber types (Sperry 1965, p. 180).

But even before this he had broadened the chemoaffinity hypothesis into a dynamic theory of nerve growth in which the chemical labels on growing axons *continuously* seek out, as it were, compatible chemical features in the substrates along which they grow and perhaps on their neighbors, and ultimately on their postsynaptic targets (Figure 2.13C):

> The results lead us to what is essentially a chemotactic view of nerve outgrowth, though without the "distance action" imputed in some definitions of chemotaxis.

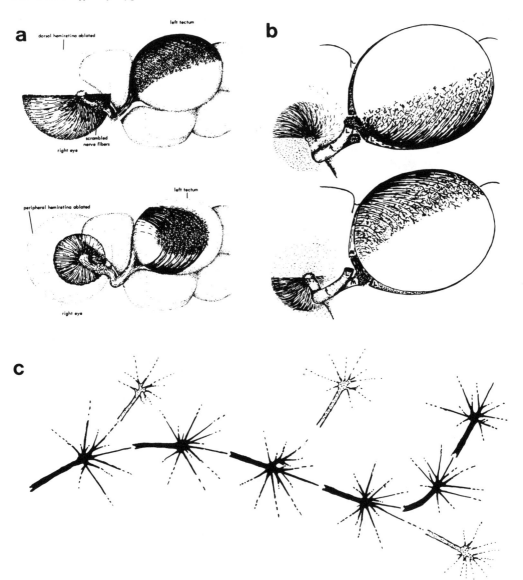

Figure 2.13. (**A**) Anatomical drawings are shown for two variants of the partial retinal ablation experiment of Attardi and Sperry (1963). (*Top*) After surgical excision of the dorsal half of the retina and after transection and regeneration of the optic nerve, the regenerated optic fibers were detected only in the medial brachium of the optic tract, and their terminals were confined to the medial half of the tectum. (*Bottom*) A second variant of this experiment demonstrated selective regeneration of optic fibers from the central retina to the central zone of the tectum. (**B**) Arora and Sperry (1962; Sperry 1965) surgically cross-sutured the medial and lateral brachia of the optic tracts in other fish. (*Top*) Following regeneration of the optic nerve, lateral tract fibers had selectively reinnervated only the lateral half of the tectum, but the course of the enduring nerve bundles was even more striking: the lateral tract fibers, although cross-united with the continuation of the medial brachium of the tract, seemed to have crossed back abruptly and taken the continuation of their own lateral tract to their target zones in the tectum. (*Bottom*) Medial tract fibers abruptly crossed back into the continuation of their own medial brachium and had selectively reinnervated the medial half of the tectum. (**C**) The refined chemoaffinity theory (Sperry 1963, 1965) included the proposal that chemical specificities on growing axon tips react selectively to the pathways and substrates enroute to the target, as is evident in this "schematic representation of sequential steps in chemotactic guidance of a growing nerve fiber.

The general principle of contact guidance is assumed to apply here as it always has. ... The same set of cytochemical factors extended from the ganglion cells of the retina into the microfilament flare at the tip of the growing optic axons and also stamped on the optic pathways could be utilized for guiding the respective fiber types into their separate proper channels at each of the numerous forks or decision points which they encounter as they make their way back through what essentially amounts to a multiple Y-maze of possible pathways. The final course laid down by any given fiber reflects the history of a continuous series of decisions based on differential affinities between the various advance filaments that probe the surroundings ahead and the diverse elements that each encounters (Sperry 1963, p. 707).

A RETURN TO THE MOTONEURON

If the development of the chemoaffinity hypothesis appears, in the main, to have drawn more heavily on Sperry's regeneration studies on the optic nerve and its vestibular and somatosensory counterparts, it is important to recall that it all began with the motoneuron. It was from the study of manipulated nerves and muscles in Urodele larvae that Weiss had described the homologous response and had recast earlier functionalist ideas into the so-called resonance-modulation model. And it was the cross-union of nerves and muscles in the rat limb that by Sperry's own account (1965) had led to the idea of chemoaffinity as an alternative to resonance as the basis of neuronal specificity. But, despite this, the motoneuron had remained as a refuge for "resonance" and "modulation" throughout the 1940s and 1950s, and it was not until 1965 that it was finally brought under the dual rubric of chemoaffinity and selective innervation.

In the first of several studies on muscle innervation in fish, Sperry again applied his favored paradigm of allowing severed nerves a choice of targets, cutting and teasing the motor trunk to three muscles innervating the pectoral fin in *Sphaeroides spengleri* (Sperry 1950b). The findings were clear, but the cautious interpretation remained surprisingly deferential to Weiss:

The random shuffling of nerve-muscle connections caused by nerve section failed to produce any corresponding disorder in muscular coordination. Three possible explanations must be considered: (1) The nerve fibers might have reestablished their motor endings in a selective manner with the original muscles. The evidence is against selective termination of this kind in other vertebrates. Furthermore the stimulation of separate fascicles proximal to the nerve scar in the present experiments indicated haphazard reestablishment of nerve-muscle connections. (2) Regeneration of atypical peripheral terminations might have been compensated by some type of functional reorganization in the centers. The fact that functional reorganization does not occur in any of the other vertebrates studied, including man [Sperry 1951a] makes its occurrence in fishes unlikely. Moreover, combined excision of both forebrain and cerebellum produced no selective impairment of the recovered coordination. Nor was recovery faster in those cases in which additional use of the fin had been favored by removal of the other fins. (3) Finally the regenerated axons might have been respecified by the muscles with which they connected, as occurs in larval

---

Multiple filopodia constantly reach out in front of the advancing fiber tip, testing the environment in all directions. The critical factors determining which filopodia will form the strongest attachments, and thereby direct the route of growth, are apparently chemical. Numerous alternative paths, like those represented by lighter terminal fans, are open, mechanically feasible, and may even be established temporarily, but fail because of differential selective adhesion." (Figures and original legend to part **C** after Sperry 1965, p. 171.)

amphibians, with consequent readjustment in the timing of their central discharge. This latter explanation appears by elimination to be the most probable (Sperry 1950b, pp. 283–4).

This experiment was repeated a few years later in *S. testudineus* and *Histrio histrio* and extended to include a variety of more radical surgical derangements (Sperry and Dupree 1956). Even when the anterior fascicles of the fin nerve were surgically excised, drastically reducing the nerve supply available for regeneration, coordinated fin movements were restored:

> That good restoration of function was also obtained after extensive reduction in the proximal supply of pectoral nerve fibers in *H. histrio* gives further indication that the recovery involves a spread of specific influences from the muscles to their motorneurons which in turn determines the incidence of central discharge as inferred to explain the comparable recoveries in amphibian limb coordination (Wiersma 1931; Weiss 1936) [Sperry and Dupree 1956, p. 155].

The 1956 paper also included experiments of the regeneration of the oculomotor nerves (where functional recoveries were poor) and on fin movements following surgical cross-union of the motor nerve trunks to the pectoral and pelvic fins. The latter was the first use of the cross-union paradigm in the fish nerve-muscle system, and interestingly yielded a permanently disturbed pattern of fin movements as had occurred in the earlier cross-unions in the rat hindlimb.

The following year both paradigms were applied to the levator and depressor branches of the mandibular nerve trunk in *Astronotus ocellatus,* with the somewhat surprising result that *both* paradigms gave rise to orderly functional recovery and the restoration of normal jaw movements. Nevertheless, in discussing these findings, Arora and Sperry (1957) were still inclined to favor "modulation" over selective innervation of the muscles by their original nerves:

> The recovery of normal vigorous movements of the mandible observed in Series

l [experiments involving transection of the mandibular nerve] . . . means either (a) that the regenerating motor-fibers must have reestablished their functional connexions selectively with their original muscles, or (b) that those fibers that connected with foreign muscles must have changed their central circuitry to suit the new terminations. The latter alternative is strongly favored by the occurrence of similar recovery in the second series in which the nerve-fibers were definitely cross-connected by surgical means to antagonistic muscles. . . .

> It is inferred (a) that the regenerating motor-fibres establish functional connexions with foreign mandibular muscles, (b) that the muscles induce a local muscle specificity in the regenerated motor axons, and (c) that this "myotypic specificity" determines in some way not yet analysed the central timing of motoneuron discharge in the trigeminal motor nucleus (Arora and Sperry 1957, pp. 261–3).

Sperry's final studies on the nerve-muscle preparation in fish, published in 1965, were an ambitious series of regeneration and cross-union experiments on the motor nerves innervating individual eye muscles in the cichlid *A. ocellatus* (Sperry and Arora 1965).

The normal innervation of the eye muscles in fish is shown in Figure 2.14B. In Sperry and Arora's first series of experiments, the oculomotor (III) nerve was transected and teased apart. After regeneration, functional recovery was excellent; coordinated eye movements were present from the outset and were indistinguishable from the movements on the unoperated side as early as two weeks after the transection. The second series of experiments consisted of four distinct cross-union maneuvers (Figure 2.14B), with the following suggestive results:

> In all cases, the crossed nerves were able to grow into the foreign muscles and to establish transmissive connexions so that the reinnervated muscles contracted both reflexly and to electrical stimulation of the regenerated nerve. However, one got the distinct impression that was difficult to

a

b

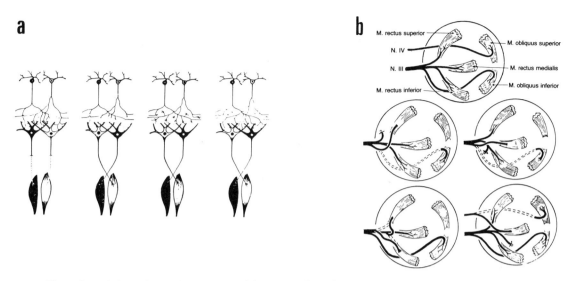

Figure 2.14. Schematic drawings showing (**A**) Sperry's (1951a) model for rewiring of central motoneuron connections secondary to myotypic respecification and (**B**) Sperry and Arora's (1965) cross-union experiments on the eye muscles of chiclid fishes that led Sperry to abandon myotypic respecification in favor of selective reinnervation of muscles by their original motor nerves. (**A**) Sperry's (1951b) model fit within the framework of "modulation" or "myotypic respecification" (Weiss, 1936), but proposed that motoneurons respond to the modulation event by changing their chemical affinities for other neurons and by altering their synaptic inputs accordingly. This sequence of induced nerve-muscle cross-union followed by the postulated synaptic adjustments is shown from left to right. (After Sperry 1951a.) (**B**) Five schematics of the eye muscles and their motor nerves in *Astronotus ocellatus* fish. The top schematic shows the normal relations: nerve III sends four identifiable motor branches to four of the eye muscles, the *superior rectus, inferior rectus, medial rectus,* and *inferior oblique*. The *superior oblique* muscle is supplied by nerve IV. The studies of Sperry and Arora (1965) included simple transection of nerve III and a variety of "competitive innervation" experiments, forcing two nerves into a single muscle – in addition to the cross-union experiments shown in the remaining four schematics. (*Center, left*) The nerve III branch to the inferior oblique muscle had been deflected into the superior rectus muscle, whose own nerve had been deflected away from the muscle (*center, right*). The nerve to the inferior oblique muscle has been deflected into the medial rectus muscle, whose own nerve again had been deflected away. (*Bottom, left*) The nerves to inferior rectus and superior rectus have been cross-united to each other's muscle. (*Bottom, right*) Nerve IV, which normally supplies the superior oblique muscle, has been deflected into the medial rectus muscle, whose normal nerve had been deflected away. (After Sperry and Arora 1965).

quantify, that the reinnervation by foreign nerves did not proceed so rapidly, so fully, nor with such good functional results as did reinnervation by the original nerve. Further, the original nerve showed a marked tendency to grow back into its own muscle in spite of the factors favoring its invasion into the foreign muscle (Sperry and Arora 1965, p. 312).

In the final series of experiments, two nerves were made to compete for the innervation of a single denervated muscle. These fish recovered normal eye movements, and histolog-ic examination confirmed that the original, or "native," nerves had taken control of the muscles. In many cases of simultaneous co-innervation, one nerve was found to innervate the muscle, while the other nerve passed through it (without contacting the muscle fibers) to reach its own muscle. Cases of delayed coinnervation were interesting because many of the fish showed *transient* maladaptive eye movements to head tilt, indicating that the foreign nerve had initially formed functional contacts before surrendering control of the muscle to the later-arriving native nerve. The implications of these findings seemed inescapable and finally led Sperry to bring the motoneuron into the dual fold of selective innervation and chemoaffinity.

> Functional recoveries of this . . . sort have been explained in the past in terms of random, nonselective reestablishment of nerve–muscle connexions followed by myotypic respecification of misregenerated fibers. In the present experiments, however, myotypic respecification effects failed to appear when individual nerve branches were separately inserted into foreign muscles. . . . Taken jointly the . . . findings suggest an explanation in terms of some kind of selectivity in the peripheral reinnervation process.
>
> . . . in those cases in which both the original and foreign nerve were inserted into the same muscle, we have further direct evidence that the original nerve is selectively favored in the reinnervation process. In general terms we can therefore infer the presence of some kind of preferential chemoaffinity in this oculomotor system that favors restoration of the original over foreign nerve-muscle connections (Sperry and Arora 1965, p. 34).

And as a postscript to more than a quarter century of experimental work, "resonance" and "myotopic specification" seemed finally laid to rest:

> That there is any such thing as myotypic specification or modulation of nerve by muscle becomes now an open question. The evidence for selective reinnervation in . . . our present findings suggests that the exclusion of such selectivity as an explanatory factor in earlier studies may have been overly hasty and that it may be well now to take another hard look at the whole question of selectivity in the growth and connexion of vertebrate peripheral nerve (Sperry and Arora 1965, p. 315).

Chemoaffinity and developmental biology

In retrospect, it appears that the chemoaffinity hypothesis was, in part, a restatement of the earlier ideas of Ramon y Cajal and Langley on the chemical matching of pre- and postsynaptic cells and of chemotropic factors in the guidance of nerve growth, and, in part, a new construction built upon the foundation laid by the ideas of Spemann and Lewis on progressive organ determination and induction, of Harrison on the progressive fieldlike differentiation of limbs and ears, and of Holtfreter on tissue affinities between early embryonic cells. But its final emergence seems to have come as the result of a long and sustained struggle with functionalist ideas developed and forcibly expressed by Weiss and his colleagues in the late 1920s and 1930s.

DECLINE OF THE FUNCTIONALIST VIEW

The shift away from the functionalist position was less the result of any single observation than a gradual tipping of the scales toward the structural view of specificity in neurogenesis. Even before Sperry began his investigations, the observations on which the functionalist hypothesis was based were being questioned; and, as his work gathered momentum, a number of other investigators began to weigh in with new observations in support of the structural-connectionist position. For example, in 1938, Ford and Woodhall reviewed an extensive body of clinical evidence drawn from patients with peripheral nerve injuries and concluded that (contrary to the then widely held view) the functional deficits experienced by many patients often persisted indefinitely, and showed no sign of improvement that could be attributed to either learning and experience. Similarly, in 1942, Piatt reported an ingenious series of experiments on peripheral nerve patterns in "aneurogenic" salamander limbs in which innervation was delayed until the limbs were near fully formed. The peripheral nerve patterns that appeared in these limbs closely matched those of normal limbs, often down to the finest branches and even to the incidence of minor variants seen in the normal adult population (Piatt 1942). These findings seriously called in question Weiss's (1941c) explanation that the structural regularities of peripheral nerves arise, after initial random innervation of the embryonic limb muscles, by mechanical "towing" of the nerves as the limb elongates and grows. And, finally, the careful studies of Speidel (1941, 1942, 1948) on the growth and modifiability of nerve patterns helped to revive the view of the growing axon as probing, sensing, and palpating its environment (see also Hamburger 1962).

The gradual shift away from the functionalist bias of the 1930s was also influenced by certain broader trends in neuroscience and cell biology. Over the quarter century from 1940 through 1965, neuroanatomical and neurophysiological data of increasing resolution served to document the regularity of ordered nerve connections in the vertebrate CNS, and provided little or no support for the notion of diffuse or random neural networks, or for the selective decoding of impulse patterns that were proposed to occur within them. At the same time, a form of chemical specificity in neurogenesis was demonstrated directly, in the selective response of particular classes of developing neurons to circulating hormones and growth factors (Weiss and Rosetti 1942; Levi-Montalcini and Hamburger 1953; Levi-Montalcini, Meyer, and Hamburger 1954; Cohen 1960; see Chapter 1 of this volume for a review). And, as we have already mentioned, there was a growing body of evidence for certain dynamic cellular properties, such as selective adhesion and recognition, that appeared to be mediated by specific recognition molecules on the surface of cells (Tyler 1947; Weiss 1947). We dwelt earlier on the neuron doctrine as a much retarded entry of the nervous system into the era of cell and molecular biology, for many of the functionalist ideas could not have been easily sustained within the framework of cell biology. Conversely, the increasing appreciation that neurons were in fact cells, with many of the same dynamic properties and cellular organelles as nonneural cells, helped to lay the groundwork for the acceptance of Sperry's ideas in the 1950s and early 1960s (Hunt and Jacobson 1974).

Historically, it is clear, however, that Sperry was the principal figure in this antifunctionalist movement. His own path had begun with the motoneuron (Sperry 1940), and, from time to time over the next twenty-five years, he was to return to it (Sperry 1945c, 1947, 1950b; Sperry and Dupree 1956; Arora and Sperry 1957; Sperry and Arora 1965). But his most formidable assault on the functionalist position undoubtedly came from his prolonged studies of the various sensory systems and especially the visual systems of teleosts and amphibians. The results of these studies led him to mount, not so much a frontal assault, as a series of flanking attacks that progressively weakened and finally destroyed the functionalist stronghold. And it is a credit to his sensitivities and his respect for his mentor that this conceptual revolution was accomplished within the framework upon which the functionalist view had been constructed. It is not without interest that it was Paul Weiss who first introduced the experimental paradigm of creating unusual patterns of connections in surgically manipulated animals when he first reported the so-called homologous response. Sperry was later to adopt the same approach, but only to show in the end that when one forces behaviorally maladaptive connections upon an animal, neither function nor experience can correct the improper circuitry. Similarly, Weiss had argued strongly against the roles of bioelectric activity and chemotropisms in neural development, advancing in their stead mechanical guidance mechanisms; and, again, Sperry was to accommodate these mechanisms within the new framework of chemoaffinity:

> No renunciation of the importance of mechanical guidance in nerve fiber growth is implied in this recognition of chemical influences. *The chemical factors merely supplement, not replace, the mechanical factors* (Sperry 1951, p. 84).

And where Weiss was to shift the focus of his *Resonanzprinzip* from muscles to the motoneurons Sperry (1940, 1941, 1943c, 1945c, 1946, 1950a, 1950b; 1951a, 1951b; Sperry and Miner 1949) was to advance as a *general* principle the notion that "end organs lead the way" in neuronal differentiation. And, for a number of years, he maintained a generous posture toward resonance – both as a possible explanation for neuronal specificity in general, and as the *accepted* explanation in the special case of the motoneuron; indeed, it was not until the evidence from one sensory system after another had made the case for the connectionist alternative so inescapable, and the role of chemical factors so overwhelming, that he finally recast the innervation of muscles and their distinctive central connections as yet another example of selective innervation and chemoaffinity (Sperry and Arora 1965, Sperry 1965).

Sperry's experiments on sensory systems had used two paradigms: (1) imposing a set of unusual or frankly maladaptive connections upon the animal and observing its later behavior, and (2) allowing regenerating axons the opportunity to "choose" between alternative pathways. In virtually every instance, the first paradigm resulted in the persistence of maladaptive behavior, and the second always led to an orderly functional recovery. His initial experiments on muscle innervation in teleosts stood as a notable exception to this generalization, since they had resulted in orderly functional recoveries after *both* paradigms (Sperry 1950b, Sperry and Dupree 1956, Arora and Sperry 1957). For a while, these results seemed most explicable on the basis of modulation and end-organ induction; but, finally, even this exception gave way when Mark (1965) and Sperry and Arora (1965) discovered that the cross-sutured motor nerves in these animals had covertly reinnervated their original muscles.

The clarity and subtlety of Sperry's thinking is also strikingly evident in an early acknowledgment that the chemoaffinity hypothesis does not preclude a role for function in shaping neural circuitry. Initially, he conceived of this as simply playing a trophic role in the growth and maintenance of neural tissue:

> The conclusion that function is not the organizing factor in the reestablishment of systematic reflex relations in these experiments in no way contradicts the possibility that function, as a generalized non-specific factor, may be of importance for the normal healthy maintenance and development of nerve structures (Sperry 1944, p. 67).

But later he was to suggest that it may also be significant for the refinement and validation of certain synapses over others:

> Learning and growth together might, through a series of irreversible steps, produce integrative structures that, when

completed, would no longer be subject to functional reorganization. However, the learning capacity of the nervous system is much more than a mere passive plasticity of a highly impressionable tissue. It is more comparable to the active functional ability of a complex machine. . . . The establishment of a central organization capable of distinguishing adaptive from nonadaptive excitation patterns must therefore precede any selective adjustment on the basis of functional effects.
>
> *The foregoing concerns functions as a patterning factor in the organization of neural connections and does not apply to function as a general condition necessary to healthy growth* (Sperry 1951a, pp. 270–1, emphasis added).

In still later papers, he was to single out the association areas of the cerebral cortex as regions where function may have an even more dramatic impact on the structural relations among neurons:

> It is possible that the unknown changes imposed on the nervous system by learning and experience are . . . similar to, or a direct derivative of, developmental features, and perhaps best understood in these terms. There are reasons to think that long-term memory in man could involve a specificity effect in the machinery for late neuron differentiation that gains behavioral expression through either a modification of the cell's fiber contacts or of its intrinsic physiological properties. . . .
>
> One can arbitrarily distinguish use effects that consist of stamping in and preserving neural organization developed in growth, from use effects that add new organization, anatomical or physiological, to the developed system. . . . The above distinction tends to break down, however, in the central association areas, where the growth pressures are more diffuse. . . . It would be no surprise to find that the neural basis of imprinting is a direct evolutionary elaboration of the physiological or biochemistry of . . . use effects in the neural networks (Sperry 1965, pp. 182–3.

In this respect, he was to anticipate by almost a decade the experimental work that has established that function is indeed involved in fine-tuning the wiring patterns of the brain. And it is interesting to see, in his references to the pendular swings from the structuralist views of Cajal and others to the functionalist notions of the 1930s and back again (Sperry, 1951a, 1963, 1965), an unusual sensitivity to the "doppelganger" relationship between structural preformism and functional modification. The functionalist ideas of the late 1920s and 1930s seemed for a while to have nudged Ramon y Cajal and Langley's ideas from center stage; but even as the chemoaffinity theory led the swing back toward their views, Sperry, almost alone, seemed to recognize that functional effects must play some role in the shaping of neural circuitry and, especially, in the long-term adaptive behavior of animals to their environments.

BUILDING BLOCKS FROM
EXPERIMENTAL EMBRYOLOGY

In contrast to Sperry's frequent citations of Harrison and of the embryonic induction school, it is difficult to identify in his writings any indication that he had been influenced consciously by Holtfreter's work. Yet it was Holtfreter who had provided the most direct evidence for some form of chemoaffinity, at the tissue level, in his identification of affinities – both positive and negative – between the cells of different embryonic germ layers and, later in development, between the cells of specific organ rudiments. It is, of course, impossible to know to what extent he was unconsciously influenced by Holtfreter's work, but what is clear is that in the end, Sperry did not simply adapt Holtfreter's ideas to the nervous system and the problem of the formation of nerve connections; rather, he extended them in at least four directions.

The first, of course, was his perception that there must be considerable chemical diversity in the nervous system as a whole, and that, in any one system, it may be rather fine-grained. It is one thing to assign specific cell-surface molecules to each of the three germ layers, or even to specific organ rudiments, but quite another matter to extend the notion of chemical differences to the level of neurons in different regions of the nervous system, or even within a given region to cells in different topographic sectors or to cells of different functional classes. This idea was not unique to Sperry: it is clearly adumbrated in the writings of earlier workers, notably Langley, but it is only in Sperry's work that the notion is spelled out as one of the implicit features of the chemoaffinity theory:

> Cell differentiation in the nervous system alone is as multifarious as that of all the other tissues of the body taken together. In addition to the diversity of the primary motor and sensory neurons, which approaches that of the tissues they innervate, there exist multiple orders of extra specificity in the complex of association neurons within the centers. . . .
> . . . although the specificity of a neuron determines what other particular cells it is able to excite, this selectivity is not restricted to a single cell type. It may encompass a variety of neurons, but always according to a precise plan . . . the developed pattern of biochemical associations within the centers is of an extremely complex and delicate design. It is in neurogenesis that the developmental processes attain their peak of refinement and complexity (Sperry 1950a, pp. 235–6).

The second direction in which Sperry extended Holtfreter's ideas was his appreciation that the same molecular labels that are used in target identification could be involved in the selective fasciculation of axons and in pathway selection. Although these ideas were not developed in detail until the early 1960s, they were first articulated much earlier (Sperry 1943b, 1951b). In 1943, he was to write:

> Another possibility is that fibers from the same region of the retina tend to adhere to each other during regeneration because of preferential surface affinities (selective fasciculation) so that the whole optic tract is normally oriented with an orderly internal arrangement as it approaches the visual centers (Sperry 1943b, pp. 47–8).

A third important contribution was the notion that categories of specificity exist and that combinations of surface labels could be used to direct the axons not only to the correct class or subclass of target cell, but also to the correct *region* within the target field. This idea initially grew out of his vestibular and somatosensory studies, but was specifically reinforced in his later visual studies (Sperry and Miner 1949; Arora and Sperry 1962, 1963).

> Consider . . . the numerous dimensions of chemical differentiation that must be present within the limited confines of the finest collaterals of the nerve fiber. In the dorsal horn of the cord, for example, a given fiber may be specified first as a pain fiber distinguishing it from fibers of other functional modalities . . . and further as a cutaneous pain fiber setting it off from fibers mediating other types of pain. In addition it must be stamped for the locus of its peripheral termination with a particular dose of one quality to mark its anteroposterior alignment and another of another quality for its dorsoventral alignment. Most fibers must be stamped with at least three such specifying properties (Sperry 1951b, p. 85).

> Applied to the visual system it means that the thousands of individual fibers in the optic nerve differ chemically among themselves according to the locus of origin in the retinal field and also according to the particular color, "on–off" and other specific physiologic functions of the fiber units (Sperry 1963, p. 92).

The idea of the combinatorial use of position markers and cell class markers was especially noteworthy, as it allowed for the potential reutilization of a common set of positional markers in many neural pathways.

The fourth advance beyond Holtfreter's tissue-affinity hypothesis was the formulation of a molecular model for how locus-specific markers may be acquired (Sperry 1965). Despite his attraction to Harrison's work on polarized fieldlike differentiation, and to the simplicity of crossed gradients of morphogens in, say, the initial development of the retina, Sperry recognized that the problems posed by the nervous system were a good deal more complex:

The nature of the gradients and their interrelations via fiber projection systems suggests a chemical basis in which some large molecule or molecular complex or unit has a long range of properties running from one extreme to another with many graded intermediate steps, each one of which is precisely controlled and precisely replicated from within a given cell. The chemical factor is then extended without loss of specificity into all the distant fiber tips of the given neuron. As a simplified hypothetical example, consider a dipole compound molecule made up of units A and P (for anterior and posterior). At the rostral pole there are 90 A units to every one of P and the reverse at the caudal pole with a 50:50 ratio in the center. Once the overall gradient is established, each unit ratio would become stamped into the differentiation machinery of the neuron and the specific factor transported throughout its arboreal fiber system. As indicated above, most neurons would also be synthesizing additional specifying molecular complexes for the dorsoventral alignment and another for the mediolateral alignment, plus further nongradient factors like those for color in the retina and for pain and temperature in the cutaneous system (Sperry 1965, p. 175).

This explicit molecular model seems as simple, powerful, and testable today as it did when it was first proposed in 1965.

In proposing how chemoaffinity labels may arise during neuronal differentiation, Sperry was, in fact, advancing a remarkably original general theory of cellular differentiation. We have noted that Harrison's (1918, 1921, 1936, 1945) studies on the fieldlike determination of limbs, ears, and other organ anlagen in salamander embryos had provided Sperry with a model for locus-specific differentiation of retinal ganglion cells, of vestibular cells, and eventually of the integument and other nonneural target organs. But in recognizing the multiplicity of chemical labels that are needed to mark a cell's class, subclass, and position, Sperry's articulation of the chemoaffinity hypothesis drew upon a much larger body of work, including that of Spemann, Lewis, and others, on the progressive determination of embryonic organs and fields:

> The over-all process of differentiation is presumed to follow a treelike pattern . . . with the gross subdivisions being set off first and these, in turn, successively subdivided to produce increasing refinement. As a result, the chemical properties of the individual neuron elements, as finally determined, are not haphazzardly arranged but exhibit systematic familial relationships . . . (Sperry 1950a, p. 236).

And later:

> Neuronal specification, as noted, may arise through induction effects imposed from without via fiber contacts as well as by intrinsic differentiation, and both processes are probably involved in many instances (Sperry 1951b, p. 85).

In the case of motoneurons and of the somatosensory and vestibular ganglion cells that have to make the correct central and peripheral connections, the idea of "end-organ induction" initially provided an important bridge between the emerging chemoaffinity hypothesis and the earlier "modulation" theory of Weiss (1936). In time, "end-organ induction" was to be abandoned as an explanation for motoneuron/muscle interaction in favor of selective outgrowth of prespecified motor axons to their correct embryonic muscles. But, while a similar process of selective outgrowth of prespecified axons was acknowledged as possible in the somatosensory and vestibular systems, end-organ induction remained the favored explanation; and Sperry continued to use his findings in these systems to illustrate the way inductive mechanisms might operate to effectively label neurons after they had formed peripheral connections. Inductive mechanisms were also invoked at various junctures in Sperry's studies of the visual system, for example, in his early suggestion that optic-nerve fibers may induce the appropriate chemoaffinity labels in the optic lobe, and when he addressed the problem of how later-formed neurons in the retina and tectum might acquire positional labels at relatively advanced developmental stages:

> It is only after the indifferent neuroblasts have migrated from the germinal layer and begun to send out axon and dendrite filaments that the specific influences affecting functional reflex relationships with which we are here concerned become effective. Specificity resulting in formation of proper synaptic associations is probably imposed upon these additional neuroblasts at an advanced stage of maturation by neurons already differentiated (Sperry 1943b, pp. 50–1).

In short, in Sperry's mind, cell–cell inductive interactions and fieldlike differentiation were conceived of as companion mechanisms for the establishment of locus-specific chemoaffinity labels.

It is arguable that it is in this latter sense that the chemoaffinity hypothesis made its most important (but perhaps least well-appreciated) contribution to developmental biology as a whole. Sperry's (1951b) proposal of crossed morphogenetic gradients, which could provide unique positional markers to each ganglion cell, anticipates much of the contemporary discussion on the question how positional information is encoded in two-dimensional cell sheets (cf. Wolpert 1971; French, Bryant, and Bryant 1976; Hunt 1976; McDonald 1977). The implied conversion of morphogen concentrations into stable ratios of surface-recognition molecules provided a plausible explanation for the acquisition of more or less permanent cellular addresses and for the translation of this positional information in the outgrowth of axons and dendrites. Sperry conceived of this as a progressive process within the nervous system, in a manner that closely paralleled pattern formation in the organism as a whole:

> . . . three basic axial gradients of differentiation – rostrocaudal, dorsoventral and radial or mediolateral – would be sufficient to impress a unique chemistry on every single cell of the CNS, and of the entire body for that matter, depending on the steepness of the gradients. As in the differentiation of the organism as a whole,

we may presume that many local fields of differentiation and subfields and subgradients are superimposed upon the three primary axial fields. These will be combined presumably with mosaic, frequency distribution and other forms of differentiation involving suppressive emanation, lateral inhibition, and the like. Differentiation within the CNS may be seen to reflect in more ways than one the differentiation of the total organism in miniature.... The body and most of its parts are represented in the nerve centers in miniature and in functional perspective, several times over in some instances (Sperry 1965, p. 173).

It is thus no exaggeration to describe the chemoaffinity hypothesis as a broad general theory to account for the spatial control of cellular differentiation and for the subsequent expression of positional information through permanent address markers on the surfaces of cells. As such, the hypothesis provides an important conceptual link between Harrison's early studies on pattern determination and fieldlike differentiation and more contemporary formulations of positional information and cell patterning (Wolpert 1971). But from the more narrow perspective of developmental neurobiology, its historical significance is to be found in its definitive overthrowal of the functionalist position and the critical return to the earlier views of Ramon y Cajal (1890, 1905, 1928) and Langley (1895, 1897). Again, Sperry expressed this best when he wrote:

Outgrowing fibers are guided by a kind of probing chemical touch system that leads them along exact pathways in an enormously intricate guidance program that involves millions and perhaps billions of different chemically distinct brain cells. By selective chemical preferences, the respective nerve fibers are guided correctly to their separate channels at each of the numerous forks or decision points which they encounter as they travel through what is essentially a multiple Y-maze of possible channels.... Each fiber in the brain pathways has its own preference for particular prescribed trails by which it lo-cates and connects with certain other neurons that have the appropriate cell flavor. The potential pathways and terminal connection zones have their own individual chemical flavors by which each is recognized and distinguished from all others in the same half of the brain and cord.

It is apparent that our current view with its emphasis on chemical selectivity, comes closer to the older ideas of Cajal and his contemporaries... (Sperry 1965, pp. 170–1).

Postscript
Our principal aim in this chapter has been to examine Sperry's work and ideas on the development of the nervous system, and, in particular, to trace the antecedents and evolution of the chemoaffinity hypothesis. It is not our intention here to consider the impact that his work has had in the two decades since 1965, but a few general comments are perhaps in order.

First, we can hardly escape noting that Sperry's ideas have endured rather well, despite repeated attempts to redefine and narrow the chemoaffinity hypothesis, or to experimentally refute it. It has also survived many attempts to supplant it by "newer" hypotheses, many of which turn out, on close examination, to be simply minor variants of the original chemoaffinity theory; and it has also survived a number of attempts to discredit it by the repeated claims that since the chemical labels it presupposes have so far eluded detection, they do not exist, or that it is incompatible with the growing body of evidence for neural plasticity. Certainly, no alternative explanation for the orderly establishment of connections, either during development or regeneration, has found general acceptance. And while contemporary neuroscientists differ in their emphases, there is now a fairly general consensus that at least in the case of the ganglion cells of the retina, some form of position-dependent differentiation must occur, and, furthermore, that the resulting chemical specification of the optic-nerve fibers is critical in enabling them to identify their correct topographic positions within the optic tectum and other visual centers. Debate continues, of course, as to the nature of the chemical labels, how they enable the fibers to find their way between the retina and the various visual centers of the brain, and, finally, how they enable the fibers to identify their proper synaptic targets within these centers. And although relatively few investigators would today subscribe to the notion that every single ganglion cell is uniquely labeled, few would nowadays question that some form of chemical labeling occurs, and that comparable labels exist upon the surfaces of the neurons to which the retina projects (rev. Gaze 1970; Meyer and Sperry 1974; Chung and Cooke 1978; Edds et al. 1979; Fraser and Hunt 1980; Trisler, Schneider, and Nirenberg 1981; Meyer 1982, see Chapter 5 in this volume; Yoon, see Chapter 4 in this volume; Hibbard, see Chapter 3 in this volume).

It is also worth noting that in his review of 1965, Sperry clearly identified the two major unresolved problems inherent in the chemoaffinity hypothesis (problems that, incidentally, still remain unresolved). The first, of course, is the nature of the chemical mechanisms underlying chemoaffinity. These include the identity of the molecules involved, their regulation, their distribution and function, whether they operate by complementarity or identity, and whether neurons are distinguished on the basis of *qualitatively* different cell-surface moieties or by more subtle differences of concentration, modulation, and/or surface distribution. The second problem concerns the way in which neurons acquire positional information? For example, how do ganglion cells "learn of their address" within the retinal field? Is this address encoded in terms of crossed axes in a cartesian coordinate system, or in some radial or other scheme? And, how is this position ultimately expressed in the outgrowth of the axons and in the formation of the retinotectal map? These are difficult questions and, despite intensive effort, most still await answers. But, again, it seems clear that Sperry's broad outline of a fieldlike differentiation in the optic cup is correct, and that patterned differentiation of retinal ganglion cells is not particularly different from the analagous processes in limbs, ears, and other organs. The recent introduction of lineage markers (rev. Conway, Fecock, and Hunt 1980) offers some promise that heritable

instructions for cell fate and address can be dissected from those arising from cell position and context, and can eventually provide clues to the molecular mechanisms underlying positional information/address assignment.

We began this essay with Sperry's 1965 account of the change that had occurred in the way that neurobiologists view the development of the nervous system in the twenty-five years that he had been studying it; and his comments to the Society for Growth and Development are perhaps an appropriate way to close:

> For a long time . . . the problem of development of nerve circuits . . . was thought to lie more properly within the province of psychology and learning theory. The brain circuits seemed to be too complicated and too precisely adapted for their functions to conceive of their being installed by the forces of growth alone without aid of functional adjustment. Accordingly, hypotheses were advanced suggesting that function somehow channels adaptive pathways out of initially equipotential nerve networks, or that synaptic hook-ups which happen to prove adaptive in function are reinforced and maintained while the others are resorbed. . . . In the widely accepted theory of "neurobiotaxis," electrical potentials generated in the nerve centers were presumed to influence the course and termination of the growing fibers. Those nuclei and tracts that happened to be activated simultaneously or in close succession were supposed to develop interconnections. . . .
>
> This tendency to favor the functional and to minimize the innate and genetic factors in the developmental patterning of brain circuits was carried to extremes during the late 20s and 30s. . . . Extreme efforts . . . were made, in some instances, to account for all of the organized behavior of the new-born mammal or newly-hatched bird or reptile on the basis of practice effects obtained from the constrained movements of the fetus in utero or of the developing chick within the egg shell. Reference was made to the "conditioning" of motor patterns under

these circumstances and to the "education" of sensory surfaces.

Today most of us are convinced we have ample proof that highly refined integrative circuits and coordination patterns can be, and are, built into the brain quite independently of functional organization.

It will be seen that our current notions involve a return in part to something like the old chemotactic theories that held favor at the turn and early part of the century. But the up-to-date picture is a compound one including phenomena like cell differentiation, determination, induction, etc. such as are recognized routinely to be operative in the ontogenetic patterning of other organ systems. In fact, if our present hypothesis is correct, the developmental organization of the brain circuits is effected in large measure through mechanisms with which the experimental embryologist is already familiar (Sperry 1951b, pp. 64–5).

The chemoaffinity theory may be viewed as marking the end of the beginning, a passageway through which the problem of development of nerve circuits passed from the province of psychology to that of cellular and molecular embryology.

Acknowledgments

We should like to thank Pat Thomas and Kris Trulock for assistance in preparation of the manuscript, Dr. Larry Swanson for his comments, and Dr. Ronald Meyer for his comments and his timely editorial help. Work by the authors is supported by Grants from the National Science Foundation (PCM–82–44490 and PCM–83–11082) and from the National Institutes of Health (NS–16980 and EY–03653).

References

Arora, H. L. 1963. Effect of forcing a regenerative optic nerve bundle toward a foreign region of the optic tectum in fishes. *Anat. Rec.* 145: 202.

Arora, H. L., and R. W. Sperry. 1957. Myotypic respecification of regenerated nerve fibres in cichlid fishes. *J. Embryol. Exp. Morph.* 5: 256–63.

–1962. Optic nerve regeneration after surgical cross-union of medial and lateral optic tracts. *Am. Zool.* 2: 389.

–1963. Color discrimination after optic nerve regeneration in the fish *Astronotus ocellatus*. *Dev. Biol.* 17: 234–43.

Attardi, D. G., and R. W. Sperry. 1963. Preferential selection of central pathways by regenerating optic fibers. *Exp. Neurol.* 7: 46–64.

Beers, D. 1929. Return of vision and other observations in transplanted amphibian eyes. *Proc. Soc. Exp. Biol., N.Y.* 26: 477–79.

Bohn, G. 1897. Uber Verwachsungsuersuchemit Amphibienlarven. *Roux' Archiv.* 4: 349–465.

Bok, S. T. 1917. The development of reflexes and reflex tracts. *Psychiat. Neurol. Biol. Amst.* 21: 281–303.

Boveri, T. 1901. Die Polaritat von Oocyte, Ei und Larve des *Strongylo centrotus lividus*. *Zool. Jahrb., Abt. f. Anat. u. Ont.* 14: 630–53.

–1902. Ueber mehrpolige Mitosen als Mittel zur Analyse des Zellkerns. *Verh. d. phys.-med. Ges. Wurzburg, NF* 35: 67–90. English translation *in* B. H. Willier and J. M. Oppenheimer (eds.) *Foundations of Experimental Embryology.* Prentice-Hall, Englewood Cliffs (NJ) 1964.

–1910. Die Potenzen der Ascaris-Blastomeren bei abgeanderten Furchung. Zugleich ein Beitrag zur Frage qualitativ ungleicher Chromosomenteilung. *In Festschrift fur Richard Hertwig,* Vol. III, Gustav Fischer, Jena (East Germany), pp. 133–214.

Child, C. M. 1915. *Individuality in Organisms.* University of Chicago Press, Chicago.

–1941. *Patterns and Problems of Development.* University of Chicago Press, Chicago.

Chung, S. H., and J. Cooke. 1978. Observations on the formation of the brain and of nerve connections following embryonic manipulation of the amphibian neural tube. *Proc. R. Soc. London, B Ser.* 201: 335–73.

Coghill, E. G. 1929. *Anatomy and the Problem of Behavior.* Cambridge University Press, Cambridge (UK).

–1930. Individuation versus integration in the development of behavior. *J. Gen. Psychol.* 3: 431–5.

Cohen, S. 1960. Purification of a nerve-growth promoting protein from the mouse salivary gland and its neurocytotoxic antiserum. *Proc. Natl. Acad. Sci. USA* 46: 302–11.

Conway, K., K. Fecock, and R. K. Hunt. 1980. Polyclones and patterns in developing *Xenopus* larvae. *Curr. Top. Dev. Biol.* 15: 216–317.

Curtis, A. S. G. 1967. *The Cell Surface: Its Molecular Role in Morphogenesis.* Logos, London.

Detwiler, S. R. 1920. On the hyperplasia of the nerve centers resulting from excessive peripheral loading. *Proc. Natl. Acad. Sci. USA* 6: 96–101.

–1936. *Neuroembryology: An Experimental Study.* Macmillan, New York.

Driesch, H. 1894. *Analytische Theorie der organischen Entwicklung.* Engelmann, Leipzig.

Edds, M. V., R. M. Gaze, G. E. Schneider, and L. N. Irwin. 1979. Specificity and plasticity of retinotectal connections. *NRP Bull.* 17: 243–375.

Fraser, S. E., and R. K. Hunt. 1980. Retinotectal specificity: Models and experiments in search of a mapping function. *Ann. Rev. Neurosci.* 3: 319–52.

French, V., P. J. Bryant, and S. V. Bryant. 1976. Pattern regulation in epimorphic fields. *Science* 193: 969–81.

Gaze, R. M. 1970. *Formation of Nerve Connections*. Academic Press, New York.

Gerard, R. W., 1941. The interaction of neurones. *Ohio J. Sci.* 41: 160–72.

Goldstein, K. 1939. *The Organism*. American Book, New York.

Grimm, L. M. 1971. An evaluation of myotypic respecification in axolotls. *J. Exp. Zool.* 178: 479–96.

Gurwitsch, A. 1922. Uber den Begriff des embryonaler Feldes. *Roux' Archiv.* 51: 383–415.

Hamburger, V. 1934. The effects of wing bud extirpation on the development of the central nervous system in chick embryos. *J. Exp. Zool.* 68: 449–94.

–1962. Specificity in neurogenesis. *J. Cell. Comp. Physiol. Suppl. I* 60: 81–92.

–1980. S. Ramon y Cajal, R. G. Harrison and the beginnings of neuroembryology. *Persp. Biol. and Med.* 23: 600–16.

–1981. Historical landmarks in neurogenesis. *Trends in Neurosci.* 4: 151–5.

Harrison, R. G. 1906. Further experiments on the development of peripherel nerves. *Am. J. Anat.* 5: 121–31.

–1907. Observations on the living developing nerve fiber. *Anat. Rec.* 1: 116–18.

–1910. The outgrowth of the nerve fiber as a mode of protoplasmic movement. *J. Exp. Zool.* 9: 787–846.

–1918. Experiments on the development of the forelimb of amblystoma, a self-differentiating equapotential system. *J. Exp. Zool.* 25: 413–61.

–1921. On relations of symmetry in transplanted limbs. *J. Exp. Zool.* 32: 1–136.

–1933. Some difficulties of the determination problem. *Am. Naturalist* 67: 306–21.

–1935. On the origin and development of the nervous system studied by the methods of experimental embryology. *Proc. Roy. Soc. London, Ser. B.* 118: 155–96.

–1936. Relations of symmetry in the developing ear of *Amblystoma punctatum*. *Proc. Natl. Acad. Sci. USA* 22: 238–47.

–1945. Relations of symmetry in the developing embryo. *Trans. Conn. Acad. Arts. Sci.* 36: 277–330.

Head. H. 1920. *Studies in Neurology*. Oxford University Press, London.

Herrick, C. J. 1930. Localization of function in the nervous system. *Proc. Natl. Acad. Sci. USA* 16: 643–50.

Herring, E. 1913. *Memory: Lectures on the Specific Energies of the Nervous System*. Open Court, Chicago.

His, W. 1886. Cited in Hamburger 1980.

Holtfreter, J. 1938. Differenzierungspotenzen isolierter Teile der Urodelen gastrula. *Arch. f. Entw.- Mech. Organ..* 138: 522–656.

–1939. Gewebeaffinitat, ein Mittel der embryonalen Formbildung. *Arch. Exp. Zellforsch* 23: 169–209.

–1943a. A study of the mechancis of gastrulation I. *J. Exp. Zool.* 94: 261–318.

–1943b. Properties and functions of the surface coat in amphibian embryos. *J. Exp. Zool.* 93: 251–323.

–1944. A study of the mechanics of gastralation, II. *J. Exp. Zool.* 95: 171–212.

Hunt, R. K. 1976. Position-dependent differentiation of neurons. *In* D. McMahon and C. F. Fox (eds.) *Developmental Biology*. Benjamin, Menlo Park (CA), pp. 227–56.

Hunt, R. K., and M. Jacobson. 1972a. Developmental stability of positional information in *Xenopus* retinal ganglion cells. *Proc. Natl. Acad. Sci. USA* 69: 780–3.

–1972b. Specification of positional information in retinal ganglion cells of *Xenopus:* Stability of the specified state. *Proc. Natl. Acad. Sci. USA* 69: 2860–4.

–1974. Neuronal specificity revisited. *Curr. Top. Dev. Biol.* 8: 203–58.

Hunt, R. K., and J. Piatt. 1974. Axial specification in salamander embryonic retina. *Anat. Rec.* 178: 515.

Huxley, J. S., and G. R. de Beer. 1934. *The Elements of Experimental Embryology*. Cambridge University Press, London.

Jacobson, M. 1968. Cessation of DNA synthesis correlated with the time of specification of their central connections. *Dev. Biol.* 17: 219–32.

Kappers, C. U. A. 1917. Further contributions on neurobiotaxis: IX. An attempt to compare the phenomena of neurobiotaxis with other phenomena of taxis and tropism. *J. Comp. Neurol.* 27: 261–98.

Langley, J. N. 1895. Note on regeneration of pre-ganglionic fibres of the sympathetic. *J. Physiol.* 18: 280–4.

–1897. On the regeneration of pre-ganglionic and post-ganglionic visceral nerve fibers. *J. Physiol.* 22: 215–30.

Lashley, K. 1929. *Brain Mechanisms and Intelligence*. University of Chicago Press, Chicago.

–1942. The problem of cerebral organization in vision. *Biol. Symp.* 7: 301–22.

Levi, G. 1934. Explanation, besonders die Struktur and die Struktur and die biologischen Eigenschaften der in vitro gezuchteten Zellen and Gewebe. *Ergeb. Anat. Entw. Gesch.* 31: 125–207.

Levi-Montalcini, R., and V. Hamburger. 1953. A diffusible agent of mouse sarcoma producing hypeplasia of sympathetic ganglia and hyperneurotization of the chick embryo. *J. Exp. Zool.* 123: 233–88.

Montalcini, R., H. Meyer, and V. Hamburger. 1954. *In-vitro* experiments on the effects of mouse sarcoma 180 and 37 on the spinal and sympathetic ganglia of the chick embryo. *Cancer Res.* 14: 49–57.

Lewis, W. H. 1903. Experimental studies on the development of the eye in amphibia. *Proc. Assoc. Am. Anat.* 3: 137–43.

–1904. Experimental studies on the development of the eye in Amphibia, I. On the origin of the lens. *Rana palustris. Am. J. Anat.* 3: 505–36.

–1906. On the origin and differentiation of the optic vesicle in amphibian embryo. *Am. J. Anat.* 6: 141–5.

–1907a. Experiments on the origins and differentiation of the optic vesicle in Amphibia. *Am. J. Anat.* 7: 259–78.

–1907b. Lens-formation from strange ectoderm in *Rana*

sylvatica. Am. J. Anat. 7: 145–69.

–1907c. Transplantation of the lips of the blastopore in *Rana palustris. Am. J. Anat.* 7: 139–41.

–1922. The adhesive quality of cells. *Anat. Rec.* 23: 387–92.

Lewis, W. H., and M. R. Lewis. 1912. The cultivation of sympathetic nerves from the intestine of chick embryos in saline solution. *Anat. Rec.* 6: 7–31.

Mark, R. F. 1965. Fin movements after regeneration of neuromuscular connections: An investigation of myotypic specificity. *Exp. Neurol.* 12: 292–302.

Matthey, R. 1926a. Recuperation de la vue apres greffe de l'oeil chez le triton adulte. *Cont. Rend. Soc. Biol.* 94: 4–5.

–1926b. La greff de l'oeil. I. Etude histologique sur la greffe de l'oeil chez la larve de salamandre (*Salamandre maculosa*). *Rev. Suisse Zool.* 33: 317–34.

–1926c. La greffe de l'oeil. Etude experimentale de la greffe de l'oeil chez le triton (*Triton distatus*). *Arch. f. Entw. Mech. d. Organ.* 109: 326–41.

McDonald, W. 1977. A polar coordinate system for positional information in the vertebrate retina. *J. Theor. Biol.* 69: 153–65.

Meyer, R. L. 1982. Ordering of retinotectal connections: A multivariate operational analysis. *Curr. Top. Dev. Biol.* 17: 101–45.

Meyer, R. L., and R. W. Sperry. 1974. Explanatory models for neuroplasticity in retinotectal connections. *In* G. Gotlich (ed.) *Plasticity and Recovery of Function in the Central Nervous System,* Vol. 3. Academic Press, New York, pp. 111–49.

Miner, N. 1951a. Cataneous localization following 180 degree rotation of skin grafts. *Anat. Rec.* 109: 326–7.

–1951b. *Integumental Specification of Sensory Neurons in the Genesis of Cutaneous Local Sign.* PhD thesis, University of Chicago, Chicago.

–1956. Integumental specification of sensory fibers in the development of cutaneous local sign. *J. Comp. Neurol.* 105: 161–70.

Miner, N., and R. W. Sperry. 1950. Observations on the genesis of cutaneous local sign. *Anat. Rec.* 106: 317.

Moscona, A. 1957. The development of *in vitro* of chimeric aggregates of dissociated embryonic chick and mouse cells. *Proc. Natl. Acad. Sci. USA* 43: 184–94.

–1962. Analysis of cell recombinations in experimental synthesis of tissues *in vitro. J. Cell. Comp. Physiol.* 60 (Suppl.): 65–80.

Moscona, A., and H. Moscona. 1952. The dissociation and aggregation of cells from organ rudiments of the early chick embryo. *J. Anat.* 86: 287–301.

Nicholas, J. S. 1924. Regulation of posture in the forelimb of *Amblystoma punctatum. J. Exp. Zool.* 40: 113–137.

–1955. Limb and girdle. *In* B. H. Willier, P. Weiss, and V. Hamburger (eds.) *Analysis of Development.* Saunders, Philadelphia, pp. 429–39.

Piatt, J. 1942. Transplantation of aneurogenic forelimbs in *Amblystoma punctatum. J. Exp. Zool.* 91: 79–101.

Ramon y Cajal, S. 1890. Sur l'origine et les ramifications des fibres nerveuses de la moelle embryonaire. *Anat. Anz.* 5: 111–19, 609–13, 631–9.

–1894. *Die Retina der Wirbelthiere.* Bergmann-Verlag, Wiesbaden. Thorpe and Glick (trans.), Thomas, Springfield (IL), 1972.

–1905. Genese des fibres nerveuses de l'embryon et observations contraires a la theorie catenaire. *Trabajos Lab. Invest. Biol. U. Madrid* 4: 219–84. *In* L. Guth (trans.) *Studies on Vertebrate Neurogenesis.* Thomas, Springfield (IL), pp. 5–70.

–1908. Nouvelles observationes sur l'evolution des neuroblasts avec quelques remarques sur l'hypothese neurogenetique de Hensen-Held. *In* L. Guth (trans.) *Studies in Vertebrate Neurogenesis.* Thomas, Springfield (IL), p. 71.

–1909–11. *Histologie du Systeme Nerveux de l'Homme et des Vertebres.* 2 Volumes. I. Azoulay (trans.). Reprinted by Instituto Ramon y Cajal del C. S. I.C., Madrid, 1952–55.

–1917. Recollections of my life. *In* H. Craigie (trans.) *Memoirs of the American Philosophical Society,* Vol. 8. Philadelphia, 1937.

–1928. *Degeneration and Regeneration of the Nervous System.* R. M. May (trans.), Hafner, New York, 1959.

Roux, W. 1881. *Der Kampf der Theile in Organismus.* Engelmann, Leipzig.

–1888. Beitrage zur Entwickelungsmechznik des Embryo. V. Ueber die kunstliche Hervorbringung "halber" Embryonen durch Zerstorung einer der beiden ersten Furchungszellen, sowie uber die Nachentwickelung (Postgeneration) der feh lenden korperhalfte. *Virchow's Archiv. Anat. Physiol.* 114: 113–53, 246–91.

–1894. Ueber den "Cytotropismus" der Furchungszellen des Grasfrosches (*Rana fusca*). *Roux' Archiv.* 1: 43–68, 161–202.

–1895. *Gesammelte Abhandlungen uber Entwickelungsmechanick der Organismen.* Engelmann, Leipzig.

Shorrey, M. L. 1909. The effect of the destruction of peripheral areas on the differentiation of the neuroblasts. *J. Exp. Zool.* 7: 25–63.

Speidel, C. C. 1933. Studies of living nerves. II. Activities of ameoboid growth cones, sheath cells, and myelin segments, as revealed by prolonged observation of individual nerve fibers in frog tadpoles. *Am. J. Anat.* 52: 1–79.

–1941. Adjustments of nerve endings. *Harvey Lectures* 36: 126–56.

–1942 Studies of living nerves VIII. Histories of nerve endings in frog tadpoles subjected to various injurious treatments. *Proc. Am. Phil. Soc.* 85: 168–82.

–1948. Correlated studies of sense organs and nerves of the lateral-line in living frog tadpoles. II. Trophic influence of specific nerve supply as revealed by prolonged observations of denervated and reinnervated organs. *Am. J. Anat.* 82: 277–320.

Spemann, H. 1901. Uber Korrelationen in der Entwicklung des Auges. *Verh. Anat. Ges.* 15: 61–79.

–1902. Entwicklungsphysiologische Studien am Triton-Ei II. *Arch. f. Entw.-Mech* 15: 448–534.

–1904. Uber experimentel er zeugte Doppelbildungen

mit optischem Defect. *Zool. Jahrb. (Suppl.)* VII: 429–70.

–1918. Uber die Determination der Ersten Organanlagen des Amphibienembryo I–VI. *Arch. f. Entw.-Mech. Organ. 43:* 448–555.

–1938. *Embryonic Development and Induction.* Yale University Press, New Haven.

Spemann, H., and H. Mangold. 1924. Uber Induktion von Embronalanlagen durch Implantation artfremder Organisatoren. *Roux' Archiv.* 100: 599–638.

Sperry, R. W. 1940. The functional results of muscle transposition in the hind limb of the rat. *J. Comp. Neurol.* 73: 379–404.

–1941. The effect of crossing nerves to antagonistic muscles in the hind limb of the rat. *J. Comp. Neurol.* 75: 1–19.

–1942. Transplantation of motor nerves and muscles in the forelimb of the rat. *J. Comp. Neurol.* 76: 283–321.

–1943a. Effect of 180 degree rotation of the retinal field on visuomotor coordination. *J. Exp. Zool.* 92: 263–79.

–1943b. Visuomotor coordination in the newt (*Triturus viridescens*) after regeneration of the optic nerve. *J. Comp. Neurol.* 79: 33–55.

–1943c. Functional results of crossing sensory nerves in the rat. *J. Comp. Neurol.* 78: 59–90.

–1944. Optic nerve regeneration with return of vision in anurans. *J. Neurophysiol.* 7: 57–69.

–1945a. Restoration of vision after crossing of optic nerves and after contralateral transplantation of eye. *J. Neurophysiol.* 8: 15–28.

–1945b. Centripetal regeneration of the 8th cranial nerve root with systematic restoration of vestibular reflexes. *Am. J. Physiol.* 144: 735–41.

–1945c. The problem of central nervous reorganization after nerve regeneration and muscle transposition. *Quart. Rev. Biol.* 20: 311–69.

–1946. Ontogenetic development and maintenance of compensatory eye movements in complete absence of the optic nerve. *J. Comb. Psychol.* 39: 321–30.

–1947. Nature of functional recovery following regeneration of the oculomotor nerve in amphibians. *Anat. Rec.* 97: 293–316.

–1948a. Patterning of central synapses in regeneration of the optic nerve in teleosts. *Physiol. Zool.* 21: 351–61.

–1948b. Orderly patterning of synaptic associations in regeneration of intracentral fiber tracts mediating visuomotor coordination. *Anat. Rec.* 102: 63–75.

–1949. Reimplantation of eyes in fishes (*Bathygobius soporator*) with recovery of vision. *Proc. Soc. Exp. Biol: Med.* 71: 80–1.

–1950a. Neuronal specificity. *In* P. Weiss (ed.) *Genetic Neurology.* University of Chicago Press, Chicago, pp. 232–9.

–1950b. Myotypic specificity in teleost motoneurons. *J. Comp. Neurol.* 93: 277–87.

–1951a. Mechanisms of neural maturation. *In* S. S. Stevens (ed.) *Handbook of Experimental Psychology.* Wiley, New York, pp. 236–80.

–1951b. Regulative factors in the orderly growth of neural circuits. *Growth Symp.* 10: 63–87.

–1951c. Developmental patterning of neural circuits. *Chicago Med. School Quart.* 12: 66–73.

–1955. Functional regeneration in the optic system. *In* W. F. Windle (ed.) *Regeneration in the Central Nervous System.* Thomas, Springfield (IL), pp. 66–76.

–1958. Physiological plasticity and brain circuit theory. *In* H. F. Harlow and C. N. Woolsey (eds.) *Biological and Biochemical Bases of Behavior.* University of Wisconsin Press, Madison, pp. 401–21.

–1963. Chemoaffinity in the orderly growth of nerve fiber patterns and connections. *Proc. Natl. Acad. Sci. USA* 50: 703–10.

–1965. Embryogenesis of behavioral nerve nets. *In* R. L. DeHaan and H. Ursprung (eds.) *Organogenesis,* Vol. 6. Holt, Rinehart and Winston, New York, pp. 161–85.

Sperry, R. W., and H. L. Arora. 1965. Selectivity in regeneration of the oculomotor nerve in the cichlid fish, *Astronotus ocellatus. J. Embryol. Exp. Morphol.* 14(3): 307–17.

Sperry, R. W., and N. Deupree. 1956. Functional recovery following alterations in nerve-muscle connections of fishes. *J. Comp. Neurol.* 106: 143–61.

Sperry, R. W., and N. Miner. 1949. Formation within sensory nucleus V of synaptic associations mediating cutaneous localization. *J. Comp. Neurol.* 90: 403–23.

Steinberg, M. 1958. On the chemical bonds between animal cells: A mechanism for type-specific association. *Am. Naturalist* 92: 65–82.

–1962. On the mechanism of tissue reconstruction by dissociated cells. I. Population kinetics, differential adhesiveness, and the absence of directed migration. *Proc. Natl. Acad. Sci. USA* 48: 1577–82.

Stone, L. S. 1944. Functional polarization in retinal development and its reestablishment in regenerating retinae of rotated grafted eyes. *Proc. Soc. Exp. Biol. N.Y.* 57: 13–14.

–1960. Polarization of the retina and development of vision. *J. Exp. Zool.* 154: 85–93.

–1966. Development, polarization and regeneration of the ventral iris clift (remnant of choroidal fissure) and protractor lentis muscle in Urodele eyes. *J. Exp. Zool.* 161: 95–108.

Stone, L. S., and N. T. Ussher. 1927. Return of vision and other observations in replanted amphibian eyes. *Proc. Soc. Exp. Biol. Med.* 25: 213–15.

Stone, L. S., I. S. Zaur, and T. E. Farthing. 1934. Grafted eyes of adult *Triturus viridescens* with special reference to repeated return of vision. *Proc. Soc. Exp. Biol. Med.* 31: 1082–4.

Stroer, W. F. 1939. Zur vergleichenden Anatomie des primaren optischen Systems bel Wirbeltieren. *Z. Anat. u. Entw.-Gesch.* 110: 301–21.

Stultz, W. A. 1936. Relations of symmetry in the head-limb of *Amblystoma punctatum. J. Exp. Zool.* 72: 317–67.

Swett, F. H. 1937. Determination of limb-axes. *Quart. Rev. Biol.* 12: 322–39.

Szekely, G. 1954. Zur Ausbildung der lokalen funktionellen specifitat der retina. *Acta Biol. Acad. Sci.*

Hung. 5: 157–67.

–1966. Embryonic determination of neural connections. *Adv. Morph.* 5: 181–219.

Townes, P. L., and J. Holtfreter. 1955. Directed movements and selective adhesion of embryonic amphibian cells. *J. Exp. Zool.* 128: 53–120.

Trinkaus, J. P., and P. W. Groves. 1955. Differentiation in culture of mixed aggregates of dissociated tissue cells. *Proc. Natl. Acad. Sci. USA* 41: 787–95.

Trisler, G. D., M. D. Schneider, and M. Nirenberg. 1981. A topographic gradient of molecules in retina can be used to identify neuron position. *Proc. Natl. Acad. Sci. USA* 78: 2145–9.

Tyler, A. 1947. An auto-antibody concept of cell structure, growth and differentiation. *Growth Suppl.* 10: 7–19.

Waddington, C. H. 1934. Morphogenetic fields. *Sci. Prog.* 114: 336–46.

–1940. *Organisers and Genes.* Cambridge University Press, London.

Weiss, P. 1924. Die Funktion transplantierfer Amphibienextremitaten. Aufstellung einer Resonanz-theorie der motorischen Nerventatigkeit auf Grund abgestimmter Endorgane. *Roux' Archiv.* 102: 635–72.

–1926. Morphodynamik. *Abh. z. Theor. Biol.* 23: 1–43.

–1928. Erregungspecifitat und Erregungsresonanz. *Ergeb. Biol.* 3: 1–151.

–1931. Das Resonanzprinzip der Nerventatigkeit. *Wien. Klin. Wochenschr.* 39: 1–17.

–1932. Verusche uber Wirkung der operativen Einleitung motorischer Nerven in das Ruckenmark (Parabioseversuche an Kroten). *Arb. d. ungar. Biol. Forschg. Inst.* 5: 131.

–1934. In vitro experiments on the factors determining the course of the outgrowing nerve fiber. *J. Exp. Zool.* 68: 393–448.

–1935. Experimental innervation of muscles by the central ends of afferent nerves (establishment of a one-neurone connection between receptor and effector organ), with function tests. *J. Comp. Neurol.* 61: 135–74.

–1936. Selectivity controlling the central-peripheral relations in the nervous system. *Biol. Rev.* 11: 494–531.

–1937a. Further experimental investigations on the phenomenon of homologous response in transplanted amphibian limbs. I. Functional observations. *J. Comp. Neurol.* 66: 181–209.

–1937b. Further experimental investigations on the phenomenon of homologous response in transplanted amphibian limbs. II. Nerve regeneration and the innervation of transplanted limbs. *J. Comp. Neurol.* 66: 481–535.

–1937c. Further experimental investigations on the phenomenon of homologous response in transplanted amphibian limbs. III. Homologous response in the absence of sensory innervation. *J. Comp. Neurol.* 66: 537–48.

–1937d. Further experimental investigations on the phenomenon of homologous response in transplanted amphibian limbs. IV. Reverse locomotion after the interchange of right and left limbs. *J. Comp. Neurol.* 67: 269–315.

–1941a. Further experiments with deplanted and deranged nerve centers in amphibians. *Proc. Soc. Exp. Biol. Med.* 46: 14–15.

–1941b. Self-differentiation of the basic patterns of coordination. *Comp. Psych. Monographs* 17: 1–96.

–1941c. Nerve patterns: The mechanics of nerve growth. *Growth Suppl.* 5:163–203.

–1947. The problem of specificity in growth and development. *Yale J. Biol. Med.* 9: 235–78.

Weiss, P., and F. Rosetti. 1942. Growth responses of opposite sign among different neuron types exposed to thyroid hormone. *Proc. Natl. Acad. Sci. USA* 37: 540–56.

Weiss, P., and A. C. Taylor. 1944. Further experimental evidence against neurotropism in nerve regeneration. *J. Exp. Zool.* 95: 233–57.

Wiersma, C. A. G. 1931. An experiment on the "resonance theory" of muscular activity. *Arch. Neurol. Physiol.* 16: 337–45.

Willier, B. H., and J. Oppenheimer. 1970. *Foundations of Experimental Embryology.* Prentice-Hall, Englewood Cliffs (NJ).

Wilson, H. V. 1907. On some phenomena of coalescence and regeneration in sponges. *J. Exp. Zool.* 5: 245–58.

Wolpert, L. 1971. Positional information and pattern formation. *Curr. Top. Dev. Biol.* 6: 183–224.

Yntema, C. L. 1955. Ear and nose. *In* B. H. Willier, P. Weiss, and V. Hamburger (eds.) *Analysis of Development.* Saunders, Philadelphia, pp. 415–28.

Yoon, M. 1976. Topographic polarity of optic tectum. Topographic plarity of the optic tectum studied by reimplantation of the tectal tissue in adult goldfish. *Cold Spring Harbor Symp. Quant. Biol.* 15: 503–19.

3 Retinotectal connections made through ecotopic nerves

Emerson Hibbard

Department of Biology
Pennsylvania State University

Introduction

Being one of the many whose interest in embryonic development and regeneration of the nervous system was directly inspired and stimulated by the work of Roger Sperry, I am delighted to have an opportunity to contribute to this publication in his honor.

More than four decades have passed since Sperry began his fascinating studies on the regeneration of retinal ganglion cell axons in fish and amphibians and the patterns of connection and behaviors after the optic nerve had been cut to alter the axial relationships between eye and brain (Sperry 1943a, 1943b, 1944, 1945, 1948a, 1948b). Those studies led to Sperry's now famous theories, first of chemospecificity, then of chemoaffinity for axial gradients in the distribution of some sort of chemical substances, to account for the fact that the regenerating fibers apparently made their way back to their original terminations in the optic lobe of the brain. The theories have been controversial and, for that very reason, provocative for numerous studies by later investigators.

Attardi and Sperry (1963) claimed anatomical evidence that after partial retinal ablations, regenerating fibers from the remaining retina preferentially terminated in those parts of the tectal lobe to which they would normally project. Subsequently, a number of investigations have shown that optic-fiber terminals can rearrange themselves for some time after they reach the brain and that the retinotectal map can expand or contract to become distributed over the available tectal space (Cronly-Dillon and Levine 1971; Yoon 1972; Cook and Horder 1974; Schmidt 1978; Schmidt, Cicerone, and Easter 1978). Such plastic readjustment of terminal endings has been presented as strong evidence in opposition to Sperry's original hypothesis of an "unadaptable rigidity of central coordination mechanisms in the visuomotor system" in lower vertebrates that required a precise chemospecificity for nerve connections (Sperry 1943b, p. 278).

Chemospecificity implies that strict one-to-one relationships are established during development between the retinal ganglion cells and the tectal sites where they may terminate. The modified theory of chemoaffinity, on the other hand (Sperry 1963), implies that regenerating axons are guided by an attraction toward a particular pathway or terminal site by chemical substrate cues distributed in graded concentrations (see Chapter 5, this volume). I shall discuss evidence that strongly supports the chemoaffinity hypothesis, notwithstanding such statements opposed to the idea as that presented in Horder and Martin's (1978) comprehensive review of the literature on this subject: "Indeed the evidence that optic fibers are subject to purely mechanical forces appears to us to be so overwhelming that it is difficult to see how other influences, such as chemospecific ones, could even play a contributory role. It is difficult to see how mechanical forces, which all fibers must always be experiencing, could be overridden by other considerations" (p. 330).

In this chapter, data is presented from

experiments in which axons of retinal ganglion cells reach the tectum and establish topographically organized retinotectal maps there in spite of the fact that the optic nerve enters the brain, not at its normal site of entry in the floor of the diencephalon, but instead at an ectopic site. The experiments involve grafting an optic rudiment to a heterotopic location in the embryo or experimentally misdirecting the optic nerves through grossly abnormal pathways. The observed course of the regenerated nerves cannot be due solely to mechanical guidance, although such forces as selective fasciculation (Horder and Martin 1978; Cima and Grant 1982), maintenance of near-neighbor relationships during growth (Gaze and Fawcett 1983), or formation of guidance channels by glial supporting cells (Silver and Sidman 1980; Silver and Sapiro 1981; Krayanek and Goldberg 1981; Bohn, Reier, and Sourbeer, 1982) may play important roles in the process.

Eye rudiments grafted to hindbrain or spinal regions of amphibian embryos

The remarkable ability of growth cones of elongating optic-nerve fibers to traverse foreign territory in the brain and establish or restore vision undoubtedly involves a stepwise process in which choices are continually being made by the elongating and retracting pseudopodial processes at the growing axon tip. Such choice of one path rather than another has been demonstrated by several instances where the appropriate branch of the optic tract has been selected by regenerating optic fibers (Jacobson 1961; Attardi and Sperry 1963; Sharma 1972; Horder 1974; Straznicky, Gaze, and Horder 1979; Bunt 1982). If they are not within "striking distance" of their normal pathway, optic fibers may fail to reach the tectum. Even in this case, there may be evidence of substrate guidance to follow the normal path into the brain.

When embryonic eye rudiments are grafted adjacent to the hindbrain or spinal cord, normal appearing eyes may develop and optic axons grow into the central nervous system of the host, but usually they do not reach the tectum. Grafts of eyes to the ear region were done more than 75 years ago to support Ramon y Cajal's theory of axonal outgrowth

(Lewis 1907). Similar grafts made by Constantine-Paton and Capranica (1976) led them to conclude that there was a consistent orientation of the growing axons in a dorsocaudal direction, and the same result was described by Harris (1982) for eyes grafted to hindbrain regions of genetically eyeless axolotls. Katz and Lasek (1978, 1979) and Constantine-Paton (1978) found that optic fibers could either ascend or descend within specific sensory spinal tracts, but ascending fibers failed to reach the tectum. Giorgi and Van der Loos (1978) reported that if the normal eyes were present and already innervating the tectal lobes, fibers from grafted eyes failed to innervate the tectum, terminating instead in the nucleus of the tractus solitarius, which normally receives taste and other sensory input from the viscera. If, on the other hand, the normal eyes had been removed, optic fibers from the grafted eyes would innervate the posterior part of the deafferented or "empty" tectum. However, the absence of normal retinal input to the tectum apparently had no such attractive influence in Harris's genetically eyeless axolotls with optic rudiments grafted to hindbrain regions (Harris 1982).

In spite of the failure of optic axons to reach the tectum in most of these experiments, the fact that they consistently follow specific sensory tracts (Katz and Lasek 1979) and terminate in sensory nuclei of the hindbrain supports the idea that they are directed by regional chemical cues in the substrate.

Eye rudiments grafted to forebrain or midbrain regions of amphibian embryos

SUPERNUMERARY EYES

My own efforts to examine questions posed by Sperry's work began with an examination of the ability of optic-nerve fibers from extra eyes grafted to the heads of frog embryos to establish functional connections with the brains of the hosts (Hibbard 1959). While these experiments were crude compared with the superb studies on similar grafts done more recently by Constantine-Paton and Law (1978), they nevertheless indicated that functional connections were made between the grafted eye and the host brain, afferent connections were indicated by visuomotor responses elicited through the grafted eye and by histological examinations, and efferent output to oculomotor muscles was shown by synchronous movements of grafted and host eyes. This behavior implied that there must be a certain amount of plasticity in the system to account for the fact that input from extra eyes had been functionally integrated into the host brain, but, at the same time, it also seemed to strongly support Sperry's ideas of chemical gradients that direct the growth of nerve fibers toward appropriate brain targets.

In these studies, there was evidence that optic fibers from the grafted eye made their way toward the optic chiasm and tract. Electrophysiological recording by Sharma (1972) has demonstrated that optic-nerve fibers from such heterotopic grafted eyes are capable of establishing a map of the visual projection in the tectum of the host. He stated that the ingrowing optic fibers behave as if they recognize the right pathway near the tectum and enter it to establish specific connections. The impression that the fibers select the optic-nerve pathway rather than growing directly toward the tectum was similar to one I had from the path taken by optic fibers regenerating through the root of the oculomotor nerve: "Unlike Mauthner's axons which showed directed growth apparently related to axial gradients, the regenerating optic fibers grew initially against their normal rostrocaudal direction of growth in order to reach the vicinity of the optic chiasm before proceeding back to the tectum in the optic tract. The tendency was therefore one of reduction of positional error relative to the normal pathway rather than to the final termination" (Hibbard 1967, p. 355).

The elegant demonstration by Constantine-Paton and Law (1978) that optic fibers from grafted supernumerary eyes can reach the tectum of the host and can compete there for terminal space with the axon terminals from the eye that normally innervates that tectal lobe would seem to require chemical cues in the tectal substrate. Remarkable longitudinally oriented alternate columns of terminal endings of fibers coming from the grafted and host eyes, which closely resemble the ocular dominance columns subserving binocular vision and depth perception in higher vertebrates (Hubel and Wiesel 1968, 1972), have also been found by these researchers when optic fibers from both normal eyes innervate one tectal lobe following ablation of the other lobe (Law and Constantine-Paton 1980). Here, as in numerous other cases of ipsilateral retinotectal projections, the map formed by the fibers from the eye on the same side as the tectal lobe being innervated is a mirror image of its normal contralateral projection. It would appear to be guided by the same gradients specifying anteroposterior and lateral position, with reversal of left and right directions.

Sperry's early study of visual restoration following cross-union of optic nerves or contralateral transplantation of eyes had demonstrated similar mirror-imaging of the retinotectal projection with consequent maladaptive responses due to erroneous localization of objects in the visual field (Sperry 1945).

Eye rudiments grafted to genetically eyeless embryos

Perhaps it should not seem remarkable that optic rudiments grafted into relatively normal eye positions in genetically eyeless embryos should be capable of becoming essentially normal eyes, showing normal vestibuloocular reflexes, providing the host with the ability to accurately localize objects in its visual field and controlling visuomotor responses (Hibbard and Ornberg 1976; Schwenk and Hibbard 1977). After all, the growth processes are the same as those occurring during normal development once the optic vesicle, which is missing as a result of the genetic defect, is restored to the embryo. However, the placement of the eye is seldom perfect, so the optic nerve usually enters the brain at an ectopic site. When this occurs, the optic fibers first grow anteriorly to the position of the normal optic tracts then turn abruptly to project posteriorly to the tectum, which suggests that biochemical cues may direct the growth of the fibers toward the tract long before they reach the tectum.

This sort of pathway taken by fibers entering the wall of the diencephalon some distance above and behind the normal entry point of the optic nerve has been beautifully demonstrated by Harris (1982), who stained the optic nerve from the grafted eye with horseradish peroxidase, cleared the tissue, and photographed it in a whole-mount preparation. Although we had shown that our eyeless axolotls having received grafted eyes were capable of accurately locating objects in their visual fields, and had recorded evoked potentials from their tectal lobes, it remained for Harris to demonstrate that the fibers from the grafted eyes were distributed in a normal visuotopic projection to the tectum. He also stated that "In all bilateral projections, optic fibers from the transplanted eyes crossed to the contralateral side of the brain at or very near the site at which the optic chiasm would have occurred in normal animals" (Harris 1982, p. 341).

Optic nerve experimentally deflected to abnormal entry sites

By cutting the optic nerve and joining that portion remaining attached to the eyeball with the cut root of another cranial nerve, the regenerating optic axons can be caused to enter the more mature brain at a grossly abnormal site. Here the growth cones must encounter and traverse already differentiated tissues, established nerve tracts, and glial elements that, under normal conditions, would be quite foreign to them.

As mentioned before, misdirected optic-nerve fibers were found, in some cases, to be capable of reaching the tectum after having been experimentally joined to the root of the oculomotor nerve (Hibbard 1967). Again the evidence for this was based on behavioral and histological studies. Beazley and Lamb (1979) carried out similar experiments and confirmed that the regenerated fibers were capable of establishing normal visuotectal projections by this route. As was stated earlier, it was my impression that most of the optic fibers that eventually reached the tectum did so through a circuitous route that carried them first to the region of the optic chiasm. In their studies, Beazley and Lamb found that the regenerating fibers took a number of different courses to reach the tectum, some passing superficially just beneath the surface of the wall of the diencephalon and a few even making a "bee line" directly toward the tectum from their entry point in the oculomotor root.

More recently, I have deflected the regenerating optic-nerve fibers to an even more distant and abnormal entry point in the brain by joining the optic-nerve stump attached to

the eye to the cut olfactory nerve (Figure 3.1). Once again, the growth cones of the elongating retinal ganglion cell axons sought out, or were guided to, the contralateral tectum, only a small complement of them projecting to ipsilateral sites. While some wandered off to other places, with part of them ending in the contralateral olfactory nerve, the majority passed over the ventrolateral surface of the telencephalon just beneath the meninges until they reached the normal site of the optic chiasm. They then penetrated into the wall of the diencephalon and followed their normal tracts back to the tectum, where they were distributed in the pattern of layers that is typical of normal optic-fiber terminations (Figure 3.2).

In this experiment, the penetration of the fibers into the brain wall when they reached the site of the optic chiasm differs from the observation of Gaze and Grant (1978) that regenerating optic fibers (entering at the normal position of the optic nerve) followed a very superficial pathway over the surface of the diencephalon, apparently not being attracted or influenced by degeneration products in their previous deeper optic tracts. Such superficial "plastering on" of newly formed fibers in subpial positions could help explain the relative positioning of older versus younger fibers in the normal optic tract with first-formed fibers lying deep and later ones lying closer to the surface (Gaze and Grant 1978; Fawcett 1981; Bunt 1982), and it also could explain the subpial position of ectopic optic fibers growing in the spinal cord (Constantine-Paton 1978). It may permit younger fibers to bypass already established tissue to reach their goal. It can, of course, be argued that these superficial positions of growing or regenerating nerves is a consequence of mechanical guidance in structural features of the substrate such as channels formed by glial endfeet at the external limiting membrane through which the fibers can pass. While that seems quite likely, there seems to be little reason to suppose that the fibers would not continue on the same trajectory along the ipsilateral surface of the diencephalon and on into the hindbrain if they were not responding to some chemical cues that alter their paths, directing them on a new course through the chiasm and tract to the contralateral tectum.

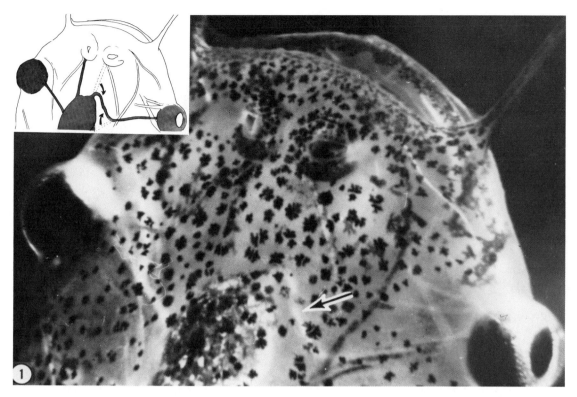

Figure 3.1. Head of a living *Xenopus* tadpole in which the cut optic nerve from the right eye has been joined to the cut olfactory nerve (arrow). The inset shows the diversion of the optic and olfactory nerves.

There does not seem to be any structural mechanical feature to explain their change of course. The fact that regenerating optic fibers in *Xenopus* took a superficial course rather than following the paths of degenerating fibers was taken by Gaze and Grant (1978) as an indication that the fibers were not being guided by place-related chemospecific cues. But, the tendency of regenerating fibers to grow toward the optic chiasm from either posterior or anterior ectopic nerves and to become organized in retinotopic order in the tectum seems to me difficult to explain in any other way.

Hypertrophy in regenerating optic cells that fail to make endings

Temporal and spatial aspects of the regeneration process must both be greatly increased when retinal axons are made to regenerate through the olfactory nerve route. The distance traversed by the regenerating growth cones is nearly double that required to reach the tectum through the normal route and obviously requires the expenditure of considerable amounts of resources and energy for extending and maintaining the greatly elongated axon.

In fact, a large increase in synthetic activity in retinal ganglion cells during the regenerative process is indicated by the marked hypertrophy of these cells in cases where they fail to establish function endings (Figure 3.3).

Changes in synthetic activity, cell morphology, and axoplasmic flow during optic-nerve regeneration have been studied by several investigators, most using goldfish. Following lesion of its axon, the retinal ganglion cell responds by increasing synthesis of nucleolar materials, increased incorporation of amino acids (Murray and Grafstein 1969), increase in the population of free ribosomes and the production of rough endoplasmic reticulum (Murray and Forman 1971), and increase in protein transport along the regenerating axon (Grafstein and Murray 1969). Ingoglia, Weis, and Mycek (1975) found large increases of radio-

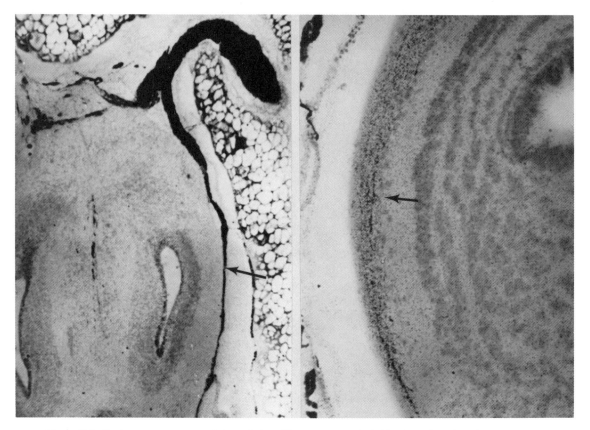

Figure 3.2. Optic axons regenerated through the olfactory nerve. *Left:* Horizontal section through the forebrain of the tadpole shown in Figure 3.1 following intraocular injection of ³H-proline. Intensely labeled optic-nerve fibers enter the brain through the olfactory nerve, a few cross to the contralateral olfactory nerve, but most pass ventrolaterally near the surface of the telencephalon to reach the optic chiasm (arrow). *Right:* Labeled terminals of the optic axons, shown on the *left,* in the stratum opticum of the contralateral tectal lobe (arrow).

active RNA in the contralateral tectum following intraocular injection of ³H-uridine during the period of time when regenerating axons were reestablishing connections in the tectum, indicating that large amounts of RNA were being transported by the regenerating fibers. Later Ingoglia (1978) and Ingoglia and Sharma (1978) identified the transported RNA as 4S RNA, not ribosomal RNA, and found that interfering with its transport could inhibit the reestablishment of the retinotectal map, although why this occurred remained unexplained. Heacock and Agranoff (1982) have found a rapidly transported protein in regenerating fibers that is barely detectable in normal fish. Most of the material produced by the ganglion cell and transported in its axon is probably utilized for extending the growth cone as the process elon-

gates, but, as suggested in Ingoglia's studies, some may be involved in a cell–cell recognition process.

Sperry's idea of regional specificities being conferred on the retina and tectum by chemical gradients organized in various axes has been challenged by several investigators who have doubted, as Horder and Martin (1978) did, whether such a model doesn't "exceed the limits on possible differentiated cell states" in relatively homogeneous tissues. However, Trisler, Schneider, and Nirenberg (1981) have obtained a monoclonal antibody that binds to cell-membrane molecules distributed in a topographic gradient in the avian retina, with a thirty-fivefold increase in antigen from ventroanterior to dorsoposterior retina, which could be used as a position marker for

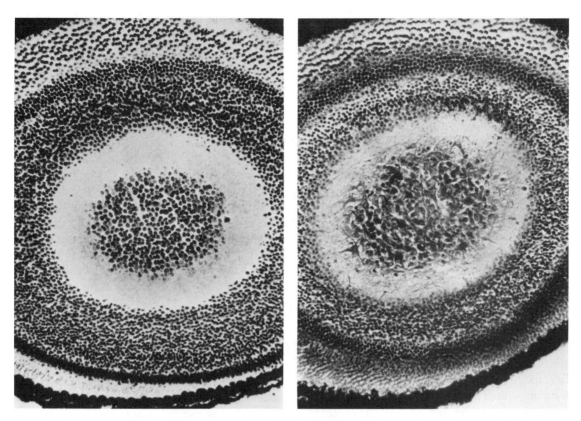

Figure 3.3. *Left:* Normal left eye of *Xenopus* tadpole. *Right:* Right eye of the same tadpole showing
marked hypertrophy of retinal ganglion cells (and their dendrites in the inner plexiform layer)
when regeneration of their optic fibers is incomplete.

retinal cells. These findings coupled with the
in-vitro studies of Barbera, Marchase, and
Roth (1973), Letourneau (1975), and Roth and
Marchase (1976) demonstrating selective adhesion either between retinal and tectal cells or
to various chemical substrates appear to reveal
a mechanism by which chemoaffinity might direct regenerating fibers toward their goals.

Once the goal of a growing axon is
reached, there must be a chemically mediated
feedback mechanism, carried by retrograde axonal transport, to inhibit the greatly increased
protein synthesis in the cell body so that further
elongation ceases. Grafstein and Murray (1969)
found that synthetic activity remained elevated
for a period of time following reconnection, the
rate of "fast" transport being about twice that
of normal two weeks after reconnection. Perhaps this protracted activity serves temporary
maintenance of collateral sprouts that are later
retracted. Murray (1982) has found a fourfold

increase in the number of myelinated axons distal to a crush lesion of the optic nerve in goldfish
and Murray and Edwards (1982) report that the
number of regenerating axons in the tectum
remains elevated for a period of time after visual function is restored. Fujisawa et al. (1982)
have also found extensive sprouting in the tectum of the newt *Cynops pyrrhogaster* with only
the fibers to normal innervation sites being retained, the extraneous ones being lost or
withdrawn.

The type of hypertrophy of retinal ganglion cells shown in Figure 3.3, if retained for
long after regeneration should be complete,
might serve as a useful indicator to determine
whether "lost" optic axons have failed to establish terminations in the brain. Some of the
abnormal sites to which "lost" optic fibers have
been traced include: posterior spinal cord
(Constantine-Paton and Capranica 1976); sensory regions of the hindbrain and posterior mid-

brain tegmentum (Constantine-Paton 1978); nucleus tractus solitarius (Giorgi and Van der Loos 1978); and tori semicircularis, nucleus isthmi, tegmental nucleus, and superior reticular nucleus (Sharma 1981). In the last case, Sharma reported that electrophysiological mapping indicated that the optic fibers were able to generate a retinotopic projection in a nonvisual part of the brain if both tectal lobes were ablated, but he could not determine whether synaptic terminations were established with cells in these areas.

Anomalous projections of optic axons following lesions of the tectum (superior colliculus) in newborn hamsters have been reported by Schneider (1973). If the more superficial layers of the tectum, where some retinal fibers would normally terminate, are removed, the projections terminate in the deeper layers of the tectum or other brain centers that normally would be receiving fibers from the tectum. If the tectum on one side of the newborn hamster's brain is lesioned and the eye on that side is removed, optic fibers that normally would have projected to the lesioned tectum will recross the midline and spread over the ipsilateral tectum in a mirror-image map (Schneider and Jhaveri 1974), causing the animal to demonstrate maladaptive responses to objects in the visual field. Mapping of anomalous projections at abnormal brain sites suggests that the chemical cues at one level in the system are carried up through the next order of neurons in the pathway.

Conclusions

Is orientation an active or passive phenomenon? What is the axon tip seeking?

The experiments reviewed describe the regenerating axons as if they were being led into particular routes, but leave uncertain how much of an active role nerve fibers play in their own orientation. We tend to talk of mechanical or chemical substrate guidance as if the nerve fibers were passively elongating and completely under the control of external forces. But a change in direction taken by an outgrowing axon requires alterations in membrane building and in the establishment of cytoskeletal elements at the growing tip to cause an asymmetry in the extension of the fiber. Time-lapse motion-picture films of axons of nerve cells in tissue culture (Pomerat 1961) give one the distinct impression that the filapodial processes of the growth cone are forcefully searching and testing their environment as the fiber elongates.

Nearly a century ago, Ramon y Cajal, referring to connections made between climbing fibers and Purkinje cells in the cerebellum, said, "The axons of the conductors referred to, upon arriving from distant centers, smell out, so to speak, the bodies of the Purkinje elements, which they embrace by means of varicose nests which are the rudiments of the future arborizations" (Ramon y Cajal 1937, p. 370). This and other references by Cajal suggest an active searching role by the developing neuron (see Chapter 2, this volume). Sperry's (1963) idea of chemoaffinity suggested that the fibers "home in" on specific nerve terminals by following chemical gradients in the tissues. It seems quite clear from the experiments on development or regeneration of ectopic optic nerves that the cells are making a real effort to reach their proper termination sites, and to do this, they must somehow be able to sense their position relative to their surroundings and to alter their course accordingly.

During ontogenetic development, or during regeneration, the neuron goes through two distinct phases, one in which the cell or a limited region of its axon, the growth cone, exhibits a considerable amount of amoeboid activity, and another in which the cell has established its terminal connections and has settled down to perform its functional role of transmitting impulses. During the motile phase, its amoeboid activity establishes its positional relationships, just as similar amoeboid activity of other cell types such as embryonic migratory neural crest cells, mesenchyme cells, Schwann cells, or presumptive germ cells brings these cells into correct spatial relationships with their neighbors in order to build a normal functional individual. Harrison (1910) stated that the activities of differentiating neurons "are of the same fundamental nature as those found not only in other embryonic cells but also in the protoplasm of the widest variety of organisms" and that the movement of the extending axon "is but a specific form of that general type of movement common to all primitive protoplasm." He suggested that in order to determine the factors that influence the paths taken by the fibers, "we are concerned, therefore, primarily with the laws which govern the direction and intensity of protoplasmic movement" (Harrison 1910, p. 840). Perhaps we should pay more attention to pseudopodial activity and amoeboid movement in unicellular organisms, which are capable of responding to a variety of environmental cues including mechanical or chemical substrate cues, diffusible chemical substances, pH gradients, oxygen tension, and even thermal, electrical, or gravitational stimuli (Allen and Haberey 1973). Growth cones of ectopic optic-nerve fibers are very likely to be capable of responding to combinations of such cues with mechanisms that have ancient evolutionary roots.

What is the axon seeking? Perhaps one reason that the answer to this question continues to elude us is that the axon may be following different cues during different periods of its growth. For example, in the case of regeneration of optic fibers through the olfactory nerve, it might initially be passively guided by the olfactory fibers already present in the stump, then might continue its trajectory but be drawn to the superficial subpial pathway over the surface of the telencephalon in order, perhaps, to take advantage of a higher oxygen tension adjacent to meningeal vasculature. Once the fiber has reached the level of the optic chiasm, it might be affected by diffusible chemical substances released by degenerative products in the tract and induced to penetrate inward and follow the normal course of the tract to the contralateral tectum. Once there, it might respond to chemical substrate cues provided by cell-membrane molecular recognition factors to establish its final positional relationships within the tectum.

Of course, it might be argued that an amoeba, being a unicellular organism, must of necessity do everything for itself and we should not ascribe to individual cells of multicellular organisms powers they may not posses. But perhaps the migratory ability of a neuron reflects a genetically mediated primitive behavior pattern built into the cell itself, providing it with more control over its own destiny than we have given it credit for.

Acknowledgments
The author wishes to thank Drs. Colwyn Trevarthen and Ronald Meyer for helpful suggestions and critical reading of the manuscript, and Mary Alice Shea for help in its preparation.

References

Allen, R. D., and M. Haberey. 1973. The behaviour of amoebae. *In* A. Pérez-Miravete (ed.) *Behaviour of Micro-Organisms*. Plenum, London and New York, pp. 157–67.

Attardi, D., and R. W. Sperry. 1963. Preferential selection of central pathways by regenerating optic fibers. *Exp. Neurol.* 7: 46–64.

Barbera, A. J., R. B. Marchase, and S. Roth. 1973. Adhesive recognition and retinotectal specificity. *Proc. Natl. Acad. Sci. USA* 70: 2482–6.

Beazley, L. D., and A. H. Lamb. 1979. Rerouted axons in *Xenopus* tadpoles form normal visuotectal projections. *Brain Res.* 179: 373–8.

Bohn, R. C., P. J. Reier, and E. B. Sourbeer. 1982. Axonal interactions with connective tissue and glial substrata during optic nerve regeneration in *Xenopus* larvae and adults. *Am. J. Anat.* 165: 397–419.

Bunt, S. M. 1982. Retinotopic and temporal organization of the optic nerve and tracts in the adult goldfish. *J. Comp. Neurol.* 206: 209–26.

Cima, C., and P. Grant. 1982. Development of the optic nerve in *Xenopus laevis*. I. Early development and organization. *J. Embryol. Exp. Morph.* 72: 225–49.

Constantine-Paton, M. 1978. Central projections of anuran optic nerves penetrating hindbrain or spinal cord regions of the neural tube. *Brain Res.* 158: 31–43.

Contantine-Paton, M., and R. R. Capranica. 1976. Axonal guidance of developing optic nerves in the frog. I. Anatomy of the projection from transplanted eye primordia. *J. Comp. Neurol.* 170: 17–31.

Constantine-Paton, M., and M. I. Law. 1978. Eye-specific termination bands in tecta of three-eyed frogs. *Science* 202: 639–41.

Cook, J. E., and T. J. Horder. 1974. Interactions between optic fibres in their regeneration to specific sites in goldfish tectum. *J. Physiol. (London)* 241(2): 89P–90P.

Cronly-Dillon, J. R., and R. Levine. 1971. Retinotectal projections in half-eyes in the adult newt *Triturus vulgaris*. *J. Physiol. (London)* 216: 62P–63P.

Fawcett, J. W. 1981. How axons grow down the *Xenopus* optic nerve. *J. Embryol. Exp. Morph.* 65: 219–33.

Fujisawa, H., N. Tani, K. Watanabe, and Y. Ibata. 1982. Branching of regenerating retinal axons and preferential selection of appropriate branches for specific neuronal connection in the newt (*Cynops pyrrhogaster*). *Dev. Biol.* 90: 43–57.

Gaze, R. M., and J. W. Fawcett. 1983. Pathways of *Xenopus* optic fibres regenerating from normal and compound eyes under various conditions. *J. Embryol. Exp. Morph.* 73: 17–38.

Gaze, R. M., and P. Grant. 1978. The diencephalic course of regenerating retinotectal fibres in *Xenopus* tadpoles. *J. Embryol. Exp. Morph.* 44: 201–16.

Giorgi, P. P., and H. Van der Loos. 1978. Axons from eyes grafted in *Xenopus* can grow into the spinal cord and reach the tectum. *Nature (London)* 275: 746–8.

Grafstein, B., and M. Murray. 1969. Transport of protein in goldfish optic nerve during regeneration. *Exp. Neurol.* 25: 494–508.

Harris, W. A. 1982. The transplantation of eyes to genetically eyeless salamanders: Visual projections and somatosensory interactions. *J. Neurosci.* 2: 339–53.

Harrison, R. G. 1910. The outgrowth of the nerve fiber as a mode of protoplasmic movement. *J. Exp. Zool.* 9: 787–848.

Heacock, A. M., and B. W. Agranoff. 1982. Protein synthesis and transport in the regenerating goldfish *Carassius auratus* visual system. *Neurochem. Res.* 7: 771–88.

Hibbard, E. 1959. Central integration of developing nerve tracts from supernumerary grafted eyes and brain in the frog. *J. Exp. Zool.* 141: 323–51.

–1967. Visual recovery following regeneration of the optic nerve through the oculomotor nerve root in *Xenopus*. *Exp. Neurol.* 19: 350–6.

Hibbard, E., and R. L. Ornberg. 1976. Restoration of vision in genetically eyeless axolotls. *Exp. Neurol.* 50: 113–23.

Horder, T. J. 1974. Electron microscopic evidence in goldfish that different optic nerve fibres regenerate selectively through specific routes into the tectum. *J. Physiol. (London)* 241: 84P–85P.

Horder, T. J., and K. A. C. Martin. 1978. Morphogenetics as an alternative to chemospecificity in the formation of nerve connections. A review of literature, before 1978, concerning the control of growth of regenerating optic nerve fibres to specific locations in the optic tectum and a new interpretation based on contact guidance. *Symp. Soc. Exp. Biol.* 32: 275–358.

Hubel, D. H., and T. N. Wiesel. 1968. Receptive fields and functional architecture of monkey striate cortex. *J. Physiol. (London)* 195: 215–43.

–1972. Laminar and columnar distribution of geniculocortical fibers in the Macaque monkey. *J. Comp. Neurol.* 146: 421–50.

Ingoglia, N. A. 1978. The effect of intraocular injection of cordycepin on retinal RNA synthesis and on RNA axonally transported during regeneration of the optic nerves of goldfish. *J. Neurochem.* 30: 1029–39.

Ingoglia, N. A., and S. C. Sharma. 1978. The effect of inhibition of axonal RNA transport on the restoration of retinotectal projections in regenerating optic nerves of goldfish. *Brain Res.* 156: 141–5.

Ingoglia, N. A., P. Weis, and J. Mycek. 1975. Axonal transport of RNA during regeneration of the optic nerves of goldfish. *J. Neurobiol.* 6: 549–63.

Jacobson, M. 1961. The recovery of electrical activity in the optic tectum of the frog during early regeneration of the optic nerve. *J. Physiol. (London)* 157: 27P–29P.

Katz, M. J., and R. J. Lasek. 1978. Eyes transplanted to tadpole tails send axons rostrally in two spinal-cord tracts. *Science* 199: 202–4.

–1979. Substrate pathways which guide growing axons in *Xenopus* embryos. *J. Comp. Neurol.* 183: 817–32.

Krayanek, S., and S. Goldberg. 1981. Oriented extracellular channels and axonal guidance in the embryonic chick retina. *Dev. Biol.* 84: 41–50.

Law, M. I., and M. Constantine-Paton. 1980. Right and left eye bands in frogs with unilateral tectal ablations. *Proc. Natl. Acad. Sci. USA* 77: 2314–18.

Letourneau, P. C. 1975. Cell-to-substratum adhesion and guidance of axonal elongation. *Dev. Biol.* 44: 92–101.

Lewis, W. H. 1907. Experimental evidence in support of the theory of outgrowth of the axis cylinder. *Am. J. Anat.* 6: 461–71.

Murray, M. 1982. A quantitative study of regenerative sprouting by optic axons in goldfish (*Carassius auratus*). *J. Comp. Neurol.* 209: 352–62.

Murray, M. and M. A. Edwards. 1982. A quantitative study of the reinnervation of the goldfish optic tectum following optic nerve crush. *J. Comp. Neurol.* 209: 363–73.

Murray, M. and D. S. Forman. 1971. Fine structural changes in goldfish retinal ganglion cells during axonal regeneration. *Brain Res.* 32: 287–98.

Murray, M. and B. Grafstein. 1969. Changes in the morphology and amino acid incorporation of regenerating goldfish optic neurons. *Exp. Neurol.* 23: 544–60.

Pomerat, C. M. 1961. *Dynamic Aspects of the Neuron in Tissue Culture* [Film]. Pasadena Medical Foundation, Pasadena.

Ramon y Cajal, S. 1937. *Recollections of My Life,* E. Horne Craigie (trans.). MIT Press, Cambridge (MA).

Roth, S., and R. B. Marchase. 1976. An *in vitro* assay for retinotectal specificity. *In* S. H. Barondes (ed.) *Neuronal Recognition*. Plenum, New York and London, pp. 227–48.

Schneider, G. E. 1973. Early lesions of superior colliculus: Factors affecting the formation of abnormal retinal projections. *Brain, Behav. Evol.* 8: 73–109.

Schneider, G. E. and S. R. Jhaveri. 1974. Neuroanatomical correlates of spared or altered function after brain lesions in the newborn hamster. *In* D. G. Stein, J. J. Rosen, and N. Butters (eds.) *Plasticity and Recovery of Function in the Central Nervous System:* Academic Press, New York, pp. 65–109.

Schmidt, J. T. 1978. Retinal fibers alter tectal positional markers during the expansion of the half retinal projection in goldfish. *J. Comp. Neurol.* 177: 279–300.

Schmidt, J. T., C. M. Cicerone, and S. S. Easter. 1978. Expansion of the half retinal projection to the tectum in goldfish: An electrophysiological and anatomical Study. *J. Comp. Neurol.* 177: 257–78.

Schwenk, G. C., and E. Hibbard. 1977. An autoradiographic study of optic fiber projections from eye grafts in eyeless mutant axolotls. *Exp. Neurol.* 55: 498–503.

Sharma, S. C. 1972. Retinotectal connexions of a heterotopic eye. *Nature, New Biol.* 238: 286–7.

–1981. Retinal projection in a non-visual area after bilateral tectal ablation in goldfish. *Nature (London)* 291: 66–7.

Silver, J., and J. Sapiro. 1981. Axonal guidance during development of the optic nerve: The role of pigmented epithelia and other extrinsic factors. *J. Comp. Neurol.* 202: 521–38.

Silver, J., and R. L. Sidman. 1980. A mechanism for the guidance and topographic patterning of retinal ganglion cell axons. *J. Comp. Neurol.* 189: 101–11.

Sperry, R. W. 1943a. Visuomotor coordination in the newt (*Triturus viridescens*) after regeneration of the optic nerve. *J. Comp. Neurol.* 79: 33–55.

–1943b. Effect of 180 degree rotation of the retinal field on visuomotor coordination. *J. Exp. Zool.* 92: 263–79.

–1944. Optic nerve regeneration with return of vision in anurans. *J. Neurophysiol.* 7: 57–69.

–1945. Restoration of vision after crossing of optic nerves and after contralateral transplantation of eye. *J. Neurophysiol.* 8: 15–28.

–1948a. Patterning of central synapses in regeneration of optic nerve in teleosts. *Physiol. Zool.* 21: 351–61.

–1948b. Orderly patterning of synaptic associations in regeneration of intracentral fiber tracts mediating visuomotor coordination. *Anat. Rec.* 102: 63–75.

–1963. Chemoaffinity in the orderly growth of nerve fiber patterns and connections. *Proc. Natl. Acad. Sci. USA* 50: 703–10.

Straznicky, C., R. M. Gaze, and T. J. Horder. 1979. Selection of appropriate medial branch of the optic tract by fibres of ventral retinal origin during development and in regeneration: an autoradiographic study in *Xenopus. J. Embryol. Exp. Morph.* 50: 253–67.

Trisler, G. D., M. D. Schneider, and M. Nirenberg. 1981. A topographic gradient of molecules in retina can be used to identify neuron position. *Proc. Natl. Acad. Sci. USA* 78: 2145–9.

Yoon, M. 1972. Reversibility of the reorganization of retinotectal projection in goldfish. *Exp. Neurol.* 35: 565–77.

4 Neural reconnection between the eye and the brain in goldfish

Myong G. Yoon
Department of Psychology
Life Sciences Centre
Dalhousie University

Topographic pattern of the visual projection

The eye tells the brain about the visual world by converting light stimuli into electric signals. These neural messages of visual information are conveyed from one neurone to another through intricate networks of neural connections. Each retinal ganglian cell processes visual information received by a small area on the retina, called its *visual receptive field,* which is located in a specific position with respect to the visual axes of the eye. The receptive fields of adjacent ganglion cells overlap in coherent order such that the topography of the external space is represented in the neural activity of the hemispheric layer of ganglion cells inside the eye. Each one of many hundreds of thousands of ganglion cells sends its axon, the *optic fiber,* to the appropriate target cells in the brain. As these optic fibers exit the posterior pole of the eyeball, they form a thick ensheathed bundle, the *optic nerve,* and course in the brain to connect with their appropriate target neurones. In goldfish, most optic fibers cross the midline and invade the contralateral lobe of the *optic tectum* in the midbrain. Entering the tectal lobe at its rostral pole, they divide into many fine fascicles that spread fanlike through a superficial layer, the *stratum opticum,* toward the caudal pole along the spheroidal circumferences of the tectum. Most ingrowing optic fibers terminate in the subjacent layer, the *stratum fibrosum et grieseum superficiale,* and selectively make functional contacts, *synapses,* with millions of visual neurones. Thus, they establish the retinotectal projection on which visuomotor coordinations depend.

The pattern of the visual projection from the eye to the brain has two essential design features. First, it is topographically coherent, in the sense that optic fibers originating from adjacent positions in the retina connect with neighboring visual neurones in the brain. Second, the projection is topographically polarized, in the sense that a temporonasal sequence of retinal positions (or a nasotemporal sequence of their corresponding receptive fields in the external visual world) is represented by a rostrocaudal sequence on the tectum, and a ventrodorsal sequence of retinal positions by a mediolateral sequence on the tectum. This topographic projection of the external visual world onto various visual areas of the brain is a general feature common to all animals so far examined.

The visual pathways of lower vertebrates (including the goldfish) have a further remarkable feature. If the original neural connections between the eye and the brain are destroyed by severing the optic nerves, the optic fibers regenerate, grow back to the visual areas in the brain and eventually restore vision. The discovery of optic-fiber regeneration and recovery of vision in adult newts by Matthey (1925, 1926) and its confirmation by Stone and Zaur (1940) provided Roger Sperry with a unique system for his pioneering experiments on neuronal connectivity (Sperry, 1943a, 1943b, 1944, 1945, 1948).

Sperry's theory of neuronal specificity

After 180° rotation of the eyes of the adult newt, leaving the optic nerves intact, Sperry (1943a) observed a complete inversion and reversal of visuomotor responses from the experimental animals. This maladaptive behavior persisted indefinitely without correction. Next Sperry (1943b, 1944) rotated the eyes by 180° and also cut the optic nerves to regenerate back to the brain. The restored visuomotor coordinations after optic-fiber regeneration in these animals were systematically inverted and reversed in the same way as those resulting from eye rotation alone. The maladaptive visuomotor coordinations that correlated with the orientation of the 180° rotated retina persisted without any sign of correction by some kind of learning process (Sperry 1943b, 1944). In further experiments in which eye transplantation from one side to the other was combined with various degrees of eye rotation or surgical cross-union of optic nerves, Sperry (1945, 1948) observed that the recovered visuomotor responses were consistently correlated with the experimental rearrangements of the retinae or optic nerves and were extremely maladaptive. Thus, he concluded that the reestablishment of functional relations between the retina and the visual centers is predetermined by growth-regulating factors irrespective of any functional readaptation process such as learning.

To explain the embryonic development and reestablishment of the orderly retinotectal projection, Sperry (1943b, 1945, 1948, 1951, 1963, 1965) formulated the chemoaffinity hypothesis of neuronal specificity. Sperry's theory is based on three assumptions: (1) The embryonic retinal ganglion cells undergo topographic differentiation (as well as cytologic and functional differentions such as "on," "off," or "on–off" type cells, etc.) along the temporonasal and ventrodorsal axes of the eye anlage. Each retinal ganglion cell acquires an axially graded differential affinity of a cytochemical nature for intercellular recognition, according to its relative position in the retina. (2) The corresponding higher-order visual neurones in the optic tectum also undergo a congruent topographic differentiation along the rostrocaudal and mediolateral axes of the tectum, and thus acquire matching or complementary differential chemoaffinities, according to their relative positions in the tectum. (3) The ingrowing optic fiber is guided chemotactically to its appropriate target zone when it enters the tectum and forms synaptic connections with just those tectal neurones whose chemoaffinity matches its own.

Retinotectal size-disparity experiments

Various experimental manipulations of the visual pathway of the adult goldfish have been carried out to test the chemoaffinity hypothesis (see Chapter 5, this volume). Attardi and Sperry (1963) reported that if a part of the retina was removed, the regenerating optic fibers from the residual retina terminated only within the predesignated target zones in the tectum, bypassing a series of empty neuron slots on their way, as predicted by the chemoaffinity hypothesis. A further support came from Jacobson and Gaze (1965): they reported that an ablation of either the medial or lateral half of the goldfish tectum resulted in a persistent partial scotoma corresponding to the retinal area that normally projected to the missing part of the tectum. They concluded that a fixed system of place specificities determined the terminal positions of regenerating optic fibers in the tectum of adult goldfish.

Soon after I entered Sperry's laboratory at Caltech, Gaze and Sharma (1970) reported an unexpected finding: when the caudal half of the goldfish tectum was ablated, the visual projection from the whole retina became compressed onto the remaining rostral hemitectum. They attributed the apparent contradiction between their result and that of Jacobson and Gaze (1965) to differences between the rostrocaudal and medolateral axes in the reinnervation of the tectum by regenerating optic fibers. These two reports intrigued me, so I began similar experiments on the goldfish visual system.

First, I repeated Gaze and Sharma's (1970) experiment by carving out the caudal half of the tectum in adult goldfish. A few months later, the remaining rostral hemitectum was found to have accepted regenerating optic fibers not only from the appropriate temporal half of the retina, but also from the inappropriate nasal half, in a correct retinotopic order (Yoon 1971). This confirmed Gaze and Sharma's (1970) finding of the field compression along the rostrocaudal axis. Why should there be axial differences then? Would it be possible to induce a field compression along the mediolateral axis as well as the rostrocaudal axis in the same tectum? To answer this, I removed only the caudal part of the medial half of the tectum (instead of the entire medial half, as in the case of Jacobson and Gaze [1965]), so that I could compare the retinal projection onto the residual posterior quarter with that onto the intact rostral area of the tectum. This surgical procedure allowed the regenerating optic fibers to enter the tectum normally via the intact rostral fascicles. A few months later, the fish showed a compression of the reestablished retinotectal projection not only along the rostrocaudal axis, but also along the mediolateral axis of the tectum (Yoon 1971).

Next I wondered whether it would be possible to induce a field compression onto the rostral half of the tectum without destroying the caudal half. The whole tectum was split into the rostral and caudal halves by an extensive transverse incision and/or insertion of a mechanical barrier (Yoon 1972a). This surgical procedure prevented the optic fibers from reinnervating the caudal tectum. The fish showed later an orderly compression of visual projection from the whole retina onto the rostral half in the presence of the caudal half (devoid of optic fibers) of the "split" tectum. When the two halves of the split tectum were allowed to rejoin by removal or absorption of the mechanical barrier, the retinotectal projection gradually decompressed, reverting back to a more or less normal pattern. Finally, the caudal part of the rejoined tectum was excised in the same fish. A few months later, the retinotectal projection was found to have compressed, again (Yoon 1972a). These results indicate that the field compression is a reversible process.

Next, a mismatch was made between the retina and the tectum by ablating the temporal half of the retina combined with ablation of the caudal half of the tectum, which normally receives projection from the remaining nasal hemiretina. After such a complementary surgical operation, the visual projection from the nasal hemiretina was found to have been transposed onto the entire remaining extent of the inappropriate rostral hemitectum in correct retinotopic order (Yoon 1972b).

"Systems-matching" hypothesis versus "topographic-regulation" hypothesis

The results of retinotectal size-disparity experiments in adult goldfish indicate that the various reorganizations of retinotectal projection such as the field compression (Gaze and Sharma 1970; Yoon 1971, 1972a), the field expansion (Yoon 1972b; Schmidt, Cicetone, and Easter 1978), and the field transposition (Yoon 1972b) cannot be accounted by the unmodifiable place-rigid chemoaffinity factors as suggested by Attardi and Sperry (1963) and Jacobson and Gaze (1965). To explain the plastic reorganizations of retinotectal projection, Gaze and Keating (1972) proposed to replace the chemoaffinity hypothesis with a radically new "systems-matching" hypothesis for the establishment of retinotopic order. The latter hypothesis assumes that the pattern of the retinotectal projection is primarily determined by competitive interactions between the ingrowing optic fibers; they make deployment of their presynaptic terminals in the tectum according to the relative positions of their retinal origins. In contrast, the postsynaptic tectal neurones are regarded as indiscriminate "passive receiver" (*my term*) of incoming optic fibers; they neither possess any differential affinities for intercellular recognition nor preferentially select any particular set of optic fibers for synaptic contacts. Thus, the optic fibers, whether originating from a whole or from a partial retina, just occupy whatever tectal space is available in a normal, compressed, expanded, or transposed pattern in correct retinotopic order.

The reorganization of retinotectal projection, resulting from readjustment of a size disparity between the retina and the tectum, may also be regarded as a "topographic regulation" analogous to the morphogenetic regulation of embryos induced by a similar surgical manipulation in a "Defect-type" experiment. To remove a rigid unmodifiability from the chemoaffinity hypothesis, I proposed the following modification (Yoon 1971, 1972a, 1972b). Partial ablation of the tectum or of the retina activates a latent regulative mechanism with respect to the topographic differentiation of individual neurones in the remaining part. The differential affinities of the remaining neurones become respecified in original topographic order by the regulative mechanism, so that these neurones acquire a new complete set of differential affinities in accord with their new relative positions with respect to the boundaries of the remaining part of the tectum or of the retina. Thus, following ablation of the caudal hemitectum, topographic regulation of the rostral hemitectum enables it to accommodate the complete set of optic fibers coming from the whole retina in a correct retinotopic order, albeit in a compressed array.

These two interpretations hold radically opposite views on the role of the optic tectum in the formation of retinotectal projection. The systems-matching hypothesis assumes that the optic tectum is a mere passive receiver submissive to the overrunning optic fibers. In contrast, the topographic-regulation hypothesis assumes that the optic tectum is an "active accommodator" that participates in the mutual selection between the presynaptic terminals of optic fibers and their appropriate postsynaptic visual neurones as postulated by the chemoaffinity hypothesis.

Is the optic tectum a passive receiver or an active accommodator of optic fibers? To answer this, I moved from the defect-type size disparity experiments to the "recombination-type" reimplantation experiments, pioneered by Hans Spemann at the turn of this century (Spemann 1906, 1912, 1938; see Chapter 2, this volume).

Tectal reimplantation after rotation or inversion

When a square piece of tectal tissue is dissected free (Figure 4.1A), rotated 90° counterclockwise about the dorsoventral axis, and then reimplanted to the same tectum (Figure 4.1B), occasionally the reimplanted tectal tissue survives such a drastic surgical manipulation and remains in place between the intact rostral and caudal parts of the same tectum (Figure 4.2, *left*). The trajectories of regener-

ating optic fibers within the tectum (traced by autoradiographic methods) reveal that the optic fibers have invaded the reimplanted tectal tissue in a systematic way. A group of the regenerating optic fibers dipped down along the cliff at the rostral edge (due to an inadvert dislocation of the horizontal layers of the reimplant from their normal level in the intact rostral tectum) and crossed the gap between the intact rostral and the reimplanted tissues. These optic fibers selectively occupied the layer of their usual passage (*the stratum opticum*) and the layer of their usual termination (*the stratum fibrosum et griseum superficiale*) within the reimplanted tectal tissue (Figure 4.2, *left*). This result suggests that the growing tips of regenerating optic fibers are able to discriminate different horizontal layers of the displaced tectal reimplant and select the appropriate layers.

How would these incoming optic fibers distribute their terminals within the 90° rotated tectal reimplant? If the optic tectum were an indiscriminate "passive receiver" submissive to any invading optic fibers, then the previous rotation of a tectal piece should not make any difference in the pattern of deployment of optic-fiber terminals from that of a normal fish. The actual pattern of the reestablished retinotectal projection, however, is far from normal, as shown in Figure 4.2, *right*. It reveals a corresponding 90° rotation within the reimplanted area of the tectum. A similar localized 180° rotation was also found in the restored retinotectal projection following reimplantation of a 180° rotated tectal tissue in adult goldfish (Yoon 1973, 1975, 1977). The ingrowing optic fibers must have recognized that a part of the tectum had been rotated and redistributed its terminals throughout the reimplanted tectal tissue according to its original orientation in the intact tectum.

These results indicate that the optic tectum of adult goldfish is *not* a passive receiver, but a discriminating *active accommodator* of ingrowing optic fibers (Yoon 1973, 1975, 1977). Throughout its extent, the tectal tissue must possess a persistent property that can direct the ingrowing optic fibers to redistribute their terminals in accordance with its original orientation. The persistence of such a property in spite of local rotation of tectal reimplants in-

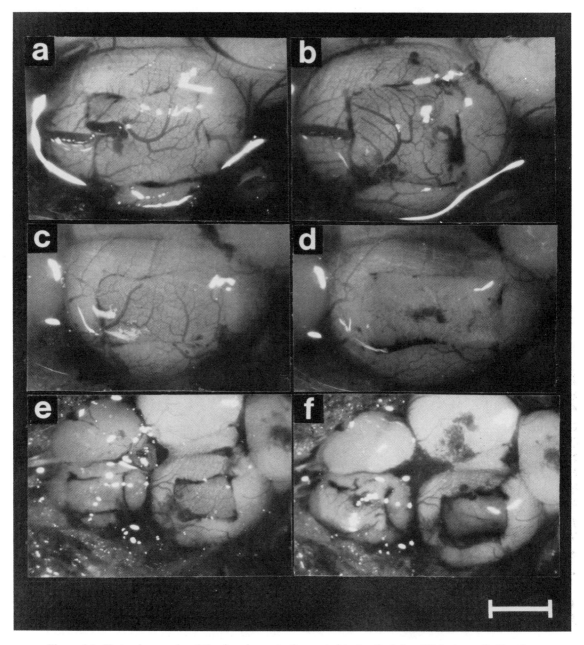

Figure 4.1. Photomicrographs of the dorsal aspect of operated tecta of adult goldfish, immediately after surgical manipulations. **(A)** A square piece of tectal tissue was excised at the central zone of the left tectum. **(B)** The dissected tectal piece was rotated by 90° counterclockwise about the dorsoventral axis and then reimplanted into the same tectum. **(C)** A rectangular piece of tectal tissue was excised at the central zone of the left tectum. **(D)** The tectal piece was inverted by 180° rotation about the mediolateral axis and then reimplanted upside down into the same tectum. The ventral surface of the inverted tectal tissue was exposed to the dorsal view. **(E)** A piece of the forebrain tissue was excised in the central zone of the left forebrain and a matching piece of tectal tissue was excised in the left tectum. **(F)** Both pieces were rotated 180° about the dorsoventral axis and the forebrain piece was transplanted into the tectum and the tectal piece into the forebrain, reciprocally. The calibration scale is 1mm for **(A)**–**(D)** and 1.6 mm for **(E)** and **(F)**.

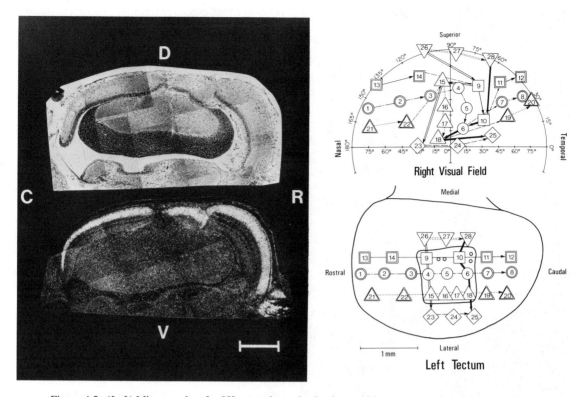

Figure 4.2. *(Left)* Micrographs of a 90° rotated tectal reimplant within an operated optic tectum. The upper micrograph shows a parasagittal section, stained by the Bodian method. The lower micrograph shows a dark field view of the autoradiogram of another parasagittal section, which was about 70 μm lateral to the upper section. R: rostral; C: caudal; D: dorsal; and V: ventral. The calibration scale is 0.5 mm. *(Right)* Reestablished retinotectal projection mapped 435 days after reimplantation of a square piece of tectal tissue following a 90° counterclockwise rotation about the dorsoventral axis. The numbers marked on the enlarged drawing of the tectum indicate the loci of microelectrodes on the dorsal surface of the tectum in the order of recording visual responses. The numbers marked on the perimetric chart show the positions of the corresponding receptive fields in the contralateral visual field for the experimental points on the dorsal tectum. The points marked by open circles gave no responses. (From Yoon 1975, p. 145.)

dicates that the optic tectum should be regarded as a topographically polarized system, composed of an unknown number of individually polarized subsystems, or *ensembles,* of visual neurones. In a normal tectum, the individual polarities of these ensembles of tectal neurones are coherently aligned.

The optic tectum of the goldfish has a very complex and delicate cytoarchitecture built by various types of cells numbering in the millions (Figure 4.3). Suppose we dissect out a rectangular piece of tectal tissue (Figure 4.1C), invert its entire laminar structure, and reimplant it to the same tectum upside down (Figure 4.1D). Such reimplantation of an inverted tectal tissue

will result in drastic discontinuities in the cytoarchitecture as well as in the topographic orientation of the tectum. Would the regenerating optic fibers recognize such changes in the operated tectum? Figure 4.4, *left,* shows an example of such an inverted tectal reimplant, which survived in place between the intact rostral and caudal parts of the tectum. The regenerating optic fibers swerved at the edge of the intact rostral tectum and dipped down along the cliff at the interface between the inverted reimplant and the intact part of the tectum. These optic fibers occupied only the deeper regions (near the optic ventricle) within the inverted tectal tissue, which corresponded to the

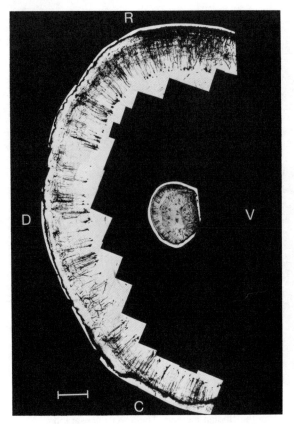

Figure 4.3. Micrograph of a parasagittal section of the optic tectum of a normal goldfish, stained by the rapid Golgi method. Calibration scale is 250 μm for the montage. R: rostral; C: caudal; D: dorsal; and V: ventral. The smaller micrograph shows an entire parasagittal section of the midbrain, stained by the Golgi method.

layers of their usual passage and termination in the superficial regions of the normal tectal tissue. The tectal cells within the reimplant remained upside down, retaining more or less normal branching patterns of their dendritic processes within the inverted cytoarchitecture of the tectal tissue (Figure 4.4, *right*).

How would the ingrowing optic fibers distribute their terminals within the inverted tectal tissue? Figure 4.5 shows a map of the restored retinotectal projection following inversion of a dissected tectal laminae by 180° rotation about the mediolateral axis. It indicates that the restored visual projection onto the inverted tectal reimplant is organized in a reverse retinotopic order along the rostrocaudal axis, whereas it is normal along the mediolateral axis. Thus, in spite of such a drastic manipulations as an in-

version of its cytoarchitecture, the reimplanted tectal tissue retains its original topographic polarity. The ingrowing optic fibers redistribute their terminals within the inverted tectal tissue to conform with its original orientation in the intact tectum.

Reciprocal transplantation between the tectum and the forebrain

What cytological factors have endowed the tectal tissue with such a persistent topographic polarity? Do other parts of the brain also possess such topographic properties that will influence the pattern of terminal distribution of ingrowing optic fibers? Let us suppose that a portion of the tectum is replaced by a similar piece of the forebrain tissue following a reciprocal transplantation after 180° rotation (Figures 4.1E and 4.1F). Can regenerating optic fibers distinguish the transplanted forebrain tissue from their normal target tectal tissue? Figure 4.6 shows an example of such a reciprocal transplantation experiment. The transplanted forebrain tissue has adhered to the intact parts of the tectum remarkably well at both the rostral and caudal interfaces. It also retains a part of the pineal body, which, having been accidentally transplanted with the forebrain tissue at the rostral interface, serves as a marker. The forebrain transplant appears to interfuse harmoniously with the surrounding tectal tissue. In spite of this healthy appearance, however, the regenerating optic fibers avoided invading the forebrain tissue. They bypassed the interfused forebrain tissue in a dramatic way. Some of the regenerating optic fibers near the rostral interface abruptly dipped down toward the optic ventricle and then coursed beneath the transplant toward their target zones in the caudal part of the operated tectum, as shown in the autoradiograph of Figure 4.6. The selective avoidance of either the forebrain transplant or a cerebellar transplant (Yoon 1979) by regenerating optic fibers contrasts with their consistent invasion into a rotated or inverted tectal reimplant, and with their orderly redistribution within the tectal tissue according to its original orientation. These results suggest that the regenerating optic fibers are continuously interacting with their cellular environments. The advancing tips of their

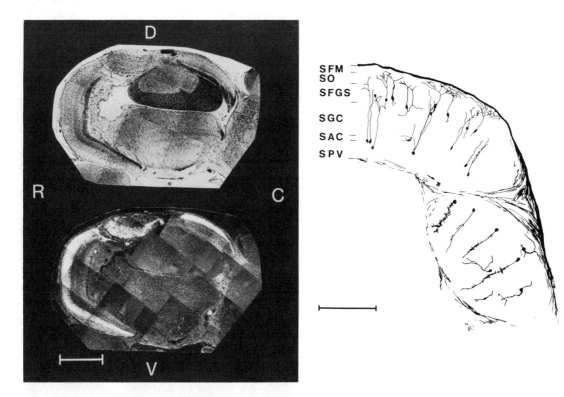

Figure 4.4. *(Left)* Micrographs of an inverted tectal reimplant within the tectum. The upper micrograph shows a parasagittal section, stained by the Bodian method. The lower micrograph shows a dark field view of the autoradiogram of another parasagittal section, which was about 70 μm lateral to the upper section. R: rostral; C: caudal; D: dorsal; and V: ventral. Calibration scale is 0.5 mm. *(Right)* Camera lucida drawing of individual cells in an operated tectum with an inverted reimplant. The upper area shows a portion of the intact rostral tectum and the lower area shows the remaining part of the inverted tectal tissue that underwent a partial degeneration. Calibration scale is 250 μm.

growth cones search for appropriate substrates to grow into, selectively choose the appropriate layer within the tectal tissue, actively avoid an interposed nonvisual neural tissue (e.g., forebrain or cerebellum), and eventually find their appropriate target neurones in the tectum.

Retention of topographic addresses and topographic polarity by reciprocally translocated and rotated tectal reimplants

Reimplantation of a single piece of tectal tissue has revealed that the tectal piece possesses an orientation property, *topographic polarity,* and that it retains the original topographic polarity regardless of whether it has been rotated or inverted. Would a piece of tectal tissue also possess a positional property, or *topographic address,* indicative of its relative position (rather than its orientation) within the

whole tectum? To accommodate the results of tectal-reimplantation experiments, Hope, Hammond, and Gaze (1976) proposed the "arrow model," which assumes that a piece of tectal tissue provides the ingrowing optic fibers with orientation information, but it does not possess any information about its relative position in the tectum. The result of their own experiment (Hope et al. 1976), however, did not support the latter assumption.

To test the possibility that a piece of tectal tissue possesses a topographic address in addition to its topographic polarity, I repeated and extended the reciprocal translocation experiment of Hope et al., as shown in Figure 4.7. Two similar well-separated pieces of tectal tissue were dissected and reciprocally translocated from one site to another within the same tectum along the rostrocaudal axis (Figures 4.7A and 4.7B) and the mediolateral axis (Fig-

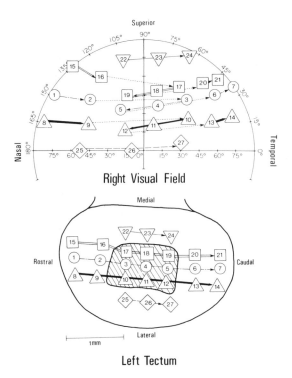

Right Visual Field

Left Tectum

Figure 4.5. Restored visual projection onto the inverted tectal reimplant. The map was obtained 397 days after reimplantation of the inverted tectal tissue along the same mediolateral axis of the tectum. The right optic nerve was also sectioned. (From Yoon 1976a, p. 509.)

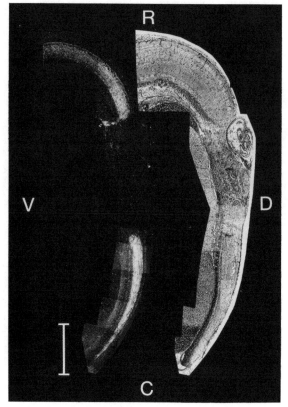

Figure 4.6. Micrographs of a transplanted forebrain tissue within an operated optic tectum. The brain was fixed three months after transplantation of an 180° rotated forebrain tissue into the left tectum, as shown in Figure 4.1(**E**) and 4.1(**F**). The micrograph on the right shows a parasagittal section, stained by the Bodian method. The transplanted forebrain tissue appeared to interfuse harmoniously with the surrounding tectal tissues. It also retained a part of the pineal body that had been accidentally transplanted with the forebrain tissue at the interface between the rostral tectum and the forebrain transplant. The micrograph on the left shows a dark field view of the autoradiogram of another parasagittal section that was about 120 μm medial to the section on the right. R: rostral; C: caudal; D: dorsal; and V: ventral. The calibration scale is 0.5 mm.

ures 4.7C and 4.7D) without rotation. If these tectal pieces did not possess any information about their relative positions, then such reciprocal translocations should not make any difference to the invading optic fibers, and, thus, a normal pattern of retinotectal projection is expected. On the contrary, however, the actual pattern of reestablished visual projection onto the operated tectum is far from normal, as shown in Figure 4.8. It shows corresponding nasotemporal translocations in the restored visual projection onto the rostocaudally translocated reimplants in the operated tectum. This indicates that ingrowing optic fibers are able to recognize the translocation of these two tectal pieces and selectively terminate at their original target zones despite their displacement in the tectum. Similar results (Yoon 1980) were obtained following a reciprocal translocation along the mediolateral axis and also in the cases where 180° rotation of tectal reimplants were

combined with their reciprocal translocation (Figures 4.7E–4.7F).

In the course of many years of work on this project, I came across an extraordinary case of an unintended experiment. One of the mediolaterally translocated tectal pieces detached from its intended site of reimplantation and, instead, adhered to an ectopic position at the rostrolateral edge of the tectum (Figure 4.9, *left* and *right*). This misplaced tectal piece was

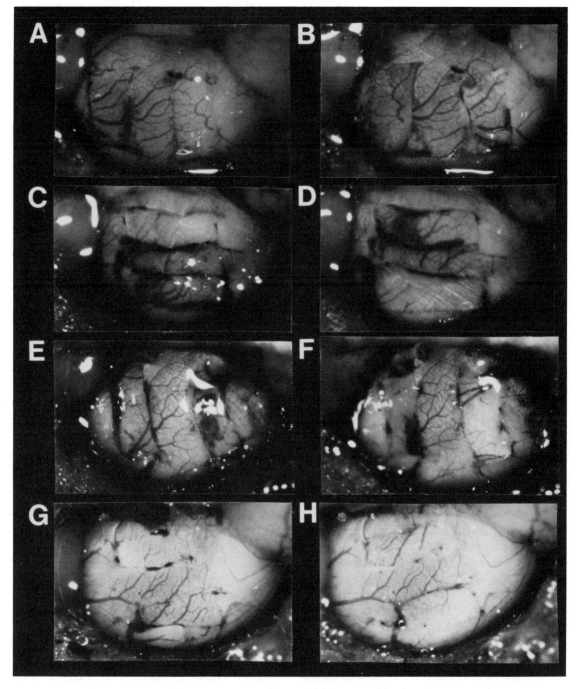

Figure 4.7. Microphotographs of the dorsal aspect of operated tecta of adult goldfish, immediately after surgical manipulations. (**A** and **E**) Two elongated rectangular pieces of the tectum were excised at the rostral and the caudal zones of the tectum. (**B**) A reciprocal translocation between the dissected tectal pieces along the rostrocaudal axis in normal orientations. (**C** and **G**) Two elongated tectal pieces were excised at the medial and the lateral zones of the tectum. (**D**) Reciprocal translocation between the two excised pieces along the mediolateral axis in normal orientation. (**F**) Reciprocal translocation of the two tectal reimplants along the rostrocaudal axis after 180° rotations about the dorsoventral axis. (**H**) Reciprocal translocation of the two tectal reimplants along the mediolateral axis after 180° rotations about the dorsoventral axis. (From Yoon 1980.)

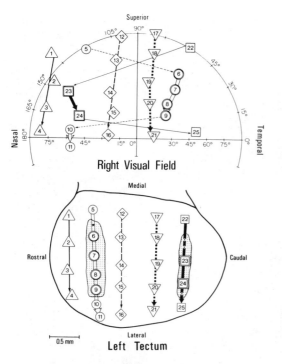

Superior

Right Visual Field

Medial

Rostral

Caudal

Lateral

0.5 mm

Left Tectum

Figure 4.8. Reestablished retinotectal projection mapped 174 days after rostrocaudal translocation of two tectal reimplants in normal orientations. The positions from which recordings were made within each tectal reimplant (nos. 6–9, connected by an open arrow; and nos. 23 and 24, connected by a solid arrow) show corresponding reciprocal transpositions of their receptive fields along the nasotemporal axis. (From Yoon 1980.)

found to have attracted a group of regenerating optic fibers that escaped the tectum proper by piercing through the pial membrane at the juncture to invade the ectopic tectal slab, as shown in Figure 4.9, *left*. The pattern of reestablished visual projection onto this misplaced tectal tissue suggests that its provenance is the medial zone of the operated tectum (Figure 4.9, *right*). This indicates that after their initial invasion into the tectum, regenerating optic fibers are not obligated to maintain their retinotopic neighborhood relations, but are able to explore a very wide range of the tectum in search of their appropriate target zones.

These results reveal that translocated pieces of tectal tissue retain their respective addresses, indicative of their original positions in the tectum as well as their polarity, indicative of their normal orientation, with respect to their selective reinnervation by particular groups of optic fibers. Thus, the optic tectum of adult goldfish is not only a *topographically polarized* system, but also a *topographically differentiated* system, composed of a number of discrete and individually polarized subsystems, or ensembles, of visual neurones (Yoon 1980). A unitary ensemble of tectal neurones carries its own topographic address, which is responsible for a mutual selection between the presynaptic terminals of ingrowing optic fibers and their appropriate postsynaptic visual neurones of the tectum in a coherent topographic order. This is exactly what Roger Sperry envisaged long ago!

Regulative modification of topographic addresses in accord with the original topographic polarity

How could we bring the plastic reorganizations of retinotectal projection (e.g., the field compression) into harmony with the retention of an apparently rigid topographic polarity in the visual pathway of adult goldfish? First, we should note that the two different phenomena are *not* so contradictory as the adjectives "plastic" and "rigid" may imply. In fact, they are compatible as follows: the reestablishment of retinotectal projection following a partial ablation of the tectum, the retina, or both occurs in a systematic way such that the topographic polarities of both the retinal tissue and the tectal tissue remain rigidly unchanged (Gaze and Sharma 1970; Yoon 1971, 1972a, 1972b). One further experiment suggests itself. Would it be possible to induce a field compression onto a rotated tectal reimplant that retains its original topographic polarity? Figure 4.10 shows such an experiment, which combines the recombination-type and the defect-type manipulations. A piece of tectal tissue was dissected free (Figure 4.10A) and reimplanted after 90° rotation (Figure 4.10B). The restored visual projection onto the reimplanted area showed later a corresponding 90° rotation (Figure 4.11, *left*. Immediately after the first mapping experiment, the caudal half of the operated tectum, including the posterior half of the 90° rotated tectal reimplant was excised (Figures 4.10C and 4.10D). Several months after the latter surgery, the reestablished visual projec-

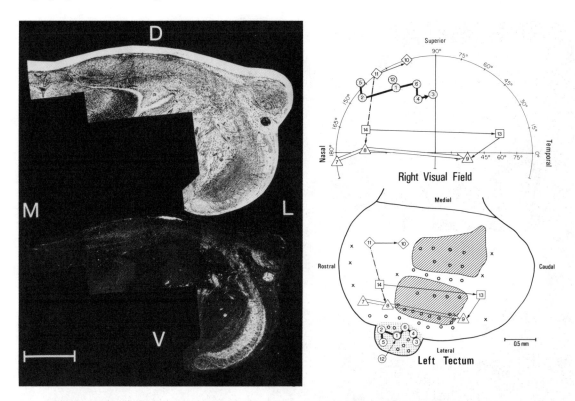

Figure 4.9. (*Left*) The upper micrograph shows a transverse section of the same operated tectum as shown in Figure 4.9, *right,* stained by the Bodian method. Some regenerating optic fibers pierced through the pial membrane of the tectum and eventually invaded the ectopic tectal tissue. The lower autoradiogram shows an adjacent section of the same tectum. ^{3}H labeling of the tectum was obtained by an intraocular injection of 7 μCi of L-[^{3}H]proline into the right eye for 10.5 hours. The dark-field micrograph indicates that the ectopic tectal tissue is labeled by [^{3}H]proline, transported from the eye along those optic fibers that have selectively regenerated into this misplaced tectal tissue. D: dorsal; V: ventral; M: medial; and L: lateral. The calibration scale is 500 μm. (*Right*) Visual projection reestablished to an ectopic tectal tissue mapped 193 days after the mediolateral translocation of two tectal reimplants in normal orientations. One of the reimplants detached from the intended reimplantation site and, instead, adhered to the tectum at an ectopic position (see Figure 4.9, *left*). The receptive fields of the recording positions on the ectopic tectal piece (nos. 5, 2, 1, 12, 5, 4, and 3; connected by a solid arrow) were located in the nasosuperior zone of the visual field. This suggests that the ectopic tectal piece came from the medial zone of the operated tectum. Recording position no. 12 is a repeated mapping for position no. 1 within the ectopic tectal tissue (about 3 hours later). (From Yoon 1980.)

tion onto the remaining part of the halved tectal reimplant revealed that a field compression occurred in a systematic way that preserved the original topographic polarity of the 90° rotated tectal reimplant, as shown in Figure 4.11, *right*. Similar results were also observed following different combinations of the recombination and defect types of surgical manipulations in adult goldfish (Yoon 1977).

These findings strongly suggest that the value of topographic address of a unitary en-

semble of tectal neurones may be modified according to its new relative position within the remaining tectal boundary following a partial ablation. Such modification of the topographic address of an ensemble of visual neurones progresses gradually (Yoon 1976b) in accord with the directive influence of its own original topographic polarity, as postulated by the topographic-regulation hypothesis (Yoon 1971, 1972a, 1972b, 1976b, 1977, 1980).

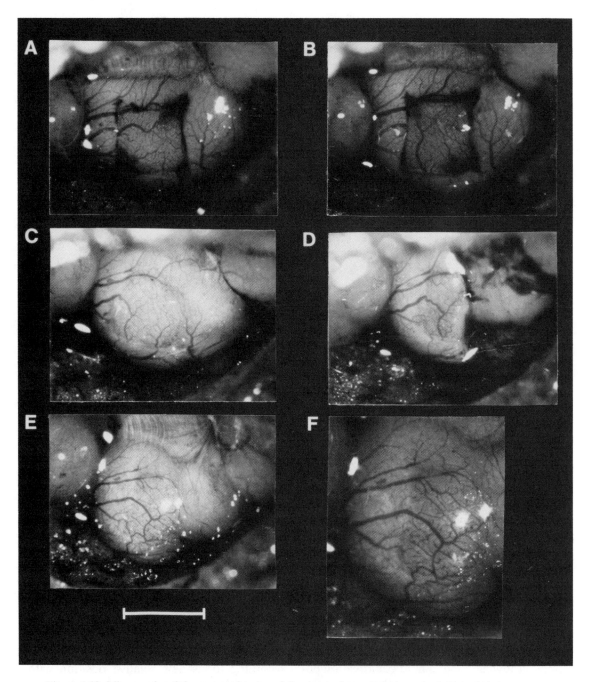

Figure 4.10. Micrographs of the operated tectum following various surgical manipulations. (**A**) A square piece of the tectal tissue was dissected from the central one of the whole left tectum. (**B**) The dissected tectal tissue was lifted intact and then reimplanted to the same tectum after a 90° counterclockwise rotation around the dorsoventral axis. (**C**) The operated whole tectum, reexposed for a mapping experiment, 85 days after the 90° rotated tectal reimplantation. (**D**) The caudal half of the same operated tectum, including the posterior half of the reimplanted area, was excised immediately after the first mapping experiment in (**C**). (**E**) The operated rostral half-tectum, which contains the remaining part of the 90° rotated reimplant. The brain was reexposed for a second mapping experiment 77 days after excision of the caudal tectum (162 days after the 90° rotated reimplantation) in the same fish. (**F**) The operated half-tectum with the 90° rotated tectal reimplant at a higher magnification. The reimplanted tectal tissue became well-healed and gave brisk visual responses in this fish. The calibration scale is 1.6 mm for (**A**)–(**E**) and 1 mm for (**F**). (From Yoon 1977.)

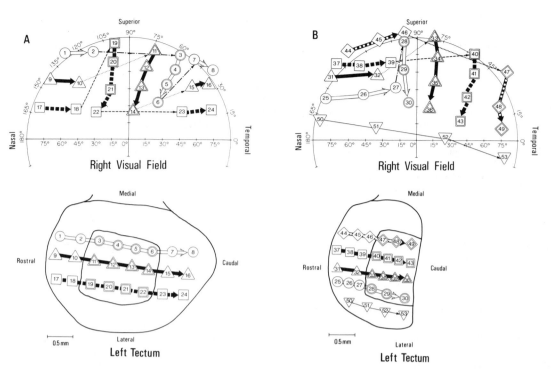

Figure 4.11. Induction of a field compression within a halved tectal reimplant. The *left* map was made 85 days after reimplantation of the 90° rotated tectal issue to the same whole tectum. The reestablished retinotectal projections show a corresponding localized 90° rotation within the replanted area. The first mapping experiment was immediately followed by excision of the caudal half of the same tectum, including the posterior part of the 90° rotated reimplant, as shown in Figures 4.10E and 4.10F. On the *right* is a second map obtained from the fish 77 days after excision of the caudal part of the previously operated tectum. The map shows that field compressions occurred in the remaining part of the halved tectal reimplant as well as in the surrounding intact area of the same half-tectum. (From Yoon 1977.)

Acknowledgments

I thank Frank Baker and Jim Stevenson for their collaboration, and Myonghae Yoon for comments on the manuscript. The research was supported by grants from the Medical Research Council and from the Natural Sciences and Engineering Research Council of Canada.

References

Attardi, D. G., and R. W. Sperry. 1963. Preferential selection of central pathways by regenerating optic fibers. *Exp. Neurol.* 7: 46–64.

Gaze, R. M., and M. J. Keating. 1972. The visual system and "neuronal specificity." *Nature (London)* 237: 375–8.

Gaze, R. M., and S. C. Sharma. 1970. Axial differences in the reinnervation of goldfish optic tectum by regenerating optic fibres. *Exp. Brain Res.* 10: 171–81.

Hope, R. A., B. J. Hammond, and R. M. Gaze. 1976. The arrow model: Retinotectal specificity and map formation in the goldfish visual system. *Proc. Roy. Soc. London, Ser. B* 194: 447–66.

Jacobson, M., and R. M. Gaze. 1965. Selection of appropriate tectal connections by regenerating optic nerve fibers in adult goldfish. *Exp. Neurol.* 13: 428–30.

Matthey, R. 1925. Recuperation de la vue apres resection des nerfs optiques chez le triton. *Cont. Rend. Soc. Biol.* 93: 904–6.

–1926. La Greffe de l'oeil. I. Etude histologique sur la greffe de l'oeil chez la larve de Salemandre (*Salamandre maculosa*). *Rev. Suisse Zool.* 33: 327–34.

Schmidt, J. T., C. M. Cicetone, and S. S. Easter. 1978. Expansion of the half-retinal projection to the tectum in goldfish: An electrophysiological and anatomical study. *J. Comp. Neurol.* 177: 257–78.

Spemann, H. 1906. Uber eine neue Methode der embryonalen Transplantation. *Ver. dt. Zool. Ges.* 16: 195–202.

–1912. Uber die Entwicklung umgedrehter Hirnteile bie

Amphibien-embryonen. *Zool. Jarb. (Suppl. 15)* 3: 1–48.

–1938. *Embryonic Development and Induction.* Yale University Press, New Haven (CT).

Sperry, R. W. 1943a. Effect of 180 degree rotation of the retinal field on visuomotor coordination. *J. Exp. Zool.* 92: 263–79.

–1943b. Visuomotor coordination in the newt (*Triturus viridescens*) after regeneration of the optic nerves. *J. Comp. Neurol.* 79: 33–55.

–1944. Optic nerve regeneration with return of vision in anurans. *J. Neurophysiol.* 7: 57–69.

–1945. Restoration of vision after crossing of optic nerves and after contralateral transplantation of eye. *J. Neurophysiol.* 8: 15–28.

–1948. Patterning of central synapses in regeneration of the optic nerve in teleosts. *Physiol. Zool.* 21: 351–61.

–1951. Regulative factors in the orderly growth of neural circuits. *Growth Symp.* 10: 63–87.

–1963. Chemoaffinity in the orderly growth of nerve fiber patterns and connections. *Proc. Natl. Acad. Sci. USA* 50: 703–10.

–1965. Embryogenesis of behavioral nerve nets. *In* R. L. Dehann and H. Ursprung (eds.) *Organogenesis,* Vol. 6. Holt, Rinehart and Winston, New York, pp. 161–85.

Stone, L., and I. Zaur. 1940. Reimplantation and transplantation of adult eyes in the salamander (*Triturus viridescens*) with return of vision. *J. Exp. Zool.* 85: 243–69.

Yoon, M. G. 1971. Reorganization of retinotectal projection following surgical operations on the optic tectum in goldfish. *Exp. Neurol.* 33: 395–411.

–1972a. Reversibility of the reorganization of retinotectal projection in goldfish. *Exp. Neurol.* 35: 565–77.

–1972b. Transposition of the visual projection from the nasal hemiretina onto the foreign rostral zone of the optic tectum in goldfish. *Exp. Neurol.* 37: 451–62.

–1973. Retention of the original topographic polarity by the 180° rotated tectal reimplant in young adult goldfish. *J. Physiol.* 233: 575–88.

–1975. Re-adjustment of retinotectal projection following reimplantation of a rotated or inverted tectal tissue in adult goldfish. *J. Physiol.* 252: 137–58.

–(1976a). Topograhic polarity of the optic tectum studies by reimplantation of the tectal tissue in adult goldfish. *"The Synapse." Cold Spring Harbor Symp. Quant. Biol.* 40: 503–19.

–1976b. Progress of topographic regulation of the visual projection in the halved optic tectum of adult goldfish. *J. Physiol.* 257: 621–43.

–1977. Induction of compression in the re-established visual projections on to a rotated tectal reimplant that retains its original topographic polarity within the halved optic tectum of adult goldfish. *J. Physiol.* 264: 379–410.

–1979. Reciprocal transplantations between the optic tectum and the cerebellum in adult goldfish. *J. Physiol.* 288: 211–25.

–1980. Retention of topographic addresses by reciprocally translocated tectal re-implants in adult goldfish. *J. Physiol.* 308: 197–215.

5 The case for chemoaffinity in the retinotectal system: Recent studies

Ronald L. Meyer

Developmental Biology Center
and
Department of Developmental and Cell Biology
University of California, Irvine

Introduction

From the time of Sperry's seminal work in the early 1940s, the development of the nervous system has been favored by an ever increasing number of investigators. After forty years, one might imagine that the original questions asked by Sperry would have long been settled. However, even a cursory reading of the literature reveals authors posing some of the same questions that Sperry asked and making lengthy discussions filled with arguments and counterarguments over the correct answers. We still ask the following questions: How do neurons become so precisely interconnected in development? Do nerve cells have unique chemical labels that direct axonal growth? Is selective axonal growth attributable to the mechanical properties of the substrate? Is neural activity important for development of patterned connections? Sperry's early papers are often cited along with the most recent work. A reader of contemporary papers may be forgiven for taking the impression that little or no progress has been made in the past forty years and that the validity of Sperry's conclusions remains entirely unsettled. And yet this is far from the truth. A careful scrutiny reveals broad support for Sperry's major inference, the chemoaffinity hypothesis. The apparent uncertainty in the literature is, in many cases, a consequence of asking much narrower and sharply focused questions than those requiring attention in the 1940s. Today's questions frequently take for granted as true what was bold hypothesis then. That we can now ask these elaborate questions

is a measure of significant progress and a testimony to Sperry's contribution.

For a detailed history, the reader is referred to Chapter 2 in this volume. We need only make a brief summary to set the context for contemporary issues. Sperry came to two important conclusions in the 1940s. The first was that a normal pattern of interneural connectivity was essential for normal function. When fibers from a frog's eye were made to connect to the wrong side of the brain, the frog reacted to visual stimuli as if it existed on the other side (Sperry 1945). The animal never learned to correct this behavior and would have starved if left unaided. Sperry concluded that individual nerves carry specific information by virtue of the positions of their cells in the retina and that each nerve must be connected to the correct postsynaptic neuron for this information to be properly interpreted. This contradicted the then prevalent notion that neural connectivity could be disordered and yet mediate normal behavior through learning. Indeed, many thought that the orderly connectivity normally found in the nervous system was merely an accident of morphogenesis and that the animal still had to learn what these connections meant. Sperry disproved this in a long series of experiments in both mammals and lower vertebrates that showed that incorrect connections always lead to inappropriate behavior (Sperry 1951a). Today, the importance of orderly nerve connections for function is taken for granted.

The second conclusion reached by Sperry

was that nerve connections are guided by chemical affinities between neurons. This followed from the regeneration experiments in lower vertebrates in which orderly function was re-established. He reasoned that if the recovery of function could not be explained in terms of learning, then it must result from the reestablishment the right pattern of connections. For the case of optic-nerve regeneration in amphibia, Sperry inferred that optic fibers had regrown back to their original sites in the optic tectum. His most direct evidence at the time was obtained with visual perimetry testing in conjunction with small tectal lesions (Sperry 1944). In a normal frog, a localized lesion to the tectum produces a localized blind spot in visual space that can be assayed by moving a small lure through the frog's visual field. When Sperry repeated this analysis on a frog with a regenerated nerve, he found that tectal lesions produced a similar pattern of blind spots. He took this as further evidence that optic fibers had reformed the original retinotopic projection onto the tectum.

In 1940, the most widely accepted explanation for orderly nerve growth was Paul Weiss's mechanical guidance. Weiss (1934) had shown in tissue culture that growing neurites selectively follow mechanical channels in the substrate, and he generalized this to explain development and regeneration. However, Sperry was led to reject this explanation. He found that surgically scrambling fibers or re-routing fibers into abnormal entry points did not, as predicted from mechanical guidance, disrupt recovery of function. Sperry (1943, 1944, 1945, 1951a, 1951b) offered the alternative chemoaffinity explanation. He supposed that each retinal ganglion cell and each tectal cell was chemically differentiated according to their position in the retina or tectum. In effect, these cells possessed an address, or intrinsic label, that denoted their position within the retina or tectum. This address was thought to be acquired during development by position-dependent cellular differentiation, positional information in today's nomenclature (Wolpert 1969). Similar labels developed along the optic pathway. The growing fiber was postulated to selectively interact with the markers along the optic pathway and in the tectum such that its

growth was directed toward its appropriate tectal site. In effect, the axon homed in on its target by following a chemical scent trail.

Sperry explained that he envisioned the interaction between the axon and subtrate as a preferential one rather than all or nothing. An axon could have the capacity to form synaptic connections with a variety of inappropriate target sites within the tectum or beyond the tectum, but had specific preferences that usually led to the establishment of the correct connections. The interaction was also considered to be nonexclusive. Other factors could also guide fiber growth and determine connectivity. Mechanical guidance, initial position, time of axonal outgrowth, presence or absence of other fibers might still be significant, depending on the particular system and particular circumstances. These two characteristics of the original version of the chemoaffinity theory, its preferential and nonexclusive nature, are important to keep in mind. They have often been forgotten, and there has been considerable confusion over what chemoaffinity is or is not. I will refer to this original version of the theory as *preferential chemoaffinity*.

The conceptual development of the chemoaffinity hypothesis continued after this early formulation. Further evidence suggested the affinity might be so strong that "growing fibers become extremely selective about the chemical identity of other cells and fibers with which they will associate" (Sperry 1965). Perhaps the most important evidence was from the study of Attardi and Sperry (1963). They surgically removed half of the retina in a goldfish and then severed the optic nerve. Using a silver stain that they had modified to be heterochromic for regenerating fibers, they were able to visualize optic fibers directly. They found that fibers followed their original route through the optic pathway and selectively invaded the half of the tectum that corresponded to the intact half of the retina. Chemoaffinity seemed to be required to explain not only selective termination, but selectivity of pathway as well. They suggested "that specific chemical affinities govern neuronal synapsis . . . (and) the patterning of central fiber pathways." Selectivity was observed even in those cases where fibers grew past denervated regions of the tectum to get to their appropriate half. This and other evidence led Sperry to believe in "the presence of strong chemical selectivity" (Sperry 1965). He suggested, "Lasting functional hookups are established only with cells to which the growing fibers find themselves selectively matched by inherent chemical affinities" (Sperry 1965).

Wisely, Sperry did not conclude that the affinities were so strong that they precluded the formation of inappropriate connections under all conceivable experimental conditions. The strength and selectivity of the affinity remained empirical questions to be decided by experiment. The evidence available did not require absolute selectivity. After the Attardi and Sperry study, Sperry wrote, "We [Sperry and Arora] are currently trying to test the strength and nature of the selective growth forces in the optic system of fishes . . ." (Sperry 1965). Attardi and Sperry (1963) had recognized that "The well-demonstrated importance of mechanical factors is not to be minimized." The possible role of neural activity was also acknowledged. Speaking of learning and memory, he stated, "Furthermore, it remains an open question whether the effects of function . . . add or subtract any actual fiber structures or synaptic contacts to the established morphology" (Sperry 1965). Chemoaffinity was not presented as an exclusive explanation for the formation of functional nerve circuits.

Sperry's caution and his concept of a preferential and nonexclusive chemoaffinity seems to have been overlooked in many of the discussions in the ensuing decades. To many, chemoaffinity has come to mean an extremely strong and selective affinity that totally dominates fiber growth. Affinity is thought to rigidly specify connectivity so that a fiber can only connect with its appropriate target cell regardless of experimental conditions. If a fiber can be shown to form a connection to an incorrect target, demonstrating plasticity, then chemoaffinity is thereby disproven. If fiber growth is shown to be affected by processes other than an affinity, such as competition between fibers and mechanical guidance, then this constitutes a counterexample to chemoaffinity. This definition of the chemoaffinity hypothesis, here referred to as *rigid chemoaffinity*, has been widely held by those expecting to obtain disproof. In

consequence, much of the argument brought against chemoaffinity has validity only with reference to a rigid form of chemoaffinity.

The discussion will focus on the role of chemoaffinity for the generation of topographic order in the retinotectal projection. However, it is important to remember that some such selective principle as chemoaffinity is clearly involved in the formation of other features of the retinal projection. Growing fibers must locate the tectum and innervate it in preference to nonoptic sites. The reader should refer to Chapter 3 for a detailed discussion of this question. Suffice it to say that a variety of experiments strongly indicate chemoaffinity in this process. Optic fibers can be forced to enter the brain at a variety of abnormal sites and yet will locate and invade the tectum. Similar evidence has come from other systems such as the CNS of grasshoppers (Raper, Bastiani, and Goodman 1983) and the neuromuscular system of vertebrates (Landmesser 1980). Another aspect of organization that almost certainly requires a chemoaffinity coding is the sorting out of fibers according to response types. In frogs, the different types of ganglion cells reinnervate their characteristic layer of the tectum following regeneration (Maturana et al. 1959) and fish recover accurate color vision following nerve section (Arora and Sperry 1963).

Macrotopography in the visual projection

In considering how the visual projection transmits retinotopic information to the brain, it is useful to make a distinction between macrotopography, which specifies the polarity and gross organization of the projection, and fine topography, which specifies the precision of local topographic order. Anatomical structures of differing scale have different functions in vision and, as will be mentioned, there is the possibility that different processes might be involved. Here we shall consider the basic orientation of the whole retinal map in the visual projection.

An obvious and straightforward test that chemoaffinity determines macrotopography is to turn an eye upside down during development or during optic-nerve regeneration. Though not the first to perform this experiment, Sperry

(1944) was the first to secure the correct answer. He rotated eyes in adult amphibians and severed the optic nerve (see Figures 5.1, 5.2A, and 5.2B). Upon recovery, his animals behaved as if their visual world were rotated. From this behavior, Sperry inferred that fibers had reconnected to their original tectal position. This experiment has been repeated with electrophysiological measurements in amphibian embryos, where the eye rotations were done prior to outgrowth of optic fibers (Jacobson 1968; Hunt and Jacobson 1972, 1974; Gaze et al. 1979). As long as the rotations are not done so early and under conditions that evoke a regulative response in the eye bud, the result is always the same. The projection of a visual field is correspondingly rotated so that fibers project to their appropriate part of the tectum, making no compensation for eye rotation. The complementary experiment, leaving the eye in place and rotating the entire tectum, has been done in frog embyros to similar effect (Chung and Cooke 1978). Large rotations of the neural plate that included the prospective tectum and the adjacent diencephalon resulted in the development of antomically rotated tecta. The

maps recorded electrophysiologically in the postmetamorphic frogs were correspondingly rotated, again showing that fibers could find their matching part in the tectum in spite of the latter's abnormal position (Figure 5.2C). In some of the operated animals, tecta formed that were mirror-image duplicates across the anterior–posterior axis; the projection to each tectal field was again oriented in accordance with the anatomical polarity. These results from rotation experiments with the eye and tectum are clearly incompatible with simple versions of mechanical guidance, where optic fibers passively preserve their relative positions along the tract between the eye and tectum. As predicted from the chemoaffinity theory, optic fibers exhibit a capacity to actively orient to central cues, thereby generating an appropriately oriented projection.

It has been suggested that fibers may become correctly oriented in the optic tract in the region of the diencephalon and that this orientation of fibers can be passively preserved as they invade the tectum to yield an appropriately oriented projection. No chemoaffinity would be required in the tectal tissue (Straz-

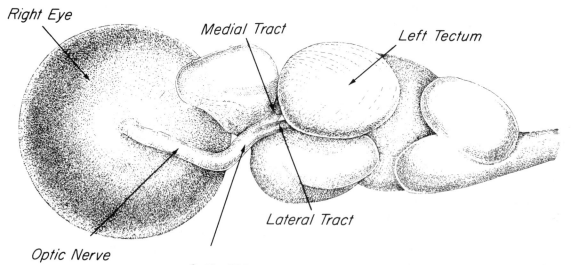

Figure 5.1. Left view of the brain and back of the right eye of a goldfish with the left eye removed. Ganglion cells, uniformly distributed across the retina, send fibers to the optic nerve, which crosses at the optic chiasma. Most fibers continue to the tectum, branching into medial and lateral tracts or brachia at the anterior end of the tectum.

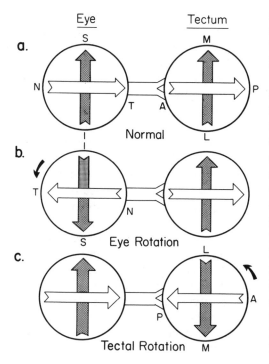

Eye   Tectum

a.   Normal

b.   Eye Rotation

c.   Tectal Rotation

Figure 5.2. (**A**) Schematic representation of the normal projection of the left eye onto the right tectum. The coordinates of the eye are presented in terms of the visual field so that the polarity arrows have the same direction in the retina and tectum. (**B**) The result of rotating an eye in development or in regeneration. (**C**) The projection resulting from rotation of the tectum and diencephalon in early development.

nicky and Gaze 1982; Fawcett and Gaze 1982). I will refer to this idea as *pathway-only cueing*. Another suggestion is that only the first few fibers that grow into the brain achieve appropriate orientation. Later fibers follow these pioneer fibers in a passive manner. This process relies on the spatiotemporal aspects of morphogenesis, called *morphogenetics* (Horder and Martin 1978), for the assembly of most of the projection. Various combinations of these and other ideas have been discussed.

On close scrutiny, these alternative hypotheses are found to require chemoaffinity guidance of proliferating nerve axons. Pathway-only cueing must postulate that optic fibers selectively respond to markers in the pathway. In essence, it requires minimum chemoaffinity that is confined to the optic tract. The morphogenetics hypothesis likewise requires the pioneer fibers to selectively orient to cues in both the pathway and target tissue. This is essentially chemoaffinity guidance that is limited to the initial group of fibers.

In fact, there is considerable evidence against both pathway-only cueing and pioneer fiber/morphogenetics. First, consider the case against the pioneer-fiber hypothesis. The most direct evidence against this concept is the oldest. It was shown in the classical studies with adult lower vertebrates that severed optic fibers will regenerate an orderly projection in spite of being surgically scrambled and growing in near synchrony with each other (Sperry 1943, 1944; Maturana et al. 1959; Gaze 1959). There is supposed to be an advantage for this pioneer-fiber explanation in development; the target lobe is close to the afferent neurons at the start of optic-nerve growth and this would reduce the navigation required from the pioneer fibers. However it has been shown a number of times by deplanting the eye rudiment that optic fibers can be forced to grow over a long circuitous route and yet will form a properly oriented projection (see Chapter 3, this volume).

It has also been possible to perturb the temporal aspects of development by surgically altering the eye rudiment *in situ*. In *Xenopus* embryos, one can remove half the eye bud and replace it with a fragment that is the mirror image of the remaining half of the eye (Gaze, Jacobson, and Szekely 1963; Straznicky, Gaze, and Keating 1974). In this way, double nasal, double temporal, and double ventral eyes have been constructed before outgrowth of optic fibers. These compound eyes, which are quite small at the time of surgery, grow like normal eyes by adding new ganglion cells to the retinal periphery (Straznicky and Tay 1977). If this morphogenetic parameter of circumferential growth is important in guiding fiber growth, then the projection formed by normal and compound eyes should all be similar. In fact, each eye forms a different projection that is predictable from the position-dependent properties of the retinal cells. Each half of the compound eye forms a map across the tectum with a polarity appropriate to the intrinsic polarity of the original eye fragments (Figure 5.3). Consequently, the pioneer fibers of first retinal ganglion cells come to project to very different

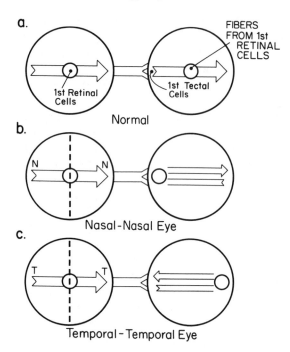

a.

FIBERS FROM 1st RETINAL CELLS

1st Retinal Cells

1st Tectal Cells

Normal

b.

N   N

Nasal-Nasal Eye

c.

T   T

Temporal-Temporal Eye

Figure 5.3. (**A**) Schematic representation of the normal relationship between retinal ganglion cells and the tectal innervation in the adult. The first ganglion cells reside in the central retina and project to the central tectum, but the first tectal cells are at the anterior end of the tectum. (**B**) Nasal-nasal compound eye of *Xenopus*. The first retinal ganglion cells project to the anterior end of the tectum. (**C**) Temporal-temporal compound eye. The first ganglion cells project to the posterior end of the tectum.

difficult to explain by assuming that later fibers follow earlier ones (Scholes 1979; Bunt 1982). In spite of considerable effort, a direct demonstration that sufficient order exists in the pathway to account for the projection in purely mechanical terms or time of growth has yet to appear.

Some of the preceding evidence is not easy to reconcile with pathway-only cueing either, and there is additional direct evidence against this model. It should be recognized from the start that existence of some pathway cueing is perfectly compatible with chemoaffinity. Sperry, himself, suggested in more recent studies that chemoaffinity cues must lie along the pathway of growing fibers as well as in the target tissue (Sperry 1963, 1965). He provided some of the first experimental evidence for pathway cueing by showing that fibers from retinal fragments prefer their appropriate half of the optic tract (Attardi and Sperry 1963). The issue is whether pathway cueing is a sufficient explanation for the macrotopography of the retinotectal projection.

Regeneration studies provide three kinds of evidence against pathway-only cueing. The first comes from simply severing the nerve and analyzing the path followed by the regenerated fibers (Udin 1978; Meyer 1980; Cook 1982). It is quite clear from studies with a variety of techniques that optic fibers invade the tectum in considerable disorder and yet eventually form an orderly projection. Some fibers follow the wrong half of the optic tract into the tectum, grow for long distances through the wrong half of the tectum, and then follow an unusual path to reach their correct locus. These fibers are not passively preserving their pathway order; they are making active choices within the tectum after having penetrated its margins in disorder.

The second type of evidence comes from experiments in which fibers from a selected part of the retina are made to regenerate into a whole vacant tectum (Figure 5.4). When part of the retina is removed and the optic nerve is crushed, fibers preferentially invade their appropriate sector of the tectum (Attardi and Sperry 1963; Meyer 1975; Sturmer 1981). In the course of regrowth, fibers are made to traverse past an inappropriate part of the tectum

tectal regions in the different eyes. First fibers eventually project to the central tectum in normal eyes (Figure 5.3A), to the anterior end of the tectum in double nasal eyes (Figure 5.3B), to the posterior end of the tectum in double temporal eyes (Figure 5.3C), and to the ventral edge of the tectum in double ventral eyes (not shown). These results are incompatible with the pioneer-fiber idea.

The pioneer-fiber hypothesis predicts that there should be a high degree of interfiber order within the optic pathway. While some early work had indicated such order might exist, most recent work gives a mixed picture. In several species, there is rather confused ordering in the optic nerve (Fawcett 1981; Scalia and Arango 1983). In others, fibers are well ordered in the nerve, but then subsequently rearrange themselves central to the chiasm in a manner

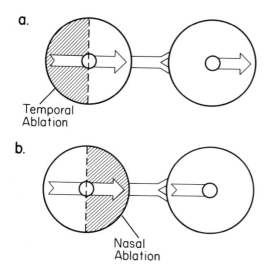

Figure 5.4. Schematic representation of the selective innervation of the tectum following retinal ablation in development and following regeneration. (A) With nasal ablation, fibers must bypass the anterior tectum to innervate the posterior half. (B) With temporal ablation, fibers stop at the anterior half of the tectum.

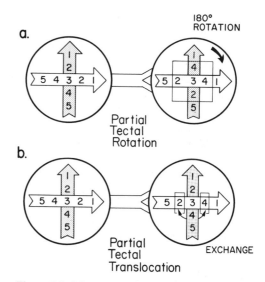

Figure 5.5. Schematic results of (A) rotation of part of the tectum and (B) translocation of part of the tectum in adult goldfish and frogs, with or without sectioning the optic nerve. The projection is correspondingly (A) rotated or (B) translocated.

to reach their appropriate position. Such by-passing directly implicates tectal cueing. More recently, it has been possible to surgically redirect selected fractions of optic fibers into specific regions of a denervated tectum (Meyer 1984). For example, when fibers normally innervating lateral posterior tectum are redirected into vacant medial anterior tectum, they grow to the lateral posterior tectum. Normally, the optic pathway through the medial anterior tectum leads to the medial posterior locations.

The third type of evidence derives from experiments in which part of tectum is surgically rotated (Figure 5.5; and Chapter 5, this volume). It has been observed in regeneration studies with both amphibians and goldfish that the rotated piece of tectum becomes reinnervated according to its intrinsic polarity (Yoon 1973; Levine and Jacobson 1974). This results in a projection onto the rotated piece that is discordant with the surrounding tectum. This is perhaps the strongest evidence against the concept of pathway-only cueing.

The proponents of pathway cueing now recognize that it cannot explain these results from regeneration. Nevertheless, they maintain that it has a role in normal development.

They propose that regenerating fibers use a very different mechanism for producing order than do fibers during development. In particular, they suggest that in normal development, fibers form an orderly projection from pathway-only cueing and then transmit to or induce on the tectum position-dependent cues. Subsequently, these cues can be subsequently read by regenerating fibers. However, the equivalent of the three types of experiments that tested this hypothesis for regeneration has been carried out for the developing system with essentially the same results.

All experiments in which the eye rudiment is deplanted to an ectopic position produce gross derangement of pathway; this argues against pathway-only cueing in development. However, in many cases, the misrouted fibers eventually find the optic tract and grow along the tract into the tectum; they may become reordered *en route*. A stronger counterexample comes from an experiment with neonatal hamsters (Finlay, Schneps, and Schneider 1979). When the superficial (optic) layers of one superior colliculus (tectum) are destroyed in the newborn just before optic fibers arrive, fibers traverse the lesioned tectum and cross the midline into the opposite intact tectum. This invasion of the wrong (ipsilateral) tectum can be nearly complete if the normal optic innervation of the latter has been eliminated by simultaneous enucleation of the corresponding eye. Whatever order these miscrossing fibers may have derived from the optic tract must be inappropriate for the intact tectum in at least one axis since each colliculus is a mirror image of the other one. In fact, the fibers appeared to be disordered on entry. Nevertheless, the final projection was retinotopic and appropriately polarized. In a similar experiment, Straznicky (1978) removed one eye of an amphibian embryo so that one tectum developed without optic innervation. After metamorphosis, fibers from the remaining eye were forced to regenerate into the "virgin" tectum. Even though regeneration is known to produce a high degree of pathway disorder (Udin 1977; Meyer 1980; Cook 1982), the projections were orderly and of the appropriate polarity.

Evidence that growing optic axons generally bypass inappropriate tectal sites following early eye lesions has been obtained from several species, including hamster newborns (Frost and Schneider 1979) and chick embryos (Crossland et al. 1974). In both these species, it was possible to remove a large proportion of retina before optic fibers grew into the tectum. Clear examples were observed of fibers tracking through an inappropriate region of tectum to terminate in the appropriate location. In hamsters, there is considerable eye growth and some retinal regeneration between the time of the retinal lesion and the anatomical analysis of the projection that made it difficult to determine the accuracy of termination. However, in chicks, the size and position of the retinal lesion could be gauged by the isthmooptic projection to the retina. Because this projection is retinotopic, the isthmooptic nucleus undergoes a position-dependent atrophy corresponding to the area of the missing retina. It was concluded that fibers innervated their appropriate area without detectable error.

The ideal tectal-rotation experiment in which a part of the tectum is rotated has not been performed on embryos, but several experiments approach this preparation. In *Xenopus,* the entire prospective tectum and diencephalon has been successfully rotated by 180° in the neural plate stage, which is well before optic innervation (Chung and Cooke 1978). The projection that formed was correspondingly rotated. This result, by itself, does not exclude the possibility of pathway cueing, as fibers entered through the rotated diencephalon. However, in some cases, only part of the tectal rudiment was rotated, giving rise to two pairs of tecta, one anterior and one posterior to the diencephalon in mirror image. In these cases, fibers formed a complete projection across every tectum. Each projection was of the correct polarity for the anatomical orientation of each tectum, so that one was rotated and the other not. It is difficult to see how one diencephalon could simultaneously provide opposite pathway cueing and the experiments indicate the existence of tectal markers. An alternate approach is to prevent the normal optic innervation from forming and then rotate the tectum. This has been done in *Xenopus* embryos by removing one eye (Straznicky 1978) or producing an eye that has a disorganized projection (Fraser and Hunt 1980). After metamorphosis, a piece of tectum was then rotated (or translocated) and fibers from the remaining good eye redirected into the tectum. Again fibers formed an appropriately rotated (or translocated) projection onto this piece of tectum.

Some results from amphibian embryos have been interpreted as supporting pathway-only cueing. However, close scrutiny shows that these are either ambiguous, or they actually give evidence of the existence of tectal cues. One such result comes from the previously mentioned study in which part of the neural plate was rotated in *Xenopus* (Chung and Cooke 1978). In addition to the results described before, it was reported that when prospective tectum but not diencephalon was rotated, the optic map onto the tectum was normal. The interpretation was made that a morphogenetic marker (organizer) in the diencephalon determined the polarity of the projection that passed through this territory and tectal markers did not exist. In reality, it is entirely possible that this "rotated" tectum was not rotated at all. Embryonic manipulations often evoke regulative responses that correct for tissue damage. No cell markers were used to monitor the result of the surgery and there were no adequate markers of tectal polarity. There is also the possibility that the recordings were not from optic fibers, but from the so-called ipsilateral projection. This is a secondary projection found in frogs and toads that relays visual responses from contralateral to ipsilateral tectum for loci within the binocular visual field (Keating and Feldman 1975). Normally, this secondary relay is confined to the ipsilateral tectum and is not a source of confusion in recording to map the direct projection. However, it was reported that often an eye in an experimental animal sent fibers to the ipsilateral tectum. These direct ipsilateral fibers would be expected to activate the relay across the midline and to drive units in the contralateral tectum. The normal polarity of the intertectal relay is such that these relayed responses would be rotated in precisely the fashion of the claimed rotation. But there is also good reason to believe that this secondary projection may have developed abnormally (Keating and Feldman 1975) and this might explain some of the reported cases of confused topography. Even if the tectum had been rotated as intended and the intertectal relay is assumed not to have confounded the result, this experiment cannot prove tectal markers do not exist. It may only mean that order produced by chemical labeling in the optic pathway can, under certain extreme conditions, dominate over tectal markers. The topographic mapping in the tecta of these animals was distinctly inferior to that of normals.

Fiber paths have been traced from compound eyes with anterograde horseradish peroxidase (Fawcett and Gaze 1982; Gaze and Fawcett 1983). Fibers from double ventral eyes grow into the medial brachia of the optic tract but not into the lateral brachia. Fibers from nasal-nasal eyes avoid the anterior end of the tectum and favor the posterior half, whereas fibers from temporal-temporal eyes invade the anterior tectum and avoid the posterior end. This was considered evidence for pathway-only cueing and against chemoaffinity. Two arguments were again raised against chemoaffinity (Gaze, Keating, and Chung 1974). One was that the expansion of the compound eye across the tectum was incompatible with tectal labels. This is a mistaken notion that will be discussed in the section on "plasticity." The other was

that the order within the optic pathway was entirely sufficient to explain the order of the projection onto the tectum; there was no "need" for tectal markers. In effect, this last statement is merely an expectation of a certain kind of behavior on the part of growing fibers and is by no means obvious. The fact that fibers appear to make active directional choices in the pathway does not mean that they are not making similar choices within the tectum. There is no clear evidence to support the assertion that a choice made in the pathway can determine the locus of tectal termination. A number of experiments have shown exactly the opposite result: the initial path taken by a fiber does not dictate the site of tectal termination and that mistakes in the pathway can be corrected by unusual growth paths within the tectum (Udin 1977; Finlay, Wilson, and Schneider 1979; Meyer 1980; Cook 1982).

In fact, some of the results from compound-eye experiments point to tectal markers. When fibers from compound eyes are made to regenerate into a virgin tectum, they follow a somewhat different route than would be expected in development. Most fibers from ventral-ventral eyes follow a diffuse medial brachia and, curiously, fibers from nasal-nasal eyes also show a strong preference for the medial route (they normally follow both brachia). If pathway cueing determined tectal innervation, one might expect double ventral and double nasal eyes to have a similar projection and for the double nasal eyes to have an abnormal projection. Neither was the case. Both projections were basically the same as those formed in normal development. The distribution of fibers from compound eyes into virgin tecta has also been examined with autoradiography (Straznicky and Gaze 1982). In contrast to the differential innervation of the normal tectum by double nasal and double temporal eyes, these researchers claimed there was no difference in innervation when these eyes were forced to regenerate into a virgin tectum. However, it is likely that the 28 days allowed for regeneration was simply too short for differential fiber growth to be adequately expressed. Quantitative autoradiography on ipsilaterally deflected fibers in goldfish (Meyer 1984) has shown that 50–80 days are required to obtain an adequate result. It is noteworthy that the few *Xenopus* that were given 42 days to regenerate in Straznicky and Gaze's experiments did show an appropriate difference.

Stability of tectal markers

Given the longstanding evidence that tectal markers do play a role in initial development, it may seem surprising that any credence was given to the notion that optic fibers induce markers in an unlabeled tectum during development. After all, it is a bit implausible to think selective regeneration is nothing more than an interesting artifact and that labels are put on the tectum after the time they are most needed when optic axons are forming initial connections in the tectum. An experiment has been cited that was thought to demonstrate such axon-induced labeling, not directly in development but in regeneration. It was reported that a surgically produced nasal half-retina in the goldfish initially innervated only its appropriate anterior half of the tectum, but after six months it expanded across the entire tectum (Schmidt, Cicerone, and Easter 1978). If this tectum was then innervated by the opposite intact eye, only its nasal half was initially represented (Schmidt 1978). This was taken to mean that the tectal markers were transformed into those of the nasal half-retina. In other fish, the tectum was denervated of optic fibers for six months and then reinnervated by a surgically formed nasal half-retina. The initial projection was reportedly expanded (Schmidt 1978). The explanation was that the tectum lost its position-dependent markers after six months.

This interpretation has serious problems. It is incompatible with the developmental studies showing selective innervation by partial retinas and the tectal rotation studies cited before. It has theoretical difficulties as well. If the tectum loses its markers following long-term denervation, then there is no obvious explanation for the appropriate polarity of the projection in regeneration since explanations in terms of pathway cueing and timing of fiber growth can be ruled out.

Two recent experiments disprove Schmidt's model. In goldfish, it is possible to surgically redirect selected optic fibers from one tectum into specific positions in the opposite host tectum (Meyer 1984). If lateral-posterior fibers are inserted into the anterior-medial end of a host tectum that had its corresponding eye removed, they will grow into the lateral-posterior quadrant. Medial-posterior fibers that are inserted at this position grow into the medial-posterior quadrant. This selectivity is as good, in fact better, in a host tectum that was denervated of optic fibers for 18 months before fiber deflection. Thus, tectal labels are maintained at least this long in the absence of optic fibers. The fiber-deflection technique was also used to test if optic fibers could relabel tectal markers. If posterior-medial fibers are inserted into the host tectum at its anterior end, which is locally denervated by a corresponding eye lesion in the host eye, deflected fibers will form a lasting innervation in the anterior tectum (Meyer 1979a). After two years, the deflected fibers were removed and the host optic nerve crushed. If deflected fibers relabeled the anterior tectum to be posterior, then some posterior fibers should project anteriorly. The actual map recorded at 40 days, however, showed normal retinotopography, indicating no relabeling of tectum (Meyer unpublished).

Although the correct interpretation of the nasal half-retina experiments is unclear, a number of alternative explanations that involve no change of tectal markers can be easily envisioned. One disturbing possibility is that the electrophysiological method on which all the data were based may not always accurately reflect the distribution of optic fibers. Autoradiographic studies indicate that the majority of optic fibers from a nasal half-retina remain in the anterior half of the tectum regardless of postoperative survival time (Meyer 1975; Schmidt et al. 1978; Sturmer 1981). Other possibilities arise because the distribution of optic fibers can be affected by other factors that may obscure effects of tectal labels. These other factors were not given adequate consideration in the previous interpretation.

Another suggested alternative to the original chemospecificity hypothesis is that the tectum is topographically labeled by nonoptic afferents that reach the tectum before optic fibers form an orderly projection. Optic fibers then use these tectal labels for forming retinotopography. By this mechanism, both optic fibers and tectal cells receive independent sets of markers, as postulated in chemoaffinity. Sperry suggested that markers might be induced by axonal contact (Sperry 1951a; Meyer and Sperry 1976). "The induction of cell differentiation through contact with other cells and tissues, common throughout development, takes on a special aspect in the nervous system. . . . It becomes possible for a group of neurons to be similarly specified through similar termination . . ." (Sperry 1951a, p. 274). Since this idea does not contradict the chemoaffinity hypothesis, it will not be discussed further.

Polarity in tectal markers

The evidence cited demonstrates the existence of position-dependent labels on optic fibers as well as local tectal cues; together, these generate the basic topography of the projection. However, it has been argued that this data alone does not prove that the tectal cues are position-dependent markers, as postulated by chemoaffinity. Instead, it has been proposed that tectal cues are merely polarity markers identical across the entire tectum. According to the *arrow model* (Hope, Hammond, and Gaze 1976), topographic order in the tectum is generated by a fiber-to-fiber interaction, fibers from the neighboring retinal regions tending to aggregate together. Regenerating fibers read the tectal polarity cue to determine which side of their neighboring fiber to be on so as to produce the proper polarity. A plausible cellular mechanism for this polarity interaction has not been forthcoming. In theory, it can explain the formation of a normal projection after disruption of timing and pathway order and the formation of a rotated projection onto a rotated piece of tectum. There are other data, however, with which this alternative model is incompatible.

The arrow model predicts that fibers from a partial retina will always expand across the entire tectum. Standing in contradiction to this prediction are clear cases of selectivity where part of the tectum is left uninnervated (Attardi and Sperry 1963; Crossland et al. 1974; Meyer 1975; Frost and Schneider 1979; Sturmer 1981). The arrow model also predicts that fibers will always compress onto a partial tectum (see the

section on "plasticity"). Again, counterexamples in which not all fibers are represented on the tectum have been observed (Meyer and Sperry 1973; Udin 1977; Finlay, Wilson, and Schneider 1979). It is noteworthy that examples of both kinds of selectivity were known well before the arrow model was presented, but have never been discussed in this context. Because these serious difficulties with the model were not appreciated, a number of experiments were undertaken to distinguish the arrow model from chemoaffinity. These generally involve translocating a piece of tectum to a foreign tectal position while preserving the polarity of the implant. The arrow model or any other model that postulates only polarity markers in the tectum predicts that an entirely normal projection would form. What is found instead is that part of the visual field is translocated as expected from chemoaffinity markers in the tectum. This result has been obtained with regenerating fiber in goldfish (Hope et al. 1976; Yoon 1979) and also in *Xenopus* in which the only previous innervation of the tectum was scrambled (Fraser and Hunt 1980), indicating that the result is valid for initial development as well as regeneration.

Plasticity

The discovery that optic fibers can be made to terminate at unusual tectal positions under certain experimental conditions, a phenomenon loosely referred to as *plasticity*, has often been taken to be the strongest evidence against chemoaffinity. I hope to show here that this problem is mainly semantic, stemming from an unrealistic and narrow definition of chemoaffinity. The contradictory evidence does not, in fact, challenge the chemoaffinity hypothesis in its classical form.

The first of the recent tests for plasticity used compound eyes of *Xenopus* made by fusing two identical half optic vesicles in early development (Gaze et al. 1963). Double nasal, double temporal, and double ventral eyes eventually formed a retinotopic projection across the entire tectum (Figure 5.3). Initially, this was taken as a clear disproof of the chemoaffinity theory, but the interpretation was made difficult by extensive growth and reorganization of the eye and tectum between the time of surgery and measurement of the projection. Exactly what kind of eye and tectum developed was debatable. These ambiguities appeared to be circumvented with the discovery of plasticity in mature lower vertebrates. When the posterior half of the tectum was ablated in adult goldfish, optic fibers were reported to eventually establish a complete retinotopic projection onto the anterior remnant without any part of the visual field missing (Gaze and Sharma 1970; Yoon 1971; see Chapter 4, this volume). This was referred to as *compression* (Figure 5.6C). It was later reported that when half of the retina was removed and the tectum left intact, again in goldfish, fibers from the retinal remnant would eventually form a retinotopic projection across the entire tectum, leaving no tectal region without optic fibers (Schmidt et al. 1978). This was called *expansion* (Figure 5.6A). Yet another example of plastic transformation in the visual projection came from the rotation of pieces of the tectum in metamorphosed frog (Jacobson and Levine 1975). Contrary to similar work in goldfish, the projection was, in a

minority of cases, completely normal. The rotation was ignored.

These observations led to the following model for guidance of the retinotectal projection: optic fibers arrange themselves in correct relative positions (and, usually, correct polarity) and fill up all available tectal sites without regard to tectal position. There is no preference by optic fibers for specific tectal loci. Instead, fibers have the capacity to form a complete topographic projection regardless of the size and origin of the available tectum. Conclusion: plasticity contradicts chemoaffinity and, therefore, the hypothesized preferential growth by chemoaffinity does not operate. This *disproof* stimulated a number of hypotheses put forward as alternatives to chemoaffinity and considerable debate has ensued. I will try to show here that the primary argument is invalid, that such demonstrations of plasticity do not contradict the chemoaffinity theory, and that the *alternatives* are either incompatible with the facts or are simply special cases of chemoaffinity.

Plasticity is sometimes discussed as if it

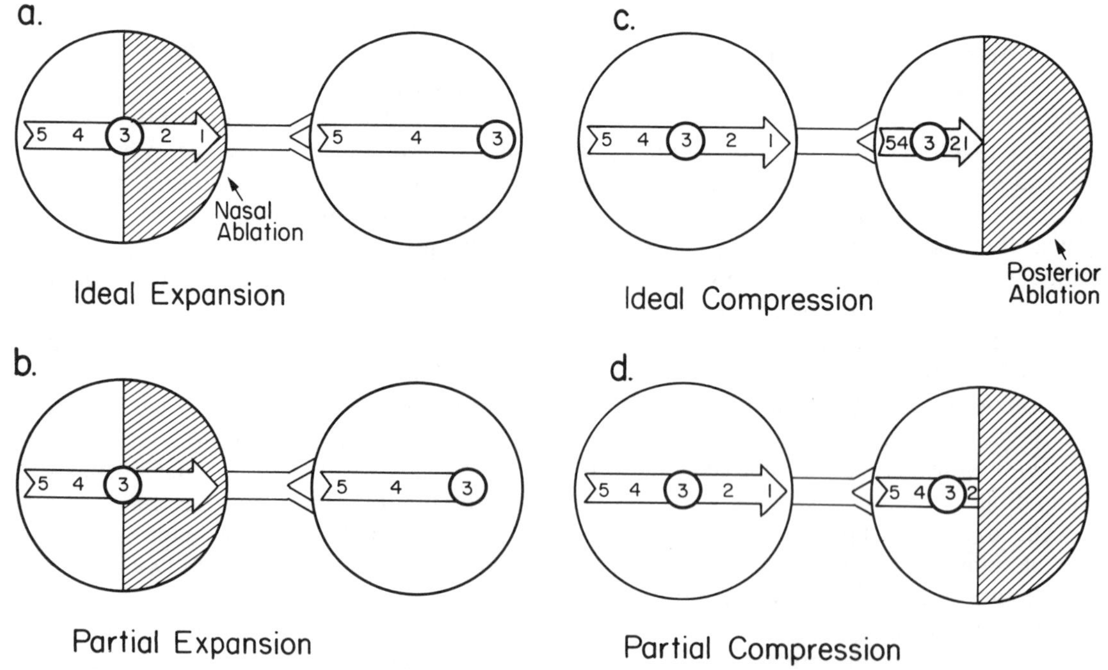

Figure 5.6. Schematic representation comparing ideal and real expansion and compression. (**A**) Ideal expansion following ablation of the nasal retina. (**B**) Actual expansion seen anatomically following nasal ablation. (**C**) Ideal compression following ablation of the posterior tectum. (**D**) Actual compression frequently seen after posterior tectal ablation.

were a universal phenomenon easily observed whenever part of the retina or tectum is removed. This is far from the case. Expansion following partial retinal ablations has never been detected in chicks (Crossland et al. 1974). In the hamster, there are cases of no apparent expansion (Frost and Schneider 1979). Where there has appeared to be some expansion, it is unclear if this is genuine because of the possibility that the ablated components of the retina had regenerated. Even in goldfish, the archetypal plastic species, the initial innervation of the tectum by fibers from most half-retinas is clearly selective for the appropriate half of the tectum (Attardi and Sperry 1963; Meyer 1975; Sturmer 1981). Only a half nasal retina may show considerable expansion from the beginning (Meyer 1975). It has been said that, given time, a half-retina expands uniformly across the whole tectum, but the evidence is weak. It is based on electrophysiological recordings, mainly from temporal half-eyes (Schmidt 1978; Schmidt et al. 1978). Autoradiography (Meyer 1975; Schmidt et al. 1978; Sturmer 1981) has not substantiated this claim, indicating instead that most fibers remain in their appropriate half and a minority expand into the foreign half (Figure 5.6B). The innervation formed by compound eyes in *Xenopus* is also not a case of simple expansion. Contrary to the early findings by electrophysiology, autoradiography has revealed a bias in the innervation toward the appropriate part of the tectum (Straznicky and Gaze 1982). In this preparation, the selectivity is weaker than in other half-retina studies, but this could be due to the presence of double the number of optic fibers in the tectum.

Compression is no less problematic. Following collicular lesions in the hamster, there is some compression, but a large area of the retina is not represented (Finlay, Wilson, and Schneider 1979). In the tree frog (*Hyla*), tectal ablations do not lead to detectable compression, even when the optic nerve is crushed and long postoperative recovery is allowed (Meyer and Sperry 1973). In *Rana* frogs, compression has been observed, but only if the optic nerve is severed and allowed to regenerate (Udin 1977). The best case for compression is, again, in goldfish, but even here it is not simple. If the projection onto an anterior half-retina is

recorded with the eye in water instead of in air, as was done in the earlier studies, the compression is found to be incomplete and inhomogeneous (Meyer 1977). The inappropriate part of the visual field is typically squeezed onto a relatively small area of the tectal remnant and its peripheral segment is usually missing (Figure 5.6D). These distortions are particularly evident when the nerve is not crushed, and the compression is sometimes nonretinotopic (Gaze and Sharma 1970; Meyer 1977). With large medial ablations, no compression (Jacobson and Gaze 1965) or a limited and inhomogenous compression (Meyer 1977) has been observed in goldfish.

It should be evident that there is more support for chemospecific selectivity in these experiments than for the contrary. Unfortunately, the complications have been overlooked and hypotheses have been formulated in terms of a universal and idealized plasticity. Data not conforming to this ideal have been ignored or dismissed as exceptional. The retinal lesion studies in chicks, for instance, have been viewed as peculiar results in an unusual species. The unfortunate consequence of such arguing of the case are theories that explain an ideal plasticity, but do not conform to the actual data. They lack generality. However, for the sake of argument and to simplify the discussion, let us suppose an ideal plasticity, that is, let us suppose that when half of the retina is removed, fibers expand retinotopically across the entire tectum; conversely, when half of the tectum is removed, fibers form a compressed retinotopic projection onto the half-tectum. What are the implications of these topographic plasticities for the chemoaffinity theory?

At first, rigid chemoaffinity is ruled out. In rigid chemoaffinity, unique fiber-to-tectum matchings are dictated without exception. However, chemoaffinity postulates a matching of cellular markers not specific cells. If these markers changed location in the cell array such that the correct match is made during compression and expansion, then even a rigid form of chemoaffinity theory could still apply. Morphollactic regulation, the reorganization of position-dependent properties without cell addition seen following ablations in embryos and the mature forms of some primitive animals, most notably hydra, would allow this to happen (Sperry 1965; Meyer and Sperry 1973; see also Chapter 4, this volume). Ablation of half of the retina or tectum could induce production of a full range of chemical markers in the remaining half. Fortunately, this particular complication would appear to be ruled out in mature lower vertebrates. Briefly, expansion of a half-retina can be reversed or prevented by the presence of fibers from an intact eye (Schmidt 1978, Sharma and Tung 1979). When fibers that normally innervate medial-posterior tectum are deflected into a denervated host tectum, they expand across the medial tectum. No retinal regulation would be expected in this case since the eye giving rise to the deflected fibers was intact (Meyer 1978b). Again this expansion is prevented if fibers from the host eye are allowed to reinnervate tectum along with deflected fibers (Meyer 1979b). Under this condition, the deflected fibers cause a compression of the host fibers away from the region occupied by the deflected fibers. Tectal regulation would not be expected since the tectum was left intact. Some studies of the time course of compression also counterindicate regulation (Cook 1979). Unfortunately, there *is* evidence for some type of regulation in embryonic amphibian eyes (Conway, Feiock, and Hunt 1980). This substantially complicates experiments involving embryonic surgery and their interpretation is currently in debate.

For simplicity, we will confine the argument to plasticity in adult lower vertebrates and will assume, in line with the majority of workers in the field, that morphollactic regulation does not occur. Other possible mechanisms for altering markers can be envisioned. Sperry suggested that during compression and expansion, fibers might modulate tectal markers so as to correspond with the markers on fibers (Meyer and Sperry 1976). This modulation was conceived as a temporary shift away from the embryonically derived baseline marker to which the cell would revert upon denervation. Another possibility is that when tectal cells are denervated, they alter their markers in a way that makes them more attractive to a wider range of fibers. These are difficult possibilities to exclude. Nevertheless, there is no evidence for changing markers either, and for the sake

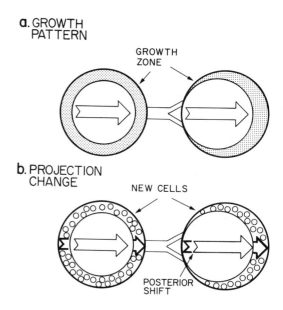

Figure 5.7. Simplified representation of (**A**) the pattern of cell addition to the retina and tectum in frogs and goldfish and (**B**) the resulting shifting connections. New ganglion cells in the temporal retina corresponding to the new tail of the arrow in (**B**) do not have a corresponding set of new tectal cells and so must displace the optic terminals previously occupying this position, represented by the original tail of the arrow, posteriorly. This preserves retinotopography.

of simplicity, let us make a worst-case assumption by asserting that markers remain unchanged during plasticity.

Given this assumption, it might be concluded that plasticity effects constitute verifiable evidence for a mismatch of any chemoaffinity markers. For this to be a valid conclusion, one has to define an appropriate match. An important difficulty that complicates such a definition comes from way the retinotectal system grows. In frogs, new neurons are added to the retina and tectum mainly during the larval period (Gaze et al. 1974), and in goldfish, such cell addition continues throughout adulthood (Johns 1978; Meyer 1978a). Although the details differ between species, the overall pattern of cell addition is the same (Figure 5.7). Retinal ganglion cells are added to the entire circumference of the retinal ciliary margin. In the tectum, cells are also added to the margin, but not at the anterior end. This means that new ganglion cells added to the edge of temporal retina do not have a corresponding set of new tectal cells at the anterior tectum on which to terminate. Instead, temporal fibers must displace the preexisting retinal fibers in a posterior direction to preserve retinotopography. A progressive posterior shift in retinotectal connections takes place during growth of the visual projection (Gaze et al. 1974, 1979; Meyer 1978a).

Since connections change normally, it is no longer a straightforward matter to define what are correct and incorrect connections. On the contrary, there is reason to think that much of the plasticity that had been thought to represent a plastic mismatch between neurons is within or at least close to the normal range of interconnectional matchings required during growth. The major direction of shift in connections during growth is along the anterior-posterior axis and most of the plasticity that has been demonstrated in adult lower vertebrates is along this same axis. Little or none has been reported mediolaterally. It is also interesting that no major shift is thought to occur in chick development and no plasticity has been detected following eye lesions in this species. If a dynamic chemoaffinity mechanism normally plays a role in the formation of orderly connections, then it must be compatible with a range of connections. It then becomes logically indefensible to conclude that plasticity contradicts chemoaffinity. The evidence for shifting connections is not evidence against chemoaffinity, but it is evidence against the assumption that plasticity can negate chemoaffinity.

It is possible that some of the connections formed in certain experimental preparations are abnormal in the sense that they involve matchings that would never form during normal growth and development. For the sake of argument, let us say that such unnatural mismatching does occur. Is this a fatal problem for the chemoaffinity theory? It does dismiss the hypothesis of rigid chemoaffinity, which permits only normal matching at all stages. However, such a reading of Sperry's theory is neither historically accurate nor theoretically justified. Sperry did not make rigid and exclusive matching a requirement of chemoaffinity matching. On the contrary, he explicity defined the affinity between nerve cells as preferential,

and, as we have pointed out, he also allowed that other factors including mechanical guidance and activity could participate as well (see also Chapter 2, this volume). He left matters of the strength and selectivity of the affinity an open question to be answered by further experiment.

In theory, the affinity could be so strong and selective that mismatching rarely or never happened under any experimental conditions. Or the affinity could be so subtle and permissive that, although it brings about the appropriate matches during normal development and under some ideal experimental conditions, it is frequently overcome by competing factors introduced in many more disruptive experiments. Demonstrations of plasticity and shifting connections give information on how strong the affinities are, how chemoaffinity may operate, and what other morphogenetic processes participate. However, it is illogical to conclude from this that chemical affinities do not exist and that they are not responsible for epigenetic regulation of connective correspondence between retinal loci and loci on the visual tectum (Meyer and Sperry 1973, 1976; Hunt and Jacobson 1974).

Chemoaffinity models allowing for plasticity

If chemoaffinity is thought of as a preferential mechanism, then plasticity and shifting connections are to be expected. Given the evidence for both chemoaffinity and plasticity, the reasonable next step is to try to incorporate these two lines of evidence into a comprehensive explanation. There are a number of models that attempt to do this. Although some of these models have been presented as alternatives to a rigid concept of chemoaffinity, they are, as we have seen, not alternatives to preferential chemoaffinity. Indeed, all the models that are compatible with the basic experimental observations, expressly or implicitly invoke preferential chemoaffinity. They all postulate the existence of retinal and tectal labels and a selective growth process directing the interaction between fibers and the tectum. It is not possible here to go through every model that has been put forward. Instead, I will discuss the two ma-

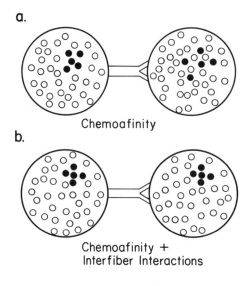

a.

Chemoafinity

b.

Chemoafinity +
Interfiber Interactions

Figure 5.8. Illustration of the "dual instruction" models. (**A**) Neighboring ganglion cells from a small region of the retina, shown as solid circles, are guided by chemoaffinity to the general area of the tectum that is appropriate. However, this guidance is low in resolution, so that their widely distributed terminals may be interspersed with nonneighboring terminals, shown as open circles. (**B**) Interfiber interactions cause fibers from the same retinal region to aggregate. This sharpens the map and produces topography independent of tectal position.

jor classes into which these models can be grouped.

The first and by far the most populous class comprises *dual instruction models* (Meyer and Sperry 1976; Willshaw and von der Malsburg 1976; Fraser 1980; Fraser and Hunt 1980; Law and Constantine-Patton 1981; Whitelaw and Cowan 1981; Meyer 1983; see Meyer 1982 for others). These postulate two ordering processes, one dependent on position in the tectum and the other position-independent (Figure 5.8). The position-dependent process is, in effect, chemoaffinity, though not always called such. Position-dependent markers within the retina and tectum are assumed, but the preferential matching between these labeled elements have been postulated to involve a variety of particular mechanisms, ranging from differential cell adhesivity to chemical interchange between terminals and tectal cells, or abstract mathematical formulations that govern segregation of elements without identifying actual cellular structures. This matching process is hy-

pothesized to be very permissive of mismatching and possibly low in resolution. It has the role of generating polarity and rough topography in the retinotectal map. Finer topography is generated by the second instructive process, which creates fiber-to-fiber retinotopography independently of tectal position. Fiber terminals carry information of the relative or absolute position of their cell bodies within the retina, and in the tectum they preferentially associate with fibers from the same retinal region. Such a process of shuffling and seeking of neighbors can theoretically generate high-resolution retinotopography without requiring further positional information from the tectal cells. It is presumed to be effective as connections shift during expansion, compression, and growth. Again the hypothesized mechanisms vary. Fiber–fiber adhesivity, impulse activity-dependent sorting, or abstract rules have been proposed. Thus, the first instruction process explains a crude selectivity and polarity in the projections. The second process explains fine retinotopography and its preservation in plastic rearrangements. The second process complements but does not replace the chemoaffinity mechanism.

A second class of models has been referred to as *best fit* (Prestige and Willshaw 1975; Meyer and Sperry 1976). The models rely on a fiber-to-tectum interaction as the sole instructive process for the generation of retinotopography (Figure 5.9). The information for this orderly interaction is derived only from position-dependent markers in the retina and tectum, but its expression is context-dependent. It depends upon other fibers and the amount of tectal space. In one model, fibers are presumed to normally terminate at intrinsically less preferred tectal sites, being constrained to do so by the presence of other fibers (Prestige and Willshaw 1975). Although this was taken to be incompatible with chemoaffinity, this conclusion does not stand. The general concept of preferential chemoaffinity does not require the site of termination to coincide with the site of maximal affinity at all times and under all circumstances, any more than an enzyme should always generate the most product from one preferred substrate regardless of chemical conditions. On the contrary, shifting connec-

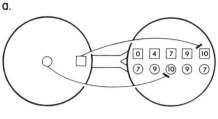

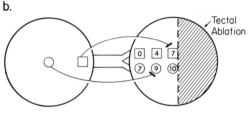

Figure 5.9. The "system optimization" model. The circle and square in the retina represent ganglion cells from the central and nasal retina, respectively. The affinity of a fiber is highest for its normal tectal site of termination and decreases nonlinearly with distance. The differential affinities of each fiber for five tectal positions along a central anterior-to-posterior strip are indicated by the corresponding numbers in circles and squares. Each vertical pair of circles and squares in the tectum is meant to designate the same single position, not two different positions. (A) In the normal projection, each fiber matches to the site of highest affinity to produce a combined affinity match of 20. (Other fiber and retinal cell locations are illustrated in Figures 5.10A and 5.11A). (B) The posterior half of the tectum is removed. Fibers make the greatest possible total affinity match. To achieve this, the fiber from the central retina moves anteriorly, allowing the nasal fiber to displace it. Any other configuration gives a combined affinity match less than 16 and so is not optimized. The optimum configuration is retinotopic compression.

tions during development tells us that there is no predetermined normal site for fibers to innervate. Unless the affinities change with growth, there must be a disparity between the site of maximal affinity that a fiber might ex-

press in isolation and the site of termination at various ages. This is obviously more complicated than the narrower version of Sperry's idea that the site of maximal affinity is where the fiber normally terminates, but it is not fundamentally at odds with a preferential chemoaffinity mechanism. The key features of position-dependent markers and selective interactions for the generation of retinotopography are retained.

In these two kinds of models, the context-dependent expression of the affinities is the result of a noninstructional process, that is, one that does not itself impart information about the retinotopography of the individual elements. Instead, it is a simple rule for matching fibers with the tectal markers. To explain expansion and compression, it is assumed that fibers use all available tectal space. With a properly chosen set of markers and rule of matching, retinotopography will be generated by the selective interaction between fibers and the tectum.

How such a model can work is perhaps best demonstrated with a concrete example. Unfortunately, previous models either lack formality (Meyer and Sperry 1976) or generality (Prestige and Willshaw 1975), so a new one, "system optimization," will be used to illustrate the concept. The model postulates a chemoaffinity system of retinal and tectal markers in which a single isolated fiber exhibits a maximum affinity for one tectal locus and a graded decrease in affinity with distance from this locus. For simplicity, it is initially assumed that the site of maximal affinity for each fiber is its normal site of termination and that the strength of maximal affinity is the same for all fibers. Figure 5.9 illustrates the affinities of two fibers, one from the central retina and one from the nasal retina for the same five tectal positions along the anterior–posterior axis. For reasons that will be evident, the starting assumptions make it necessary to assign these affinities in a nonlinear fashion. In the example, the rate of decrease (affinity gradient) increases arithmetically with distance from the site of maximum affinity. The rule of matching is that the individual fibers project to the tectal locus that optimizes the matching for the system as a whole. This is computed by summing the *affinity matches* formed by the individual fibers to give the *system optimum*.

For an intact retina and tectum, as shown in Figure 5.9A, fibers will grow to their normal locus to produce the system optimum, here 10 + 10 for the affinity matches made by the two fibers shown, and the affinity matches from all the other fibers not shown. For simplicity, the system optimum will be given in terms of two fibers, but the results to follow hold when properly computed for a complete one-dimensional array. In Figure 5.9B, the posterior half of the tectum is removed, thereby forcing the corresponding fibers to seek sites on the anterior remnant. The system optimum is obtained when the fiber from the central retina moves anteriorly from its individual site of maximum affinity to one of lesser affinity and is replaced at its normal site by the fiber from the nasal retina. This configuration yields a combined affinity match of 9 + 7. If the central fiber had not moved, the next best set of affinity matches would be only 10 + 4. Thus, the system is optimized when compression is retinotopic. The model will similarly generate retinotopic expansion following ablation of a half-retina, as shown in Figure 5.10. If it is assumed that fibers from a half-retina expand uniformly across the tectum, affinity matching will generate retinotopographic order in the expanded projection because this arrangement again yields the system optimum.

Note that the occurrence of plasticity involves an entirely separate assumption from the process that generates order. This assumption can be thought of in terms of the number of different fibers that can be accommodated onto the existing tectal area, the fiber–tectum ratio. Full plasticity effectively assumes this ratio is always maximized. If the ratio is assumed instead to be fixed so that only half of the retina will be accommodated onto a surgically formed half-tectum or if a surgically formed half-retina will occupy only the area of half a tectum, then system optimization will produce selectivity with no plasticity. A half-tectum would receive fibers only from the appropriate half-retina and a half-retina will project only to its appropriate half-tectum. Incremental increases in the fiber–tectum ratio result in limited plasticity where regions adjacent to the appropriate part of the

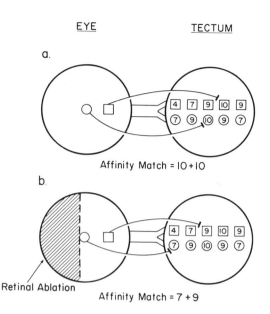

Figure 5.10. Conventions are the same as in Figure 5.9 except that a fiber from the middle nasal retina instead of the far nasal retina is illustrated. (**A**) Normal projection. (**B**) The temporal half of the retina that had projected to the anterior half of the tectum has been removed. The remaining fibers expand uniformly across the tectum. To make the greatest total affinity match, the fiber from the central retina moves to the anterior end of the tectum and the fiber from the middle nasal retina moves to the middle tectum. Under this condition, the system is optimized for a total contribution of 16 from the two fibers.

retina are increasingly represented. Thus, the observed species difference can be easily accommodated.

System optimization can also explain how retinotopography is maintained during shifting connections during growth. Again it is assumed that ganglion cells will compete for tectal space. At the anterior end of the tectum, no new cells are generated to accommodate the new ganglion cells added to the temporal retina. A new temporal cell must somehow prefer the anterior end of the tectum and cause the posterior displacement of the preexisting fiber at that position. It is not sufficient to postulate that the new fiber has a higher affinity for the anterior end. A steeper affinity gradient must also be postulated, otherwise retinotopography will not be preserved. In fact, as illustrated in Figure 5.10, the new fiber can have the same affinity for the anterior end as the preexisting fiber and only a steeper affinity gradient. The system will be optimized when the new fiber is anterior. At the posterior end of the tectum, new cells are added. In this case, the new nasal retinal cell must project to the most posterior part of the new tectal region and the preexisting nasal fiber must move into the anterior part of the newly added posterior crescent. This posterior shift will occur if both preexisting and new nasal fibers have their highest affinity for the new posterior end. To make this scheme work for successive growth cycles, it is useful to assume the new fiber has the highest affinity. However, a higher affinity is alone not sufficient to generate the correct topography. (The reader can see this by replacing triangle 12 of Figure 5.11 with a triangle numbered 14.) The gradient of affinity for the new fiber must also be steeper, though it can be linear as illustrated in Figure 5.11. Again retinotopography represents the system optimum.

The system can grow in this fashion indefinitely. With each growth cycle, older fibers move farther from their site of maximal affinity. Only the newest fibers are temporarily positioned at their site of maximal affinity. Eventually, all temporal retina cells, except the original starting ones, will have a maximal affinity for the anterior end of the tectum, and nasal cells will have maximum affinity for the posterior end; peripheral ganglion cells will have a higher affinity gradient than central cells. Such a system lacks the point-to-point normal preference originally postulated; yet it will still exhibit retinotopic expansion and compression or selectivity as before, depending on the assumed fiber–tectum ratio. Since most retinal and tectal cells are added postembryonically, this scenario seems the more likely.

A possible cellular mechanism by which affinity matching might work in growing nerve networks is "vector affinity" (Meyer 1984): the cellular markers responsible for topography are postulated to produce nothing more than the directional growth of nerve fibers. A fiber compares the local environment at its different filopodia or branches and selectively elongates some and retracts others. The direction and magnitude of the resulting growth, the growth vector, results from the specific interaction between the retinal and tectal markers. Thus, dif-

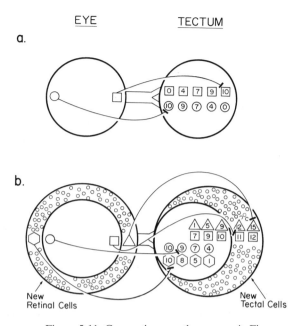

Figure 5.11. Conventions are the same as in Figures 5.9 and 5.10. (**A**) Normal projection showing a fiber from the temporal retina (circle) and a fiber from the nasal retina (square). (**B**) The projection following a round of retinotectal growth. New cells, represented by the area with many small circles, are added to the retina and tectum. The tectal affinities of a new ganglion cell in the temporal retina (hexagon) destined for the anterior end of the tectum are denoted by the numbers enclosed in the hexagons. The affinities of the new nasal cell (triangle) destined for the posterior end of the tectum are designated by the numbers in the triangles. Again note that all the vertically arranged sets of numbers are meant to apply to single tectal positions along the anterior-to-posterior axis. As illustrated, the best affinity match is made when the preexisting projection shifts posteriorly across the tectum and retinotopography is preserved. The reader can determine that this shift represents the system optimum.

ferent fibers can exhibit differential growth when at the same tectal site. This vector can be considered to be generated by the affinity gradient postulated for system optimization. Specifically, a fiber that finds itself at any given place in the tectum will compare its affinity values for adjacent tectal sites. It will move toward the higher value with a magnitude proportional to the difference in affinity values being sampled. Termination is not governed by any recognition of a *correct* or *best* site on the part of a fiber, but is a probalistic function of the time in contact with any given tectal cell. Consequently, a large growth vector away from a tectal site will discourage termination at that site, whereas a weak or absent vector will encourage it. Termination is also affected by the presence of other fibers. It is presumed that tectal cells regulate the number of synapses, so that potential synaptic sites are limited. This produces local competition between fibers that, for any given tectal region, favors the fiber spending the most time there. The fiber that has the smallest growth vector directed away from a tectal region will preferentially terminate there to the exclusion of other fibers. The result of such competition can be calculated like system optimization and can likewise produce retinotopography. Plasticity versus selectivity in size-disparity experiments, leading to expansion or compression, will depend on the intrinsic constraints on the size of the terminal arbor of the nerve fiber. On the one hand, arbor size could be entirely regulated by competition. If so, reduction in the fiber number would lead to enlarged arbors and, hence, expansion. Increase in fiber number would cause shrinkage of arbors, allowing fibers to be accommodated in a given tectal volume as in compression. On the other hand, arbor size could be fixed, with selectivity the result. Arbor size is, in effect, the fiber–tectum ratio.

As for the case of system optimization (see the preceding discussion on shifting connections during growth), appropriate retinotopic ordering of fibers can be generated by a vector-affinity process with a simple system of labels: nasal fibers and temporal fibers exhibit growth vectors directed toward posterior and anterior tectum, respectively, and peripheral ganglion cells show progressively greater overall growth vectors. Under these conditions, any two fibers in a given tectal site will exhibit growth vectors that are suitably different in direction, or magnitude, or both. At first, this appears quite different from the original chemoaffinity hypothesis. However, like the original, vector affinity postulates refined retinotectal markers and selective marker-mediated growth. It differs only in the assignment of these markers and in the details of how fibers interact with tectal cells and with each other.

The future of chemoaffinity

The preceding discussion can be boiled down to two main points. First, it is apparent that the case for chemoaffinity is now strong, indeed stronger than at any time in the past. Well-formulated counterproposals to chemoaffinity have proved inconsistent with the evidence and appear implausible. The other point is that much of the argument against chemoaffinity is semantic. It stems from the assumption of a narrow definition of chemoaffinity in which matching is taken to be rigid and in which no other factors are allowed to participate. A more realistic and more historically accurate representation of the hypothesis conceives chemoaffinity between cells of the retina and tectum to be preferential and permissive of other factors. Preferential chemoaffinity is actually an integral part of all of the plausible "alternative" hypotheses to chemoaffinity.

There is another side to this coin. If the affinities had turned out to be very strong and selective and worked in a simple one-to-one matching fashion, then we would have, at least at one level of analysis, a fairly complete understanding of the development of selective nerve connections. No doubt this was Sperry's hope. It may well turn out to be the case for some aspects of connectivity like laminar termination of optic input within the tectum (see Chapter 4, this volume), but, in general, development of retinotopography is not so simple. This means that what the chemoaffinity hypothesis can provide is an outline for an explanation, but, in its present form, not the complete answer to retinotectal mapping. A number of basic questions about chemoaffinity remains to be answered. We know that chemoaffinity is responsible for at least the gross organization of the map, but its role could be considerably more pervasive. We simply do not know what its limits are. We are also surprisingly ignorant about the kind of information chemoaffinity conveys. For example, is chemoaffinity providing a lock-and-key recognition system or just a directional growth cue?

Though it is evident that chemoaffinity plays a major role in ordering the retinotectal projection, other processes clearly contribute. What the relationship is between chemoaffinity and these other processes remains murky.

There is also little firm data on the biochemical basis for the retinal and tectal markers or on the cellular mechanisms that mediate the affinity. While markers are almost certainly arranged in some kind of position-dependent fashion, just how they are organized, whether as a gradient or mosaic, and how many dimensions they have, whether 2, 3, or more markers per cell, are open questions. There is reason to think that the affinity is a short-range interaction, but it cannot be said that it is a purely cell-contact phenomenon. It could be instead mediated by short-range diffusion of marker molecules.

Fortunately there are some questions that were burning issues in the 1940s that we no longer ask. We do not ask whether nerve connections are genetically determined. Rather, we now ask how genetics determines connectivity through the process of development. We do not try to explain all neural functions in terms of learning theory. Instead, we look for cellular mechanisms of brain development that can explain learning. We no longer think of all neurons as being chemically equivalent, but look for subtle differences in surfaces properties that we believe exist. We do not view nerve function in terms of networks in which precise connectivity is unimportant, but invest considerable resources into analyzing the intricate pattern of connectivity we know must be responsible. The modern view of the nervous system is based on cellular identities and refined specificities of connections. We have Roger Sperry and his theory of specific connective affinities between neurons to thank for bringing us so far toward an understanding of how structure is created in the nervous system.

References

Arora, H. L., and R. W. Sperry. 1963. Color discrimination after optic nerve regeneration in the fish *Astronotus ocellatus*. *Dev. Biol.* 7: 234–43.

Attardi, D. G., and R. W. Sperry. 1963. Preferential selection of central pathways by regenerating optic fibers. *Exp. Neurol.* 7: 46–64.

Bunt, S. M. 1982. Retinotopic and temporal organization of the optic nerve and tracts in the adult goldfish. *J. Comp. Neurol.* 206: 209–26.

Chung, S. H., and J. Cooke. 1978. Observations on the formation of the brain and of nerve connections following embryonic manipulation of the amphibian neural tube. *Proc. Roy. Soc. London, Ser. B*, 201: 335–73.

Conway, K., K. Feiock, and R. K. Hunt. 1980. Polyclones and patterns in growing *Xenopus* eye. *Curr. Top. Dev. Biol.* 15: 217–317.

Cook, J. E. 1979. Interactions between optic fibres controlling the locations of their terminals in the goldfish optic tectum. *J. Embryol. Exp. Morph.* 52: 89–103.

Cook, J. E. 1982. Errant optic axons in the normal goldfish retina reach retinotopic tectal sites. *Brain Res.* 250: 154.

Crossland, W. J., W. M. Cowan, L. A. Rogers, and J. P. Kelly. 1974. The specification of the retino-tectal projection in the chick. *J. Comp. Neurol.* 155: 127–64.

Fawcett, J. W. (1981). How axons grow down the *Xenopus* optic nerve. *J. Embryol. Exp. Morphol.* 65: 219–33.

Fawcett, J. W., and R. M. Gaze. 1982. The retino-tectal fibre pathways from normal and compound eyes in *Xenopus*. *J. Embryol. Exp. Morphol.* 72: 19–37.

Finlay, B. L., S. E. Schneps, and G. E. Schneider. 1979. Orderly compression of the retinotectal projection following partial tectal ablation in newborn hamster. *Nature (London)* 280: 153–5.

Finlay, B. L., K. G. Wilson, and G. E. Schneider. 1979. Anomalous ipsilateral retinotectal projections in Syrian hamsters with early lesions: Topography and functional capacity. *J. Comp. Neurol.* 183: 721–40.

Fraser, S. E. 1980. A differential adhesion approach to the patterning of nerve connections. *Dev. Biol.* 79: 453–64.

Fraser, S. E., and R. K. Hunt. 1980. Retinotectal specificity: Models and experiments in search of a mapping function. *Ann. Rev. Neurosci.* 3: 319–52.

Frost, D. O., and G. E. Schneider. 1979. Plasticity of retinofugal projections after partial lesions of the retina in newborn Syrian hamster. *J. Comp. Neurol.* 185: 517–68.

Gaze, R. M. 1959. Regeneration of the optic nerve in *Xenopus laevis*. *Quart. J. Exp. Physiol.* 44: 290–308.

Gaze, R. M., and J. W. Fawcett. 1983. Pathways of *Xenopus* optic fibres regenerating from normal and compound eyes under various conditions. *J. Embryol. Exp. Morph.* 73: 17–38.

Gaze, R. M., J. D. Feldman, J. Cooke, and S.-H. Chung. 1979. The orientation of the visuo-tectal map in *Xenopus*: Developmental aspects. *J. Embryol. Exp. Morphol.* 53: 39–66.

Gaze, R. M., M. Jacobson, and G. Szekely. 1963. The retinotectal projection in *Xenopus* with compound eyes. *J. Physiol. (London)* 165: 484–99.

Gaze, R. M., M. J. Keating, and S.-H. Chung. 1974. The evolution of the retinotectal map during development in *Xenopus*. *Proc. Roy. Soc. London, Ser. B* 185: 301–30.

Gaze, R. M., and S. C. Sharma. 1970. Axial differences in the reinervation of the goldfish optic tectum by regenerating optic nerve fibers. *Exp. Brain Res.* 10: 171–81.

Hope, R. A., B. J. Hammond, and R. M. Gaze. 1976. The arrow model: Retinotectal specificity and map formation in the goldfish visual system. *Proc. Roy. Soc. London, Ser. B* 194: 447–66.

Horder, T. J., and K. A. C. Martin. 1978. Morphogenetics as an alternative to chemospecificity in the formation of nerve connections. *Symp. Soc. Exp. Biol.* 32: 275–358.

Hunt, R. K., and M. Jacobson. 1972. Development and stability of positional information in *Xenopus* retinal ganglion cells. *Proc. Natl. Acad. Sci. USA* 69: 780–3.

–1974. Neuronal specificity revisited. *Curr. Top. Dev. Biol.* 8: 203–59.

Jacobson, M. 1968. Development of neuronal specificity in retinal ganglion cells of *Xenopus. Dev. Biol.* 17: 202–18.

Jacobson, M., and R. M. Gaze. 1965. Selection of appropriate tectal connections by regenerating optic nerve fibers in adult goldfish. *Exp. Neurol.* 13: 418–30.

Jacobson, M., and R. L. Levine. 1975. Plasticity in the adult frog brain: Filling the visual scotoma after excision or translocation of parts of the optic tectum. *Brain Res.* 88: 339–45.

Johns, P. R. 1978. Growth of the adult goldfish eye. III. Source of the new cell. *J. Comp. Neurol.* 176: 343–58.

Keating, M. J., and J. D. Feldman. 1975. Visual deprivation and intertectal neuronal connections in *Xenopus laevis. Proc. Roy. Soc. London, Ser. B* 191: 467–74.

Landmesser, L. 1980. The generation of neuromuscular specificity. *Ann. Rev. Neurosci.* 3: 279–302.

Law, M. I., and M. Constantine-Patton. 1981. Anatomy and physiology of experimentally produced striped tecta. *J. Neurosci.* 1: 741–59.

Levine, R. L., and M. Jacobson. 1974. Deployment of optic nerve fibers is determined by positional markers in the frog's tectum. *Exp. Neurol.* 43: 527–38.

Maturana, H. R., J. Y. Lettvin, W. S. McCulloch, and W. H. Pitts. 1959. Evidence the cut optic nerve fibers in a frog regenerate to their proper places in the tectum. *Science* 130: 1709–10.

Meyer, R. L. 1975. Tests for field regulation in the retinotectal system of goldfish. *In* D. McMahon and C. F. Fox (eds.) *Developmental Biology, Pattern Formation, Gene Regulation.* Benjamin, Menlo Park, (CA), pp. 257–75.

–1977. Eye-in-water electrophysiology mapping of goldfish with and without tectal lesions. *Exp. Neurol.* 56: 23–41.

–1978a. Evidence from thymidine labelling for continuing growth of retina and tectum in juvenile goldfish. *Exp. Neurol.* 59: 99–111.

–1978b. Deflection of selected optic fibers into a denervated tectum in goldfish. *Brain Res.* 155: 213–27.

–1979a. Retinotectal projection in goldfish to an inappropriate region with a reversal in polarity. *Science* 205: 819–21.

–1979b. "Extra" optic fibers exclude normal fibers from tectal regions in goldfish. *J. Comp. Neurol.* 183: 883–902.

–1980. Mapping the normal and regenerating retinotectal projection of goldfish with autoradiographic methods. *J. Comp. Neurol.* 189: 273–89.

–1982. Tetrodotoxin blocks the formation of ocular dominance columns in goldfish. *Science* 218: 589–91.

–1983. Tetrodotoxin inhibits the formation of refined retinotopography in goldfish. *Dev. Brain Res.* 6: 293–8.

–1984. Target selection by surgically misdirected optic fibers in the tectum of goldfish. *J. Neurosci.* 4: 234–50.

Meyer, R. L., and R. W. Sperry. 1973. Tests for neuroplasticity in the anuran retinotectal system. *Exp. Neurol.* 40: 525–39.

–1976. Retinotectal specificity: Chemoaffinity theory. *In* G. Gottlieb (ed.) *Studies on the Development of Behavior and the Nervous System. Vol. 3: Neural and Behavioral Specificity.* Academic Press, New York, pp. 111–49.

Prestige, M. C., and D. J. Willshaw. 1975. On a role for competition in the formation of patterned neural connections. *Proc. Roy. Soc. London, Ser. B* 190: 77–98.

Raper, J. A., M. Bastiani, and C. S. Goodman. 1983. Pathfinding by neuronal growth cones in grasshopper embryos. I. Divergent choices made by the growth cones of sibling neurons. *J. Neurosci.* 3: 20–30.

Scalia, R., and V. Arango. 1983. The anti-retinotopic organization of the frog's optic nerve. *Brain Res.* 266: 121.

Schmidt, J. T. 1978. Retinal fibers alter tectal positional markers during the expansion of the retinal projection in goldfish. *J. Comp. Neurol.* 177: 279–300.

Schmidt, J. T., C. M. Cicerone, and S. S. Easter. 1978. Expansion of the half retinal projection to the tectum in goldfish: An electrophysiological and anatomical study. *J. Comp. Neurol.* 177: 257–78.

Scholes, J. H. 1979. Nerve fiber topography in the retinal projection to the tectum. *Nature (London)* 278: 620–4.

Sharma, S. C., and Y. L. Tung. 1979. Interactions between nasal and temporal hemiretinal fibers in adult goldfish tectum. *Neurosci.* 4: 113–19.

Sperry, R. W. 1943. Visuomotor coordination in the newt (*Triturus viridescens*) after regeneration of the optic nerve. *J. Comp. Neurol.* 79: 33–55.

–1944. Optic nerve regeneration with return of vision in anurans. *J. Neurophysiol.* 7: 57–69.

–1945. Restoration of vision after crossing of optic nerves and after contralateral transposition of the eye. *J. Neurophysiol.* 8: 15–28.

–1951a. Regulative factors in the orderly growth of neural circuits. *Growth Symp.* 10: 63–87.

–1951b. Mechanisms of neural maturation. *In* S. S. Stevens (ed.) *Handbook of Experimental Psychology.* Wiley, New York, pp. 236–80.

–1963. Chemoaffinity in the orderly growth of nerve fiber patterns and connections. *Proc. Natl. Acad. Sci. USA* 50: 703–10.

–1965. Embryogenesis of behavioral nerve nets. *In* R. L.

Dehaan and H. Ursprung (eds.) *Organogenesis,* Vol. 6. Holt, Rinehart and Winston, New York, pp. 161–85.

Straznicky, K. 1978. The acquisition of tectal positional specification in *Xenopus. Neurosci. Lett.* 9: 177–84.

Straznicky, K., and R. M. Gaze. 1982. The innervation of a virgin tectum by a double-temporal or a double-nasal eye in *Xenopus. J. Embryol. Exp. Morph.* 68: 9–21.

Straznicky, K., R. M. Gaze, and M. J. Keating. 1974. The retinotectal projection from a double-ventral compound eye in *Xenopus laevis. J. Embryol. Exp. Morph.* 31: 123–37.

Straznicky, K., and D. Tay. 1977. Retinal growth in normal double dorsal and double ventral eyes in *Xenopus. J. Embryol. Exp. Morph.* 40: 175–85.

Sturmer, C. 1981. Modified retinotectal projection in goldfish: A consequence of the position of retinal lesions. *In* H. Flohr and W. Precht (eds.) *Lesion-Induced Neuronal Plasticity in Sensorimotor Systems.* Springer-Verlag, Berlin, pp. 369–76.

Udin, S. B. 1977. Rearrangement of the retinotectal projection in *Rana pipiens* after unilateral caudal half-tectum ablation. *J. Comp. Neurol.* 173: 561–82.

–1978. Permanent disorganization of the regenerating optic tract in the frog. *Exp. Neurol.* 58: 455–70.

Weiss, P. 1934. In vitro experiments on the factors determining the course of the outgrowing nerve fiber. *J. Exp. Zool.* 68: 393–448.

Whitelaw, V. A., and J. D. Cowan. 1981. Specificity and plasticity of retinal connections: A computational model. *J. Neurosci.* 1: 1369–87.

Willshaw, D. J., and C. von der Malsburg. 1976. How patterned neural connections can be set up by self-organization. *Proc. Roy. Soc. London, Ser. B* 194: 431–45.

Wolpert, L. 1969. Positional information and pattern formation. *Curr. Top. Dev. Biol.* 6: 183–224.

Yoon, M. 1971. Reorganization of retinotectal projection following surgical operations on the optic tectum in goldfish. *Exp. Neurol.* 33: 395–411.

–1973. Retention of the original topographic polarity by the 180° rotated tectal reimplant in young adult goldfish. *J. Physiol.* 233: 575–88.

–1979. Reciprocal transplantations between the optic tectum and the cerebellum in adult goldfish. *J. Physiol.* 288: 211–25.

PART II
Split-brain studies of perception, motor coordination, and learning in cats and monkeys, and comparisons to humans

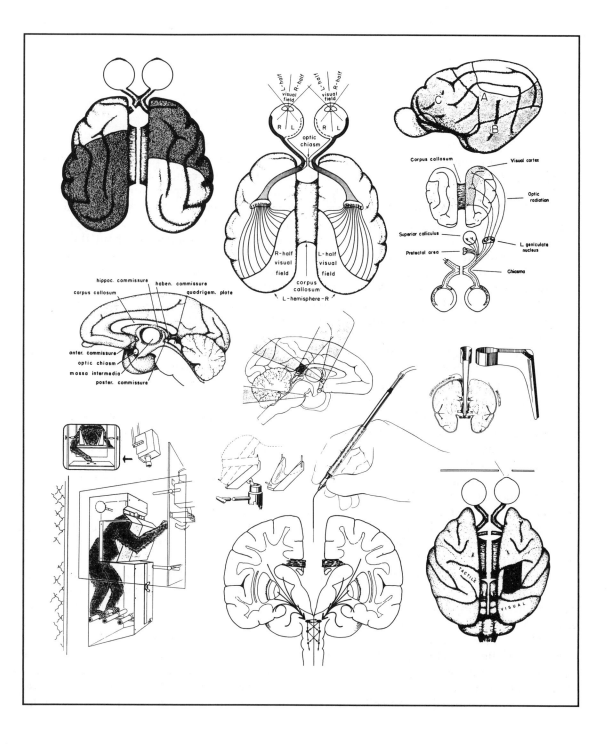

After the historic announcement of split-brain learning by Ron Meyers and Roger Sperry in 1953, Sperry directed a vigorous research activity that explored an astonishing range of questions about perception, learning, and motor coordination in the divided mammalian brain. All efforts were at understanding localization of function in the cerebral cortex. The pace of this voyage of discovery can be judged from the results and ideas for future research projects that were discussed in Sperry's 1961 *Science* review.

We have chapters from some of the participants in the first ten years and from others who came later to follow the same paths. The findings had far-reaching consequences, not only in comparative physiological psychology, but also in clinical neuropsychology. Highly original techniques were used to operate on the optic chiasma and neocortical commissures, sometimes combined with cortical ablations. Both the findings and the methods devised to demonstrate behavioral consequences were to be of crucial importance in tests made later with human commissurotomy patients. Sperry always encouraged imaginative exploration of the brand new opportunities that his surgical innovations opened up for observing the cerebral control of behavior. This is what he calls his "problem oriented" approach – it allows methods to change to suit changing questions. The fruits of this flexibility are only partly represented in the following pages, but the selection we have is, nonetheless, impressive.

Giovanni Berlucchi and his colleague An-
tonella Antonini from Padova discuss anatomical discoveries concerning the cortical visual system that arose from work Berlucchi did in Sperry's lab in the 1960s. Although the visual field is mapped, in the striate cortex, in halves that are mirror symmetric about the vertical meridian through the fovea, the subject has to perceive one world. How the two halves of information are brought together poses a classic problem that has long puzzled anatomists. Sperry proposed a solution that recent physiological work supports.

John Robinson and Theodore Voneida teamed up in Sperry's lab to explore the lower levels of visuomotor coordination in cats, and their work helps elucidate subcortical mechanisms that are capable of regulating a balance of attention, perception, and learning in the two halves of the cerebrum, even when the latter is split by commissurotomy. The degree of unity depends on what the animal is asked to do, and great ingenuity is required to devise a sufficient variety of tasks.

Mitchell Glickstein was an ebullient and friendly presence at Caltech from the very early days. His first abstracts with Sperry, on transfer of somesthetic learning in commissurotomized monkeys, came out in 1959. He explored effects of unilateral prefrontal ablations and removals of somatic cortex, and studied delayed-response learning with optic tract sections, unilateral frontal lesions, and commissurotomy, receiving valuable support in surgical operations from Harbans Arora. Here he discusses the implications of his experiments for understanding of visual guidance of movements and discusses recent research that directs attention to the cerebellum. Glickstein has carried out physiological studies in cats that prove the cerebellum to be a major center for visuomotor coordination, capable of partially compensating for the divisive effects of a split forebrain.

Bruno Preilowski from Germany carried out an important study at Caltech of the abilities of commissurotommy patients, partial and complete, to coordinate actions of the two hands, showing that the anterior part of the corpus callosum, the genu, has an important role in bimanual coordination. Here he reports experiments he has carried out on monkeys since returning to Germany that elucidate part of the baffling complex mechanisms for voluntary manual coordination.

Charles Hamilton moved across from the genetics and microbiology side of Caltech to Sperry's lab in the early 1960s to study effects of split-brain surgery on eye–hand coordination in monkeys. After a postdoctoral at Stanford, he returned to Caltech to continue the monkey research when Sperry was fully occupied with studies of commissurotomy patients. Hamilton has carried out many carefully controlled tests to see if the visual awareness and learning of split-brain monkeys are the same in the two hemispheres, or if some glimmer of the complementarity of function seen in human beings can be found in the monkey, too. Recently, the research has become more hopeful, but interpretation of the differences seen between left and right halves of a monkey brain is still exceedingly difficult.

Mortimer Mishkin and his colleague Raymond Phillips are not Caltechers. However, Mishkin is an undisguised admirer of Sperry's work. They give us a sample of the brilliant studies, directed by Mishkin at the Laboratory of Neurophysiology of the National Institutes of Mental Health, of the mechanisms by which the monkey performs visual learning. By using a reciprocal ablation technique combined with commissurotomy, the advantages of which were described a quarter of a century ago by Sperry, Mishkin and Phillips demonstrate that limbic inputs are essential to the function of visual memories. This opens up a whole new world of memory research in which notions of reward or reinforcement have much richer connotations.

6 The role of the corpus callosum in the representation of the visual field in cortical areas

Giovanni Berlucchi
and
Antonella Antonini
Istituto di Fisiologia Umana
Università di Verona

The striking disconnection syndromes shown in the classical split-brain animals and humans by Myers (1962) and Sperry (1974) leave no doubt about the primary importance of the corpus callosum in the transfer of perceptual information between the cerebral hemispheres. However, many years later, it must be admitted that the anatomical and physiological bases for this role of the corpus callosum in interhemispheric perceptual communication are still incompletely understood. In an early discussion, Sperry (1962a) underlined a difficulty in interpreting the functional significance of the predominantly homotopic callosal connections that appear to join the cortical representations of identical loci in the right and left halves of the visual fields or of corresponding points on the right and left sides of the body. He gave his preference to a "principle of supplemental complementarity" that envisaged, for example, a representation of the whole visual field in each hemisphere – the contralateral field being projected through the direct thalamocortical pathway and the ipsilateral field being transmitted by a second projection through the corpus callosum in a continuous and complementary fashion (Figure 6.1). Sperry thought that such a principle would require a heterotopic patterning of callosal connections to link noncorresponding cortical sites of the two hemispheres; however, subsequent research showed that complementary transfer of functions could be reconciled, at least partly, with a fundamentally homotopic distribution of the callosal system. We discuss this research in the following.

Callosal connections and the representation of the vertical meridian of the visual field

Sperry's scheme assumed that an orderly side-by-side arrangement of the direct projection and the indirect callosal projection to the visual cortex could result in a continuous map of the entire visual space in each hemisphere, in spite of the fact that the organization of the primary or direct visual pathways provides exclusively for the representation of each half of the visual field in the opposite hemisphere. However, a wealth of anatomical studies has revealed that the interhemispheric projections arising from and terminating in the primary visual cortex of most mammals are limited to the boundary region between areas 17 and 18 (Berlucchi 1981; Innocenti 1980). Each of these areas contains a representation of the opposite visual hemifield, and the border between them corresponds to the projection of the vertical meridian (Hubel and Wiesel 1965). This finding, along with the electrophysiological evidence that visual receptive fields of single callosal neurons are centered on the vertical midline of the field of vision (Berlucchi, Gazzaniga, and Rizzolatti 1967; Hubel and Wiesel 1967; Shatz 1977b), led to the conclusion that the representation of the visual field through the corpus callosum is limited to regions adjoining the vertical meridian and does not in-

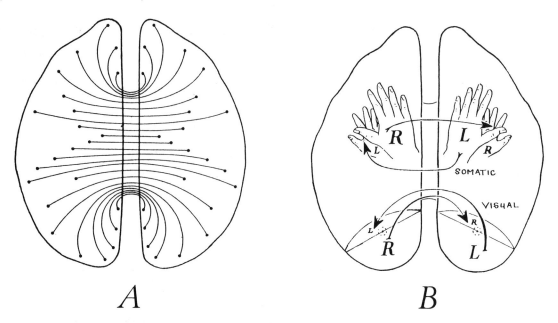

A   *B*

Figure 6.1. Sperry's principle of "supplemental complementarity" suggests that, rather than linking corresponding loci of the right and left hemispheres (**A**), the callosal function may be devoted to supplement, in a continuous and complementary fashion, the direct intrahemispheric projections (**B**) in such a way that an uninterrupted map of the whole visual field is represented in each half of the brain. (From Sperry 1962a.)

clude the more peripheral portions of the visual space along the horizontal meridian. The electrophysiological analysis made it appear as though Sperry's hypothesis of a supplemental complementarity could be supported only insofar as some neurons at the 17–18 border proved to receive both a direct and a callosal visual input, and the convergence between these two inputs was such as to build up receptive fields that straddled the vertical meridian and extended a few degrees into both halves of the visual field (Berlucchi and Rizzolatti 1968, Lepore and Guillemot 1982). This meaningful convergence could involve both homotopic (i.e., 17 to 17) and heterotopic (i.e., 17 to 18) callosal connections, provided the information conveyed by such connections was spatially and structurally congruent with that transmitted by the matching direct projection (Figure 6.2).

Over the past ten years or so, it has been shown that the brain of higher mammals possesses many retinotopically organized cortical visual areas in addition to 17 and 18 (Van Essen 1979), and the callosal connections of these areas have been reported to be less selectively distributed than those of areas 17 and 18 (Van Essen and Zeki 1978; Newsome and Allman 1980; Van Essen, Maunsell, and Bixby 1981; Segraves and Rosenquist 1982a). Does this more diffuse character of the callosal connections mean that they carry information from a larger expanse of the visual field to provide a widespread complementary input, comparable to the vertical midline-bound callosal connections of the primary visual cortex? And if this is the case, what is the relation between the callosal connections, the intrahemispheric visual projections, and the retinotopic map in these higher-order cortical areas?

Detailed anatomical maps of the distribution of callosal neurons and their terminals in several higher-order visual cortical areas of the cat have now been obtained, and their relationship to electrophysiologically determined visuotopic representations has been established. Based on these studies, Segraves and Rosenquist (1982a, 1982b) estimated that the portion of the visual field representation that receives and sends callosal projections increases progressively from areas 17, 18, and 19

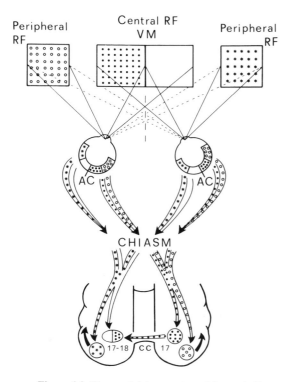

Peripheral RF | Central RF VM | Peripheral RF

Figure 6.2. The partial decussation of the optic fibers originating from the retinas of the two eyes results in a binocular representation, in each hemisphere, of the contralateral field of vision. Binocular and *bilateral* receptive fields result from a combination of intrahemispheric and callosal inputs, both of which are related to the representation of the central portion of the visual field. Cortical neurons having peripherally located receptive fields detached from the vertical meridian are not involved in the interhemispheric transfer of visual information. AC: area centralis; CC: corpus callosum; RF: receptive field; and VM: vertical meridian.

the corpus callosum, it confronts the physiologist with the old puzzle of the functional significance of connections between cells concerned with a particular region of the right field and cells concerned with the symmetrical region in the left field. Are the two regions separated by a large territory of visual field around the vertical meridian? As jocularly remarked by Sperry (1962b), at first glance, the purpose of such connections "would seem to be about as helpful as a double exposure in photography."

Our recent experiments on split-chiasm cats (Antonini, Berlucchi, and Lepore 1983) indicate that the increase of the visual-field representation through the callosum in the suprasylvian cortical areas of the cat and the apparent extension of interhemispheric interconnections to cortical points representing the peripheral visual field in these areas do not necessarily entail a departure from the rule associating callosal connections and the representation of the vertical meridian. As in areas 17 and 18 (Berlucchi and Rizzolatti 1968; Lepore and Guillemot 1982), a precise convergence of thalamic and callosal visual inputs is instrumental in ensuring a continuous and homogeneous representation of the two halves of the visual field in receptive fields of single neurons in lateral suprasylvian visual areas.

Experiments with "split-chiasm" cats and the representation of the periphery by callosal connections

The split-chiasm preparation (Berlucchi and Rizzolatti 1968) is optimally suited for studying the organization of the callosal visual input to cortical or subcortical centers. Since all of the crossed retinal fibers are transected, each hemisphere receives a direct visual input entirely from the ipsilateral (temporal) retina. Responses of neurons in one hemisphere to visual stimuli presented to the contralateral eye must be indirectly mediated by interhemispheric connections, and they disappear after section of the posterior half of the corpus callosum. Recordings from the suprasylvian visual area PMLS of Palmer, Rosenquist, and Tusa (1978) on one side in split-chiasm cats (Antonini et al. 1983) showed that more than 50% of the neurons responded to stimulation of either

to the more lateral suprasylvian visual areas. In the latter areas, homotopic callosal projections, although densest in the region that represents the vertical meridian, are present in all portions of each area and, therefore, by inference, at cortical sites representing portions of the visual field considerably more distant, indeed up to 60° from the vertical meridian. Thus, homotopic interhemispheric connections of suprasylvian visual areas are likely to link up cortical points representing mirror-symmetrical peripheral regions along the horizontal meridian of the visual field. While this pattern of interconnections could explain how each hemisphere obtains information from at least a large part of the ipsilateral visual field through eye; these binocular neurons had two receptive fields either side of the vertical meridian, one in the contralateral visual field (through the ipsilateral eye) and one in the ipsilateral visual field (through the contralateral eye). All the remaining neurons in the sample were monocular in that they were activated only through the ipsilateral eye and the contralateral visual field.

Both monocular receptive fields of binocular neurons were apposed to or lay in the close vicinity of the vertical meridian, and they matched each other for response properties and elevation relative to the horizontal meridian. If the vertical meridians of the two eyes were exactly superimposed, as it must occur under conditions of normal visual fixation, these binocular receptive fields proved to be composed of two adjacent monocular half-fields lying on opposite side of the vertical meridian.

By contrast, the receptive fields of monocular neurons could occupy any position within the contralateral visual field. Binocular neurons tended to be concentrated in the lower parts of PMLS, corresponding to the representation of the vertical meridian, and monocular neurons tended to be concentrated in the upper part of PMLS, corresponding to the representation of the peripheral visual field (Figure 6.3); however, the two types of neurons could be found in all portions of this cortical area. This is hardly surprising, since receptive fields in PMLS are usually very large (on the average about 15° across), and even in those portions of the area that are predominantly concerned with the periphery of the visual field, there are neurons whose receptive fields are wide enough to come close to or meet the vertical meridian.

It is our contention that the callosal neurons and afferents described by Segraves and Rosenquist (1982b) in the zones predominantly connected with the peripheral visual field are provided with large receptive fields extending from the periphery to the vertical meridian. This contention is supported by the disappearance, after a posterior callosal section, of the receptive field in the contralateral eye, but not that in the ipsilateral eye, for all binocular neurons in PMLS, whether they lie in the zone predominantly concerned with the vertical meridian or in that predominantly concerned with

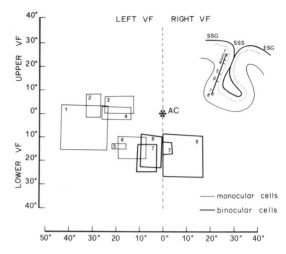

Figure 6.3. Binocular interactions in the postero-medial suprasylvian visual cortical area (area PMLS of Palmer et al. 1978) of split-chiasm cats occur only for neurons whose receptive fields in the two eyes are spatially related to the representation of the central portion of the visual field. As the two receptive fields of each binocular neuron are apposed to the vertical meridian and are matched for elevation relative to the area centralis, their combination results in an uninterrupted responsive area, including the vertical meridian and extending on both sides of it. AC: area centralis; VF: visual field; ESG: ectosylvian gyrus; SSG: suprasylvian gyrus; and SSS: suprasylvian sulcus. (From Antonini et al. 1983.)

the peripheral visual field. We concur with the claim that the callosal representation of the visual field increases from area 17, where it probably does not extend more than 10° from the vertical meridian, to the lateral suprasylvian areas, where it can encompass 50° or more to the ipsilateral side of the vertical meridian (Antonini et al. 1983). However, this increase in visual-field representation through the corpus callosum in higher-order visual cortical areas is not the result of callosal connections that selectively unite sites representing the peripheral visual field, which would be hard to understand in functional terms, but rather because receptive fields in these cortical areas are considerably larger than those in the primary visual cortex: to such a degree, indeed, that they may extend from the vertical meridian almost to the extreme periphery of the visual field. This conclusion is in full agreement with the extensive binocular representation of the ipsilateral visual field normally found in the lateral suprasylvian visual areas of cats with intact optic pathways (Hubel and Wiesel 1969, Marzi et al. 1982). At the receptive field level, this representation is continuous with that of the contralateral field, and it is largely suppressed by a posterior callosal section (Marzi et al. 1980, Marzi et al. 1982). There is no evidence for the existence of bilateral receptive fields with large gaps along the vertical meridian, as would be expected if their function were to link mirror-symmetrical representations of the peripheral fields in the two hemispheres (Hubel and Wiesel 1969, Marzi et al. 1982).

Callosal connections and visual maps in the superior colliculus

A similar complementary and continuous representation of both halves of the visual field is found upon examination of the receptive fields of single neurons in the anterior part of the superior colliculus of the cat (Antonini, Berlucchi, and Sprague 1978). Here, too, the representation of the ipsilateral visual field is primarily due to the corpus callosum, which can transmit visual information from cortical areas in one hemisphere to the opposite superior colliculus by driving neurons of the uncrossed corticotectal pathways (Antonini et al. 1979). As in the visual lateral suprasylvian areas, the representation of the ipsilateral visual field in the superior colliculus through the corpus callosum is very extensive, even though it is limited to neurons concerned with the vertical meridian, because of the generally large size of the receptive fields.

Visual maps and callosal connections in the monkey

Work on the visual system of primates (Van Essen and Zeki 1978; Newsome and Allman 1980; Van Essen et al. 1981; Van Essen, Newsome and Bixby 1982) fits in with the findings on the cat, showing that callosal connections become more diffuse as one moves from the primary visual cortex to other visual areas in the occipital, temporal, parietal, and frontal lobes. This anatomical pattern is accompanied, as in the cat, by an increase in the representation of the ipsilateral visual field (Gross Rocha-Miranda, and Bender 1972; Mohler, Goldberg, and Wurtz 1973; Robinson, Gold-

berg, and Stanton 1978). We submit that in all these areas, callosal connections are limited to neurons with receptive fields that include the vertical meridian, and that the apparent irregularity in the distribution of the callosal connections ("callosal fingerprints," see Van Essen et al. 1982) is simply a consequence of the patchy and irregular representation of the visual field in visual areas other than 17 and 18 (Van Essen and Zeki 1978, Newsome and Allman 1980, Van Essen et al. 1981, Van Essen et al. 1982).

In extrastriate areas, neurons with receptive fields including or abutting the vertical meridian can be scattered in many separate territories rather than being concentrated in a neatly delimited sector. A seemingly diffuse pattern of callosal projections, which probably depends on an irregularity of the topographic map, is present even in area 18 of the cat (Sanides and Albus 1980). An extreme example of the diffuseness of the callosal connections is the macaque's inferotemporal cortex, where a retinotopic organization is apparently lacking; in this area, all receptive fields include the vertical meridian, and most of them are large and bilateral (Desimone and Gross 1979, Gross et al. 1972). The widespread interhemispheric connections of the inferotemporal cortex appear to subserve the function of providing the input for the ipsilateral component of the bilateral receptive fields (Gross, Bender, and Mishkin 1977). In these bilateral fields, the striking selectivity for visual patterns shown by inferotemporal neurons is the same for the contralateral (intrahemispheric) and the ipsilateral (interhemispheric) components, in keeping with the findings on the homogeneous response properties of similarly constructed bilateral receptive fields in the cat cortex (Antonini et al. 1983).

An apparent exception to the continuity across the midline of visual bilateral receptive fields has been described with parietal neurons in the monkey (Motter and Mountcastle 1981). Some of these neurons respond to visual stimuli presented on the right and the left of the vertical meridian, but not to stimuli presented in between. While the response to stimuli in the ipsilateral field is most likely to be mediated by interhemispheric afferents, the lack of continuity between the two responsive areas on different sides of the vertical meridian need not be taken as evidence for a dissociation between such interhemispheric afferents and territories representing the vertical meridian. The central area of unresponsiveness may be due to a temporary attentional suppression of activity in response to foveal information, regardless of whether this is relayed by intrahemispheric or interhemispheric projections. This interpretation is suggested by the observation that, in the same area, there are other neurons with two disjoint receptive fields, one above and the other below the horizontal meridian, as well as neurons with an annular receptive field sparing the fovea.

The corpus callosum and binocular interaction

The previous description emphasizes the role of the corpus callosum in providing an input from the ipsilateral visual field to cortical or subcortical neurons that receive an input from the contralateral visual field via direct intrahemispheric projections. In animals with partially crossed optic pathways, this convergence of matching intrahemispheric and interhemispheric afferents, building up homogeneous receptive fields balanced across the vertical midline, usually applies to both eyes, since the overwhelming majority of neurons with bilateral receptive fields are also binocular. A second role in perceptual processing for convergence of intrahemispheric and interhemispheric visual afferents may arise from the formation of receptive fields that permit binocular comparison when the direct inputs to the primary areas in the two hemispheres originate from different eyes. As described before, this situation is artificially created in the split-chiasm cat by cutting the crossed optic projections.

An exclusive or predominant channeling of the optic input from each eye into the *contralateral* half of the brain occurs naturally not only in submammalian vertebrates, but also in albino mutants of several mammalian species that suffer from a genetically determined excessive crossing of the retinal projections in the optic chiasm (Hubel and Wiesel 1971, Marzi 1980). Several studies have contrasted the absence or paucity of binocular interactions in

several visual centers of albino mammals, with the wealth of such interactions in the same centers of normally pigmented animals of the same species (Hubel and Wiesel 1971; Marzi, Simoni, and Di Stefano et al. 1976; Shatz 1977a, 1977b). However, it is now clear that binocular interactions can take place in at least some visual centers of albino mutants due to the convergence of intrahemispheric and interhemispheric visual projections. In the Siamese cat, for example, most neurons in the visual-lateral suprasylvian areas respond to stimulation of either eye, exactly as they do in ordinary cats. This binocular reactivity has a different anatomofunctional basis in the two breeds, since a callosal section leaves it unaffected in ordinary cats, whereas it eliminates the input from the ipsilateral eye in the Siamese cat (Marzi et al. 1980, Zeki and Fries 1980). The corpus callosum has also been shown to be important, though not totally indispensable, for transmitting information from each eye to the ipsilateral superior colliculus in Siamese cats, thus enabling collicular neurons to integrate this information with that arriving from the other eye (Antonini et al. 1981). Comparable results have recently been obtained for the primary visual-cortical areas of albino rats (Diao, Wang, and Pu 1983).

The question is often raised whether callosal connections contribute to the binocular interactions that characterize the physiological responses of visual cells in cortical areas of animals with partially crossed optic pathways. The fact that each retina sends projections into both hemispheres would seem to make interhemispheric connections unnecessary for the convergence of information onto cortical and subcortical neurons. However, Dreher and Cottee (1975) and, more recently, Blakemore et al. (1983) reported a reduction in the number of binocularly driven neurons at the 17–18 border of cats submitted to removal or cooling of the contralateral corresponding areas. Elberger (1981) and Payne et al. (1980) described a drastic drop in the percentage of binocular neurons in the same areas of cats that had undergone a section of the corpus callosum either at birth or as adults. In the adult animal, at least, this effect develops several days after the section (Payne et al. 1980); it must, therefore, be different from that which immediately follows contralateral cortical removal or cooling (Dreher and Cottee 1975, Blakemore et al. 1983). Attempts to replicate these results in our laboratory have consistently met with failure. We have not observed a loss of binocular interaction in areas 17 and 18 of adult cats in which the corpus callosum had been cut from one hour to seven weeks before the experiment (Minciacchi and Antonini 1984). Elberger and Smith (1985) have recently reported that section of the corpus callosum reduces binocular interactions in the cat visual cortex only when performed before two weeks of age.

In spite of these conflicting results, the hypothesis that the callosal connections of the primary visual cortex may intervene in some binocular processes remains entirely plausible. For example, binocular stereopsis along the midsagittal plane requires either some overlap along the vertical meridian of the projections from the nasal and temporal hemiretinae, or a set of interhemispheric connections limited to the vertical meridian representation, or both. The existence of a nasotemporal overlap in the retinal projections has been demonstrated for several species, but its functional significance has not been determined (Stone, Leicester, and Sherman 1973; Stone and Fukuda 1974; Bunt, Minckler, and Johanson 1977). Section of the corpus callosum is accompanied by a loss of coarse stereopsis along the midsagittal plane in man (Blakemore 1969, Mitchell and Blakemore 1970). According to Bishop (1971) fine stereopsis along the midsagittal plane would be subserved solely by the nasotemporal overlap in the retinal projections. The recent results of Blakemore et al. (1983) suggest that rather than extending the receptive fields of neurons of areas 17 and 18 into the ipsilateral visual field, callosal connections of these areas may be involved in forming binocular receptive fields with interocular disparity in the cortical regions that correspond to the nasotemporal overlap. Receptive fields with binocular disparity in this region would thus depend both on incomplete crossing of optic fibers in the chiasm and on the interhemispheric links provided by callosal connections (Whitteridge and Clarke 1982).

It is obvious that any contribution of the callosal connections to stereoscopic vision must be restricted to receptive fields with a transverse diameter of at most 10° that lie in the immediate vicinity of the vertical meridian. It is unlikely that the large receptive fields found in the lateral suprasylvian visual areas could subserve this function; they are more probably involved in the capacity of the visual systems in each hemisphere to cross-integrate visual information originating from the two hemifields. Presumably, they provide the neural basis for equivalence of perceptual experience across the two eyes or the two hemifields, and for interocular transfer of learning in chiasm-sectioned animals (Berlucchi et al. 1979, Gross and Mishkin 1977).

Is the callosal pathway involved in inhibitory interactions between cells in the two hemispheres?

This particular aspect of the callosal function may be deduced from the presence of excitatory receptive fields that have suppressive surrounds extending into the ipsilateral visual field. In the monkey's cortical area V4, such receptive fields do exist and the corpus callosum seems in part responsible for this interhemispherically mediated suppression of neuronal activity (Moran et al. 1983). The important feature of this inhibition is that it can be evoked by visual stimuli presented in the ipsilateral hemifield even at large distances from the vertical meridian. However, these callosum-dependent inhibitory surrounds are continuous with the excitatory portion of the receptive field lying on the other side of the vertical meridian, supporting once more the evidence that callosal influences are compatible only with an uninterrupted visuotopic representation of the visual space on both sides of the vertical meridian.

The across-the-midline inhibition is probably subserved by callosal-projecting neurons with large receptive fields, extending from the vertical meridian to the periphery of the visual field. As callosal fibers appear to be excitatory in nature (Naito et al. 1970), the ipsilateral inhibitory surrounds of these cortical receptive fields must rely on local inhibitory interneurons activated by the callosal input. The presence of these broad inhibitory surrounds in the ipsilateral visual field of a size much exceeding that of the contralateral excitatory portion of the receptive field can be related to the anatomical finding of a rather diffuse pattern of callosal projections in this area (Zeki 1978). These large inhibitory surrounds appear, in all cases, to adjoin the vertical meridian and their function is most likely identical to that of similar inhibitory surrounds of cells with receptive fields lying entirely in the contralateral visual field.

Plasticity in the development of the callosal system

A striking anatomical difference between the adult and the newborn cat is the restriction of callosal connections to the 17–18 border in the adult animal as compared to the widespread callosal connectivity in the same areas in the newborn (Innocenti, Fiore, and Caminiti 1977). This postnatal reduction of interhemispheric connections raises the question of whether the definitive adult anatomy depends on inherent morphogenetic principles alone or on selective environmental factors as well (Innocenti 1981). There is strong evidence that while the projections concerned with the representation of the vertical meridian are scarcely affected by the animal's visual experience, since they are retained even if the animal is raised in the dark (Innocenti and Frost 1979, 1980; Lund and Mitchell 1979), the fate of callosal connections outside the 17–18 border in the adult cat depends on the pattern of early visual stimulation.

In the normal adult cat, loss of callosal projections from regions remote from the representation of the vertical meridian may result from the incongruence between the visual messages carried by the inter- and intrahemispheric pathways to these regions. It is, in fact, highly unlikely that in normal everyday visual experience, the peripheral portions of the right and left hemifields contain the same stimuli at the same time. It may be that the mismatch between the callosal and noncallosal inputs upsets the balance in competition between terminals of the intra- and interhemispheric pathways, so that only the intrahemispheric projections coming from corresponding points of the two retinas are left. The situation is different near the vertical meridian, where symmetrical targets extending on both sides of the vertical meridian could provide identical stimuli to the cortex via

inter- and intrahemispheric pathways, and this might allow both to be retained.

This hypothesis is supported by the observation that in animals with an anomalous correspondence between the two retinas, such as cats rendered strabismic from birth or squinting animals like Siamese cats, the callosal system retains its neonatal diffuse organization (Shatz 1977c; Lund, Mitchell, and Henry 1978). This persistence of diffuse callosal connections can be ascribed to the fact that due to the strabismus, noncorresponding points in the retinas may receive an identical stimulation, thereby favoring abnormal connections between their cortical representations both within and between the hemispheres (Shatz 1977c, Shatz and Levay 1979). An alternative explanation of the maturation of the visual callosal connections would emphasize the importance of the correlation between the *spontaneous* activities of the ganglion cells in the retinal strip projecting to both hemispheres (Rhoades and Fish 1983). A similar hypothesis has been advanced to explain development of convergent retinotectal maps in lower vertebrates (Willshaw and von der Malsburg 1976).

These features of the callosal connectivity that we have discussed are concerned exclusively with the visual system. Other studies suggest that callosal connections of the cortical areas that serve other modalities may also be arranged according to an orderly selective pattern. For example, the somatoesthesic and auditory systems possess multiple cortical representations of the peripheral receptors (Stone and Dreher 1982), and their callosal connections are limited to specific areal portions or neuronal groups (see references in Berlucchi 1981). Further investigations on callosal connectivity in those various cortical areas may reveal common properties of interhemispheric connections, and this knowledge may, in turn, help the understanding of cortical circuitry in general.

Conclusions

The fact that the two halves of the visual field are projected to different hemispheres has consistently posed a problem for theories about the neural substrates of visual perception. Sperry was well aware of this problem when, many years ago, he presented his first detailed account of the possible relations between neurology and the mind-brain problem (Sperry 1952). Although he conceded that "when a visual figure is perceived as a unified whole, it is natural to suppose that the brain pattern also possesses a corresponding unity," he also pointed out that such a unity ought to be searched not in a compact unified pattern of neural discharge, but rather in an overall cerebral organization that predisposes the organism to deal with the perceived object as a unit. He viewed topographic projections from sense organs to the cortex as the reflections of the developmental processes of neurogenesis, rather than the bases of isomorphic representation of the external world. "If topographic projection could be eliminated by random displacement of neurons, at the same time maintaining all the original synaptic connections and the conduction-time intervals, . . . little or no disturbance would be expected from the standpoint of orthodox circuit theory" (Sperry 1952).

We feel that a similar reasoning can be applied to the organization of the callosal connections of visual areas that we have described here. It does not matter for the unity of visual perception that the two halves of the visual field are initially projected to different hemispheres, and that neurons "looking at" one-half of the visual field lie in cerebral structures widely separated from those that contain neurons concerned with the other half of the visual field. Due to the organization of the callosal connections, there are in each hemisphere neurons that "look at" both halves of the visual field, thus supporting the complementary pattern for callosal integration that Sperry suggested long ago (Sperry 1962a). We submit that the normal conjoint action of the two hemispheres in visual perception and memory depends crucially on these neurons, and that the disconnection syndrome shown in visually guided behavior by split-brain animals and humans is directly caused by the elimination of bilateral receptive fields of neurons normally integrating intra- and interhemispheric visual inputs.

While this scheme leaves much unanswered and fails to address important questions, such as the distinction between the interhemispheric transfer of sensory material

and that of memories, at least it can be offered as an initial attempt to describe the neural events that underlie interhemispheric communication in vision.

References

Antonini, A., G. Berlucchi, M. Di Stefano, and C. A. Marzi. 1981. Differences in binocular interactions between cortical areas 17 and 18 and superior colliculus of Siamese cats. *J. Comp. Neurol.* 200: 597–611.

Antonini, A., G. Berlucchi, and F. Lepore. 1983. Physiological organization of callosal connections of a visual lateral suprasylvian cortical area in the cat. *J. Neurophysiol.* 49: 902–21.

Antonini, A., G. Berlucchi, C. A. Marzi, and J. M. Sprague. 1979. Importance of corpus callosum for visual receptive fields of single neurons in the cat superior colliculus. *J. Neurophysiol.* 42: 137–52.

Antonini, A., G. Berlucchi, and J. M. Sprague. 1978. Indirect, across-the-midline retinotectal projections and the representation of ipsilateral visual field in the superior colliculus of the cat. *J. Neurophysiol.* 41: 285–304.

Berlucchi, G. 1981. Recent advances in the analysis of the neural substrates of interhemispheric communication. *In* O. Pompeiano, and C. Ajmone Marsan (eds.) *Brain Mechanisms and Perceptual Awareness.* Raven Press, New York, pp. 133–52.

Berlucchi, G., M. S. Gazzaniga, and G. Rizzolatti. 1967. Microelectrode analysis of transfer of visual information by the corpus callosum. *Arch. Ital. Biol.* 105: 583–96.

Berlucchi, G., and G. Rizzolatti. 1968. Binocularly driven neurons in visual cortex of split-chiasm cats. *Science* 159: 308–10.

Berlucchi, G., J. M. Sprague, A. Antonini, and A. Simoni. 1979. Learning and interhemispheric transfer of visual pattern discriminations following unilateral suprasylvian lesions in split-chiasm cats. *Exp. Brain Res.* 34: 551–74.

Bishop, P. O. 1971. Neural mechanisms for binocular depth discrimination. *In* E. Grastyan, and P. Molnar (eds.) *Advances in Physiological Sciences. Sensory Functions.* Pergamon, Oxford (UK), pp. 441–9.

Blakemore, C. 1969. Binocular depth discrimination and the nasotemporal division. *J. Physiol. (London)* 205: 471–97.

Blakemore C., Y. C. Diao, M. L. Pu, Y. K. Wang, and Y. M. Xiao. 1983. Possible functions of the interhemispheric connections between visual cortical areas in the cat. *J. Physiol. (London)* 337: 331–49.

Bunt, A., D. S. Minckler, and G. W. Johnson. 1977. Demonstration of bilateral projection of the central retina of the monkey with horseradish peroxidase neuronography. *J. Comp. Neurol.* 171: 619–80.

Desimone, R., and C. G. Gross. 1979. Visual areas in the temporal cortex of the macaque. *Brain Res.* 178: 363–80.

Diao, Y. G., Y. K. Wang, and M. L. Pu. 1983. Binocular responses of cortical cells and the callosal projection in the albino rat, *Exp. Brain Res.* 49: 410–18.

Dreher, B., and L. J. Cottee. 1975. Visual receptive-field properties of cells in area 18 of cat's cerebral cortex before and after acute lesion in area 17. *J. Neurophysiol.* 38: 735–50.

Elberger, A. J. 1981. Ocular dominance in striate cortex is altered by neonatal section of the posterior corpus callosum in the cat. *Exp. Brain Res.* 41: 280–91.

Elberger, A. J., and E. L. Smith. 1985. The critical period of corpus callosum section to affect cortical binocularity. *Exp. Brain Res.* 57: 213–23.

Gross, C. G., D. B. Bender, and M. Mishkin. 1977. Contributions of the corpus callosum and the anterior commissure to visual activation of inferior temporal neurons. *Brain Res.* 131: 227–39.

Gross, C. G., and D. B. Mishkin. 1977. The neural basis of stimulus equivalence across retinal translation. *In* S. Harnad (ed.) *Lateralization of the Nervous System.* Academic Press, New York, pp. 109–22.

Gross, C. G., C. E. Rocha-Miranda, and D. B. Bender. 1972. Visual properties of neurons in inferotemporal cortex of the macaque. *J. Neurophysiol.* 35: 96–111.

Hubel, D. H., and T. N. Wiesel. 1965. Receptive fields and functional architecture in two nonstriate visual areas (18 and 19) of the cat. *J. Neurophysiol.* 28: 229–89.

–1967. Cortical and callosal connections concerned with the vertical meridian of visual fields in the cat. *J. Neurophysiol.* 30: 1561–73.

–1969. Visual area of the lateral suprasylvian gyrus of the cat. *J. Physiol. (London)* 202: 251–60.

–1971. Aberrant visual projections in the Siamese cat. *J. Physiol. (London)* 218: 33–62.

Innocenti, G. M. 1980. The primary visual pathway through the corpus callosum: Morphological and functional aspects in the cat. *Arch. Ital. Biol.* 118: 127–88.

–1981. The development of interhemispheric connections. *Trends in Neurosci.* 4: 142–4.

Innocenti, G. M., L. Fiore, and R. Caminiti. 1977. Exhuberant projection into the corpus callosum from the visual cortex of newborn cats. *Neurosci. Lett.* 4: 237–42.

Innocenti, G. M., and D. O. Frost. 1979. Effects of visual experience on the maturation of the efferent system to the corpus callosum. *Nature (London)* 280: 231–4.

–1980. The postnatal development of visual callosal connections in the absence of visual experience or of the eyes. *Exp. Brain Res.* 39: 365–75.

Lepore, F., and J. P. Guillemot. 1982. Visual receptive field properties of cells innervated through the corpus callosum in the cat. *Exp. Brain Res.* 46: 413–24.

Lund, R. D., and D. E. Mitchell. 1979. The effect of dark rearing on visual callosal connections of cats. *Brain Res.* 167: 172–5.

Lund, R. D., D. E. Mitchell, and G. H. Henry. 1978. Squint-induced modification of callosal connections in cats. *Brain Res.* 144: 169–72.

Marzi, C. A. 1980. Vision in Siamese cats. *Trends in Neurosci.* 3: 165–9.

Marzi, C. A., A. Antonini, M. Di Stefano, and C. R. Legg. 1980. Callosum-dependent binocular interactions in the lateral suprasylvian area of Siamese cats which lack binocular neurons in areas 17 and 18, *Brain Res.* 197: 230–5.

–1982. The contribution of the corpus callosum to receptive fields in the lateral suprasylvian visual areas of the cat. *Behav. Brain Res.* 4: 155–76.

Marzi, C. A., A. Simoni, and M. Di Stefano. 1976. Lack of binocularly driven neurones in the Siamese cat's visual cortex does not prevent successful interocular transfer of visual form discriminations. *Brain Res.* 105: 353–6.

Minciacchi, D., and A. Antonini, 1984. Binocularity in the visual cortex of the adult cat does not depend on the integrity of the corpus callosum. *Behav. Brain Res.* 13: 183–92.

Mitchell, D. E., and C. Blakemore. 1970. Binocular depth perception and the corpus callosum. *Vis. Res.* 10: 49–54.

Mohler, C. W., M. E. Goldberg, and R. Wurtz. 1973. Visual receptive fields of frontal eye field neurons. *Brain Res.* 61: 385–9.

Moran, J., R. Desimone, S. J. Shein, and M. Mishkin, 1983. Suppression from ipsilateral visual field in area V4 of the macaque, *Abs. Soc. Neurosci.* 9: 953.

Motter, B. C., and V. B. Mountcastle, 1981. The functional properties of the light-sensitive neurons of the posterior parietal cortex studied in waking monkeys: Foveal sparing and opponent vector organization. *J. Neurosci.* 1: 3–26.

Myers, R. E. 1962. Transmission of visual information within and between the hemispheres: A behavioral study. *In* V. B. Mountcastle (ed.) *Interhemispheric Relations and Cerebral Dominance.* The Johns Hopkins Press, Baltimore, pp. 51–73.

Naito, H., K. Nakamura, T. Kurosaki, and Y. Tamura. 1970. Transcallosal excitatory postsynaptic potentials of fast and slow pyramidal tract cells in cat sensorimotor cortex. *Brain Res.* 19: 299–301.

Newsome, W. T., and J. M. Allman. 1980. Interhemispheric connections of visual cortex in the Owl monkey, *Aotus trivirgatus,* and the bushbaby, *Galago senegalensis. J. Comp. Neurol.* 194: 209–34.

Palmer, L. A., A. C. Rosenquist, and R. J. Tusa. 1978. The retinotopic organization of the lateral suprasylvian visual areas in the cat. *J. Comp. Neurol.* 177: 237–56.

Payne, B. R., A. J. Elberger, N. Berman, and E. M. Murphy. 1980. Binocularity in the cat visual cortex is reduced by sectioning the corpus callosum. *Science* 207: 1097–9.

Rhoades, R. W., and S. E. Fish. 1983. Bilateral enucleation alters visual callosal but not corticotectal or corticogeniculate projections in hamsters. *Exp. Brain Res.* 51: 451–62.

Robinson, D. L., M. E. Goldberg, and G. B. Stanton. 1978. Parietal association cortex in the primate: Sensory mechanisms and behavioral modulation, *J. Neurophysiol.* 41: 910–32.

Sanides, D., and K. Albus. 1980. The distribution of interhemispheric projections in area 18 of the cat: A coincidence with discontinuities of the representation of the visual field in the second visual area (V2). *Exp. Brain Res.* 38: 237–40.

Segraves, M. A., and A. C. Rosenquist. 1982a. The distribution of the cells of origin of callosal projections in cat visual cortex. *J. Neurosci.* 2: 1079–89.

–1982b. The afferent and efferent callosal connections of retinotopically defined areas in the cat cortex. *J. Neurosci.* 2: 1090–1107.

Shatz, C. 1977a. A comparison of visual pathways in Boston and Midwestern Siamese cats. *J. Comp. Neurol.* 171: 205–28.

–1977b. Abnormal interhemispheric connections in the visual system of Boston Siamese cats: A physiological study. *J. Comp. Neurol.* 171: 229–46.

–1977c. Anatomy of interhemispheric connections in the visual system of Boston Siamese cats and ordinary cats. *J. Comp. Neurol.* 173: 497–518.

Shatz, C., and S. LeVay. 1979. Siamese cats: Altered connections of the visual cortex. *Science* 204: 328–30.

Sperry, R. W. 1952. Neurology and the mind-brain problem. *Am. Scientist* 40: 291–312.

–1962a. Orderly function with disordered structure. *In* H. von Foerster and G. W. Zopf, Jr. (eds.) *Principles of Self-Organization.* Pergamon Press, New York, pp. 279–90.

–1962b. Some general aspects of interhemispheric integration *In* V. B. Mountcastle (ed.) *Interhemispheric Relations and Cerebral Dominance.* The Johns Hopkins Press, Baltimore, pp. 43–9.

–1974. Lateral specialization in the surgically separated hemispheres. *In* F. O. Schmitt and F. G. Worden (eds.) *The Neurosciences: Third Study Program.* The MIT Press, Cambridge, pp. 5–19.

Stone, J., and B. Dreher. 1982. Parallel processing of information in the visual pathways. *Trends in Neurosci.* 5: 441–6.

Stone, J. and Y. Fukuda. 1974. The naso-temporal division of the cat's retina re-examined in terms of Y-, X- and W-cells. *J. Comp. Neurol.* 155: 377–94.

Stone, J., J. Leicester, and S. M. Sherman. 1973. The naso-temporal division of the monkey retina. *J. Comp. Neurol.* 150: 333–348.

Van Essen, D. C. 1979. Visual cortical areas. *Ann. Rev. Neurosci.* 2: 227–73.

Van Essen, D. C., H. R. Maunsell, and J. L. Bixby. 1981. The middle temporal visual area in the macaque: Myeloarchitecture, connections, functional projections and topographic organization. *J. Comp. Neurol.* 199: 293–366.

Van Essen, D. C., W. T. Newsome, and J. L. Bixby. 1982. The pattern of interhemispheric connections and its relationship to extrastriate visual areas in the macaque monkey. *J. Neurosci.* 2: 265–83.

Van Essen, D. C., and S. M. Zeki. 1978. The topographic organization of rhesus monkey prestriate cortex. *J. Physiol. (London)* 227: 193–226.

Whitteridge, D., and P. G. H. Clarke. 1982. Ipsilateral visual field represented in the cat's visual cortex. *Neurosci.* 7: 1855–60.

Willshaw, D. J., and C. von der Malsburg. 1976. How patterned neural connections can be set up by self-organization. *Proc. Roy. Soc. London, Ser. B* 194: 431–45.

Zeki, S. M. 1978. Uniformity and diversity of structure and function in rhesus monkey prestriate visual cortex. *J. Physiol. (London)* 277: 273–90.

Zeki, S. M., and W. Fries. 1980. A function of the corpus callosum in the Siamese cat. *Proc. Roy. Soc. London, Ser. B* 207: 249–58.

7 Studies of visual perception and orienting in cats with fore- and midbrain commissure section

John S. Robinson
Formerly of the Department of Psychiatry
Brain-Behavior Research Center
University of California
and
Theodore J. Voneida
Department of Neurobiology
Northeastern Ohio Universities College of Medicine

Introduction

The split-brain research of Roger Sperry and his co-workers is a remarkably successful application of experiments with animal subjects to man's pursuit of an understanding of himself. The animal studies served not only as an inspiration for the investigations of human commissurotomy patients, they served also as important controls, providing for a clearer interpretation of the human findings.

Initial experiments demonstrated the isolation of cognitive processes in the two hemispheres of cats and monkeys following section of the forebrain commissures. They provided an exciting prediction of what would be found if patients with hemispheres separated for the surgical control of life-threatening epilepsy were carefully tested, using methods patterned after the animal experiments. At the same time they provided a key for interpretation of the momentous discovery of the isolation of two consciousnesses in the separated brain halves of operated patients. They indicated that this mental division was caused by the interruption of commissural pathways and was not some peculiar consequence of brain pathology or of medication for epilepsy.

We will review our early work with split-brain cats and present some studies completed recently. The latter raise and, we hope, help to answer further questions about the role of cross-midline connections in animal and human behavior.

Our earlier studies of cognitive processing in the split-brain animal

Our joint research of interhemispheric mechanisms began in the early sixties when we came to Sperry's laboratory with dissimilar though complementary interests and a shared enthusiasm for his psychobiological approach to brain-behavior problems. One of us (JSR) arrived with a strong behavioristic background, whereas the background of the other (TJV) was as strongly biological. The unifying factor that led us to collaborate was Sperry's attempt to understand and explain behavior in biological terms. Our complementary backgrounds engendered the psychobiological collaboration that we have enjoyed for nearly a quarter of a century.

BIHEMISPHERIC COORDINATION IN PERCEPTION

Initially, we studied the completeness of hemispheric functional separation following commissurotomy. Specifically, we wanted to know if isolation of percepts in the separate brain halves was as complete as had been demonstrated earlier for the isolation of memory traces in the split-brain cat (Myers 1955, 1956; Stamm, Miner, and Sperry 1956).

We designed a problem that required cats to make cross-midline comparison of visual inputs presented simultaneously on either side of the vertical meridian and thus to the separate hemispheres (cf. Chapter 6, this volume). Subjects had to cross-integrate vertical and horizontal stripe components of compound stimuli in a two-choice discrimination. They secured a reward by selecting the compound that had nonmatching components (VH or HV); the alternative choice compounds (HH or VV) were negative.

Performance on this task was near normal following optic chiasm section, dividing input from the two eyes and the two halves of the visual field. Following subsequent section of the caudal two-thirds of the corpus callosum, accuracy of choices dropped but remained above chance. This combined surgery did, however, achieve complete memory trace isolation; opposing discriminations ($\triangle +$, O$-$ versus $\triangle -$, O$+$) could be learned by the separate hemispheres concurrently without conflict, as shown earlier in Myers' pioneering study (1956). These results have been interpreted as showing that the caudal corpus callosum is needed for efficient cross-integration of visual-pattern perception in the chiasm-sectioned cat. When this portion of the corpus callosum is divided, the cat can still cross-integrate some visual information, but this residual capacity seems to be lost when the remaining rostral third of the callosum is sectioned (Voneida and Robinson 1970). We must make such an interpretation with caution, however, in view of studies demonstrating the importance of such variables as motivation and different methods employed in testing for the outcome of interhemispheric transfer (Doty and Negrão 1973).

In an earlier study, complete forebrain commissurotomy (corpus callosum, hippocampal and anterior commissures) had proved ineffective in blocking cross-comparison of brightness inputs (Robinson and Voneida 1964). The addition of midbrain commissurotomy merely increased performance variability in the latter task. We suggested that, under these circumstances, cross-integration for brightness discrimination had taken place via midbrain tegmental pathways.

The studies of cross-midline communication revealed an hierarchy of fore- and midbrain systems that appear to vary greatly in the stimulus complexity that they can handle and in their ability to mediate reliable response coordination.

CAPACITY FOR PERCEPTION IN SEPARATED HEMISPHERES

A primary prerequisite for evaluating interhemispheric communication in the previous experiments is the demonstration that each hemisphere can make the required perceptual comparison on its own. If the ability to do this is not maintained at a high level, one cannot be sure that failure of the animal to make interhemispheric comparison is due to impaired cross-conduction.

We found that after chiasm and callosum were sectioned, subjects with one eye-hemisphere occluded were unable to maintain precommissurotomy 90+% response levels on comparison tests similar to the one described before. Performance remained high, however, for the bilateral concurrent intrahemispheric condition, that is, when both hemispheres worked simultaneously on the same comparisons. We also found that the deficit with unilateral input was more severe on one side than on the other. In subsequent experiments, we explored these effects more directly and discovered that in most cases, cognitive capacity of the cat's single hemisphere is indeed significantly less than that of the whole brain (Robinson and Voneida 1970, 1975; Voneida and Robinson 1971). We used complex-task performance (Robinson and Voneida 1970, 1975) or learning (Voneida and Robinson 1971) to reveal the cat's single-hemisphere deficit. Sechzer (1970), moreover, showed that the split-brain cat's learning of even a simple pattern discrimination was greatly prolonged if the stimuli were confined to one hemisphere. In addition, Hamilton (1977b) reported that unilateral visual-pattern-discrimination learning in monkeys required nearly three times as long per problem (about 1000 trials) as bilateral learning of the same discriminations.

These findings were not what one would have predicted on the basis of Sperry's earlier review of studies with split-brain animals, in which he emphasized the functional interchangeability of the half and the whole brain (Sperry 1961).

EQUALITY OF PERCEPTION IN THE TWO HEMISPHERES

The early studies of commissurotomized patients from Sperry's laboratory showed how the surgery created two independent, isolated mental spheres within a single brain (Gazzaniga 1967; Sperry 1967, 1968; Sperry, Gazzaniga, and Bogen 1969). As time went on, the completeness of this isolation continued to be a subject of keen interest and intense study. In much of the later work, however, this isolation was simply accepted and was exploited for the study of what is perhaps the most outstanding aspect of human brain organization, i.e., the lateralization of specific capacities in one or the other hemisphere, with a given function tending to be found on the same side in most individuals. This characteristic of human cerebral organization is illustrated abundantly in later chapters of this volume.

In our comparison of the cognitive capacities of right and left hemispheres of individual split-brain cats, it was relatively easy to show differences in capacity if we used performance on a cognitively demanding task (Robinson and Voneida 1973). This finding of hemisphere differences gained substantial support from a study by Gulliksen and Voneida (1975) that rigorously examined the question of equality of learning ability in the individual cat's separated hemispheres. Here, too, Sperry's comments in the previously mentioned review article did not prepare us for the differences we obtained; he asserted that the brain-bisected monkey's two hemispheres are not only genetically equal, but, up to the time of splitting, experientially equal as well (Sperry 1961, p. 5).

Concurrently with our work on the cat, Hamilton was attempting to bridge the gap between animals and humans by trying to see if, after all, there was not some asymmetry of function in what had first appeared to be the equivalent hemispheres of the monkey (see Chapter 10, this volume). Such asymmetry has been reported for baboons by Trevarthen (1978), who found evidence for a dominant and a subordinate hemisphere in his study of right- and left-handed animals. These subjects learned a manipulative skill, using primarily the preferred hand; following subsequent bisection of chiasm and forebrain commissures, he found that control of the skill was concentrated in the hemisphere contralateral to the preferred hand.

In our report of hemisphere differences, we were careful to point out that the superior hemisphere was equally often on the right and left in different cats. We cautioned against identifying our finding with the kind of inherent and consistent hemisphere dominance that occurs in humans. In a review of his own and others' work, Hamilton (1977a) concluded that the existence of hemispheric specialization in nonhumans had little experimental support. His more recent work, however, shows that such specialization can be demonstrated for the monkey (see Chapter 10, this volume).

The following pages include a presentation of our recently completed unpublished work related to visually guided behavior in the unencumbered fore- and midbrain commissurotomized animal.

Recent studies of changes in orienting and attending behavior resulting from commissurotomy

During the past several years, we have shifted our attention to the direct effects of commissurotomy on free behavior. We have attempted to design experiments that will provide a clear view of the effects of midline surgery on cats that are unencumbered by experimental behavioral constraints. It is hoped that these data may provide some insight into what effect commissurotomy might have in humans without brain disease or medication.

GENERAL DESCRIPTION
OF THE EXPERIMENTS

Tests of performance were given in three separate settings: orientation to live prey; vision-duration thresholds for discrimination of targets differing in brightness, orientation, size and form; and latency of response to the same targets. We will present the orientation study first and then the visual threshold and response latency experiments for the insight they may provide for interpreting the results obtained in the orientation problem.

All cats in the orientation study were selected on the basis of their aggressive attack behavior toward mice in preliminary observations made in the orientation test apparatus to be described (Figure 7.1). The visual-threshold and response latency measurements employed

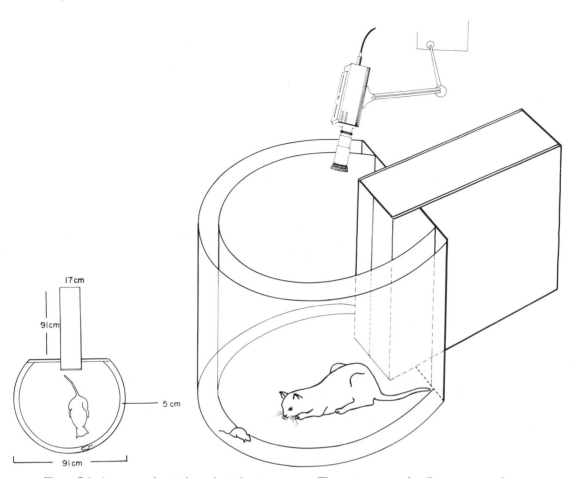

Figure 7.1. Apparatus for testing orientation to a mouse. The outer surround wall was opaque; the inner, transparent. A split curtain of sheet rubber covered the starting tunnel exit. The experimenter prepared for a trial by introducing a mouse into the display space and a cat into the starting tunnel. A trial was begun when the cat entered the arena, at which time a video recorder and timer were started.

a task that had been mastered previously to a high level of proficiency. Stimuli were projected onto a tangent screen facing the open front of a test cage (Figures 7.2 and 7.3).

Surgery was performed under sterile conditions with the aid of a stereoscopic microscope, as described by Voneida (1963). Convalescent periods of at least two weeks were allowed prior to testing. Surgery was checked histologically upon termination of testing, and all commissurotomies were confirmed to be complete except in one animal (Bby) in which the rostral tip of the corpus callosum remained unsectioned. Four subjects (Bby, Mtt, Trp, Spk) underwent section of the corpus callosum, anterior and hippocampal commissures as a first operation. Subsequent to post-

operative testing, each of these underwent section of the commissure of the superior colliculus. Four others (Brt, Rgo, Sek, and Arn) underwent superior collicular commissurotomy only.

COMMISSUROTOMY AND ORIENTING

In this experiment, we studied the effect of midbrain (CSC) commissurotomy on orientation to live prey. We selected 11 cats from our colony (nine unoperated, two with forebrain commissures sectioned) for aggressive attack behavior toward mice. The subjects' responses to live but inaccessible mice were recorded in two tests of four daily sessions each (T1 and T2). Initial test performances of the animals with forebrain commissures cut were not significantly different from those of the nine unoperated subjects (NS = 9 and 2, Mann-Whitney U = 6; p > 0.05). After the first test, the superior colliculi were surgically disconnected in the five experimental animals (three intact and two forebrain-sectioned cats, see Table 7.1). Following a minimal recovery period of two weeks, we tested all cats in T2.

Figure 7.1 shows the perimeter surround in which we presented a live mouse. A trial was initiated by introducing a mouse into the space between the perimeter surround and the transparent plastic barrier, releasing the cat from the starting tunnel and starting a timer and video recorder. Initially, all subjects bumped against the barrier in attempts to capture the mouse. They adapted readily, however (usually early in T1), by staying some distance from the barrier, apparently to obtain a clearer view of the mouse (Bloom and Berkley 1977). All subjects provided measurable amounts of orientation to the unobtainable prey throughout both pre- and postoperation tests (motivation was maintained by giving a live mouse to the cat in the arena at the end of each daily session). The cat was considered to be oriented to the prey during the period in which he faced the mouse and "bracketed" it with his ears (as seen from above and behind, Figure 7.1). This period is subsequently called *orientation time*. The validity of this criterion was attested to by the cat's "locking on" to the mouse and moving when it moved, so that bracketing was maintained. Videotape records were analyzed daily and the data compiled. The percent orientation time to (1) motionless or (2) moving prey in T1 and T2 provided us with a total of four test scores for each subject.

We found that all experimental subjects with colliculi disconnected oriented less in T2 than they did in T1, with mean percent decrements of 66 and 42 for the moving and

Table 7.1. *Subjects, operations, and tests*

	Normal	Forebrain	Midbrain	Fore- & Midbrain
Orientation	Csc[a]	Bby[b]	Brt	Bby
	Brt	Trp[b]	Rgo	Trp
	Rgo		Sck	
	Frn[a]			
	Sck			
	Rdy[a]			
	Arn[a]			
	Sym[a]			
	Gln[a]			
Visual threshold	Bby	Bby	Brt	Bby
	Mtt	Mtt	Arn[c]	Mtt
	Trp	Trp		Trp
	Spk	Spk		Spk
	Brt			
	Arn[c]			
Response latency	Brt	Bby	Brt	Bby
	Arn	Mtt	Arn	Mtt
		Trp		Trp
		Spk		Spk

[a]Control subjects: tested twice with time between tests equal to duration of experimental subjects' convalescence period.
[b]Experimental subjects: received initial orientation test with forebrain commissures sectioned. Scores were within the range of normal subjects' scores.
[c]Attempts to measure thresholds after midbrain surgery were not successful.

motionless prey, respectively. For both decrements w = 15, p = 0.03 (Wilcoxon's signed rank test). The control subjects showed mean decrements of 28.5 and 2.8 for the moving and the motionless mouse, respectively, with p >0.1 for both by the Wilcoxon test, but some subjects showed an increased orientation time in T2 for one or both stimuli.

How are we to interpret these findings? The majority of fibers in the commissure of the superior colliculi arise from neurons that occupy the deeper layers of each superior colliculus and terminate on reticular nuclei within the mid- and hindbrain and the spinal cord (Edwards and de Olmos 1976; Edwards 1977, 1980; Magalhães-Castro et al. 1978). It has been suggested that these polymodal neurons are active in the integration of orienting behavior (Anderson and Symmes 1969, Casagrande et al. 1972, Harting et al. 1973) and, indeed, that the superior colliculus, traditionally assumed to be primarily visual in function, is perhaps more appropriately considered as an integrator of multimodal sensorimotor activity. It follows that section of the collicular commissure might be expected to have a greater effect on sensorimotor integrative functions than on purely visual ones. Further evidence for this motor integrative function of the superior colliculus and midbrain tegmentum is provided by Voneida's report (1970) of profound visuomotor disturbance following midline section of the mesencephalic tegmentum in cats.

Sprague (1966); Robert and Cuenod (1969); Hoffman and Straschild (1971); Goodale (1973); Saraiva, Aragao, and Magalhães-Castro (1976); and Mascetti and Arriagada (1981) have shown that cross-midline pathways between the colliculi contribute a largely inhibitory component to the modulation of the rostrocaudal neural activity down the two sides of the cat's brain. When both brain halves are intact and can compete for guidance of the animal, such a component may play an important role. Indeed, its section might very well be expected to produce significant behavioral loss. It appears to ensure the proper balance of activation and suppression on the two sides. This balance may be required for mediation of unified goal-directed behavior since goal attainment frequently requires shifts of attention to one side or the other in an unpredictable sequence, as in the animal's pursuit of prey. If, indeed, this proves to be a correct interpretation of the role of the superior collicular commissure in the cat's behavior, it is reasonable to attribute the reduction in prey orientation to collicular deconnection.

COMMISSUROTOMY AND
VISUAL THRESHOLDS

In this experiment, we studied the effect of fore- or midbrain commissurotomy (or the two combined) on visual exposure duration thresholds, utilizing the tangent screen task illustrated in Figures 7.2 and 7.3. Thresholds were determined in six unoperated subjects. Four of these were tested three separate times: prior to surgery, after section of forebrain commissures, and then again after a second operation in which the superior colliculi were disconnected by midline section. One of the other two subjects was tested prior to surgery, then after colliculi separation; the other was tested only before any surgery (thresholds could not be obtained on this subject following the midbrain operation because behavior was too unstable).

Subjects learned to orient to the center of the tangent screen when the shade was raised, to wait for presentation of the target, and to respond promptly and accurately upon appearance of the target (which signaled the baited door). A modified single-staircase method was used to measure duration thresholds for the eight targets in Figure 7.3. Twenty-four median thresholds were determined for each subject, one for each of the eight targets at each of the three degrees of eccentricity: near (N), intermediate (I), and far (F), illustrated in Figure 7.2.

A detailed description of preparatory training is given in Robinson, Murray, and Voneida (1978). We present a brief description here. Subjects were trained initially on the individual problems (Figure 7.3) to a 20/30 correct criterion and then on a composite schedule of eight trials/problem/day, with a trial-to-trial randomized alternation of all combinations of the 18 target doors and eight problems. Training was continued until there was concurrent

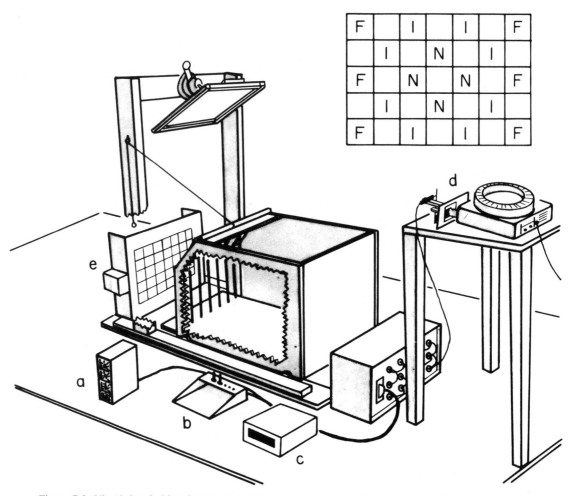

Figure 7.2. Visual-threshold and response latency apparatus. In the figure, a: interval timer; b: control panel; c: response timer; d: solenoid-operated shutter; and e: voice key. In the response latency study, the response timer starts when the target is presented and is stopped by tangent screen vibration when the cat strikes the target. The inset shows the 18 possible target doors on the tangent screen. Angular distances from the subject's straight-ahead visual axis: near (N), 20 degrees; intermediate (I), 40 degrees; and far (F), 50 degrees to 55 degrees (distances are approximate because of small trial-to-trial differences in the unrestrained cat's distance from the screen).

performance on all problems at the 95% level (38/40 correct).

A trial in the test of thresholds for discrimination was initiated by raising the shade. When the subject faced the center of the screen, the target was presented. Initially, exposures were well above threshold; much longer times were allowed for the targets in the multiple-figure discrimination arrays than for the single-figure detection targets. Times were increased on the trial following an error and decreased after correct response. Subjects were

not allowed to correct following an error, there being only one presentation of the stimulus per trial. Changes in exposure duration ranged from 500-ms steps up or down above 1 s, to 20–30-ms steps downward from 150 ms to the 40-ms lower limit of the shutter speed.

All targets were presented on all doors (8 targets × 18 doors: 144 configurations) in two-day test blocks of 72 trials/day, with random trial-to-trial variation of configurations. Subjects were run for 36 days so that each target-door combination was presented 18 times. The

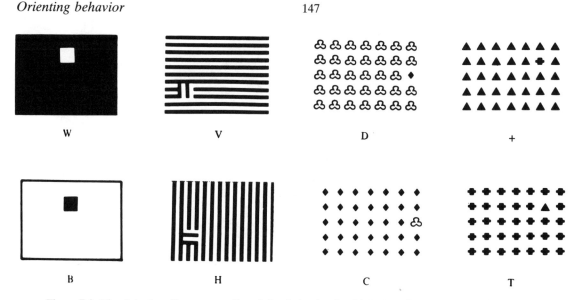

Figure 7.3. The detection (figure-ground) and discrimination (multiple-figure) arrays. The clover and diamond shapes differed in several dimensions; the triangle and cross differed in form only. A target would appear on one of the 18 tangent screen doors in a given trial (see text).

threshold for a combination was defined as the median of the three shortest of the 18 durations at which it was presented and responded to correctly.

To obtain median thresholds, the 144 target-door thresholds for each subject were reduced to 24 by assigning a given one of these thresholds to one of three target eccentricities: near (N), intermediate (I), or far (F) (Figure 7.2). The median threshold was then determined for each of the eight targets in each of the eccentricities (8 targets × 3 positions = 24 thresholds).

Figure 7.4 shows the thresholds for the 24 target-position combinations before surgery, after section of forebrain commissures, and after superior collicular commissurotomy. There is little evidence of visual loss; in fact, some thresholds are lowest after the combination of both operations.

Table 7.2 summarizes the data for the four cats subjected to both operations and the single subject (Brt) with collicular commissurotomy only. Median thresholds for a given target-distance combination before and after surgery were compared to see if the operation had an effect. For the four subjects, median thresholds were compared. Percent changes for the eight targets in the three positions (near,

intermediate, and far) were calculated and the average percent change for the separate positions is shown in the table. The results of significance tests (Wilcoxon Paired Replicates) made of the eight target threshold changes are also shown.

The effects of forebrain commissurotomy are evident in Table 7.2, if one compares forebrain and normal scores; whereas there are negligible mean percent changes found in group visual thresholds, the pattern of threshold gains and losses in the individual subjects is not random. It appears that the operation did produce functionally significant injury. A subject accommodated itself to the injury within the limits set by its capacity for adaptation and the relative eccentricity of the stimulus. Note the improvement–loss gradient corresponding to the latter factor in rows 1 and 2 of Table 7.2.

The subject's "adaptation capacity" can be estimated by the rate of its preoperative learning of the visual search task and from the findings of the threshold testing procedure. The three subjects who showed average (Mtt and Trp) or superior (Bby) preoperative learning showed improvements or only small losses in thresholds postoperatively (mean threshold change = −15.0%). The one subject (Spk) whose preoperative learning was much below

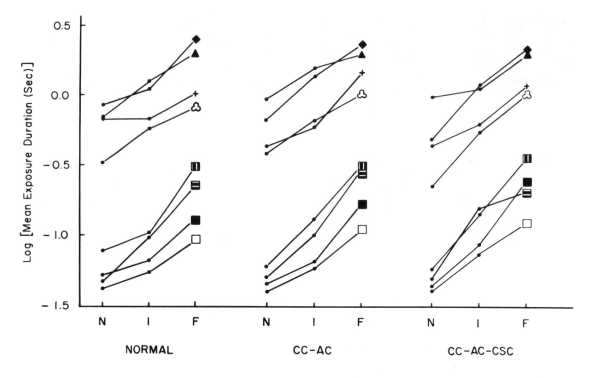

Figure 7.4. Mean exposure-duration thresholds for six normal subjects, and for four of the six who had forebrain commissures and then the commissure of the superior colliculus sectioned in separate operations. The points represent the means of the thresholds across subjects and across target positions with a given angular distance.

Table 7.2. *Effects of fore- and midbrain (CSC) commissurotomy on visual thresholds[a]*

	Near		Intermediate		Far	
	M% Diff.	P	M% Diff.	P	M% Diff.	P
Forebrain – normal[b]	− 5.6	NS	4.5	NS	7.8	NS
Forebrain & CSC – normal	− 17.7	0.031	10.5	NS	15.0	< 0.012
Forebrain & CSC – forebrain only	− 8.2	NS	21.1	NS	9.2	NS
CSC – normal[c]	− 24.4	0.031	− 11.5	NS	− 24.5	< 0.05

[a]Mean percent differences are the averages of the percent differences for the eight targets. P values show the likelihood of obtaining the given differences by chance. See text. Note that negative values designate improvement and positive values losses.
[b]Group median pre- and postoperative thresholds (Bby, Mtt, Trp, and Spk) are compared in rows 1–3; pre- and postoperative thresholds for one subject (Brt) are compared in row 4.
[c]Thresholds were established prior to surgery in an additional subject (Arn), but attempts to secure postoperative thresholds were unsuccessful.

average showed large threshold losses for all three positions (mean threshold change = 33.2%). All subjects tended to show threshold changes reflecting variations in eccentricity of the stimuli.

When the effects of forebrain and CSC commissurotomies combined were measured, postoperative test thresholds after the first and second operations did not differ significantly (Table 7.2, forebrain and CSC versus forebrain only). With the addition of the second operation, the near-distance thresholds tended to improve; intermediate and far thresholds showed increased losses (forebrain and CSC versus normal).

Two subjects (Brt and Arn) received CSC commissurotomy alone. Brt's preoperative learning was well above average. Arn was a poor learner, there being a considerable gap between his (as well as Spk's) and the other four subjects' preoperative mastery of the experimental tasks.

Table 7.2 shows postoperative improvement for all three positions for Brt (CSC versus normal). Arn completed the preoperative threshold testing, but all postoperative attempts to get him to respond to targets at shortened exposure durations were unsuccessful.

There are behavioral and physiological data suggesting that forebrain commissurotomy should have deleterious effects on visual thresholds as we measured them. This is apart from the well-known observations establishing that such an operation abolishes the ability of cats, monkeys, and humans to transfer most forms of visual experience (Doty and Negrão 1973; Sperry et al. 1969) and the ability of a human to cross-integrate components of a form (or word) that are to the left and right of the vertical meridian (Gazzaniga, Bogen, and Sperry 1965). Apparently, the deficits may represent, as well as the interhemispheric disconnection effect, losses in intrahemispheric mechanisms that render the relatively isolated half-brains less able to process unilateral visual inputs.

Behavioral evidence that a perceptual loss does in fact occur is provided by Trevarthen (1974). He concludes, on the basis of studies of visual perception in split-brain patients he has made with Sperry and colleagues at Caltech, that forebrain commissurotomy has a marked effect on their perceptual capacity, resulting in reduced readiness to perceive throughout the visual field and decreased attentional ability for orienting perception selectively (Trevarthen 1974, p. 198). Physiological studies provide abundant reasons for expecting forebrain commissurotomy to produce the kind of perceptual loss reported by Trevarthen. The callosum is known to play an important role in the intrahemispheric integration of the visual

field in both cats and monkeys. Early studies of bilateral visual-field representation in a given hemisphere have reported projection of the ipsilateral field in the region of the vertical meridian of area 17 via circuits that could be silenced by callosal section (Choudhury, Whitteridge, and Wilson 1965; Hubel and Wiesel 1967; Berlucchi and Rizzolatti 1968). This indirect projection complements the projection of the contralateral hemifield via the familiar (direct) geniculocortical pathways.

More recently, as discussed by Berlucchi and Antonini in Chapter 6, this volume, a much wider intrahemispheric representation of the complementary ipsilateral hemifield, in suprasylvian cortex, has been reported for the cat (Heath and Jones 1972; Spear and Baumann 1975; Camarda and Rizzolatti 1976; Palmer, Rosenquist, and Tusa 1978; Sanides 1978; Marzi et al. 1980). Antonini, Berlucchi, and Sprague (1978) and Antonini et al. (1979) have shown that callosal circuits are involved not only in cortical visual-field representation, but in the field's projection on the superior colliculi as well. For example, they have shown the substantial survival of binocular cells on a given side in cats with both the chiasm and superior collicular commissure cut, and their virtual disappearance when the callosum was then cut.

Our visual-threshold task required operated subjects to see test stimuli at exposure durations that were at the normal cats' limit of performance. They did not, however, require cross-integration – all of our large mirror-symmetrical targets provided a properly oriented subject, looking at the center of each stimulus, with enough information to mediate a correct response from either half of the brain. However, one might expect that commissurotomized subjects, since they are "hemianopic" in each hemisphere, *would* show significant impairment of task performance.

Subjects in our experiment who were normal or superior learners did show visual-threshold deficits following forebrain commissurotomy, but these deficits were relatively small. Losses increased with increases in eccentricity of the targets, which suggests that ipsilateral projection, eliminated by the operation, is more important for perception of distant than central targets. The same visual hemifield has direct projection to the other hemisphere, which provides greater cortical representation for the perception of more central targets (Talbot and Marshall 1941).

The subject that was a poor learner, however, showed the kind of perceptual loss Trevarthen (1974) observed in human subjects with split-brain surgery. There was profound impairment across the entire field. This response to the surgery suggests that, in addition to the specific sensory loss, there was a general disruption of behavior. The commissurotomy may have interrupted corticotectal circuits between association cortex and the midbrain involved in the maintenance of attention and arousal (Sprague et al. 1977, p. 468). The slow learner may be especially vulnerable to disturbances in this system, and after the operation, no longer enjoys the requisite stimulus persistence or motor control to attain preoperative threshold levels. However, when given tests of retention prior to testing thresholds, this subject responded reliably to targets in all parts of the field as long as there were no constraints on stimulus duration. The split-brain patients' profound loss of perceptual capacity may also have been the result of the commissurotomy combined with abnormalities of attention-arousal mechanisms produced by the extracallosal damage known to exist in most patients and/or by medication for control of residual symptoms of epilepsy.

Addition of the section of the commissure of the superior colliculi to the forebrain operation results in an increase in the size of the graded losses observed after the latter. The double surgery destroys some of the pathways playing a role in the functioning of the corticomidbrain system that Berlucchi et al. (1972, p. 124) described as "... the complex neural mechanism by which patterns are perceived and discriminated." In the forebrain operation, transcallosal projection of the ipsilateral visual field to important association areas is interrupted. The midbrain operation destroys fibers connecting these areas with the midbrain via inferior and medial pulvinar nuclei.

When commissurotomy of the midbrain to separate the superior colliculi was the only operation, the superior learner, Brt, showed no deficit. He had not undergone the potentiating forebrain surgery and still possessed an intact functionally equivalent pretectum (cf. Berlucchi et al. 1972, p. 167). The same operation did, however, have a profound effect on the poor learner, Arn. This subject, like Spk, appears to have been especially vulnerable to disruption of attention-arousal circuits, possibly as a result of preexisting deficiencies in his own mechanisms for these processes. With postoperative retraining, he was eventually able to respond reliably to continuously present targets.

COMMISSUROTOMY AND LATENCY OF RESPONSE

The previous results, which provide so little evidence of sensory loss related to midline section in most subjects, led us to look for disruption of motor expression in a response latency test following commissurotomy.

The same apparatus was used, appropriately modified (see Figure 7.2). We also used the same test schedule used for thresholds. The target durations were greater than, but close to, the visual threshold values attained earlier, so that a premium was placed on prompt response. We did not differentially reward fast responses as in traditional reaction-time training; as long as the subject's first response on a given trial was correct, it was reinforced; an incorrect response resulted in termination of the trial.

Preoperative exposure durations were also used postoperatively. The response latency for a given target-door combination was defined as the median latency for the first five correct responses.

Response latencies were determined for all six of the subjects who had been given visual-threshold testing (see Table 7.1). Four of them were tested initially after forebrain commissurotomy and then again after midbrain surgery; the other two were tested prior to any surgery and then after collicular separation. These two groups were well matched for learning and performance (see the visual-threshold results and conclusions given before). The two subjects tested before surgery and after collicular separation included a good (Brt) and poor performer (Arn); the four with forebrain commissurotomy were made up of one good

Table 7.3. *Effect of fore- and midbrain commissurotomy on response latency*[a]

	Near		Intermediate		Far	
	M% Diff.	P	M% Diff.	P	M% Diff.	P
Forebrain – normal	5.3	NS	12.4	NS	33.9	< 0.012
Forebrain & CSC – forebrain only	20.0	< 0.012	21.4	< 0.012	9.0	NS
CSC – normal	35.6	< 0.012	35.2	< 0.012	24.1	NS
Forebrain & CSC – normal	24.1	0.027	36.0	< 0.012	42.3	< 0.012

[a]Column entries are defined in footnote *a*, Table 7.2. Comparisons are between median thresholds for Bby, Mtt, Trp, and Spk (forebrain, forebrain & CSC) and Brt and Arn (normal) in rows 1 and 4, and between these two groups' pre- and postoperative scores in rows 2 and 3.

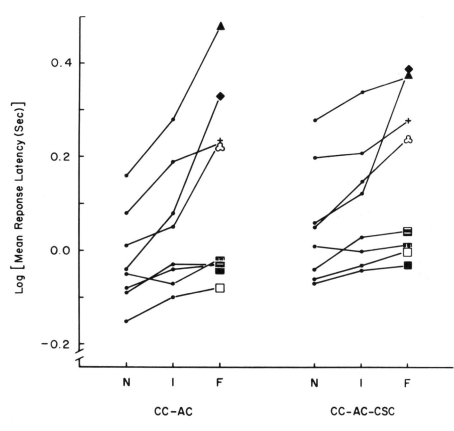

Figure 7.5. Response latencies for the four subjects with the forebrain and midbrain operations. The points represent means of latencies across subjects and across targets with a given angular distance.

(Bby) and one poor (Spk) performer and two of intermediate ability (Trp and Mtt). Evaluation of the effects of surgery, shown in Table 7.3 and Figure 7.5, were made using the 24 latencies calculated for each subject (8 targets × 3 positions – N, I, and F).

The latencies of the two normal subjects were compared with the other four subjects' latencies (Table 7.3: forebrain – normal and forebrain and CSC – normal) and with their own latencies after collicular bisection (CSC – normal). Comparison was also made between the four subjects' first and second postoperative latencies (forebrain and CSC, forebrain only). Appropriate median latencies served for calculation of the mean percent differences and significance values as for the visual-threshold task.

The latencies of forebrain commissurotomized subjects are consistently longer than those of the normal subjects, but the differences only attain a substantial size and statistical significance for the far (F) position (mean percent difference = 33.9, w = 36, p < 0.01). Superior collicular commissurotomy, when it is the only operation, produces substantial latency loss over a wider range than that produced by the forebrain operation. There are sizeable increases in latency for the near (N) and intermediate (I) distances, both of them statistically significant, and a smaller nonsignificant but still positive difference for the far (F) position. The same pattern of latency increases following midbrain surgery is found when the operation is superimposed on forebrain commissurotomy. The increases are not so large, but there are still significantly longer latencies for the N and I positions.

Comparison of the latencies of the normal and twice-operated subjects (forebrain and CSC) shows the combined effect of the two operations, those of the operated group being significantly longer for all three positions. The largest mean percent difference in the table appears precisely where one would expect it, namely, between the thresholds for the far position of subjects who have had no surgery and those who have had both operations.

Our conclusions are as follows: postoperative latencies of responses to peripheral (far) targets were substantially longer for all subjects with forebrain commissurotomy. This finding parallels an observation made by Trevarthen and Sperry in a study of ambient vision in split-brain patients. They report an overall drop in peripheral awareness that they ascribe to the commissurotomy's impairment of the patients' attention, amounting to a contraction of the effective visual fields (Trevarthen and Sperry 1973, pp. 553, 559). The latter consequence, for both cats and the human patients, might result from the loss of stimulus enhancement normally provided by the indirect projection of the ipsilateral field via the callosum, as discussed before (see the section on commissurotomy and visual thresholds).

Both subjects with midbrain commissurotomy and deconnection of the superior colliculi as the only operation showed consistent substantial response latency losses postoperatively. This is consistent with our interpretation of the loss of orienting ability following this operation as the result of motor-integrative impairment rather than visual loss. Results of this kind are to be expected in the light of the many studies reviewed by Sprague, Berlucchi, and Rizzolatti (1973) that show the important role played by the colliculi in the mediation of postural movements, especially those of eyes and head involved in the fixation of visual targets.

The selective loss on near and intermediate targets may be accounted for in the following way. The total response latency has *decision-time* and *movement-time* components (Jensen 1980). The more central decision time, required for organization of the response, is lengthened by the midline surgery. This component is proportionately larger for near and intermediate than for far positions, so that changes in it are less easily obscured by the movement-time component, which is concerned with peripheral aspects of response execution that are unaffected by the surgery. Presumably, if decision time had been measured separately, losses for all three positions would have been observed.

When the midbrain operation was added to the forebrain surgery (Table 7.3, row 2), deficits appeared that were identical to those obtained with collicular deconnection only. Thus, near and intermediate losses were observed in all six subjects with this operation. The midbrain operation appeared to potentiate the latency increase for far targets produced by the forebrain commissurotomy. This effect may be a consequence of further reduction in visual afference, and interruption of tectopulvinar pathways to association cortex may have been responsible.

General discussion

In our discussions of the individual experiments, we have attempted to account for our consistent results in the orientation and response latency studies and the more variable results in the visual-threshold experiment. In the following section, we attempt to rule out alternative explanations for various aspects of the data.

The failure to find substantial visual-threshold losses in some subjects following the fore- and midbrain commissurotomy cannot be explained in terms of incomplete surgery. Histology showed that target structures in all except one brain were completely sectioned. Nor can response to nonvisual cues be the answer: although the baited screen was accessible to the cat at the beginning of a trial, the response did not occur until a visual target was presented. Also, subjects invariably responded to the target door on occasions when another door was inadvertently baited or when other doors were baited deliberately as a control for unintentional cues.

Consistent impairment of response to stimuli in more central parts of the visual field in the orientation and response latency experiments following the midbrain surgery, and impairment of response to more distant stimuli after forebrain section, constitute a double dissociation of the effects of the surgery. The results suggest that section of specific cross-midline connections at the two levels is the critical factor, rather than some simple peripheral motor loss or a more general factor such as surgical shock. Sprague et al. have reported, in commenting on the latter, that even such an extensive operation as ablation of areas 17 and 18 did not disturb attention and orientation to stimuli in tests of "visually guided behavior characteristic of the species" (Sprague et al 1977, p. 454). Finally, histological examination of the brains also rules out interpretation of the loss in terms of unintentional destruction of nonmidline structures.

The previous two kinds of deficit may be related to the different roles played by forebrain and midbrain in their mediation of the animal's efficient response to its environment. Commissurotomy produced some impairment of the forebrain's capacity as analyzer of complex visual information, so that it could no longer process the difficult far targets reliably. Section of the commissure of the superior colliculi, on the other hand, destroyed tecto-reticular pathways, so that the midbrain's

mediation of sensorimotor-integrative functions required for orienting to stimuli was no longer optimal.

Five of the six Ss with the midbrain operation (Arn excepted) performed well on their first postoperative tangent screen tests 10–30 days after surgery. They made no, or very few, errors when presented with figure-ground targets in any of the 18 positions. Consistent deficits only became evident when pre- and postoperative time measurements were compared in the response latency and prey orientation studies. Matelli et al. (1983) report obtaining quite different results following section of the midbrain commissures. Their cats showed long-lasting neglect of stimuli in upper visual space, failing to retrieve food baits presented above the horizontal meridian. Our Ss, unlike those of Matelli et al., were highly overtrained in retrieving food baits from all screen positions prior to surgery. This may account for their accuracy in tests of retention after the operation. Of course, other explanations for the discrepancy are possible.

Forebrain commissures and midbrain decussations: Differing effects of midline section

In these recent experiments, we have focused on the behavioral effects of separating the brain halves of cats tested without further sensory or motor constraints, such as eye occlusion, chiasm section, or limb restraint. Results clearly demonstrate that an animal's orientation to live prey is significantly affected when its superior colliculi are disconnected. The deficit cannot be explained simply as the result of visual loss. The largest deficit observed was obtained with a subject (Brt) who showed no visual threshold loss following this operation. It might be explained, however, by our finding that midline surgery results in an increase in latency of response to visual cues.

We showed in a separate series of tests that, for all cats, there was a significant increase in latency of response to visual cues following midbrain commissurotomy. Thus, we attribute the orientation losses to increases in latency of response and explain the latter by noting that the midbrain operation destroys connections between the deep layers of the superior colliculi (subserving polysensory, motor, and integrative functions) and the reticular core of the tegmentum and spinal cord. We suggest that it is these (decussating, noncommissural) connections that play a key role in orienting behavior, rather than those that interconnect the superficial collicular cells, which are more directly related to visual function.

Following forebrain commissurotomy, most subjects showed a center–periphery gradient of small visual threshold losses, which we attribute to the hemianopsia produced in each hemisphere by callosum section. One of the two subjects (Brt) with the midbrain surgery as the only operation showed no visual threshold loss at all. Cats that were poor learners, before operation, however, showed profound visual-threshold loss across the entire visual field after either operation. We attributed the loss to the vulnerability of these individuals to disturbances of midbrain attention-arousal mechanisms. These subjects' extremely slow learning of the experimental tasks suggests that their cerebral mechanisms mediating these functions must have been deficient, thus providing the basis for the special vulnerability. The forebrain operation may then have triggered the behavior loss by severing callosal connections to suprasylvian and other association areas known to have reciprocal connections with the tectum. The midbrain operation would have precipitated loss by interrupting tectoreticular pathways directly.

Perhaps the forebrain operation by itself only produces serious consequences in those species with greater degrees of lateralization and greater dependency on interhemispheric integration. Sperry has described the behavior of the unrestricted split-brain patient as showing a lowering of "overall mental potential" (Sperry 1974, p. 16). He points out that experience with these patients gives one the impression that it is the commissurotomy that has affected them in this way, producing symptoms that are enhanced by extracallosal damage. The symptoms described by Sperry appear to involve an inability to handle novelty and abstractness. This notion could be tested by comparing normal and commissurotomized

cats on the acquisition of a complex problem. We have (unpublished) evidence, for example, suggesting that the unencumbered cat's mastery of a same/different problem is much easier if training precedes callosal section than if it follows, but we have not studied this matter formally.

Conclusions

We have provided a brief summary of our collaborative studies after our fortuitous meeting in Sperry's laboratory in the early sixties. There is no question that it was his approach that drew us into our analyses of interhemispheric mechanisms and that has continued to exert a profound influence on our thinking.

Our early work took the studies of interhemispheric transfer of a learned response as a point of departure and, influenced also by our own backgrounds in psychology and biology, led us into a series of experiments related to the interhemispheric comparison of percepts. This soon led us anatomically beyond the forebrain commissures into the domain of the mesencephalon, to examination of the effects of section of posterior and tectal commissures and of surgery carried ventrally into the tegmental midline. The results raised more questions than they answered, and we soon found ourselves embracing unconventional views of split-brain cats. We became convinced that neither of this creature's isolated hemispheres was equal to its whole brain, nor were the hemispheres equal to each other.

It became increasingly apparent to us that a limiting factor of some importance in all such studies may be the restrictions imposed on the experimental animal by the investigator, namely, the masks, suits, and limb restraints so commonly employed in split-brain studies of animals. We therefore designed a series of tests that examined the effect of fore- and midbrain surgery on sensory and sensorimotor processes in the experimental animal unencumbered by such devices. We have discussed the results of these studies in terms of their implications for future work and in relation to the interpretation of earlier studies on split-brain humans, themselves encumbered by medications and brain pathology. Processes that govern the orientation of attention and the control of motor activity require brainstem and neocortical circuits in intimate reciprocal relations, both vertically and across the midline via decussations and commissures. Effects of commissurotomy must be assessed in this context.

Acknowledgments

Our research was supported in part by Public Health Service Grants NS 11779 and MH 07051. We would like to thank Mr. Robert Cummins and Dr. Stephen Fish for their very competent assistance in various phases of these studies. Preparation of the manuscript was supported by funds from the Northeastern Ohio Universities College of Medicine.

References

Anderson, K. V., and D. Symmes. 1969. The superior colliculus and higher visual functions in the monkey. *Brain Res.* 13: 37–52.

Antonini, A., G. Berlucchi, C. A. Marzi, and J. M. Sprague. 1979. Importance of corpus callosum for visual receptive fields of single neurons in cat superior colliculus. *J. Neurophysiol.* 42: 137–52.

Antonini, A., G. Berlucchi, and J. M. Sprague. 1978. Indirect, across-the-midline retino-tectal projections and representation of ipsilateral visual field in superior colliculus of the cat. *J. Neurophysiol.* 41: 285–304.

Berlucchi, G., and G. Rizzolatti. 1968. Binocularly driven neurons in visual cortex of split chiasm cats. *Science* 159: 308–10.

Berlucchi, G., J. M. Sprague, J. Levy, and A. C. DiBerardino. 1972. Pretectum and superior coliculus in visually guided behavior and in flux and form discrimination in the cat. *J. Comp. Physiol. Psychol. Monograph* 78: 123–72.

Bloom, M., and M. A. Berkley. 1977. Visual acuity and the near point of accommodation in cats. *Vis. Res.* 17: 723–30.

Camarda, R., and G. Rizzolatti. 1976. Visual receptive fields in the lateral suprasylvian area (Clare-Bishop area) of the cat. *Brain Res.* 101: 427–43.

Casagrande, V. A., J. K. Harting, W. C. Hall, and I. T. Diamond. 1972. Superior colliculus of the tree shrew: A structural and functional subdivision into superficial and deep layers. *Science* 177: 444–7.

Choudhury, P. B., D. Whitteridge, and M. E. Wilson. 1965. The function of the callosal connections of the visual cortex. *Quart. J. Exp. Physiol.* 50: 214–19.

Doty, R. W., and N. Negrão. 1973. Forebrain commissures and vision. *In* R. Jung (ed.) *Handbook of Sensory Physiology. Vol. VII/3B.* Springer-Verlag, New York, pp. 543–82.

Edwards, S. B. 1977. The commissural projection of the superior colliculus in the cat. *J. Comp. Neurol.* 173: 23–40.

–1980. The deep cell layers of the superior colliculus: Their reticular characteristics and structural organization. *In* A. Hobson and M. Brazier (eds.) *The Reticular Formation Revisited.* Raven Press, New York, pp. 193–209.

Edwards, S. B., and J. S. de Olmos. 1976. Autoradiographic studies of the projections of the midbrain reticular formation: ascending projections of nucleus cuneiformis. *J. Comp. Neurol.* 165: 417–32.

Gazzaniga, M. S. 1967. The split brain in man. *Sci. Am.* 217: 24–9.

Gazzaniga, M. S., J. E. Bogen, and R. W. Sperry. 1965. Observations on visual perception after disconnexion of the cerebral hemispheres in man. *Brain* 88: 221–36.

Goodale, M. A. 1973. Cortico-tectal and intertectal modulation of visual responses in the rat's superior colliculus. *Exp. Brain Res.* 17: 75–86.

Gulliksen, H., and T. J. Voneida. 1975. An attempt to obtain replicate learning curves in the split-brain cat. *Physiol. Psychol.* 3: 77–85.

Hamilton, C. R. 1977a. An assessment of hemispheric specialization in monkeys. *Ann. N.Y. Acad. Sci.* 299: 222–32.

–1977b. Investigations of perceptual and mnemonic lateralization in monkeys. *In* S. Harnad, R. Doty, L. Goldstein, J. Jaynes, and G. Krauthamer (eds.) *Lateralization in the Nervous System.* Academic Press, New York, pp. 45–62.

Harting, J. K., W. C. Hall, I. T. Diamond, and G. F. Martin. 1973. Anterograde degeneration study of the superior colliculus in *Tupaia glis*: Evidence for a subdivision between superficial and deep layers. *J. Comp. Neurol.* 148: 361–86.

Heath, C. J., and E. G. Jones. 1972. The anatomical organization of the suprasylvian gyrus of the cat. *Ergeb. Anat. Entw. Gesch.* 45: 1–64.

Hoffman, K. P., and M. Straschild. 1971. Influences of corticotectal and intertectal connections on visual responses in the cat's superior colliculus. *Exp. Brain Res.* 12: 120–31.

Hubel, D. H., and T. N. Wiesel. 1967. Cortical and callosal connections concerned with the vertical meridian of visual fields in the cat. *J. Neurophysiol.* 30: 1561–73.

Jensen, A. R. 1980. Chronometric analysis of intelligence. *J. Social Biol. Struc.* 3: 103–22.

Magalhães-Castro, H. H., A. Dolabela de Lima, P. E. S. Saraiva, and B. Magalhães-Castro. 1978. Horseradish peroxidase labeling of cat tectotectal cells. *Brain Res.* 148: 1–13.

Marzi, C. A., A. Antonini, M. DiStefano, and C. R. Legg. 1980. Callosum-dependent binocular interactions in the lateral suprasylvian area of Siamese cats which lack binocular neurons in areas 17 and 18. *Brain Res.* 197: 230–35.

Mascetti, G. G., and J. R. Arriagada. 1981. Tectotectal interactions through the commissure of the superior colliculi: An electrophysiological study. *Exp. Neurol.* 71: 122–33.

Matelli, M., M. F. Olivieri, A. Saccani, and G. Rizzolatti. 1983. Upper visual space neglect and motor deficits after section of the midbrain commissures in the cat. *Behav. Brain Res.* 10: 263–85.

Myers, R. E. 1955. Interocular transfer of pattern discrimination in cats following section of crossed optic fibers. *J. Comp. Physiol. Psychol.* 48: 470–3.

–1956. Function of corpus callosum in interocular transfer. *Brain* 79: 358–63.

Palmer, L. A., A. C. Rosenquist, and R. J. Tusa. 1978. The retinotopic organization of lateral suprasylvian visual areas in the cat. *J. Comp. Neurol.* 177: 237–56.

Robert, F., and M. Cuenod. 1969. Electrophysiology of the intertectal commissures in the pigeon. II. Inhibitory interaction. *Exp. Brain Res.* 9: 123–36.

Robinson, J. S., D. M. Murray, and T. J. Voneida. 1978. The cat's response to stimulus difference as attention focus and cue. *Perception* 17: 437–47.

Robinson, J. S., and T. L. Voneida. 1964. Central cross-integration of visual inputs presented simultaneously to the separate eyes. *J. Comp. Physiol. Psychol.* 57: 22–8.

–1970. Quantitative differences in performance on abstract discriminations using one or both hemispheres. *Exp. Neurol.* 26: 72–83.

–1973. Hemisphere differences in cognitive capacity in the split-brain cat. *Exp. Neurol.* 38: 123–34.

–1975. Visual processing in the split-brain cat: Analysis of the single hemisphere deficit. *Exp. Neurol.* 49: 140–9.

Sanides, D. 1978. The retinotopic distribution of visual callosal projections in the suprasylvian visual areas compared to the classical visual areas (17, 18, 19) in the cat. *Exp. Brain Res.* 33: 435–43.

Saraiva, P. E. S., A. S. Aragao, and B. Magalhães-Castro. 1976. Recovery of depressed superior colliculus activity in neodecorticate opossum through the destruction of contralateral superior colliculus. *Brain Res.* 112: 168–75.

Sechzer, J. A. 1970. Prolonged learning and split-brain cats. *Science* 169: 889–92.

Spear, P. D., and T. P. Baumann. 1975. Receptive field characteristics of single neurons in lateral suprasylvian visual area of the cat. *J. Neurophysiol.* 38: 1403–20.

Sperry, R. W. 1961. Cerebral organization and behavior. *Science* 133: 1749–57.

–1967. Split-brain approach to learning problems. *In* G. C. Quarton, T. Melnechuk, and F. O. Schmitt (eds.) *The Neurosciences: A Study Program.* Rockefeller University Press, New York, pp. 714–22.

–1968. Mental unity following surgical disconnection of the hemispheres. *In The Harvey Lectures, Series 62.* Academic Press, New York, pp. 293–323.

–1974. Lateral specialization in the surgically separated hemispheres. *In* F. O. Schmitt and F. G. Worden (eds.) *The Neurosciences: Third Study Program,* The MIT Press, Cambridge, pp. 5–19.

Sperry, R. W, M. S. Gazzaniga, and J. E. Bogen. (1969). Interhemispheric relationships: The neocortical commissures; syndromes of hemisphere disconnection. *In* P. J. Vinken and G. W. Bruyen (eds.) *Handbook of Clinical Neurology,* Vol. 4. North-Holland, Amsterdam, pp. 273–90.

Sprague, J. M. 1966. Interaction of cortex and superior colliculus in mediation of visually guided behavior in the cat. *Science* 153: 1544–7.

Sprague, J. M., G. Berlucchi, and G. Rizzolatti. 1973. The role of the superior colliculus and pretectum in vision and visually guided behavior. *In* R. Jung (ed.) *Handbook of Sensory Physiology. Vol. VII/3B.* Springer-Verlag, New York, pp. 27–101.

Sprague, J. M., J. Levy, A. DiBerardino, and G. Berlucchi. 1977. Visual cortical areas mediating form discrimination in the cat. *J. Comp. Neurol.* 172: 441–8.

Stamm, J. M., N. Miner, and R. W. Sperry. 1956. Relearning tests for interocular transfer following division of optic chiasm and corpus callosum in cats. *J. Comp. Physiol. Psychol.* 49: 529–33.

Talbot, S. A., and W. H. Marshall. 1941. Physiological studies on neural mechanisms of visual localization and discrimination. *Am. J. Opthal.* 24: 1255–64.

Trevarthen, C. B. 1974. Functional relations of disconnected hemispheres with the brainstem, and with each other: Monkey and man. *In* M. Kinsbourne and W. L. Smith (eds.) *Hemisphere Disconnections and Cerebral Function.* Thomas, Springfield (IL), pp. 187–207.

–1978. Manipulative strategies of baboons and origins of cerebral assymetry. *In* M. Kinsbourne (ed.) *Asymmetrical Function of the Brain.* Cambridge University Press, Cambrídge, pp. 329–91.

Trevarthen, C. B., and R. W. Sperry. 1973. Perceptual unity of the ambient visual field in human commissurotomy patients. *Brain* 96: 547–70.

Voneida, T. J. 1963. Performance of a visual conditioned response in split-brain cats. *Exp. Neurol.* 8: 493–504.

–1970. Behavioral changes following midline section of the mesencephalic tegmentum in the cat and monkey. *Brain, Behav. Evol.* 3: 241–60.

Voneida, T. J., and J. S. Robinson. 1970. Effect of brain bisection on capacity for cross-comparison of patterned visual input. *Exp. Neurol.* 26: 60–71.

–1971. Visual processing in the split-brain cat: One versus two hemispheres. *Exp. Neurol.* 33: 420–31.

8 Brain pathways in the visual guidance of movement and the behavioral functions of the cerebellum

Mitchell E. Glickstein
Department of Anatomy
University College, London

Preliminaries

I finished my PhD in Psychology at Chicago in 1958. Because I started as a clinical student, I only discovered brain research in my last year in graduate school, working with Garth Thomas. That year gave me a keen interest in brain mechanisms in learning, and Sperry's laboratory at Caltech was an obvious choice for postdoctoral work. I was delighted when Sperry accepted my application to work with him.

My two years with Sperry introduced me to thinking about psychological functions in terms of connectionist anatomy of the brain. Sperry had already ruled out intracortical fiber systems as necessary for normal functioning, since there was little or no detectable deficit in vision or movement after cross-hatching of the visual or motor cortex in experimental animals (Sperry 1958). The analysis of the role of the corpus callosum in interhemispheric transfer of learning, which Sperry had begun with Ronald Myers at Chicago, was still being actively studied when I came to the Caltech laboratory in 1958. I was pleased to join that effort, studying intermanual transfer in split-brain monkeys in collaboration with Sperry (Glickstein and Sperry 1963).

Sperry's approach had revealed a major function for the corpus callosum in the transfer of information between the hemispheres (Sperry 1961). But the role of commissural fibers in motor control was still unclear. How could split-brain animals with vision restricted to one hemisphere and movement controlled from the other guide their movements under visual control? In this chapter, I argue that one pathway for such guidance may involve the cerebellum. In addition to its role in the visual guidance of movement, the cerebellum probably has other functions, and I also review some of the increasing evidence for the role of the cerebellum in motor learning. Many of the ideas had their beginnings in my work with Sperry, and I remain grateful to him for the start he gave me in thinking about brain mechanisms in behavior.

Introduction

The second half of the nineteenth century saw a major advance in our understanding of the localization of functions in the cerebral cortex. By 1850, the sensory and motor specializations of the spinal roots were known, but there was little or no understanding of the functions of different parts of the brain. In particular, there was no answer to the question of whether different regions of the cerebral cortex might play a specialized role in sensation or in movement. The single experiment that is most responsible for initiating the modern view of cortical localization was that done by Fritsch and Hitzig in 1870. They stimulated a dog's brain electrically and found that there is a unique region of the cerebral cortex that, when stimulated, produces movement on the opposite of the body.

After Fritsch and Hitzig's (1870) discovery of a motor area, the search was on for other regions of the cortex that might have other specialized functions. Eleven years later, Munk (1881) reported that unilateral lesions of a monkey's occipital lobe cause contralateral hemianopia and that bilateral lesions cause blindness. Although the interpretation of Fritsch and Hitzig's and of Munk's experiments was at first controversial, by 1900, most authorities agreed that a portion of the frontal lobe is motor in function and that a portion of the occipital lobe is visual.

The behavior of most mammals is under almost constant visual guidance. Many human movements, like picking up a pencil, or sewing a button, probably involve a continuous sequence of activity, first in the visual, and then in the motor cortex. Insofar as these two cortical areas are sequentially active in the control of behavior, it is reasonable to ask about the pathways that connect them. How is information relayed from the visual to the motor cortex? This form of question can be extended to embrace subcortical structures as well. For example, if a visually guided task involves sequential activation of the superior colliculus and the red nucleus, what neural pathways relay information between these two structures?

The anatomical basis for the connections between the visual and the motor cortex seemed, at first, to be straightforward. Abundant U fibers connect adjacent gyri, and conspicuous long-association bundles unite distant lobes in the human cerebral cortex. These are part of an elaborate corticocortical fiber system that can be revealed by simple dissection. It seemed only reasonable to earlier authors that visually guided movements must involve a series of corticocortical relays beginning in the visual cortex and proceeding via a chain of association fibers to end, finally, in the motor cortex. The corpus callosum would serve for those tasks that require interaction between the two sides of the brain, such as cooperation between the two hands, or guiding the right hand to an object in the left visual field.

But when the function of the corticocortical fibers was tested directly by cutting them, the results were often negative or equivocal. Cutting commissural fibers does not obviously impair bimanual coordination; severing the long-association bundles between the occipital and the frontal lobes does not impair severely the visual guidance of movement.

Ettlinger and Morton (1963) and Mark and Sperry (1968) trained monkeys to perform tasks that require cooperation between the two hands. They found that the execution of such bimanual tasks was not affected by cutting the forebrain commissures. Additional section of the midbrain commissures does impair bimanual coordination (Mark and Sperry 1968), but even these animals improved with time. Midline cuts in the cerebellar white matter produced no further deficit. How did the animals recover?

Myers, Sperry, and McCurdy (1962) cut corticocortical fibers between visual and motor areas, and tested the ability of cats and monkeys to guide their body and limbs under visual control. Some visumotor coordination was preserved in all cases, whether the fibres were severed by making deep subcortical cuts within each hemisphere, or by ablating the visual cortex on one side, the motor cortex on the other, and cutting the forebrain commissures. As expected, monkeys in which the motor cortex has been ablated on one side are impaired in use of the opposite hand, but the unaffected hand can still grasp or pursue objects in the intact visual field. Similarly, Schrier and Sperry (1959) had noted that split-brain cats can use any combination of eye and forepaw in learning or performing a visual discrimination task.

Preferential and forced eye–hand coordination in split-brain monkeys

Although monkeys with section of the optic chiasm and the corpus callosum can use any combination of eye and hand, Downer (1959) had found that they prefer to use the hand contralateral to the open eye. I replicated this hand-preference effect in split-brain monkeys in experiments that I began in Sperry's lab. The preference did not appear if the most caudal fibers of the corpus callosum were spared, but it appeared immediately when these remaining splenial fibers were cut; see Figure 8.1.

But the preference for using one or the other hand does not mean that monkeys in which the forebrain commissures have been cut

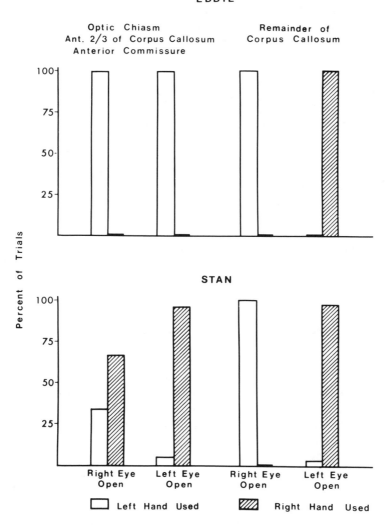

Figure 8.1. Hand preference of monkeys before and after section of the posterior third of the callosal fibers. There was no systematic hand preference following the midline section of the optic chiasma, anterior two-thirds of the corpus callosum, and the anterior commissure. A preference for using the hand contralateral to the open eye emerged after splenial fibers (posterior one-third) were cut. (After Glickstein and Sperry 1963.)

cannot use the nonpreferred hand. Sperry and I (Glickstein and Sperry 1963) trained monkeys to pick up a small bit of food from a rotating disc. We then restricted vision to one hemisphere by sectioning the optic tract unilaterally. After tract section, all of the animals could still perform the task using either hand. When we cut the corpus callosum and anterior commissure as well, performance with the hand ipsilateral to the surviving optic tract was mildly impaired for a few days, but the animals could be retrained quickly to their preoperative levels of performance and agility. These results suggested that the motor cortex might still have had access to visual information even though there was no visual input to that side of the brain.

Trevarthen (1962, 1965) approached the same problem by a somewhat different route. He also found that split-brain monkeys could learn to use any combination of eye and hand. But if the animals were trained to perform a visual discrimination task in which conflicting information was presented simultaneously to the two eyes, they typically attended to and learned the information that was arriving at the eye contralateral to the preferred hand. When vision was restricted to the other eye, the animals often shifted to using the other hand.

How does a split-brain monkey control the ipsilateral limb? Some authors (e.g., Brinkman and Kuypers 1973) believe that control over the limb on the same side of the visual input may be by way of uncrossed motor pathways. Kuypers (personal communication) argues that even after a unilateral hemispherectomy, humans can control movement of the ipsilateral arm. According to this view, the monkey might simply reach under visual control using an ipsilateral descending pathway and then control its fingers and wrist under somatosensory guidance. An alternative is that there are residual uncut pathways between the hemispheres. But although interpretation may differ as to mechanism, many studies (e.g., Gazzaniga 1963; Lund, Downer, and Lumley 1970; Brinkman and Kuypers 1973; Keating 1973) confirm that when vision is restricted to one hemisphere and the forebrain commissures are cut, monkeys can still recover the ability to guide movements of the limb ipsilateral to the open eye.

Finger use in split-brain monkeys

Gazzaniga (1963) confirmed that split-brain monkeys can use any combination of eye and hand in solving a visual discrimination task. But his animals were clumsy when they were required to use the ipsilateral eye–hand combination, and there was typically a "fanning out of the fingers" at the termination of a movement. Kuypers and his collaborators studied the problem of hand and finger use by such monkeys in great detail. In one experiment (Brinkman and Kuypers 1973), monkeys were tested after the optic chiasm and corpus callosum were cut. Although the animals could still guide either arm with either eye, they failed completely if they were required to guide their hand or fingers by sight when using the hand ipsilateral to the open eye. Haaxma and Kuypers (1975) in similar experiments cut the intrahemispheric fibers between the occipital and frontal lobes and found that although the monkeys could still guide whole arm movements, they were unable to orient their wrist and fingers under visual control.

The experiments of Kuypers and his collaborators make the important point that visual control of movements of the distal extremities is more severely affected by cortical disconnection than the control of proximal muscles. But the entire pathway for the visual guidance of the wrist and fingers may not necessarily be corticocortical. In almost all of Haaxma and Kuypers (1975) cases, the intracortical fiber cuts were made at the level of the caudal parietal lobes. Such cuts would interfere with connections from the banks of the superior temporal fissure and the adjacent regions of the parietal lobe. These cortical areas contain a high concentration of visually responsive cells (Hyvarinen and Poranen 1974; Mountcastle et al. 1975; Robinson, Goldberg, and Stanton 1978; Hyvarinen and Shelpin 1979; Zeki 1980), and lesions of the parietal lobe have been known since Ferrier (1876, 1886) to impair visually guided movements (Denny-Brown and Chambers 1958; Bates and Ettlinger 1960; Ettlinger and Kalsbeck 1962; Hartje and Ettlinger 1973; Faugier-Grimond, Frenois, and Stein 1978; Lamotte and Acuna 1978).

If the pathway from the visual to the motor cortex is exclusively corticocortical, then interruption at any point along the route should block visually guided movement. The principal cortical target of the parietal lobe visual areas is the cortex in the region of the arcuate fissure (Pandya and Kuypers 1969; Chavis and Pandya 1976), hence, removal of this periarcuate cortex might be expected to disrupt visually guided movement of the hands and fingers. But lesions in the region of the arcuate fissure produce only a mild and transient impairment of visually guided finger movements (Buchbinder et al. 1980). If the entire pathway from striate to motor cortex were corticocortical, the impairment would be expected to have been more severe and permanent.

Visual-motor connections and conditioning

The neural circuits through which vision may influence movement can be studied in another way. Voneida (1963) trained cats to withdraw their forepaw at the onset of a flashing light. The animals were first adapted to resting in a hammock with a small cuff positioned on one forepaw. When a light began to flash, the cat could avoid a shock by promptly flexing its forepaw. Voneida first established that the motor cortex is probably involved in performance of this task, since the conditioned response was abolished and could not be relearned if the motor cortex opposite the trained paw was ablated. Voneida then studied commissurotomized cats in an attempt to trace connections between a visual input that was restricted to one-half of the brain and a motor output originating in the opposite half. When vision was restricted to the hemisphere opposite the intact cortex, the cats could still respond to the flash with the unaffected paw even after forebrain, diencephalic, and midbrain commissures were cut. How did visual information that was channeled to one hemisphere reach the other side?

In a review article, Sperry (1961) pointed out that there were many puzzling results in studies of interhemispheric motor control and he concluded that "the neural pathways for these volitional movements have yet to be determined." One possible explanation for the observed effects was proposed by Voneida (1963), who suggested that a pathway involving the superior colliculus, dorsolateral pontine nuclei, and the cerebellum might have allowed interhemispheric integration of a visual signal with a conditioned limb response in his split-brain cats. Subsequent anatomical and physiological experiments have provided increasing support for this suggestion.

Visual input to the pontine nuclei and cerebellum

One possible alternative or parallel pathway from visual to motor areas of the brain involves the cerebellum. A principal circuit through the mammalian brain originates in the cerebral cortex and projects to the cerebellum by way of the pontine nuclei. There are also projections to the cerebellum via the pons from the diencephalic and midbrain structures. Cells in the pontine nuclei project via the middle cerebellar peduncle to terminate as mossy fibers in the cerebellar cortex. It is now clear that there is abundant transmission of visual information along this cortico-ponto-cerebellar path (Brodal 1972a, 1972b; Glickstein, King, and Stein, 1972; Baker et al. 1976; Burne, Mihailoff, and Woodward 1978; Gibson et al. 1978; Sanides, Fries, and Albus 1978; Glickstein et al. 1980; Albus et al. 1981; Cohen et al. 1981; Glickstein and May 1982), and to the pons from the superior colliculus (Altman and Carpenter 1961; Kawamura and Brodal, 1973; Harting, 1977; Mower, Gibson, and Glickstein 1979; Mower et al. 1980; Burne et al. 1981), the ventral lateral geniculate nucleus (Edwards, Rosenquist, and Palmer 1974; Graybiel 1974), and the pretectum (Mower et al. 1979). Pontine cells that receive cortical (Baker et al. 1976) and collicular (Mower et al. 1979) input can be driven readily by appropriate visual targets. The axons of visual cells in the pons must relay visual information to the cerebellar cortex. A complete review of some of these studies of pontine transmission of visual information to the cerebellum has been published recently (Glickstein and May 1982). Here I will discuss some of the relevant experiments and conclusions insofar as they bear on the question raised by the studies of visually guided behavior in brain-lesioned animals.

Pontine receptive fields, laterality, and the visual guidance of movement

There is a major projection from the mammalian visual cortex to the pontine nuclei. The cells of origin of this pathway have been determined using retrograde transport of horseradish peroxidase (HRP) in cats (Albus et al. 1981; Cohen et al. 1981) and monkeys (Glickstein et al. 1980). In both species corticopontine fibers arise from layer V pyramidal cells. In cats, area 18 and the lateral suprasylvian visual areas are the major sources of cortical visual input to the pontine nuclei. In monkeys, the corticopontine visual projection arises principally from cells on both banks of the superior temporal fissure, the rostral banks of the parietooccipital fissure, and the parietal lobe adjacent to these fissures anteriorly. The cortex within these areas contains a high percentage of visually activated cells (Hyvarinen and Poranen 1974, Robinson et al. 1978, Zeki 1980).

In cats, pontine cells upon which visual cortical fibers terminate can be driven by appropriate visual targets, and they do not respond to other types of sensory input (Baker et al. 1976). Pontine visual cells code a wide range of direction and velocity of moving targets and are relatively insensitive to differences in the orientation or shape of those targets. These receptive field properties are consistent with the suggestion that they may play a role in guiding movement.

The superior colliculus of cats (Mower et al. 1979) and of other mammals (Harting 1977; Burne et al. 1981) projects to the dorsolateral pontine nuclei. In cats, unlike other mammals, the majority of the projections from the colliculus and visual cortex to the pons do not overlap. Cells in the cat dorsolateral pontine nucleus that receive a projection from the superior colliculus can be activated by appropriate visual targets (Mower et al. 1979). Like the visual cells activated from the cortex, they are sensitive to the direction and velocity, and often the size, of moving targets, and they are relatively indifferent to the particular orientation or shape of those targets. Dorsolateral pontine visual cells may also be concerned with the visual guidance of some classes of movements.

Cortical cells that project to the pons have receptive fields that are different from those of cortical cells that are involved in form or color vision. Corticopontine cells have been identified antidromically by stimulation of their terminals in the pontine nuclei (Gibson et al. 1978). The responses of corticopontine visual cells are similar to those of the pontine visual cells upon which they terminate. Unlike most cortical visual cells, they are relatively uninfluenced by orientation, but are highly sensitive to the direction and velocity of moving targets. The receptive field properties of dorsolateral pontine visual cells are similar to those of cells in the superficial laminae of the superior colliculus from which they receive an input (Wickelgren and Sterling 1969; Mower et al. 1979).

Thus, there are cells both in the cortex and the superior colliculus that relay visual motion information to the cerebellum by way of the pontine nuclei.

Nearly all of the efferent fibers from the cerebral cortex and the colliculus terminate ipsilaterally in the pontine nuclei. Consistent with this anatomical arrangement, the receptive fields of nearly all pontine visual cells are centered in the contralateral visual field (Baker et al. 1976; Mower et al. 1979). Although the axons of most pontine cells decussate, a sizeable minority remain uncrossed, projecting to the cerebellum on the same side via the middle cerebellar peduncle. Many dorsolateral pontine cells are retrogradely labeled following HRP injections into the ipsilateral cerebellar cortex (Mower et al. 1980; Rosina et al. 1980) and a high percentage can be activated antidromically by electrical stimulation of the ipsilateral cerebellar vermis or hemisphere (Mower et al. 1980).

As Voneida (1963) suggested, a pathway via the dorsolateral pons and ipsilateral cerebellum and then to motor pathways on the contralateral side may have been the anatomical basis for the preservation of responses to flash in his cats. The same anatomical pathway via the superior colliculus, dorsolateral pons, and ipsilateral cerebellum could account for the preservation of visually guided paw use in the experiments of Schrier and Sperry (1959) and of Myers et al. (1962). Such a pathway might also account for the successful visually guided paw and whole-body movements in split-brain monkeys, and the bilateral visuomotor coordination in human commissurotomy patients when visual information is restricted to one hemisphere. Since in monkeys, cortical as well as collicular visual information reaches the dorsolateral pons (Harting 1977; Glickstein et al. 1980), cortical visual information may be relayed in part to the ipsilateral cerebellum, and, hence, be available for guiding the ipsilateral limbs in a split-brain monkey or person. Since split-brain monkeys cannot use vision to control the ipsilateral wrist and fingers, it is possible that only decussating pontocerebellar fibers contribute to the visual control of distal muscles.

The cerebellum and bimanual control

In the experiments of Mark and Sperry (1968), the monkeys left hand had to know where the object was that the right hand was feeling, and it seemed difficult to understand how this could be possible in the absence of the corpus callosum and midbrain commissures. Perhaps a sort of "corollary discharge" may play a role in preserving bimanual coordination in such cases, signaling the locus of one hand to the other (see Chapter 9, this volume)

Sperry (1950) coined the term *corollary discharge* to refer to the idea that if a voluntary movement of the eyes, the head, or the body displaces the image of objects on the retina, there should be a central signal from the motor pathways that feeds into the sensory system and can null the apparent movement of the image (see the foreword, this volume). Such a mechanism was also invoked by Von Holst and Mittelstaedt (1950) to account for the stability of the visual world as we move about in it and for the jiggling of the visual world if we tap gently on our eyeball.

A mechanism similar to corollary discharge might serve as the anatomical basis for cooperation between the two hands. What would the anatomical basis of this sort of corollary discharge look like? The classical description of corticopontine anatomy by Ramon y Cajal (1909–11) may provide a clue. Many of the pyramidal tract axons that arise in the motor cortex bifurcate as they course through the pontine nuclei. The parent axon continues on to the pyramidal tract in the medulla and beyond; the branch terminates on a pontine cell. If some of the pontine cells that receive pyramidal tract collaterals project to the ipsilateral cerebellum, such a circuit might serve as the anatomical basis for bimanual coordination, signaling to the command system of the left arm about an intended movement by the right; see Figure 8.2.

The cerebellum and motor learning

In addition to its possible role in the sensory guidance of movement and in coordination between the limbs, the cerebellum is probably involved in motor learning as well. Although there have been theoretical suggestions for such a role for the cerebellum (e.g., Marr 1969), there has, until recently, been little direct experimental evidence to support this idea. But now there are at least two kinds of motor learning that seem to depend on the cerebellum: adaption of the vestibuloocular reflex (VOR) and conditioning of the nictitating membrane response (NMR) in rabbits.

If you turn your head to the right, there is a tendency for your eyes to move to the left, thus stabilizing the visual world on the retina. The basic anatomic circuitry involved in the VOR is relatively simple, involving only a three-neuron arc from the inner ear to the extraocular muscles (Lorente de No 1935; Szentagothai 1950). If you wear a magnifying lens or an inverting prism in front of your eye, the normal VOR becomes inappropriate. In the case of an inverting prism, if you turned your head to the right and your eyes moved left, the reflex eye movement would produce an increase, not a decrease, in the motion of the objects on the retina. The visual world would be even less stable.

It is now clear that the VOR is modifiable and can adapt to such optically induced changes in the direction or size of the visual image. Gonshor and Melville-Jones, (1973, 1976) studied objects who wore inverting prisms for several days. As they wore the prisms, the amplitude of the VOR decreased, and with sufficient exposure to the prismatic reversal, even the direction of the VOR could be altered. Miles and Fuller (1974) and Miles and Eighmy (1980) showed that if monkeys look through a lens that increases or decreases the size of the retinal image, the strength of the VOR is increased or decreased, respectively, appropriate to the change in magnification. All of these adaptive changes in the VOR would tend to decrease retinal image slip when the head is turned.

Rabbits (Ito 1974, 1975) and cats (Robinson 1976) lose the adaptive modification of the VOR after lesions are made in the cerebellum. Although the exact locus within the cerebellum and the mechanism for these plastic changes in the VOR is still controversial (Lisberger 1982), the evidence is convincing that the cerebellum

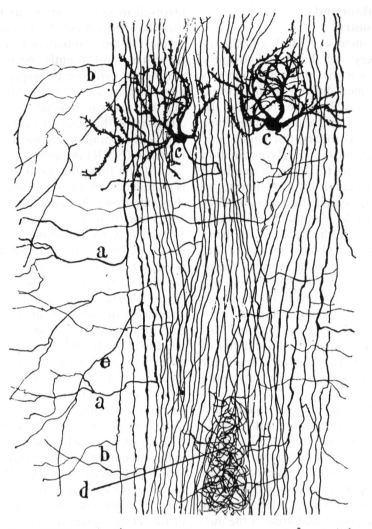

FIG. 440. — Coupe longitudinale du pont de Varole ; chat âgé de huit jours.
Méthode de Golgi.

a, collatérales pyramidales épaisses représentant des fibres terminales en raison de leur diamètre;
— *b*, collatérales ordinaires ; — *c*, cellules du pont de Varole placées entre les faisceaux des
fibres pyramidales ; — *d*, plexus des collatérales de la voie pyramidale ; — *e*, collatérales des-
cendantes.

Figure 8.2. Cajal's drawing from Golgi-stained material showing bifurcation of cortico-spinal fibers as
they course through the pontine nuclei. The branch within the pons synapses on a pontine cell. (From
Ramon y Cajal 1909–11.)

is necessary for the acquisition and for retention of a modified VOR.

The cerebellum is necessary for another
form of motor learning: the conditioned nictitating membrane response (NMR) in rabbits.
If a neutral stimulus such as a light or tone is
presented repeatedly and immediately followed by a puff of air to the cornea or a mild

electric shock across the orbit, the animal will
learn to blink and to sweep its nictitating membrane across the cornea when the neutral stimulus alone is presented (Gormezano 1972). The
NMR is simple, and, hence, it has unique advantages for studying physiological mechanisms in learning. Thompson and his colleagues
(McCormick et al. 1981) demonstrated that le-

sions of the cerebellum, including its deep nuclei, abolish a previously learned NMR and prevent its reacquisition. Yeo et al. (1982) in this laboratory and Clark et al. (1982) in Thompson's laboratory found that small lesions that are restricted to the cerebellar nuclei can abolish completely the rabbits' ability to retain or to reacquire the NMR.

Acquisition and retention of the conditioned NMR requires the cerebellum, but until recently, it was not certain whether the response required the cerebellar cortex or nuclei or both. The main input to the cerebellar nuclei is from Purkinje cells in the cerebellar cortex. But since the nuclei also receive fibers from other structures as well, they could conceivably function autonomously. It is now clear that the cerebellar cortex as well as the nuclei are necessary for the conditioned NMR. Yeo and Hardiman in this laboratory recently found that small lesions confined to the hemispheric portion of lobule VI of the rabbit cerebellum completely abolish a preoperatively learned NMR and prevent the animal from reacquiring the responses. The unconditioned responses to shock is unaffected, and the animals can readily acquire the conditioned NMR when tested on the other eye. This preparation should prove a fruitful one for further analysis of the neural basis of motor learning.

Conclusions

The cerebellum may provide the anatomical basis for the preservation of visually guided movement and bimanual coordination found in the disconnection studies of Sperry, his students, and other investigators. In addition to its probable role in the sensory guidance of movement and in motor coordination, there is increasing evidence for the role of the cerebellum in reflex plasticity and motor learning.

Acknowledgments

I am grateful to Doctors H. J. G. M. Kuypers, C. Trevarthen, T. Voneida, and P. Wall and Mr. Michael O'Donaghue for their critical reading of an earlier draft of this paper.

References

Albus, K., F. Donate-Oliver, D. Sanides, and W. Fries. 1981. The distribution of pontine projection cells in visual and association cortex of the cat: An experimental study with HRP. *J. Comp. Neurol.* 201: 175–89.

Altman, J., and M. Carpenter. 1961. Fiber projections of the superior colliculus in the cat. *J. Comp. Neurol.* 116: 157–78.

Baker, J., A. Gibson, M. Glickstein, and J. Stein. 1976. Visual cells in the pontine nuclei of the cat. *J. Physiol. (London).* 255: 415–33.

Bates, J., and G. Ettlinger. 1960. Posterior biparietal ablations in the monkey: Changes to neurological and behavioural testing. *Arch. Neurol.* 3: 177–92.

Brinkman, J., and H. Kuypers. 1973. Cerebral control of contralateral and ipsilateral arm, hand, and finger movements in the split-brain Rhesus monkey. *Brain* 96: 653–74.

Brodal, P. 1972a. The cortico-pontine projection from the visual cortex in the cat. I: The total projection from area 17. *Brain Res.* 39: 297–317.

–1972b. The cortico-pontine projection from the visual cortex in the cat. II: The projection from areas 18 and 19. *Brain Res.* 39: 319–35.

Buchbinder, S., B. Dixon, Y. W. Hwang, J. G. May, and M. Glickstein. 1980. The effects of cortical lesions on visual guidance of the hand. *Soc. Neurosci. Abst.* 6: 675.

Burne, R. A., S. A. Azizi, G. A. Mihailoff, and D. J. Woodward. 1981. The tectopontine projection in the rat. With comments on visual pathways to the basilar pons. *J. Comp. Neurol.* 202: 287–307.

Burne, R. A., S. A. Mihailoff, and D. J. Woodward. 1978. Visual cortico-pontine input to the paraflocculus; A combined autoradiographic and horseradish peroxidase study. *Brain Res.* 143: 139–46.

Chavis, D., and D. Pandya. 1976. Further observations on corticofrontal connections in the Rhesus monkey. *Brain Res.* 117: 369–86.

Clark, G.A., D. A. McCormick, D. G. Lavond, K. Baxter, W. J. Gray, and R. F. Thompson. 1982. Effects of electrolytic lesions of cerebellar nuclei on conditioned behavioral and hippocampal neuronal responses. *Soc. Neurosci. Abst.* 8: 22.

Cohen, J. L., F. Robinson, J. May, and M. Glickstein. 1981. Cortico-pontine projections of the lateral suprasylvian cortex: De-emphasis of the central visual field. *Brain Res.* 219: 239–48.

Denny-Brown, D., and R. Chambers. 1958. The parietal lobe and behavior. *Res. Publ. Assoc. Nerv. Ment. Dis.* 36: 35–117.

Downer, J. de C. 1959. Changes in visually guided behaviour following mid-sagittal division of optic chiasm and corpus callosum in monkey (*Macaca mulatta*) *Brain.* 82: 251–9.

Edwards, S. B., A. C. Rosenquist, and L. A. Palmer. 1974. An autoradiographic study of ventral lateral geniculate projections in the cat. *Brain Res.* 72: 282–7.

Ettlinger, G., and F. E. Kalsbeck. 1962. Changes in tactile discrimination and in visual reaching after successive and simultaneous bilateral posterior parietal ablations in the monkey. *J. Neurol. Neurosurg. Psychiat.* 25: 256–68.

Ettlinger, G., and H. B. Morton. 1963. Callosal section: Its effect on performance of a bimanual skill. *Science* 139: 485–6.

Faugier-Grimond, S., C. Frenois, and D. Stein. 1978. Effects of posterior parietal lesions on visually guided behaviour in monkeys. *Neuropsychol.* 16: 151–68.

Ferrier, D. 1876. *The Functions of the Brain.* Smith, Elder & Co., London.

–1886. *The Functions of the Brain,* 2nd Ed. Smith, Elder & Co., London.

Fritsch, G. T., and E. Hitzig. 1870. Uber die elektrische Erregbarkeit des Grosshirns. *Arch. f. Anat., Physiol. u. Wiss. Med.* 300–32.

Gazzaniga, M. 1963. Effects of commissurotomy on a preoperatively learned visual discrimination. *Exp. Neurol.* 8: 14–19.

Gibson, A., J. Baker, G. Mower, and M. Glickstein. 1978. Cortico-pontine cells in area 18 of the cat. *J. Neurophysiol.* 41: 484–95.

Glickstein, M., J. L. Cohen, B. Dixon, A. Gibson, M. Hollins, E. La Bossiere, and F. Robinson. 1980. Cortico-pontine visual projections in macaque monkeys. *J. Comp. Neurol.* 190: 209–29.

Glickstein, M., R. King, and J. Stein. 1972. Visual input to the pontine nuclei. *Science* 178: 1110–11.

Glickstein, M., and J. May. 1982 Visual control of movement: The circuits which link visual to motor areas of the brain with special reference to the visual input to pons and cerebellum. *In* W. D. Neff (ed.) *Contributions to Sensory Physiology.* Academic Press, New York, pp. 103–45.

Glickstein, M., and R. W. Sperry. 1963. Visual-motor co-ordination in monkeys after optic tract section and commissurotomy. *Fed. Proc.* 22: 456.

Gonshore, A., and G. Melville-Jones. 1973. Changes of human vestibulo-ocular response induced by vision reversal during head rotation. *J. Physiol.* 234: 102–3.

–1976. Extreme vestibulo-ocular adaptation induced by prolonged optical reversal of vision. *J. Physiol.* 256: 381–414.

Gormezano, I. 1972. Investigations of defence and reward conditioning in the rabbit. *In* A. H. Black and W. F. Prokasy (eds.) *Classical Conditioning.* Appleton-Century-Crofts, New York.

Graybiel, A. 1974. Visuo-cerebellar and cerebellar-visual connections involving the ventral geniculate nucleus. *Exp. Brain Res.* 20: 303–6.

Haaxma, R., and H. G. J. M. Kuypers. 1975. Intrahemispheric cortical connections and visual guidance of hand and finger movements in the Rhesus monkey. *Brain* 98: 239–60.

Harting, J. K. 1977. Descending pathways from the superior colliculus: An autoradiographic analysis in the Rhesus monkey (*Macaca mulatta*). *J. Comp. Neurol.* 173: 583–611.

Hartje, W., and G. Ettlinger. 1973 Reaching in light and dark after unilateral posterior parietal ablations in the monkey. *Cortex* 9: 346–54.

Hyvarinen, F., and A. Poranen. 1974. Functions of the parietal association area 7 as revealed from cellular discharge in alert monkeys. *Brain* 97: 637–92.

Hyvarinen, F., and Y. Shelpin. 1979. Distribution of visual and somatic functions in the parietal association area 7 of the monkey. *Brain* 102: 561–4.

Ito, M. 1974. Visual influence on rabbit vestibulo-ocular reflex presumably effected via the cerebellar flocculus. *Brain Res.* 65: 170–4.

–1975. Learning control mechanisms by the cerebellum investigated in the flocculo-vestibulo-ocular system. *In* D. B. Tower (ed.) *The Nervous System. Vol. 1: The Basic Neurosciences.* Raven Press, New York, pp. 245–52.

Kawamura, J., and A. Brodal. 1973. The tectopontine projection in the cat: An experimental anatomical study with comments on pathways for teleceptive impulses to the cerebellum. *J. Comp. Neurol.* 149: 371–90.

Keating, E. G. 1973. Loss of visual control of the forelimb after interruption of cortical pathways. *Exp. Neurol.* 41: 635–48.

Lamotte, R. H., and C. Acuna. 1978. Defects in accuracy of reaching after removal of posterior parietal cortex. *Brain Res.* 139: 309–26.

Lisberger, S. G. 1982. Role of the cerebellum during motor learning in the vestibulo-ocular reflex. Different mechanisms in different species? *Trends in Neurosci.* 5: 437–41.

Lorente de Nó, R. 1933. Vestibulo-ocular reflex arc. *Arch. Neurol. Psychiat.* 30: 245–91.

Lund, J. C., J. L. de C. Downer, and J. S. P. Lumley. 1970. Visual control of limb movements following section of optic chiasma and corpus callosum in the monkey. *Cortex* 6: 323–46.

Mark, R. F., and R. W. Sperry. 1968. Bimanual co-ordination in monkeys. *Exp. Neurol.* 21: 92–104.

Marr, D. 1969. A theory of cerebellar cortex. *J. Physiol.* 202: 437–70.

McCormick, D. A., D. G. Lavond, G. A. Clark, R. G. Kettner, C. Rising, and R. F. Thompson. 1981. The engram found? Role of the cerebellum in classical conditioning of nictitating membrane and eyelid responses. *Bull. Psychonom. Soc.* 18: 103–5.

Miles, F. A., and B. B. Eighmy. 1980. Long-term adaptive changes in primate vestibulo-ocular reflex. I: Behavioral observations. *J. Neurophysiol.* 43: 1406–25.

Miles, F. A., and J. H. Fuller. 1974. Adaptive plasticity in the vestibulo-ocular responses of the rhesus monkey. *Brain Res.* 80: 512–16.

Mountcastle, V. B., J. C. Lynch, A. Georgopoulos, H. Sakata, and C. Acuna. 1975. Posterior parietal association cortex of the monkey. Command functions for operations within extrapersonal space. *J. Neurophysiol.* 38: 871–908.

Mower, S., A. Gibson, and M. Glickstein. 1979. Tecto-pontine pathway in the cat: Laminar distribution of cells of origin and visual properties of target cells in dorsolateral pontine nucleus. *J. Neurophysiol.* 42: 1–15.

Mower, S., A. Gibson, F. Robinson, J. Stein, and M. Glickstein. 1980. Visual pontocerebellar projections in the cat. *J. Neurophysiol.* 43: 355–66.

Munk, H. 1881. *Uber die Functionen der Grosshirnrinde.* A. Hirschwald, Berlin, pp. 28–53. English translation in G. Von Bonin (ed.) *The Cerebal Cortex.* Thomas, Springfield (IL), 1960, pp. 97–117.

Myers, R. E., R. W. Sperry, and N. M. McCurdy. 1962. Mechanisms in visual guidance of limb movements. *Arch. Neurol.* 7: 195–202.

Pandya, D. N., and H. G. J. M. Kuypers. 1969. Cortico-cortical connections in the Rhesus monkey. *Brain Res.* 13: 13–36.

Ramon y Cajal, S. 1909–11. *Histologie du Systeme Nerveux.* C.S.I.C., Madrid. (Trans. into French by L. Azoulay; reprinted 1952.)

Robinson, D. A. 1976. Adaptive gain control of vestibulo-ocular reflex by the cerebellum. *J. Neurophysiol.* 39: 954–69.

Robinson, D. L., M. E. Goldberg, and G. Stanton. 1978. Parietal association cortex in primate: Sensory mechanisms and behavior modulations. *J. Neurophysiol.* 41: 91–132.

Rosina, A., L. Provini, M. Bentivoglio, and H. G. J. M. Kuypers. 1980. Ponto-neocerebellar axonal branching as revealed by double fluorescent retrograde labeling techniques. *Brain Res.* 195: 461–6.

Sanides, D., W. Fries, and K. Albus. 1978. The cortico-pontine projection from the visual cortex of the cat: An auto-radiographic investigation. *J. Comp. Neurol.* 179: 77–87.

Schrier, A. M., and R. W. Sperry. 1959. Visuo-motor integration in split-brain cats. *Science* 129: 1275–6.

Sperry, R. W. 1950. Neural basis of the spontaneous optokinetic responses produced by visual inversion. *J. Comp. Physiol. Psychol.* 43: 482–9.

–1958. Physiological plasticity and brain circuit theory. *In* H. F. Harlow and C. N. Woolsey (eds.) *Biological and Biochemical Bases of Behavior.* University of Wisconsin Press, Madison, pp. 401–21.

–1961. Cerebral organization and behavior. *Science* 133: 1749–57.

Szentagothai, J. 1950. The elementary vestibulo-ocular reflex arc. *J. Neurophysiol.* 13: 395–407.

Trevarthen, C. B. 1962. Double visual learning in split-brain monkeys. *Science* 136: 258–9.

–1965. Functional interactions between cerebral hemispheres of the split-brain monkey. *In* E. G. Ettlinger (ed.) (Ciba Foundation Study Group) *Functions of the Corpus Callosum.* Churchill, London, pp. 24–40.

Voneida, T. J. 1963. Performance of a visual conditioned response in split-brain cats. *Exp. Neurol.* 8: 493–504.

Von Holst, E., and H. Mittelstaedt. 1950. Das Reafferenzprinzip. *Naturwissenschaften* 37: 256–72.

Wickelgren, B. S, and P. Sterling. 1969. Receptive fields in the superior colliculus of the cat. *J. Neurophysiol.* 32: 16–23.

Yeo, C. H., M. J. Hardiman, M. Glickstein, and I. S. Russell. 1982. Lesions of cerebellar nuclei abolish the classically conditioned nictitating membrane response. *Soc. Neurosci. Abst.* 8: 22.

Zeki, S. 1980. The responses of cells in the anterior bank of the superior temporal sulcus in macaque monkeys. *J. Physiol.* 308: 116.

9 Intermanual transfer, interhemispheric interaction, and handedness in man and monkeys

Bruno Preilowski
Department of Psychology
University of Tübingen

I would like to preface this account of some of my work at Sperry's laboratory, and of other ventures that followed directly from it, by a somewhat apologetic note of debt.

With my formal application to Sperry for a postdoctoral position, I submitted a proposal to study memory in monkeys using partial reversible interruptions of commissural functions. However, when I first met Sperry in 1970, he pointed out that, while monkey work could be done anywhere in the world, at Caltech, I had the unique opportunity to study patients in whom the neocommissures had been partially or completely sectioned for the treatment of intractable epilepsy. I was easily persuaded to study "split-brain" patients. Nevertheless, some unrelieved ambition must have remained that later made me invest 10 years in setting up two labs at two different universities in Germany for research with monkeys.

My association with Sperry was a major influence in my choice of a career in research and teaching in physiological psychology, as well as a tremendous help to this day in pursuing it. But it has left me with a nagging feeling of not having delivered enough for all the possibilities he made available and the personal and professional support he gave me. I like to tell myself, however, that this guilty feeling derives, at least partly, from the fact that one enters into research with "split-brain" patients hoping to get the answers to the great psychological riddles presented by phenomena that we describe with terms like consciousness, will, attention, emotion, cognition, etc. only to find

that the experimental results constantly pose new perplexing questions of a different nature instead. Around the time that I had completed my first experiments in Sperry's lab in 1971, most of the questions and problems arising from their results, leading away from the primary goals first aimed at, surely must have appeared quite secondary to what Sperry had then come to see of overriding importance, namely, the consciousness and value issue. No, I have not been able to follow Sperry's admonitions to look for the answers to the really important questions.

I did get "hooked" by the problem of consciousness in the split-brain patients, just like everyone else has who has worked with them. However, remembering Gustav Theodor Fechner's advice that there are no problems involved in the psychophysics of the soul except those that we create for ourselves, I cautiously operationalized consciousness in terms of facial self-recognition. By using skin-resistance measures, it was possible to show that both separated hemispheres, actually the right even more clearly than the left, could recognize a picture of the patient's own face. Self-recognition was indicated because repeated presentations of pictures of the subject's own face elicited consistently large skin electric responses, whereas those to pictures of friends and relatives, as well as to pictures of emotionally stimulating subjects such as surgical scenes or erotic pictures, habituated rather rapidly (Preilowski, Gray, and Sperry 1972; Preilowski 1979a, 1979b).

For the most part, however, my ventures

have been in the less hotly disputed area of sensorimotor functions, and I was led to concentrate more on such interhemispheric interactions as remained after commissurotomy, rather than interhemispheric differences.

Coordination of the two hands in split-brain patients

The most fascinating aspect of the "split brain" to me has always been the apparent normality of the patients' behavior despite the destruction of such massive bundles of nerve fibers in their brains. While deficits in the transfer of information between the hemispheres had been demonstrated under laboratory conditions in patients with complete section of the corpus callosum and the anterior commissure ("complete split brain"), the motor activities of these people in everyday life appeared to be normal (e.g., Sperry, Gazzaniga, and Bogen 1969). Still more puzzling was the complete absence of demonstrable deficits in two "partial split-brain" patients in whom only the posterior third of the corpus callosum was spared (Gordon, Bogen, and Sperry 1971).

As it turned out, the apparent normality of bilateral sensorimotor integration in the patients applied only to skills that had been highly overlearned preoperatively. If new bimanual coordination skills had to be acquired, in which the action of one hand had to be taken continuously into account for appropriate actions of the other hand, deficits due to the surgery did appear (Preilowski 1972, 1977).

The apparatus used to investigate the learning of a new two-hand coordination skill consisted of an *x-y* recorder fitted with crank handles. Turning of one handle registered as horizontal movement, turning of the other produced vertical displacement of the recorder pen, and, by simultaneous movements of both handles, the pen could be moved in any direction. The task was to draw a straight line within a strip 2.5 mm wide and 155 mm long as fast as possible, without touching the boundary lines. The required ratio of right-hand to left-hand input was varied by changing the angle of the line to be drawn. Three years later, the same type of performance was tested with a system requiring linear instead of rotary movements of the two extremities.

In the "complete split-brain" patients, although not all to the same extent, a deficit in bimanual coordination in this situation was quite obvious. The "partial anterior split-brain" patients showed much more subtle deficits that, at first, were almost indistinguishable from difficulties experienced by normal and unoperated epileptic controls; compared with single-hand performance (straight vertical or horizontal lines), two-hand performance took 5 to 10 times longer. With continued practice, however, the controls eventually became as fast working with both hands simultaneously as when they worked with only one hand, whereas the split-brain patients, even with more extended practice, still needed more than twice the time for two-hand work in comparison to single-hand speed, and they depended on vision to maintain unequal inputs from the two hands. The tracings produced by the controls were relatively smooth, whereas those of the split-brain patients showed steplike waves, reflecting the lack of mutually timed simultaneous movements and the typical effect of reactions to delayed feedback. These deficits, which have been confirmed (Zaidel and Sperry 1977), have remained essentially unaltered in 1984, when I last repeated the tests with some of the same patients, 13 years after the first tests (Figure 9.1).

MOTOR SKILL AND MOTOR
COROLLARY DISCHARGE

It can be concluded from motor-learning studies in normal subjects that in the successive phases of a developing skill, different control mechanisms dominate (e.g., Fleishman 1957; Fleishman and Rich 1963). It appeared possible that these shifts in control mechanisms would be reflected in shifts of the relative contributions of different brain areas in the performance of the two-hand coordination task I had employed. It may be hypothesized that, during the first stages, error corrections by posterior visual and tactile-kinesthetic functions dominate, whereas advanced performance must rely more heavily on information monitoring the motor action as an output program, with more perfect prediction, and this would entail a shift toward more involvement of frontal cortical regions. With partial or complete destruction of

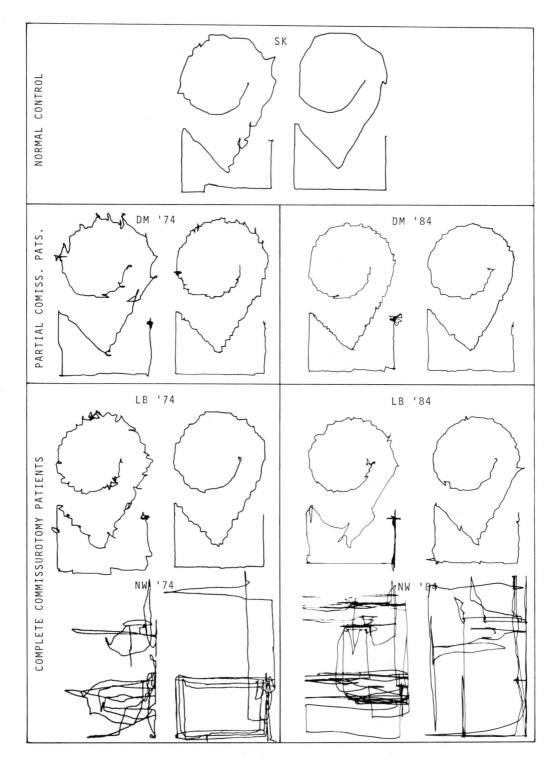

Figure 9.1. Performance samples of a normal control, a partial commissurotomy patient (DM) and two complete commissurotomy patients (LB, NW). In 1974, three years after having been tested on the Rotary Two-Hand-Coordination Task, the patients' performance was measured with a Linear Two-Hand-Coordination Task (Preilowski 1977). The latter test was repeated in 1984. The samples show first and last attempts.

the corpus callosum, some, at least, of these mechanisms must be interfered with.

The deficits of the split-brain patients described before coincide nicely with the qualitative characteristics of performance predictable on the basis of missing control mechanisms, or missing interhemispheric links between those cortical areas thought to be involved in such mechanisms. The partial frontal split-brain patients have lost the means for direct exchange of motor corollary discharges, and, thus, they remain dependent on slower visual and tactile-kinesthetic feedback, which prevents them from reaching higher levels of skill. The additional loss of posterior parts of the callosum, and, presumably, with it, the loss of the ability to exchange tactile-kinesthetic information, would explain the even worse performance of the complete split-brain patients. However, the extreme difficulties of some of the complete split-brain patients with the two-hand coordination tests appear to result from more than the simple addition of deficits in the direct interhemispheric exchange of sensory feedback and motor corollary discharges. These difficulties consisted of persisting jerky, almost athetotic motions, blocking, and alternation, as well as compulsory coaction of both hands. They are probably a consequence of the fact that only one side at a time is under direct motor control.

The idea of a direct intracerebral source of information to the coordinative centers of the brain about ongoing motor actions or intentions, of course, came directly from Sperry's corollary discharge theory (Sperry 1950) and von Holst and Mittelstaedt's reafference principle (Holst and Mittelstaedt 1950), which Teuber cited in connection with frontal lobe functions (Teuber 1964; see also the foreword, this volume).

The previous set of experiments points to an important general aspect of brain and behavior studies that Sperry already addressed over 40 years ago in his research on the effects of transposition of nerves and muscles. He called it an "erroneous assumption that [the] ability to use a limb in seemingly normal fashion implies the presence of normal muscular coordination" (Sperry 1945, p. 323). It would be equally erroneous to draw conclusions about motor functions of the brain from tests that

yield only gross and summary performance scores, and consist of only a few trials. During the early phase of testing, performance is too variable, and too many ways exist to achieve the same mediocre level of performance. Reliable and meaningful performance differences become visible only with extended testing. Only then does motor control become dependent upon specific functions, and substitutions for them by other less efficient mechanisms are reflected in the performance. Similar arguments pertain, of course, to the neuropsychological study of other behaviors as well.

Returning to the problem of corollary discharges and frontal cortex, I present further data from a task rarely used nowadays in neuropsychological research, namely, weight discrimination.

MOVEMENT PLANNING AND WEIGHT COMPARISONS

Assessing the weight of an object involves an evaluation not only of particular sensations from skin, muscle, and joint receptors, but also of motor processes (Müller and Schumann 1889, Payne and Davis 1940). That such motor processes are influenced by qualities of the object other than its weight has been well known since the first descriptions of the size–weight illusion (Charpentier 1890).

In a preliminary study (Preilowski 1971), two complete and two partial commissurotomy patients, as well as two normal controls, were tested for their ability to discriminate between weights under three conditions: judgments as to which of two unseen weights was heavier had to be made after successive lifting of the weights with the same hand, after lifting with both hands simultaneously, and, finally, after lifting first one weight with one hand and then the second weight with the other hand. The weights were placed on the fingers of the subjects by the experimenter, and, after the weights were removed, the subjects gave a signal by flexing the finger of the hand that had held the heavier weight, or, in the unimanual condition, by moving the finger once or twice.

The results showed no differences between the three groups of subjects when they compared weights with the same hand, which was to be expected, since all subjects should be able to make intrahemispheric comparisons normally. When judgments were made after lifting with both hands simultaneously, the decisions of the complete split-brain patients fell to chance levels. The performance of the partial split-brain subjects was not significantly different from that of the unoperated controls under this condition, but both groups of operated subjects made judgments at chance when comparisons had to be made after successive lifting of the weights by two hands.

As with the previously described two-hand coordination test, the performance differences between partial and complete split-brain patients in weight discrimination can be explained in terms of differentially affected posterior sensory and frontal motor functions. The complete split-brain patients performed badly because they have lost all neocortical connections and could make no direct interhemispheric comparisons. The partial split-brain patients, on the other hand, lacking frontal cortical connections and thus the possibility to directly compare preparatory motor settings, were still able to compare somatic sensory feedback via posterior preserved parts of the corpus callosum. They could make a correct estimate of weight as long as the motor output was equal to both hands. Equal motor output to the hands is most probable when the weights are lifted simultaneously. With successive lifting of weights, however, it is less likely that motor effort is precisely equal; hence, the partial split-brain subjects, having lost the basis to evaluate differences in motor effort from the two hands, made larger errors comparing the sensory information under this condition.

COMPLICATIONS FROM
ATTENTIONAL FACTORS

A few years later, I repeated the weight-lifting experiment, testing five patients with completely split brains, the same two partial commissurotomized patients, and 12 normal controls. During this experiment, some of the complete split-brain patients exhibited problems already during single-hand testing. A considerable number of trials could not be analyzed because the patients emitted confused finger signals. They would signal once, then follow with a double signal, or vice versa. When

reminded of the instructions, they would often proceed to signal consistently only once (or only twice) throughout a block of trials. During bimanual lifting, double signals were also frequent, lifting the fingers first of one hand and then of the other. Sometimes the patients were aware of the double signals and explained that they were trying to correct a judgment made earlier.

When the ranges of error were compared with those of the normal controls, all of the complete split-brain patients were significantly worse in both two-hand conditions. For the partial split-brain patients, only successive comparisons were impaired. This result seemed to confirm the findings of the preliminary study. An analysis of the errors committed by the patients showed that there was a tendency for more errors to be made in successive comparisons when the second weight was heavier than the first weight. Also, there were errors related to the subjects' hand preference. It is possible that these systematic errors occur because some sort of information was exchanged interhemispherically, i.e., subcortically, in the patients. Alternatively, they may be indicative of a deficit in the allocation of attention or activation between hemispheres, to which also some of the previously mentioned confusion in signaling during intermanual weight comparisons could be attributed. Attentional factors could influence either the perceptual or the response part of the task, or both, complicating the rather simple logic used so far to interpret the findings. Indeed, unstable attentional processes complicate all studies of cognitive functions in commissurotomy patients (as is discussed in Chapter 13, this volume).

It is not possible within the scope of this chapter to go into a discussion of further details of this study, some of which have stimulated additional experiments with normal subjects. For the present purpose, it is sufficient to point out that the main conclusion, namely, that a comparison of motor output, perhaps as an exchange of motor corollary discharges, is dependent upon the anterior portions of the corpus callosum, is not threatened by any detail of the error analysis. Indeed, this conclusion is supported by the fact that the normal controls showed an influence of hand preference only in the successive condition and not when simultaneous intermanual comparisons were made, whereas both patient groups showed such systematic errors under both successive and simultaneous response conditions.

COROLLARY MOTOR DISCHARGE, THE SUPPLEMENTARY MOTOR CORTEX, AND SUBCORTICAL COORDINATIVE STRUCTURES

The supplementary motor cortex appears as a possible candidate for a territory within the frontal cortex where motor corollary discharges could be generated. This region, first identified by the Vogts (Vogt and Vogt 1919), recently has become the focus of increased attention. It is here that the earliest onset and maximum amplitude of the Bereitschaftspotential preceding voluntary movements can be localized (e.g., Deecke and Kornhuber 1978; Libet, Wright, and Gleason 1982). It is a part of the paralimbic region, which has been identified as an important pathway of motivation to the motor system (e.g., Kornhuber 1980; for a recent discussion, see Goldberg 1985). More direct evidence for the involvement of the supplementary motor cortex in bimanual coordination comes from studies with monkeys. Electrophysiological studies showed neurons of this area, in contrast with those of the primary motor cortex, to be related to ipsilateral as well as contralateral movements (Brinkman and Porter 1979). Furthermore, unilateral lesions of the supplementary motor cortex produced deficits in bimanual activities (Brinkman 1981) that could be ameliorated by sectioning the corpus callosum (Brinkman 1982). If the commissural pattern of man is similar to that of the monkey, then fibers connecting the supplementary cortices (Pandya and Rosene 1985) certainly would be completely cut in both groups of split-brain patients discussed here.

At present, it is not known to what extent an interaction between both hemispheres, for example, between the supplementary motor areas, can take place without the cortical commissures. Subcortical routes via the ipsilateral striatum, thalamus, red nucleus, or the pontine nuclei (e.g., Wiesendanger, Séguin, and Künzle 1973) could be involved. So far, however, a more direct pathway in the form of commissures in the massa intermedia has been demonstrated only in the monkey (Glees and Wall 1948) and also implicated in bilateral motor functions (Lumley 1972). In man, the massa intermedia is a highly variable structure and contains no commissures (Toncray and Krieg 1946).

The supplementary motor cortex has also been proposed as a control area for highly overlearned motor skills (Goldberg 1985). This is in contrast with the almost classical, albeit never proven, idea (but see Chapter 8, this volume) that highly automatized skills descend to subcortical levels (Lashley 1921). As has been pointed out frequently (Sperry et al. 1969, Preilowski 1975), preoperatively overlearned skills such as buttoning clothes, tying shoelaces, shuffling cards, riding a bicycle, etc. are not significantly influenced by commissurotomy. On the other hand, a closer analysis of these behaviors in the split-brain patients, still lacking so far, may show that performance is not as normal as it appears to be. Sperry's warning "that the descent of central reorganization to subcortical levels, if it occurs at all, is not sufficient to make an acquired habit independent of its cortical organization" (Sperry 1945, p. 359) is still to be heeded.

Before experimental or clinical data indicate otherwise, I would think that subcortical processes, such as pyramidal collaterals to the cerebellum (see Chapter 8, this volume) or to other perhaps even spinal targets (Preilowski 1975), would play only a minor role during the acquisition of fine motor skills. It seems more likely that they would be important in the context of stabilizing the whole of the sensorimotor organism, for example, in coordination of eye, head, and body movements, or in movements of the extremities, which would require coordinated adjustments of body posture. For instance, the interference observed during asymmetric arm movements (in comparison with easier mirror-image movements) is not due to interactions via callosal pathways, as has been suggested (Cohen 1971), since split-brain patients experience the same difficulties with such movements as normal controls (Preilowski 1975). Considering that asymmetric movements of the arms would shift the center of gravity, the need for posture adjustment and a tendency to inhibit such movements in subcortical integrative mechanisms appear likely.

Intermanual transfer in monkeys and handedness

As exciting and important as studies of the behavior of split-brain patients are, limitations inherent in what are essentially single case studies of persons of different age, cognitive and sensorimotor abilities, as well as different etiology and severeness of extracallosal lesions, are quite obvious. Experiments with intact healthy human subjects, as well as animal studies, which allow for a control of some factors uncontrollable in humans, are necessary complements. In the following, I describe some of the animal research that grew out of questions posed by my previous work with the split-brain patients.

DEFICITS IN INTERMANUAL
TRANSFER OF NORMAL MONKEYS

One problem with the experiments on motor coordinations of humans was the uncertainty concerning the extent to which the various factors involved in the bimanual tasks were confined to one-half of the brain. When I undertook animal experiments to examine functions of the corpus callosum in interhemispheric and intermanual sensorimotor interactions, it appeared desirable to find not only a task that a monkey could do, but also one that would maximize the contribution of unilateral cortical processes. The pioneering work of Sperry and his co-workers, as well as other investigators, on visually guided movements, bimanual coordination, and learning transfer in split-brain cats and monkeys had already demonstrated that different results could obtain with varied involvement of vision and proximal limb movements (for review, see Chapter 8, this volume). By choosing a task that Wiesendanger and Hepp-Reymond (1970) had described for the study of pyramidal tract functions in control of finger movements, I hoped to avoid some of these problems.

In this task, the monkey has to produce a specific force for a defined length of time between the fingertips of one hand. The diffi-

culty of the task can be varied by adjusting the lower and upper limits of force required, as well as changing the duration for which the force has to be kept at that level. In practice, the required duration was increased first until 1.5 s of continuous pressure was produced, then the gap between the minimum and maximum-level of acceptable force was narrowed in successive steps with the aim of training the monkeys to the highest possible delicacy of performance.

At the beginning, we provided no feedback except for a reward in form of a 190-mg banana-flavored pill, delivered when the monkey had produced just the right amount of force for the required length of time. As the difficulty of the task was increased, it turned out that the animals were unable to learn with this type of terminal feedback. I finally had to give up the strategy to completely lateralize all factors involved in the response and resorted to binaural auditory feedback. Figure 9.2 gives a schematic account of the events during a trial.

A trial lasted for 10 s and was signaled by a 300-Hz tone. This trial on tone was switched to 500 Hz as long as the force produced by the monkey was within the acceptable limits. If the correct force was held continuously for 1.5 s, a 1000-Hz tone was sounded, the trial terminated, and the reward delivered. Four blocks of maximally 36 trials each were run. A block was terminated after 18 trials were successfully concluded. I decided on an all-or-none feedback signal, so that the lateralized tactile-kinesthetic feedback would remain essential for monitoring the fine adjustments of force production that the task required.

In the first study, we used four intact subadult rhesus monkeys. They had been subjects in several behavioral experiments before, but were naive for the finger-pressure discrimination task. Two of the animals were first trained to the highest possible level of difficulty with their preferred hand and then tested for transfer of learning to the other hand. The remaining two monkeys were trained with both hands, switching hands from day to day, letting each hand progress at its own speed. Somewhat to our surprise, the two animals that had been trained with one hand showed no signs of transfer; they had to be completely retrained with

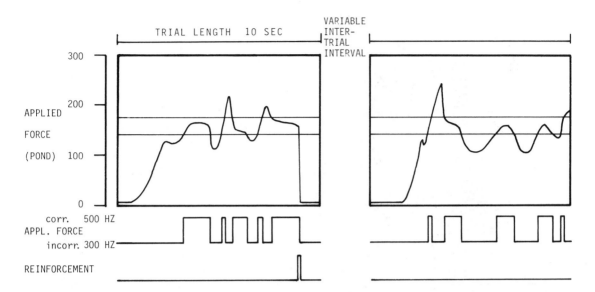

Figure 9.2. Schematic representation of two trials of a force-discrimination experiment. The animal has to produce a force within the lower and upper limits (indicated by the two parallel lines) and hold it continuously for 1.5 s to obtain a reward. A trial lasts for maximally 10 s and is signaled by a 300-Hz tone, which is replaced by a 500-Hz tone whenever the force is within the specified limits.

the other hand, including the shaping of finger use at the manipulandum.

Several interpretations might be offered for this first result: perhaps our task, which required the animals to use a finger-thumb opposition to reach the middle of a donut-shaped manipulandum housing the tiny pressure transducer, was too artificial or unnatural. Furthermore, since the transducer was fastened to the end of a flexible metal gooseneck dangling in front of the experimental cage, it may have been much more natural for the monkey to grasp it and pull on it, as the animals, in fact, did at the start of transfer testing. This would interfere with the trained habit. Another possibility was that some sort of "situation-specific learning" had occurred during training, in the sense that use of one particular arm had obtained a critical stimulus function and prevented adequate reproduction of the required response to a new stimulus (i.e., sensations from the other hand). The third and most intriguing possibility was that learning had remained lateralized within one hemisphere despite intact commissures. Several considerations seemed to favor the last explanation: for example, the animals trained with both hands on alternate days appeared slower in learning

and their final performance remained far below that of the animals trained with only one and the same hand. They did not seem to profit with one hand from work done with the opposite hand, learning appearing to progress independently with each hand. For both the other two explanations, in terms of response interference or situation-specific learning, a high level of delayed transfer should have been visible during retraining. This, however, was not obtained.

In the next experiment, with six more monkeys, all, with the exception of one, different from those used previously, we employed a new manipulandum. It required that a force be applied to squeeze together two metal lips placed in a slot such that they were accessible only with a pincer grasp of the fingers of one hand (see Figure 9.3). The device was suspended in a loose universal-joint assembly in front of the test cage to discourage use of whole-arm movements. Thus, the manipulandum had to be steadied with the wrist of the same hand in order to apply force between two fingers. The minimal effort required to shape the appropriate behavior in monkeys supports the idea that this manipulandum provided more of an incentive for adequate manipulations and

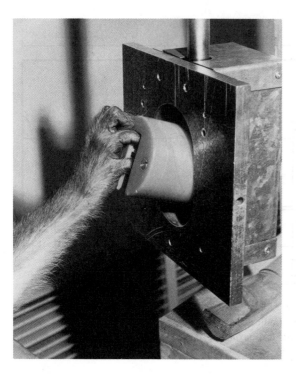

Figure 9.3. Force-discrimination manipulandum, requiring a pincer grasp to press together two metal lips within the vertical slot.

less for behaviors that would interfere with the trained habit than was the case for the device previously used. As a further precaution, three of the animals were trained again with both hands at the lower levels of difficulty before continuing training with one hand. The other three monkeys were trained with one hand from the beginning. Following single-hand training, transfer testing took place at various levels of difficulty.

The results of this study supported the idea of lateralized learning of the force discrimination between fingers of one hand. During the two-hand training, the monkeys needed as many, or more, trials with each hand to reach criterion than monkeys trained with one hand only. Performance appeared to be developing quite independently for the right and left hand of each animal. After single-hand training, there was no immediate transfer, whether previous two-hand pretraining had been given or not. Only with transfer at lower levels of difficulty were some savings in the training with the other hand observed. Transfer at a higher level of difficulty was absent. Most striking in

these cases was the lack of transfer of the previously used finger posture. The results of this experiment raised the question whether or not lack of transfer at higher levels of difficulty was due to the increased demands of the task, i.e., whether the commissures were sufficient for transfer of learning in a less demanding task, but not for learning of a more difficult one. An alternative explanation was that prolonged work with one hand, necessary to reach criterion at higher levels of difficulty, compared to relative short pretransfer training at lower levels of difficulty, would reduce intermanual transfer of learning. We do have several indications from other experiments that extensive unimanual training may actually reduce intermanual transfer. The details of these experiments, however, which differ from the previously mentioned ones in many respects, must be reserved for publication elsewhere.

Instead, I shall just briefly describe a final experiment in which the animals were required to produce a specific force by pulling on a lever, the idea being to have a task comparable with the previous one, but needing movements of the arm. If transfer deficits in the previous experiments were due only to factors like situation-specific learning, then the same effects should be apparent in this experiment. If transfer deficits were due to an anatomical lateralization specific for finger control, no deficit should be found in the transfer between arms, which are known to have extensive ipsilateral sensorimotor innervations in addition to the dominant contralateral control. Unfortunately, the results were not as clear cut as one would have predicted on the basis of either one of these hypotheses alone. There was no immediate transfer in any of the six animals tested, but there was extensive delayed transfer so that, within a rather short time, adequate performance levels were reached using the previously untrained arm. Transfer of training was stronger for the arm movement than it had been for the finger movement.

It is realistic to assume that a number of factors other than those discussed here play a role in the observed failure, or partial failure, of intermanual and interarm transfer. Nevertheless, it can be tentatively concluded that the development of a fine sensorimotor skill dependent on control of the distal extremities can remain lateralized to the opposite hemisphere in the presence of intact commissures. As an additional hypothesis, it might be proposed that, with extended training of only one hand in such a task, an active interhemispheric inhibition might preclude the bilateral establishment of skill.

Although the situation is not directly comparable, it is worth pointing out that after one hemisphere has been rendered dysfunctional by cortical spreading depression, learning in the rat remains lateralized after the restitution of normal function for long periods, with no evidence for passive transfer despite the fact that all interhemispheric connections are intact (e.g., Russell and Ochs 1963). A similar phenomenon is the suppression of interocular transfer in normal rabbits (Van Hof and Russell 1977), fish (Ingle 1968), and birds (Palmers and Zeier 1974), which is thought to prevent conflict in the case of different visual inputs to the two eyes. Suppression of interocular transfer appears to be linked to a certain degree of functional independence of the visual fields of the two eyes. Similarly, an increased independence of function in the anterior extremities may be correlated with an increased capacity for interhemispheric suppressive actions with regard to these limbs.

The hypothesis of lateralized learning in subjects with intact neocortical commissures and an active role of the corpus callosum in *preventing* interhemispheric transfer carries important implications for the development of handedness and perhaps of laterality in general. It would provide a mechanism by which a weak asymmetric tendency, caused by some systematic influence or by chance, could develop into a consistent functional asymmetry.

HANDEDNESS IN MONKEYS

The study of handedness as an expression of cerebral asymmetry requires precautions similar to those of the study of interhemispheric transfer. The most important precaution is to make sure that the handedness tests tap lateralized cerebral functions directly. Tests of human handedness are, for the most part, indirect. They usually measure preferences, which may be epiphenomena of some other underlying

sensorimotor asymmetry. Preference tests are useful to predict the direction of cerebral asymmetry, but they do not give a reliable indication of the degree of the cerebral asymmetry, which might be reflected more directly in tests of asymmetry in speed and efficiency of performance (performance handedness).

One can study manual performance differences unconfounded by cognitive reflections of the subjects about possible consequences of choosing a particular hand for a particular task, and uninfluenced by cultural pressures or by overtrained lifelong tool-using habits in monkeys, using a measure of sensorimotor coordination, as in our finger-pressure discrimination task. We have measured performance of both hands of our subjects with this task and we have also measured preference handedness in a large variety of more natural tests, ranging from simple food retrieval under various conditions to quite demanding manipulations or productions of large efforts of force to obtain a reward.

To summarize the results very briefly, we found that the expression of hand preferences in rhesus monkeys increased with the amount of sensorimotor effort expended in a task. Sensorimotor effort is used here in the broad common sense of both amount of force exerted by hands and arms as well as general adjustments of body posture or body parts made by the animal to gain the reward. Thus, preferences were also influenced by individual differences of the subjects, for example, by the ways in which they would try to solve a task. The direction of a preference for different subjects varied under some as yet unknown influence. However, individual animals could be characterized by both consistency and degree of expression of a preference, and by the way in which they reacted toward attempts to influence preferences, for example, by manipulating the ease with which one or the other hand could be used.

In one experiment, we used a two-choice delayed alternation task. The manipulanda were two identical drawers that had to be pulled out to let a reward drop out from a hole in the bottom of the drawer into a food cup. In one condition, the drawers were side by side; in another condition, they were mounted one above the other. The monkey had to reach through a hole in the test cage, equidistant from both manipulanda, with one hand to pull out one of the drawers. When the drawers are mounted one above the other, both can be reached with equal facility by using either hand; when they are mounted side by side, each drawer is more easily manipulated with the contralateral hand. There were basically four types of reactions, which, incidentally, did not correlate with speed of learning or quality of performance. One type was characterized by consistent use of the same hand, a second type by an immediate switch from the consistent use of one hand in the vertical to consistent alternations of hand use in the horizontal condition, a third showed gradual systematic changes between single-hand and dual-hand use when conditions were changed, and the fourth type showed no systematic use of hands under either condition. Performance differences between hands were also found in some animals in a test of gross motor strength and in the fine-force discrimination task. But we were unable to predict from preference tests whether performance with the right or left hand would be better. These preliminary results are sufficiently interesting to encourage a further critical reexamination of the data on handedness in monkeys and man.

With regard to human handedness, it is worth stressing the difference between "preference handedness" and "performance handedness," and it is necessary to take account of the expression of individual differences in sensorimotor coordinative strategies, especially when trying to relate handedness to other manifestations of cerebral asymmetry. As far as the comparative study of laterality and the search for an animal model is concerned, I consider the present results to be consonant with an evolutionary rationale of the phenomenon of cerebral asymmetry that would predict that hemispheric specialization in different species may have taken different forms due to different evolutionary pressures.

The existing work on laterality in monkeys (e.g., Hamilton 1977, Lehman 1978, LeMay and Geschwind 1981, Warren 1981) and the resurgent discussion about it (e.g., MacNeilage, Studdert-Kennedy, and Lindblom 1984) is preoccupied with finding some lateralized precursor of gestural sign language,

speech, or other human-type asymmetry. I maintain that we should not expect humanlike functions or structures to be lateralized in the same way in animals, but should find asymmetry, or complementarity of hand use, in functions of importance for the survival of each species. By the same token, the expression of a hemispheric specialization, such as appears possible, for example, to control use of the fingers in precision grip, may have taken different forms in different species. An evolutionary theory would thus allow for a consistent predominance of one hemisphere for some specialized functions as well as a higher degree of left–right variability for others.

Consequently, while Warren (1981) may be right in claiming that hand preferences in nonhuman primates are subject to change through experience and, hence, will show wide interindividual variation, I do not agree with his conclusion that this means that we should expect no asymmetries of hand use in primates other than man. However, this does not lead me to see the necessity for a consistent asymmetric distribution of laterality throughout a series of primate species; the state of affairs in humans may have been brought about by additional evolutionary pressures irrelevant to monkeys. For example, new requirements for communication associated with the evolution of human social behavior, culture, and education of the young may have favored a new consistent division of function between the hands. Finally, I do not accept that preferences for hand use give the best information about laterality of function and the cerebral asymmetry that lies behind it. Indeed, in human beings, hand "preference" for certain acts appears to be but one consequence of complementary roles of the two hands in the coordination and sensory regulation of bimanual movements.

Conclusions as to the role of the corpus callosum in motor coordination of the hands

If the rather heterogeneous, subjectively selected, and, in some cases, still preliminary results presented before may be condensed to apparent coherence, they suggest the following: (1) the corpus callosum has a major role in the exchange of information on motor planning for the two hands; (2) despite the presence of intact commissures, lateralization of learning may occur in normal monkeys or human beings; and (3) this may be a mechanism for the development of adaptive cerebral asymmetry of functions. It is unlikely that such a simple conception will long survive further examination. It becomes more and more likely that the corpus callosum has many different functions in support of a delicately balanced perceptuomotor and cognitive system, with different subdivisions playing complementary roles. These roles may change over time as a result of maturation and experience, or according to different stages of processing that are taking place, and they may be influenced, in turn, by variable states of the other parts of the brain. It is one measure of the importance of the split-brain studies initiated by Sperry and his collaborators that so many fundamental questions raised by this work are still being busily explored.

Acknowledgments

I am indebted to Professor Roger Sperry for his support of the studies with the patients through NIMH Grant MH 03372. The animal work was performed at the Universities of Konstanz and Tübingen with major financial assistance of the Deutsche Forschungsgemeinschaft. The help of H.-C. Engele, M. Reger, M. Tanaka, and E. Weber in running the experiments is gratefully acknowledged. Finally, I must thank Colwyn Trevarthen for many helpful remarks.

References

Brinkman, C. 1981. Lesions in supplementary motor area interfere with a monkey's performance of a bimanual coordination task. *Neurosci. Lett.* 27: 267–70.

–1982. Callosal section abolishes bimanual coordination deficit resulting from supplementary motor area lesion in the monkey. *Soc. Neurosci. Abst.* 8: 734.

Brinkman, C., and R. Porter. 1979. Supplementary motor area in the monkey: Activity of neurons during performance of a learned motor task. *J. Neurophysiol.* 42: 681–709.

Charpentier, A. 1890. Influence des efforts musculaires sur les sensations des poids. *Cont. Rend. Soc. Biol.* 42 (Series 10, Vol. 2): 212.

Cohen, L. 1971. Synchronous bimanual movements performed by homologous and nonhomologous muscles. *Perc. Motor Skills* 32: 639–44.

Deecke, L., and H. H. Kornhuber. 1978. An electrical sign of participation of the mesial "supplementary" motor area in human voluntary finger movement. *Brain Res.* 159: 473–6.

Fleishman, E. A. 1957. A comparative study of aptitude patterns in unskilled and skilled psychomotor performances. *J. Appl. Psychol.* 41: 263–72.

Fleishman, E. A., and S. Rich. 1963. Role of kinesthetic and spatial-visual abilities in perceptual motor learning. *J. Exp. Psychol.* 66: 6–11.

Glees, P., and P. D. Wall. 1948. Commissural fibers of the macaque thalamus. *J. Comp. Neurol.* 88: 129–37.

Goldberg, G. 1985. Supplementary motor area structure and function: Review and hypotheses. *Behav. Brain Sci.* 8: 567–616.

Gordon, H. W., J. E. Bogen, and R. W. Sperry. 1971. Absence of deconnexion syndrome in two patients with partial section of the neocommissures. *Brain* 94: 327–36.

Hamilton, C. R. 1977. An assessment of hemispheric specialization in monkeys. *In* S. J. Dimond and D. A. Blizard (eds.) *Evolution and Lateralization of the Brain. Annals of the New York Academy of Sciences.* New York Academy of Sciences, New York, pp. 222–32.

Holst, E. von, and H. Mittelstaedt. 1950. Das Reafferenzprinzip (Wechselwirkungen zwischen Zentralnervensystem und Peripherie). *Die Naturwissen.* 37: 464–76.

Ingle, D. 1968. Interocular integration of visual learning by goldfish. *Brain, Behav. Evol.* 1: 58–85.

Kornhuber, H. H. 1980. Introduction. *In* H. H. Kornhuber and L. Deecke (eds.) *Motivation, Motor and Sensory Processes of the Brain: Electrical Potentials, Behaviour and Clinical Use. Progress in Brain Research,* Vol. 54. Elsevier, Amsterdam, pp. IX–XII.

Lashley, K. S. 1921. Studies of cerebral function in learning. II: The effects of long continued practice upon cerebral localization. *J. Comp. Psychol.* 1: 453–68.

Lehman, R. A. W. 1978. The handedness of rhesus monkeys. I: Distribution. *Neuropsychol.* 16: 32–42.

LeMay, M. J., and N. Geschwind. 1981. Morphological cerebral asymmetries in primates. *In* B. Preilowski and H.-C. Engele (eds.) *Is There a Cerebral Hemispheric Asymmetry in Non-Human Primates?* University of Tuebingen, Tuebingen, pp. 9–25.

Libet, B., E. W. Wright, Jr., and C. A. Gleason. 1982. Readiness-potentials preceding unrestricted "spontaneous" vs. pre-planned voluntary acts. *Electroenceph. Clin. Neurophysiol.* 54: 322–35.

Lumley, J. S. P. 1972. The role of the massa intermedia in motor performance in the rhesus monkey. *Brain* 95: 347–56.

MacNeilage, P. F., M. G. Studdert-Kennedy, and B. Lindblom. 1984. Functional precursors to language and its lateralization. *Am. J. Physiol.* 246: R912–14.

Müller, G. E., and F. Schumann. 1889. Ueber die psychologischen Grundlagen der Vergleichung gehobener Gewichte. *Arch. f. die gesamte Physiol.* 45: 37–112.

Palmers, C., and H. Zeier. 1974. Hemispheric dominance and transfer in the pigeon. *Brain Res.* 76: 537–41.

Pandya, D. N., and D. L. Rosene. 1985. Some observations on trajectories and topography of commissural fibers. *In* A. G. Reeves (ed.) *Epilepsy and the Corpus Callosum.* Plenum Press, New York, pp. 21–39.

Payne, B., and R. C. Davis 1940. The role of muscular tension in the comparison of lifted weights. *J. Exp. Psychol.* 27: 227–42.

Preilowski, B. 1971. Movement planning and weight comparisons. *Caltech Biol. Ann. Rep.*, p. 116.

–1972. Possible contribution of the anterior forebrain commissures to bilateral coordination. *Neuropsychol.* 10: 267–77.

–1975. Bilateral motor interaction: Perceptual-motor performance of partial and complete "split-brain" patients. *In* K. J. Zuelch, O. Creutzfeldt, and G. C. Galbraith (eds.) *Cerebral Localization.* Springer, Berlin, pp. 115–32.

–1977. Phases of motor-skills acquisition: A neuropsychological approach. *J. Human Move. Stud.* 3: 169–81.

–1979a. Self-recognition as a test of consciousness in left and right hemisphere of "split-brain" patients. *Act. Nerv. Sup.* 19 (Suppl. 2): 343–4.

–1979b. Consciousness after complete surgical section of the forebrain commissures in man. *In* I. S. Russell, M. W. van Hof, and G. Berlucchi (eds.) *Structure and Function of Cerebral Commissures.* Macmillan, London, pp. 411–20.

Preilowski, B., G. G. Gray, and R. W. Sperry. 1972. An attempt to test for self-recognition in the right hemisphere of split-brain patients. *Caltech Biol. Ann. Rep.,* p. 81.

Russell, S. I., and S. Ochs. 1963. Localization of a memory trace in one cortical hemisphere and transfer to the other hemisphere. *Brain* 86: 37–54.

Sperry, R. W. 1945. The problem of central nervous reorganization after nerve regeneration and muscle transposition. *Quart. Rev. Biol.* 20: 311–69.

–1950. Neural basis of the spontaneous optokinetic response produced by visual inversion. *J. Comp. Physiol. Psychol.* 43: 482–9.

Sperry, R. W., M. S. Gazzaniga, and J. E. Bogen. 1969. Interhemispheric relationships: The neocortical commissures; syndromes of hemisphere disconnection. *In* P. J. Vinken and G. W. Bruyn (eds.) *Handbook of Clinical Neurology,* Vol. 4. North-Holland, Amsterdam, pp. 273–90.

Teuber, H. L. 1964. The riddle of the frontal lobe function in man. *In* J. M. Warren and K. Akert (eds.) *The Frontal Granular Cortex and Behavior.* McGraw-Hill, New York, pp. 410–44.

Toncray, J. E., and W. J. S. Krieg. 1946. The nuclei of the human thalamus: A comparative approach. *J. Comp. Neurol.* 85: 421–59.

Van Hof, M. W., and I. S. Russell. 1977. Binocular vision in the rabbit. *Physiol. Behav.* 19: 121–8.

Vogt, C., and O. Vogt. 1919. Allgemeinere Ergebnisse unserer Hirnforschung 4. Die physiologische Bedeutung der architektonischen Rindenfelderung auf Grund neuer Rindenreizungen. *J. f. Psychol. Neurol. (Leipzig)* 25: 339–462.

Warren, J. M. 1981. Handedness and laterality in monkeys and man. *In* B. Preilowski and H.-C. Engele (eds.) *Is There a Cerebral Hemispheric Asymmetry in Non-Human Primates?* University of Tuebingen, Tuebingen, pp. 27–49.

Wiesendanger, M., and M. C. Hepp-Reymond. 1970. Cerebrale Organisation der Motorik und Fertigkeitsbewegungen. *In* K. Baettig (ed.) *Psychologische Experimente.* Huber, Bern, pp. 110–16.

Wiesendanger, M., J. J. Séguin, and H. Künzle. 1973. The supplementary motor area – a control system for posture? *In* R. B. Stein, K. G. Pearson, R. S. Smith, and J. B. Redford (eds.) *Control of Posture and Locomotion.* Plenum Press, New York, pp. 331–46.

Zaidel, D., and R. W. Sperry. 1977. Some long-term motor effects of cerebral commissurotomy in man. *Neuropsychol.* 15: 193–204.

10 Hemispheric specialization in monkeys

Charles R. Hamilton
Division of Biology
California Institute of Technology

Roger Sperry is famous as a generator of innovative ideas and as a challenger of traditional beliefs in biology and psychology. He has developed simple yet elegant methods for studying key problems in neural specificity, interhemispheric communication, and cerebral function. Most remarkable is his ability to construct theories that continue to guide our thinking in these areas and to initiate productive programs of research to test his ideas. He is so successful at this that it is surprisingly difficult to recall any experiments he has undertaken that did not work!

By contrast, most of us have accumulated a considerable collection of results that, despite careful planning and execution of the experiments producing them, ended up contrary to expectation or inconclusive. Usually, they are forgotten because journal editors and reviewers understandably favor publishing our supposedly more productive positive findings rather than our equally valid negative ones. Unfortunately, this bias can lead to a false impression of the importance of the positive findings because of the lack of a suitable frame of reference. For this reason, we chose to summarize here all of our experiments on hemispheric specialization in monkeys regardless of whether or not the findings were statistically significant. In this way, we hoped to generate a more general feel for the extent and character of hemispheric specialization in monkeys than could be obtained from reading just the published positive studies. But, first, we will briefly comment on the importance and present status of work on hemispheric specialization in animals.

Statement of the problem

During the past 20 years, the most intensely investigated area of neuropsychology has become the study of hemispheric specialization in the human brain. This is evident from even casual inspection of the major journals and of recent books that review this work (e.g., Harnad et al. 1977, Gazzaniga 1979, Bryden 1982, Bradshaw and Nettleton 1983). Much of the impetus for this surge of activity came from the dramatic studies with split-brain patients by Roger Sperry and his colleagues (Bogen 1969a, 1969b; Levy 1974; Sperry 1974; Gazzaniga and Le Doux 1978; Sperry 1982; Zaidel 1983). The bold conclusion that the left half of most human brains is specialized for analytic, sequential, and linguistic processing, whereas the right half is superior in holistic, parallel, and spatial abilities, has revolutionized research in neuropsychology and cognitive psychology. Although aspects of cerebral laterality had been recognized for well over a century, a clear and effective statement of its nature and extent, capable of interpreting and directing experimental studies, was not available until Sperry's remarkable findings and global interpretations. In particular, the specialized abilities of the right hemisphere had gone largely unnoticed. The initial necessary phase of describing and categorizing the types of hemispheric differences is now well underway and the study of the biological and psychological mechanisms that subserve these lateralized functions is beginning to flourish (reviewed in: Harnad et al. 1977; Corballis and Morgan 1978; Moscovitch 1979; Bryden 1982; Bradshaw and Nettleton 1981, 1983; Hellige 1983).

Do similar specializations in hemispheric function exist in nonhuman brains? An answer would be extremely valuable for both theoretical and experimental purposes. Theoretically, it is often thought that capacities for language, abstract thought, or even conscious experience in human beings are dependent on hemispheric specialization, which, in turn, is frequently claimed to be a uniquely human characteristic. Studies of the extent and nature of lateralized processing in other animals would provide information necessary for evaluating the validity of these conjectures as well as for understanding the basic evolutionary development of hemispheric differences. Experimentally, a convincing example of humanlike lateralization in other animals would make possible investigations that could not be done with human subjects. We could, for example, study the development of hemispheric specialization in young animals under controlled conditions of rearing; explore the neural mechanisms of laterality with surgical, electrical, or pharmacological techniques; and examine the effects of neurological disease or damage on behavioral function and recovery. Indeed, the development of a robust animal model is probably essential to an adequate understanding of laterality at levels more basic than those of functional localization. We believe, accordingly, that research with animals represents a necessary step toward the long-range goals of understanding the advantages conferred upon creatures by the evolution of lateralized cognitive mechanisms and of discovering how the mechanisms in the two hemispheres differ at neural levels.

Relatively few findings of hemispheric specialization have been reported for species other than man. Fortunately, most of these reports have been reviewed recently (Glick, Jerussi, and Zimmerberg 1977; Hamilton 1977a, 1977b; Warren 1977; Nottebohm 1979; Walker 1980; Warren 1980; Denenberg 1981; Glick and Ross 1981) for only a brief critique can be given here.

Evidence for hemispheric specialization in animals

The evidence for hemispheric specialization in animals to date is weak in several respects. First, very few of the reported results have been replicated by other laboratories. Second, several of the reports seem contradictory, although with the diverse procedures used, their findings are often difficult to compare. Third, many of the proposed examples of laterality seem obscure or trivial, at least when compared with the cognitive asymmetries reported for human subjects. Not every asymmetric structure or function in the body is necessarily related to hemispheric specialization in humans! Fourth, the criteria for judging whether or not an observed asymmetry reflects hemispheric specialization vary enormously from study to study. In order to be convincing as evidence for hemispheric specialization, we feel that asymmetric functions must be consistently represented in either the left or the right hemisphere, or else linked to another readily identifiable asymmetry such as handedness or an asymmetric neural structure. In particular, findings based on "significantly lateralized" individuals from a population without an identifiable net bias become very hard to interpret unless preidentified functional or structural asymmetries are correlated with the asymmetry of the function in question. The interpretive difficulties arise because a host of unrecognized asymmetries in experimental procedures, or even random fluctuations in the results, can lead to false appearances of lateralized behavior. In summary, while few would deny that animals may show behavioral, biochemical, or physical characteristics that are lateralized, the extent to which such findings in animals are relevant to hemispheric specialization as found in humans remains unknown. For all these reasons, it is difficult to accept the view that hemispheric specialization in animals is already an established fact (cf. Denenberg 1981).

The most convincing evidence for hemispheric specialization in animals comes from studies of the control of birdsong (Nottebohm 1980). In several species, this ability appears lateralized to the left hemisphere, and it is thought to resemble the production of human speech in other respects as well. A few points, however, argue against the immediate acceptance of birdsong as a model for humanlike hemispheric specialization: (1) There are no apparent anatomical differences between neural components on the two sides of the avian brain as there are in the human brain. (2) Physiological studies suggest that song production is bilateral in the brain and that peripheral asymmetries in the syrinx can explain the functional lateralization observed experimentally (McCasland 1983). (3) There is no evidence yet that song comprehension is also lateralized. (4) The distant evolutionary relationship between birds and humans, without intervening examples of vocal lateralization, raises the possibility of parallel development of nonhomologous mechanisms for these behaviors.

Other researchers have suggested that the left hemisphere of chicks is better at discriminating visual stimuli, such as grains from pebbles, and that the right is more reactive to emotionally charged stimuli (Rogers and Anson 1979; Andrew, Mench, and Rainey 1982; Gaston 1983). These results lead to the plausible but revolutionary inference that a bird more effectively searches for food with its right eye while it watches for danger with its left! On the other hand, informal field observations suggest that birds do not normally suffer from hemineglect while looking for food or predators. For example, parrots often give a characteristic vocal response to flying hawks seen through either eye.

A flood of research with rodents has indicated that certain motoric, spatial, and emotional behaviors are lateralized, often in conjunction with asymmetrically distributed neurotransmitters. The basic difficulties with accepting these findings as models for human laterality are the apparent lack of agreement among them and the remoteness of the behaviors studied from those commonly tested with human subjects. For example, Glick (Glick et al 1977, Glick and Ross 1981) found significant but very small population biases when female rats circled (55% turned to their right) or chose one of two levers to depress (58% picked the right), although individual rats did have consistent preferences that correlated with asymmetries in dopamine distribution. Using another measure, Robinson (1979) found a strong, although transient, effect at the population level of left, but not right, hemispheric

damage on overall activity levels of male rats, with correlated changes in noradrenalin levels. By contrast, Denenberg (1981) reported no differential effect of unilateral lesions on activity or directional preferences of normally reared male rats. However, Denenberg (1981) did find differential effects of unilateral lesions on a variety of behaviors in rats if they were systematically handled shortly after birth (an unnatural amount of stimulation for a rat). Behaviors differentially affected by unilateral lesions included spatial preference (opposite in direction to those observed by Glick), taste aversion, and mouse killing. Until these results with rodents, drawn from studies differing in subjects (sex, strain, handling) and techniques (type of test, type of lesion), are replicated and compared under similar experimental conditions, it is difficult to accept a conclusion more specific than the following: interesting effects of unilateral manipulations may be obtained, but the underlying reasons and interpretations are obscure.

Nonhuman primates are the obvious subjects of choice for investigations of hemispheric specialization because of their close phylogenetic relationship to human beings and because their behavioral repertoire resembles that of human beings in several respects. These similarities maximize the chances of finding homologous hemisphere specialization in animals and humans and simplify the problem of selecting appropriate tests for lateralized function. Furthermore, anatomical asymmetries are known to be present in the brains of apes, although their existence is questionable in monkeys (LeMay and Geschwind 1975; Wada, Clarke, and Hamm 1975; Yeni-Komshian and Benson 1976; Falk 1978). Unfortunately, reports of lateralized cognitive behaviors in apes so far have not appeared, and, in any event, apes are too rare and precious to provide an appropriate model for widespread use in comparative studies.

Several investigators have tested monkeys, with clearly negative results, for hemispheric differences in the learning, memory, and performance of simple pattern discriminations (reviewed in: Hamilton 1977a, 1977b; Warren 1977, 1980). On the other hand, positive findings have been reported from experiments using stimuli that would be expected to reveal lateralized processing in humans, such as variations in species-specific calls, facial features, sequences, orientation, and movement. Most of the studies finding laterality have reported better performance by the left hemisphere (Hamilton and Lund 1970; Hamilton, Tieman, and Farrell 1974; Dewson 1977; Beecher et al. 1979; Hamilton 1983; Hamilton and Vermeire 1983). Two of them, however, found a right hemispheric superiority (Vermeire, Erdmann, and Hamilton 1983; Ifune, Vermeire, and Hamilton 1984), and two found the superior hemisphere to be the one contralateral to the preferred hand (Garcha, Ettlinger, and Maccabe 1982; Hamilton and Vermeire 1982). It should be noted that using stimuli such as just mentioned does not ensure finding laterality in monkeys (Hamilton, 1977a, 1977b; Overman and Doty 1982). The principal objections to these studies with positive results are the relatively small effects reported, the small number of subjects tested, and the fact that most of them have not been replicated.

In summary, the prospect of finding credible examples of hemispheric specialization in animals now seems encouraging, a significant change from the prevalent opinion when we began studying this question over a decade ago. However, it also appears that, except possibly for birdsong, no example of lateralized ability is established well enough to justify a concerted attack on the mechanisms of its development and operation, particularly if our primary interest is in hemispheric specialization in human beings. Thus, considerable effort continues to be directed toward finding convincing, exploitable examples of laterally specialized functions in the brains of animals.

Our experiments with monkeys

The approach of most of our experiments is conceptually simple. Split-brain monkeys are surgically prepared by dividing the cerebral commissures, which effectively separates the cognitive mechanisms of the two cerebral hemispheres, and by sectioning the optic chiasm, which allows visual input to be lateralized to one hemisphere by simply occluding the contralateral eye (Sperry 1968, Hamilton 1982). With this preparation, each hemisphere may be tested independently for its ability to learn or

perform any visual task we wish to study. A variety of discriminations are then taught to each side and examined for asymmetries in learning, memory, or performance. We look for hemispheric differences between the left and right hemispheres, between the hemispheres ipsi- and contralateral to the preferred hand, and with each of these as related to the sex of the subjects. Particular care is taken to balance the experimental designs for procedural asymmetries such as the hemisphere and discriminations trained first and the side of the brain retracted during surgery.

Thirty-eight split-brain monkeys have completed enough experiments to warrant inclusion in this overview. Their pertinent characteristics are given in Table 10.1. All but two were rhesus monkeys (*Macaca mulatta*); the exceptions (FRD and HPJ) were pigtail macaques (*M. nemestrina*). Each monkey was tested for hand preferences in reaching for food placed on a tray or in a bottle (Warren, Abplanalp and Warren 1967) soon after arriving at the laboratory and before formal training or surgery. A handedness index [HI = $100 (R - L)/(R + L)$, where R equals the number of reaches with the right hand, and L the number of reaches with the left hand] was calculated for each subject. As shown in Table 10.1, handedness preferences ranged from completely left handed (-100) to strongly right handed ($+95$). All subjects then had the optic chiasm, corpus callosum, and anterior and hippocampal commissures divided in one or two stages using neurosurgical techniques developed at Caltech (Sperry 1968). Five subjects (DPE, IRW, MNX, RYE, and ZLD) had additional midsagittal division of the midbrain cross-connections (habenular, posterior, and collicular commissures) for other reasons. The hemisphere retracted during each surgical procedure is also indicated in Table 10.1. All subjects were tested on a variety of experiments for many years; only the experiments that test for hemispheric specialization are indicated in Table 10.1.

Three paradigms for examining discrimination learning were employed: two-choice, top-only, and go/no-go. For two-choice problems, two stimuli were presented simultaneously, one above the other, on separate stimulus-response screens that each subtended about 7° in visual angle. The monkey's task was to learn to push the one we chose as correct in order to obtain a food reward. The top-only method was identical except that only the top screen was used for stimulus presentation. When the positive stimulus was presented, the top screen should be pushed; when the negative stimulus was presented, the bottom screen should be pushed. A symmetrically rewarded go/no-go paradigm was used when large 30° stimuli were presented or when successively presented stimuli were to be compared. Either a push to the positive stimulus, or withholding a push to the negative stimulus, was rewarded. Both of the latter two methods required comparing the stimulus presented to representations in memory rather than directly to another stimulus, a procedure thought to increase the likelihood of revealing hemispheric specialization (Moscovitch 1979). These problems were taught in training boxes with adjustable eye and hand openings that allowed us to determine easily which hemisphere was being tested (Sperry 1968).

The number of trials-to-criterion and errors-through-criterion required to achieve a performance of 90% correct in four successive blocks of ten trials was determined for each hemisphere. A dominance index [DI = 100 $(R - L)/(R + L)$, where R and L equal the number of trials or errors made by the right and left hemispheres, respectively] was calculated for each discrimination learned and the average DI for each monkey on a set of similar problems was then obtained. The grand mean of these average DIs was calculated for all of the monkeys tested in a given experiment and this mean DI tested for significance by appropriate two-tailed t-tests. To see if the hemispheric asymmetries for learning problems were related to handedness of the monkeys, the correlation between DIs and HIs was determined for each experiment and tested for significance. When the data from different experiments were combined for additional statistical tests, the DIs from individual problems for each monkey were first averaged and then the mean of these averages calculated across monkeys. In this case, the number of problems learned by each monkey differs according to

which experiments it had completed, as indicated in Table 10.1.

The most important variable in these experiments is the type of stimuli used. We tried to select stimuli that would tap perceptual abilities normally present in monkeys and that would be similar to stimuli that elicit lateralized processing reliably in human beings. Patterns that would not be expected to evoke lateralized cognitive processing in humans were chosen as control stimuli. Examples of the stimuli used in the various experiments are pictured in Figure 10.1, grouped according to the category they were intended to represent. The labels describing the particular sets of stimuli are the same as in the tables, which allows the stimuli to be easily paired with the corresponding results. All the stimuli used have been depicted in the figure except for those comprising the facial discriminations; two complete series of faces are pictured in Hamilton and Vermeire (1983).

RESULTS FROM INDIVIDUAL EXPERIMENTS

To date, we have substantially completed 4 experiments that use control patterns and 15 experiments that test for lateralized ability in learning or performing discriminations with the stimuli categorized as spatial, facial, or sequential. The overall results (Table 10.2) are reported separately for female and male subjects, and again for all subjects combined. Both the mean DIs comparing left and right hemispheres and the correlations of DIs and HIs are given for each experiment; their levels of statistical significance are also indicated.

A glance at Table 10.2 reveals that there are no large or significant DIs for the experiments using control patterns, which shows that on the average, there were no differences between the hemispheres in learning these problems. In addition, there were no significant correlations between DIs and HIs, which indicates that neither the hemisphere contralateral nor ipsilateral to the preferred hand was better able to learn these discriminations. Thus, the learning of these patterns was equally good with either hemisphere, as expected.

For the experiments using the spatial, facial, and sequential tasks selected with the hope

Table 10.1. *Characteristics of 38 split-brain monkeys and the experiments they completed*

Sex	Subject	HI[a]	Ret.[b]	Pattern					Orientation					Movement					Faces			Sequence
				1	2	3	4	5	6	7	8	9	10	11	12	13	14	15	16	17	18	19
Female	DPE	−87	LRL	×	×	×	×			×	×	×	×		×	×	×		×	×	×	×
	PHL	−84	L	×	×								×						×			
	KIP	−83	R	×	×				×				×						×			×
	BRN	−77	RL	×		×	×			×	×	×				×				×	×	×
	AMY	−41	R	×	×	×				×	×	×					×			×	×	
	ETH	−15	L	×	×	×				×		×										
	POT	−5	L	×	×				×				×		×							
	MNX	6	LR	×	×	×	×			×		×			×	×	×			×	×	×
	YAM	7	L	×	×				×				×		×	×	×		×			
	RYE	26	RL	×	×					×			×		×				×	×	×	×
	BOO	35	R	×	×	×	×		×	×	×		×		×				×	×	×	
	ZLD	46	LR		×	×				×		×				×	×					
	UNA	66	R	×	×					×		×			×	×	×			×		
	NED	68	R	×					×			×	×						×			
	BNN	72	L	×	×				×				×						×			
	HSH	84	LR	×	×	×			×	×	×	×	×		×	×	×		×			
	LMN	93	R	×	×	×	×				×	×			×	×	×		×	×	×	
	WED	95	L					×	×	×	×	×	×		×	×	×		×			×
	FRD	?	L					×						×				×				
	MLL	?	LR					×						×				×				
	SCN	?	L					×						×				×				
	HPJ	?	L					×						×								

Table 10.1. (*continued*)

Sex	Subject	HI[a]	Ret.[b]	Pattern				Orientation						Movement				Faces				Sequence
				1	2	3	4	5	6	7	8	9	10	11	12	13	14	15	16	17	18	19
Male	MRV	−100	RL	×	×	×	×		×	×	×	×	×		×				×			
	TEA	−97	R	×	×	×	×		×	×	×	×	×	×	×	×			×	×	×	×
	IRM	−82	RL	×	×				×				×						×	×	×	
	ZOR	−73	L	×		×	×			×		×		×		×	×					×
	OZZ	−37	RL	×	×				×			×			×				×			×
	EDN	−20	L		×																	
	IRW	−9	RLR	×	×	×			×	×		×	×	×	×	×	×		×	×	×	×
	CRN	3	LR		×	×	×			×		×			×	×	×			×	×	
	CHT	4	R	×	×		×		×				×			×	×		×			×
	SOL	13	LR	×	×				×				×						×			
	KEF	28	R	×	×	×	×			×	×	×		×	×	×	×			×	×	
	DOE	32	LR	×	×	×	×		×	×	×	×	×	×	×	×	×		×	×	×	×
	EDG	52	L	×	×	×			×	×			×	×	×	×			×			×
	ADM	?	L					×								×		×				
	BND	?	L					×								×		×				
	HLM	?	LR					×								×		×				

[a]HI, handedness index.
[b]Ret., hemisphere retracted in the one to three operations performed on each monkey.

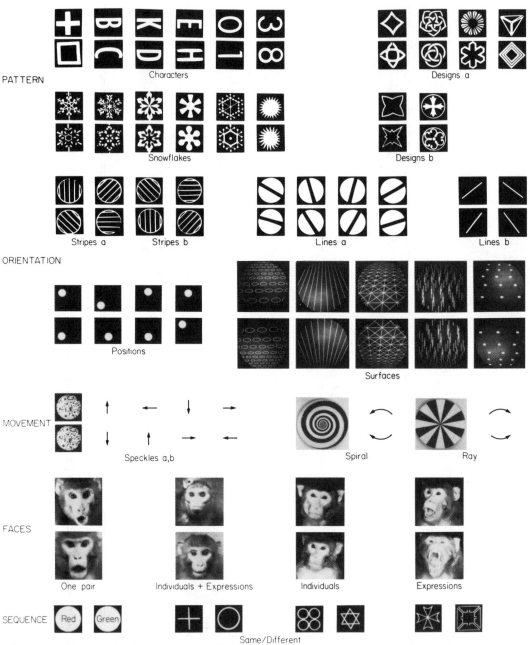

Figure 10.1. Photographs of the stimuli used in the 19 experiments are grouped according to the categories described in the text and tables. The smaller stimuli subtended about 7° and the larger ones about 30°. Most experiments consisted of several discriminations, each of which is pictured with the positive stimulus above the negative one. The stimuli for "lines b" and "position" are pictured as seen by one hemisphere; the other hemisphere was tested with the left–right mirror image to control for possible asymmetries resulting from hemianopia. The moving stimuli are pictured once with the discriminations of directions of movement indicated by arrows. Only representative photographs of faces are pictured; there were four discriminations in each experiment, and except for the experiment labeled "one pair," each discrimination consisted of five positive poses and five negative ones. For the sequential discriminations, the positive sequence was defined as a sequence of two different stimuli; the negative stimulus was a repetition of the same stimulus.

Table 10.2. *Average dominance indices (DI) and their correlations (r) with handedness indices for each experiment*

Category	Experiment	Stimulus	Number	Paradigm	Reference[a]	Female Subjects N	DI	r	Male Subjects N	DI	r	All Subjects N	DI	r
Pattern	1	Characters	6	Two-choice	3,4,5,9	14	2	0.39	11	−3	−0.05	25	0	0.27
	2	Snowflakes	6	Two-choice	3,4,9	13	7	0.29	10	2	0.43	23	5	0.34
	3	Designs a	4	Top-only	8,9	9	−6	0.25	8	−10	0.08	17	−8	0.21
	4	Designs b	2	Top-only	9	6	15	−0.55	6	−22	0.14	12	−3	−0.15
Orientation	5	Stripes a	2	Go/no-go	2	4	36+		3	17		7	28**	0.20
	6	Stripes b	2	Go/no-go	3,4	9	13	0.04	9	−5	0.35	18	4	−0.01
	7	Lines a	4	Top-only	8,9	10	26*	0.08	8	11	−0.42	18	20**	−0.12
	8	Lines b	2	Top-only	9	5	6	−0.90*	5	2	0.24	10	4	0.59*
	9	Positions	4	Top-only	9	10	16	0.91**	7	4	−0.27	17	11+	−0.17
	10	Surfaces	1	Go/no-go	3,4,6	10	−13	−0.19	9	12	−0.05	19	−1	
Movement	11	Speckles a	4	Top-only	1	4	39+					4	39+	−0.14
	12	Speckles b	4	Top-only	2,9	10	8	−0.14	9	−4	−0.40	19	2	0.00
	13	Spiral	1	Go/no-go	3,4,9,10	11	10	−0.13	13	14	0.25	24	12	−0.52*
	14	Ray	1	Go/no-go	9,10	9	−6	−0.37	6	15	−0.92**	15	2	
Faces	15	One pair	4	Top-only	2	4	−3		3	−5		7	−4	0.23
	16	Ind. + exp.	4	Go/no-go	4,6	9	20*	0.10	9	−6	0.13	18	7	0.28
	17	Individuals	4	Go/no-go	7,9	9	−1	0.29	7	1	0.34	16	0	0.28
	18	Expressions	4	Go/no-go	7,9	8	−20**	0.87**	7	3	0.18	15	−9	0.77**
Sequence	19	Same/different	4	Go/no-go	4,5	6	−3	0.83*	6	8	0.70	12	2	

[a]The references to these experiments are: 1, Hamilton and Lund 1970; 2, Hamilton, Tieman, and Farrell 1974; 3, Hamilton 1977a; 4, Hamilton, Tieman, and Farrell 1974; 3, Hamilton 1977b; 5, Hamilton and Vermeire 1982; 6, Hamilton and Vermeire 1983; 7, Vermeire, Erdmann, and Hamilton 1983; 8, Hamilton 1983; 9, Hamilton and Vermeire unpublished; 10, S. B. Tieman unpublished.

Significance levels: +, < 0.1; *, < 0.05; **, < 0.01.

of revealing lateralized processing, there are several examples of DIs and correlations that differ significantly from zero. Looking at the combined results for all subjects, we see that there are about 3.7 times ($\chi^2 = 10.39$, p < 0.005) as many significant DIs and correlations as would be expected by chance at the 5% significance level, which suggests we are not just observing random fluctuations in our experiments. Furthermore, if just the signs of the DIs are considered, there is a significant general tendency for the DIs to be positive(12/15, p < 0.02, sign test), which indicates an overall left hemispheric superiority. In general, there is no significant tendency for the direction of the correlations of DIs with HIs to be significant.

There is a tendency for the DIs and correlations to be larger and more often significant for our sample of female monkeys than for male monkeys. This finding was statistically significant within two of the experiments with facial features (Hamilton and Vermeire 1983, Vermeire et al. 1983). While we feel that this result is probably real, it is premature to speculate on the interpretation of greater laterality for facial discrimination by female monkeys.

Although several significant findings emerged, it is evident that the number of non-significant results outweighs the number of significant ones. At least three kinds of interpretations of this fact are possible. According to one interpretation, the significant cases just represent random fluctuations in the data, a view we argued against on statistical grounds before. A second interpretation would question the appropriateness of some of the individual experiments and would suggest that only the tasks that revealed hemispheric specialization really tapped lateralized mechanisms effectively. In fact, this is the interpretation usually implicit in any survey of results reported in journals because of the tendency to publish only positive findings. However, we cannot claim realistically that our significant results came from experiments that were better suited to revealing lateralized processing than were the ones that gave nonsignificant outcomes. A third interpretation would be to accept all the data as valid and view the frequent lack of significant results as representing the existence of a real but relatively small effect embedded in

a rather variable sample of data. We will explore this third view for the rest of this chapter.

POOLING RESULTS BY CATEGORIES

If the various experiments are viewed as equally valid, then it makes sense to combine the data from all experiments within a particular category of stimuli and evaluate their overall significance. We, therefore, looked for lateralization of learning for the pooled categories of orientation, of direction of movement, and of facial features. We also combined the data for discriminations of orientation and of moving stimuli in order to get a more general estimate of the lateralization of "spatial" abilities; both of these categories require discriminating spatially relevant cues, namely, tilt, position, or direction of movement. For each category, the average DI of individual monkeys is plotted against that monkey's HI in Figure 10.2. The average DIs and the correlation of DIs with HIs for various groups are given in Table 10.3 along with their statistical significance. Because only one set of sequential discriminations has been completed, the corresponding data shown in Table 10.2 are simply repeated in Table 10.3 for ease of comparison.

The combined data (Table 10.3) for the pattern discriminations again display no significant lateral asymmetries as measured by the average DI or the correlation of DIs with HIs, thereby confirming the lack of cerebral specialization for discriminating geometrical patterns. This is also evident in Figure 10.2A in which DIs for individual monkeys scatter around the horizontal zero axis and there is no clear correlation of DI with HI.

In contrast, the combined DI for orientation (Table 10.3) is highly significant (p < 0.001). This is also evident in Figure 10.2B, where the individual data for the 36 monkeys lie largely above the horizontal zero axis. The correlation with handedness is not significant. These results indicate that hemispheric asymmetries exist for discriminating orientation. A similar tendency is found for the experiments that use moving stimuli (Figure 10.2C), although conventional levels of significance are not quite reached (Table 10.3). When we combine the categories of orientation and movement into a more general spatial cat-

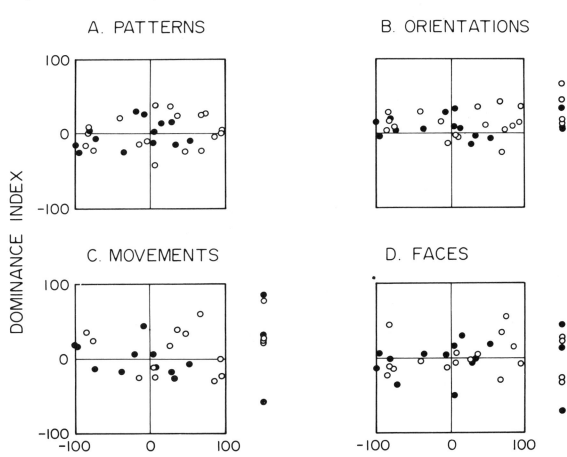

Figure 10.2. The average dominance index for each monkey is plotted against that monkey's handedness index for four categories of experiments. The indices are defined quantitatively in the text. Positions above the horizontal zero axis represent better learning by the left hemisphere; those below the axis represent better learning by the right side. Positions to the right of the vertical zero line refer to monkeys that are right handed; those to the left refer to left-handed subjects. Open symbols represent female monkeys; closed symbols signify male monkeys. The symbols to the right of the plots are for seven monkeys that were not tested for handedness before surgery.

Table 10.3. *Weighted average dominance indices (DI) and their correlations (r) with handedness indices for categories of stimuli*

Category	Female Subjects				Male Subjects				All Subjects			
	N	DI	N	r	N	DI	N	r	N	DI	N	r
Pattern	18	1	18	0.17	13	−2	13	0.29	31	0	31	0.22
Orientation (0)	21	17**	17	0.03	15	8*	12	−0.21	36	13***	29	0.01
Movement (M)	16	16+	12	−0.19	14	4	11	−0.39	30	10+	23	−0.18
Spatial (O + M)	22	15**	18	−0.13	16	9*	13	−0.21	38	12***	31	0.09
Faces	19	2	15	0.23	15	−2	12	0.27	34	0	27	0.26
Sequence	6	−3	6	0.83*	6	8	6	0.70	12	2	12	0.77**

Significance levels: +, < 0.1; *, < 0.05; **, < 0.01; ***, < 0.001.

egory (Table 10.3) and test the results, we again find a highly significant cerebral asymmetry in favor of the left hemisphere (p <0.001), with no significant correlation with handedness. We tentatively conclude, therefore, that the left hemisphere is better able to distinguish stimuli that differ in spatial relationships than is the right. It should be noted that the superior side is opposite to that usually found with human subjects.

The combined results for all the facial discriminations are decidedly in favor of equal ability for the two hemispheres (Table 10.3, Figure 10.2D). However, in two of these experiments (Table 10.2), we found significant DIs for female subjects, although they favored opposite hemispheres. It is possible that different basic aspects of facial discriminations were tapped in these two experiments, perhaps analogous to the different strategies employed by split-brain human subjects when viewing faces (Levy, Trevarthen, and Sperry 1972). However, until we can replicate these results or determine if different cues were processed in these experiments, we must be conservative and conclude, with some reservations, that there is no overall tendency for facial processing to be better lateralized to one hemisphere of our monkeys.

The results for the experiment using sequentially presented stimuli also indicate no overall advantage for the left or right hemisphere, but the significant correlation of DIs with HIs does suggest that the hemisphere opposite the preferred hand learns this task more readily. We also have seen significant correlations with handedness in a few other experiments (Table 10.2) as have Garcha et al. (1982).

The overall picture

What have we learned by examining collectively over 2,000 learning curves from 38 split-brain monkeys in 19 sets of experiments?

First, although no task requiring discrimination of simple patterns ever demonstrated significant cerebral asymmetries of function, discrimination of stimuli drawn from categories that should reveal asymmetries in human subjects produced significant findings of lateralized processing in a considerably larger number of experiments than would be expected by chance.

This result indicates that, for monkeys, there is something fundamentally different about discriminating types of stimuli that demonstrate hemispheric differences in human beings. In addition, it shows that possible, unrecognized asymmetries in testing or surgery did not produce artifacts that mimic cerebral laterality, for they would affect learning of both control patterns and laterality problems equally.

Second, when the individual experiments that tested discriminations based on stimuli differing in spatial cues were combined, a highly significant tendency was found for the left hemisphere to learn more readily than the right. This occurred even though all the experiments, whether or not they had significant results, were included, which reinforces the suggestion that a basic hemispheric difference in lateralized ability was being observed. It should be recognized, however, that even the highly significant DIs for the combined spatial discriminations were not large. They represent an average ratio of learning ability for the two hemispheres of only 1.3 in favor of the left, with the largest ratio being 2.6 (Hamilton 1983). Also, the result that spatial discriminations are more lateralized to the left hemisphere is opposite to the usual finding with human beings (De Renzi, Faglioni, and Scotti 1971; Berlucchi 1974; Benton, Hannay, and Varney 1975), suggesting that monkeys have reversed laterality from that found for humans for this type of discrimination. This possibility (Hamilton 1983) is supported by a recent report of greater participation of the left hemisphere of monkeys in the discrimination of differences in the position of a dot within a frame (Jason, Cowey, and Weiskrantz 1984), a discrimination similar to the ones in experiment 9 (Table 10.2). However, we cannot rule out the possibility that our monkeys processed the spatial stimuli in an unrecognized way, appropriate to analytical abilities often attributed to the left hemisphere, as sometimes happens in humans (Berlucchi 1974).

Third, the results from categories based on facial and sequential cues, while including significant findings in individual experiments, did not indicate a simple scheme of lateralization to the left or right hemisphere. While this complication does not obviate the interest of these individual experiments, it does require additional hypotheses to encompass the more diverse set of results and, therefore, makes these findings less compelling as examples of humanlike hemispheric specialization.

Despite the qualifications, there seems to be sufficient evidence to conclude that some kind of nonartifactual lateralization of function is present in the brains of monkeys even though the specific factors controlling the direction of laterality are not completely clear. We may now ask whether our results better fit the older concept of left cerebral dominance or the more modern idea of complementary hemispheric specialization.

Our results immediately invite an explanation in terms of left hemispheric dominance for cognitive processing. We will examine this idea first, recognizing its regression to ideas from earlier times and its present unpopularity. When data from all our experiments were considered, we found that all DIs significant at $p < 0.1$ or better (Table 10.2) showed the left hemisphere to be superior even though most of the tests had used stimuli and procedures that should favor the right hemisphere of human subjects. Furthermore, 12 of the 15 ($p < 0.05$, sign test) laterality experiments produced a left hemispheric advantage if only the direction of laterality was examined, and 27 out of 38 ($p < 0.05$, sign test) monkeys favored the left hemisphere when all the DIs for the experimental problems learned by each monkey were combined. The three experiments mentioned before from other laboratories (Dewson 1977, Beecher et al. 1979, Jason et al. 1984) also suggested left hemispheric superiority. In other words, all of the significant experiments in Table 10.2 as well as those of other researchers have demonstrated left hemispheric superiority. Perhaps the left hemisphere of monkeys really is better at solving complex problems such as those commonly used to test for dominance. If so, its intellectual superiority might become increasingly evident as the problems it solves become more difficult, independent of whether the task appears left or right hemispheric according to human data. This resembles the older interpretations of cerebral dominance in humans that considered the left hemisphere to be more intelligent, perceptive, rational, and aware, a view that is still held by some (Eccles 1980, Gazzaniga 1983).

If this interpretation were correct, we would expect a correlation between magnitude of laterality, as measured by DI, and task difficulty, as measured by the errors made during learning. This correlation, in fact, is significant ($r = 0.58$, $p < 0.01$) for the 19 experiments summarized in this chapter. We can almost hear Roger Sperry muttering something like "resurrecting the idea of general left dominance ought to set psychobiology back about 25 years."

For those who favor instead the newer concept of hemispheric specialization, with its emphasis on complementary superiorities of the two sides of the brain, we offer two supporting observations. First, a significant right hemispheric superiority was found for females in our experiments that required discrimination of facial expression (Table 10.2; Vermeire et al. 1983), a predominantly right hemispheric ability in humans. In fact, in our most recent experiments completed after this chapter was submitted, a right hemispheric advantage for learning, remembering, and generalizing facial discriminations was significant for the entire group of male and female monkeys (Hamilton and Vermeire 1985). Second, in a recent study of hemispheric preferences of split-brain monkeys watching videotape recordings, the right hemisphere watched longer and responded by making significantly more facial expressions than did the left hemisphere (Ifune et al. 1984). Thus, in at least two types of experiments, a right hemispheric superiority was found in the same population of subjects that showed left hemispheric advantages in other experiments. This leaves open the possibility that with more adequate testing, the right hemisphere of monkeys may convincingly emerge as superior in its own right, a situation that would be reminiscent of the delayed recognition of right hemispheric abilities in human beings. We might even imagine Sperry voicing a restrained sigh of approval!

References

Andrew, R. J., J. Mench, and C. Rainey. 1982. Right–left asymmetry of response to visual stimuli in the domestic chick. *In* D. J. Ingle, M. A. Goodale, and R. J. W. Mansfield (eds.) *Analysis of Visual Behavior.* The MIT Press, Cambridge, pp. 197–209.

Beecher, M. D., M. R. Petersen, S. R. Zoloth, D. B. Moody, and W. C. Stebbins. 1979. Perception of conspecific vocalizations by Japanese macaques: Evidence for selective attention and neural lateralization. *Brain Behav. Evol.* 16: 443–60.

Benton, A., H. J. Hannay, and N. R. Varney. 1975. Visual perception of line direction in patients with unilateral brain disease. *Neurol.* 25: 907–10.

Berlucchi, G. 1974. Cerebral dominance and interhemispheric communication in normal man. *In* F. O. Schmitt and F. G. Worden (eds.) *The Neurosciences: Third Study Program.* The MIT Press, Cambridge, pp. 65–9.

Bogen, J. E. 1969a. The other side of the brain. I: Dysgraphia and dyscopia following cerebral commissurotomy. *Bull. L.A. Neurol. Soc.* 34: 73–105.

–1969b. The other side of the brain. II: An appositional mind. *Bull. L.A. Neurol. Soc.* 34: 135–62.

Bradshaw, J. L., and N. C. Nettleton. 1981. The nature of hemispheric specialization in man. *Behav. Brain Sci.* 4: 51–91.

–1983. *Human Cerebral Asymmetry.* Prentice-Hall, Englewood Cliffs, NJ.

Bryden, M. P. 1982. *Laterality: Functional Asymmetry in the Intact Brain.* Academic Press, New York.

Corballis, M. C., and M. J. Morgan. 1978. On the biological basis of human laterality. I: Evidence for a maturational left–right gradient. II: The mechanisms of inheritance. *Behav. Brain Sci.* 2: 261–336.

Denenberg, V. H. 1981. Hemispheric laterality in animals and the effects of early experience. *Brain Behav. Sci.* 4: 1–49.

DeRenzi, E., P. Faglioni, and G. Scotti. 1971. Judgment of spatial orientation in patients with focal brain damage. *J. Neurol. Neurosurg. Psychiat.* 34: 489–95.

Dewson, J. H., III. 1977. Preliminary evidence of hemispheric asymmetry of auditory function in monkeys. *In* S. Harnad, R. W. Doty, L. Goldstein, J. Jaynes, and G. Krauthamer (eds.) *Lateralization in the Nervous System.* Academic Press, New York, pp. 63–71.

Eccles, J. C. 1980. *The Human Psyche.* Springer-Verlag, Berlin.

Falk, D. 1978. Cerebral asymmetry in old world monkeys. *Acta Anat.* 101: 334–9.

Garcha, H. S., G. Ettlinger, and J. J. Maccabe. 1982. Unilateral removal of the second somatosensory projection cortex in the monkey: Evidence for cerebral predominance? *Brain* 105: 787–810.

Gaston, K. E. 1983. Evidence for left hemisphere dominance of visual discrimination learning in the chick. *Soc. Neurosci. Abst.* 9: 651.

Gazzaniga, M. S., (ed.). 1979. *Handbook of Behavioral Neurobiology, Vol. 2.* Plenum Press, New York.

–1983. Right hemispheric language following brain bisection – A 20 year perspective. *Am. Psychol.* 38: 525–37.

Gazzaniga, M. S., and J. E. LeDoux. 1978. *The Integrated Mind.* Plenum Press, New York.

Glick, S. D., T. P. Jerussi, and B. Zimmerberg. 1977. Behavioral and neuropharmacological correlates of nigrostriatal asymmetry in rats. *In* S. Harnad, R. W. Doty, L. Goldstein, J. Jaynes, and G. Krauthamer (eds.) *Lateralization in the Nervous System.* Academic Press, New York, pp 213–49.

Glick, S. D., and D. A. Ross. 1981. Lateralization of function in the rat brain: Basic mechanisms may be operative in humans. *Trends Neurosci.* 4: 196–9.

Hamilton, C. R. 1977a. Investigations of perceptual and mnemonic lateralization in monkeys. *In* S. Harnad, R. W. Doty, L. Goldstein, J. Jaynes, and G. Krauthamer (eds.) *Lateralization in the Nervous System.* Academic Press, New York, pp. 45–62.

–1977b. An assessment of hemispheric specialization in monkeys. *Annu. N.Y. Acad. Sci.* 299: 222–32.

–1982. Mechanisms of interocular equivalence. *In* D. J. Ingle, M. A. Goodale, and R. J. W. Mansfield, (eds.) *Analysis of Visual Behavior.* The MIT Press, Cambridge, pp. 693–717.

–1983. Lateralization for orientation in split-brain monkeys. *Behav. Brain Res.* 10: 399–403.

Hamilton, C. R., and J. S Lund. 1970. Visual discrimination of movement: Midbrain or forebrain? *Science* 170: 1428–30.

Hamilton, C. R., S. B. Tieman, and W. S. Farrell, Jr. 1974. Cerebral dominance in monkeys? *Neuropsychol.* 12: 193–7.

Hamilton, C. R., and B. A. Vermeire. 1982. Hemispheric differences in split-brain monkeys learning sequential comparisons. *Neuropsychol.* 20: 691–8.

–1983. Discrimination of monkey faces by split-brain monkeys. *Behav. Brain Res.* 9: 263–75.

–1985. Complementary hemispheric superiorities in monkeys. *Soc. Neurosci. Abst.* 11: 869.

Harnad, S., R. W. Doty, L. Goldstein, J. Jaynes, and G. Krauthamer (eds.). 1977. *Lateralization in the Nervous System.* Academic Press, New York.

Hellige, J. R., (ed.). 1983. *Cerebral Hemisphere Asymmetry.* Praeger Press, New York.

Ifune, C. K., B. A. Vermeire, and C. R. Hamilton. 1984. Hemispheric differences in split-brain monkeys viewing and responding to videotape recordings. *Behav. Neurol. Biol.* 41: 231–5.

Jason, G. W., A. Cowey, and L. Weiskrantz. 1984. Hemispheric asymmetry for a visuo-spatial task in monkeys. *Neuropsychol.* 22: 777–84.

LeMay, M., and N. Geschwind. 1975. Hemispheric differences in the brains of great apes. *Brain, Behav. Evol.* 11: 48–52.

Levy, J. 1974. Psychobiological implications of bilateral asymmetry. *In* S. J. Dimond and J. G. Beaumont (eds.) *Hemispheric Dominance and the Human Brain.* Elek Science, London, pp. 121–83.

Levy, J., C. B. Trevarthen, and R. W. Sperry. 1972. Perception of bilateral chimeric figures following hemispheric deconnexion. *Brain* 95: 61–78.

McCasland, J. S. 1983. Neuronal control of bird song production. Doctoral dissertation, Caltech, Pasadena, CA.

Moscovitch, M. 1979. Information processing and the cerebral hemispheres. *In* M. S. Gazzaniga (ed.) *Handbook of Behavioral Neurobiology, Vol. 2.* Plenum Press, New York, pp. 379–446.

Nottebohm, F. 1979. Origins and mechanisms in the establishment of cerebral dominance. *In* M. S. Gazzaniga, (ed.) *Handbook of Behavioral Neurobiology, Vol. 2.* Plenum Press, New York, pp. 295–344.

–1980. Brain pathways for vocal learning in birds: A review of the first 10 years. *Prog. Psychobiol. Physiol. Psychol.* 9: 85–124.

Overman, W. H., Jr., and R. W. Doty. 1982. Hemispheric specialization displayed by man but not macaques for analysis of faces. *Neuropsychol.* 20: 113–28.

Robinson, R. G. 1979. Differential behavioral and biochemical effects of right and left hemispheric cerebral infarction in the rat. *Science* 205: 707–10.

Rogers, L. J., and J. M. Anson. 1979. Lateralisation of function in the chicken fore-brain. *Pharmacol. Biochem. Behav.* 10: 679–86.

Sperry, R. W. 1968. Mental unity following surgical disconnection of the cerebral hemispheres. *In The Harvey Lectures,* Series 62. Academic Press, New York, pp. 293–323.

–1974. Lateral specialization in the surgically separated hemispheres. *In* F. O. Schmitt and F. G. Worden (eds.) *The Neurosciences: Third Study Program.* The MIT Press, Cambridge, pp. 5–19.

–1982. Some effects of disconnecting the cerebral hemispheres. *Science* 217: 1223–6.

Vermeire, B. A., A. L. Erdmann, and C. R. Hamilton.

1983. Laterality in monkeys for discriminating facial expression and identity. *Soc. Neurosci. Abst.* 9: 651.

Wada, J. A., R. Clarke, and A. Hamm. 1975. Cerebral hemispheric asymmetry in humans. *Arch. Neurol.* 32: 239–46.

Walker, S. F. 1980. Lateralization of functions in the vertebrate brain: A review. *Brit. J. Psychol.* 71: 329–67.

Warren, J. M. 1977. Handedness and cerebral dominance in monkeys. *In* S. Harnad, R. W. Doty, L. Goldstein, J. Jaynes, and G. Krauthamer (eds.) *Lateralization in the Nervous System.* Academic Press, New York, pp. 151–72.

–1980. Handedness and laterality in humans and other animals. *Physiol. Psychol.* 8: 351–9.

Warren, J. M., J. M. Abplanalp, and H. B. Warren. 1967. The development of handedness in cats and rhesus monkeys. In H. W. Stevenson, E. H. Hess, and H. L. Rheingold (eds.) *Early Behavior: Comparative and Developmental Approaches.* Wiley, New York, pp. 73–101.

Yeni-Komshian, G. H., and D. A. Benson. 1976. Anatomical study of cerebral asymmetry in the temporal lobe of humans, chimpanzees, and rhesus monkeys. *Science* 192: 387–9.

Zaidel, E. 1983. Disconnection syndrome as a model for laterality effects in the normal brain. *In* J. B. Hellige (ed.) *Cerebral Hemisphere Asymmetry: Method, Theory and Application.* Praeger Press, New York, pp. 45–151.

11 A corticolimbic memory path revealed through its disconnection

Mortimer Mishkin
and
Raymond R. Phillips
Laboratory of Neuropsychology
National Institutes of Mental Health

We have recently proposed that visual memory in the monkey depends on a flow of stimulus-evoked neural activity through both the visual and limbic systems (Mishkin 1982). According to our neural model, the visual perception of an object depends on the processing of its physical attributes through a succession of cortical visual areas that leads from the striate cortex through the prestriate complex to an area called TE, a cytoarchitectonic division that occupies approximately the anterior two-thirds of the inferior temporal cortex (Bonin and Bailey 1947). Stimulus-evoked neural activity as far as area TE, considered to be the final cortical visual station, is taken to represent the visual configuration of the object and to be sufficient for perception. Subsequent recognition of that object, however, is thought to require, in addition, that the object's configural representation be stored within area TE (and perhaps others of the visual areas); in this way, recognition could occur whenever the stored representation was reactivated. The circuit responsible for bringing about such storage is still unknown, but a central link in the circuit is presumed to be the temporal-lobe limbic system. Visual area TE projects heavily to this system, sending efferents directly to the amygdala and indirectly to the hippocampus via the entorhinal cortex (Van Hoesen and Pandya 1975; Herzog and Van Hoesen 1976; Turner, Mishkin, and Knapp 1980).

Functional evidence suggesting that the pathway from neocortex to limbic structures is critical for object recognition comes from studies demonstrating severe recognition losses following bilateral removal of either area TE (Mishkin and Oubre 1976) or the amygdalo-hippocampal complex (Mishkin 1978; Zola-Morgan, Squire, and Mishkin 1982). By itself, however, this evidence is inadequate to establish that the temporal-lobe limbic structures participate in recognition memory by virtue of the inputs they receive from area TE. In an attempt to gather adequate evidence, we undertook a series of crossed-lesion disconnection experiments.

More than 25 years ago, Sperry and Myers combined their split-brain technique with unilateral or reciprocal cortical ablations in attempts to localize some of the neural mechanisms of perceptuomotor coordination and memory. Sperry repeatedly discussed the advantages of this crossed-lesion disconnection strategy for untangling the contributions of different zones of the cortex in the coordination of sensory and motor processes as well as in the formation of engrams (Sperry 1958, 1961a, 1961b, 1967) (Figure 11.1A). He even broached the possibility of using this technique to investigate the contribution to learning and memory made by the limbic structures of the brain (Sperry 1961b, p. 613). The present study is thus, in large measure, an attempt to realize one of Sperry's early visions.

The crossed-lesion design was used previously (Mishkin 1958, 1966) in an experiment that tested the functional dependence of area TE on inputs that this area was thought to receive from the striate cortex via the prestriate.

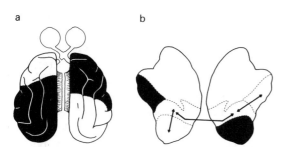

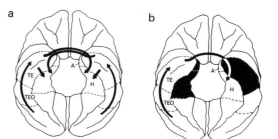

Figure 11.1. (**A**) Crossed-lesion disconnection technique applied by Sperry and Myers to the study of visuomotor coordination in the cat. (From Sperry 1961b.) (**B**) Crossed-lesion disconnection technique applied to the study of visual discrimination learning in the monkey. (From Mishkin 1966.)

Figure 11.2. (**A**) Postulated flow of visual information from cortex to limbic system in the monkey brain seen in ventral view. Information passes from the occipital lobe to the inferior temporal visual areas TEO and TE, and from there to the temporal-lobe limbic structures, including amygdala (A) and hippocampus (H). In this scheme, interaction between area TE and the limbic system is postulated to be direct both within and between the hemispheres, the interhemispheric interaction being mediated by heterotypic connections crossing the anterior commissure. This scheme was shown to be incorrect by the results obtained in animals given the crossed lesion illustrated in (**B**). (**B**) Crossed corticolimbic lesion in Experiment I. The lesion consisted of an amygdalohippocampal ablation in one hemisphere and an ablation of area TE in the other. (For convenience in comparing these schematics with the actual coronal sections through the lesions illustrated in Figure 11.4, the left temporal limbic lesion has been placed on the left in this figure, and the right temporal cortical lesion has been placed on the right.) Following the crossed lesion, visual memories could no longer be formed, suggesting that the heterotypic connection depicted here crossing the anterior commissure is either nonexistent or insufficient to sustain corticolimbic interaction.

In that earlier study, a unilateral inferior temporal resection was combined with a contralateral occipital lobectomy. If corticocortical connections were actually arranged as proposed, then such a combination of lesions should have left a transcallosal pathway through which the intact striate area of one hemisphere could transmit visual information to the intact area TE of the other (Figure 11.1B). That this postulated remaining route was now in fact essential was demonstrated by the finding that transection of the splenium of the corpus callosum completely disrupted visual discrimination performance. Indeed, the disconnection appeared to render the intact area TE totally inactive in visual learning and memory. The isolation of area TE from visual inputs by this disconnection technique was corroborated subsequently in studies demonstrating that the intact but disconnected cortical tissue could no longer be visually activated, whether the visual activation was measured electrophysiologically (Rocha-Miranda et al. 1975; Gross, Bender, and Mishkin 1977) or metabolically (Macko et al. 1982).

In the experiments to be described here, combinations of lesions analogous to those that effectively disconnected area TE from striate cortex were made in a series of attempts to disconnect the limbic system from area TE.

Experiment I: Memory failure after crossed corticolimbic lesions, without commissurotomy

In the first attempt, a unilateral amygdalohippocampal resection was combined with a contralateral ablation of area TE. Assuming the existence of a heterotypic pathway crossing from the intact area TE in one hemisphere, through the anterior commissure, to the intact limbic system in the other hemisphere (Figure 11.2A), we would expect the asymmetrical combination of lesions to yield substantial sparing of visual recognition ability (Figure 11.2B). If this ability were indeed largely spared, then the effect of adding a transection of the anterior commissure to the crossed TE-limbic lesion could be assessed in a later stage. As it turned out, however, a profound loss of visual recognition memory was produced by the crossed lesion alone, thereby preventing assessment of the effects of commissural transection and necessitating a redesign of the disconnection experiment. Since the rationale for the later attempt arose from this initial one, this initial attempt will be described in detail first.

Three experimentally naive rhesus monkeys (*Macaca mulatta*), weighing 4.0 to 5.0 kg at the time of surgery, were trained preoperatively in delayed nonmatching-to-sample (DNMS) after which they were given the crossed lesion described before (AH × TE) and then retrained. Their performance was compared with that of nine identically trained monkeys from previous studies (Mishkin and Oubre 1976, Mishkin 1978); three of these animals had received bilateral amygdalohippocampal lesions (AH), three had received bilateral TE lesions (TE), and three had served as normal controls (N).

All testing was conducted in a Wisconsin General Testing Apparatus (WGTA) inside a darkened sound-shielded room. The stimuli were presented on a stationary tray that contained a row of three food wells spaced 14 cm apart and located 12 cm in front of the monkey. The procedure, detailed previously (Mishkin and Delacour 1975, Mishkin 1978), can be summarized as follows. Preoperatively, monkeys were trained to displace an object covering one of the three wells to uncover a half-peanut reward. When an animal had learned to do this consistently with single objects, it was trained in DNMS with a set of approximately 1,000 objects that differed in size, shape, texture, and color. After each object had been used once, it was set aside and not used again until every other object had been used. Each DNMS trial consisted of an acquisition phase, in which a baited sample object was presented over the central well, followed 10 s later by a test phase. In the test phase, the sample object, now unbaited, was paired with a baited novel object, each of which was presented over a lateral well, the novel object appearing over the left or right well in a balanced order. The opaque screen was lowered for both the 10-s within-trial delay and a 30-s intertrial interval. Testing continued in this manner at the rate of 20 trials per day until the animals reached a criterion of 90 correct responses in ten consecutive blocks of ten trials each, after which all three animals were operated. Following a two-week recovery pe-

riod, the monkeys were retrained on DNMS either to criterion or for a maximum of 1,500 trials. The animals were then given a performance test (Gaffan 1974) in which, first, the delay between acquisition and test was increased in stages from the original 10 s to 30 s, 60 s, and 120 s, in blocks of 100 trials each; and then, the number, or list, of sample objects presented successively in acquisition before pairing each with a novel object in the test phase was increased in stages from the original single object to three, five, and finally ten objects, in blocks of 150 trials each.

The areas intended for surgical removal in this and the succeeding experiments are illustrated in Figure 11.3. (For reasons that will become clear later, area TE in this figure is shown divided into an anterior and a posterior portion, TEa and TEp, respectively). The lesion in this experiment AH × TE, was performed in one stage via three surgical approaches. First, the amygdaloid complex and surrounding periamygdaloid cortex, i.e., the cortex medial to the rhinal sulcus, were removed from the left hemisphere via an orbitofrontal approach. Second, the hippocampal formation and subjacent parahippocampal gyrus were removed from the same hemisphere, i.e., the left, via an occipitotemporal approach. Finally, in the right hemisphere, area TE was resected via a temporal approach after removal of the zygomatic arch. The posterior boundary of area TE, i.e., the boundary between areas TE and TEO, was defined as a line parallel and 1 cm rostral to the ascending portion of the inferior occipital sulcus.

Animals in this and the later experiments were anesthetized with ketamine hydrochloride (10 mg/kg) and sodium pentobarbital (30 mg/ kg) and secured in a head holder. With the use of aseptic microsurgical technique, the appropriate area was exposed and removed by aspiration with a small-gauge sucker. Wounds were closed in anatomical layers with silk sutures, and Bicillin was administered as a prophylactic measure. Following completion of behavioral testing, all animals were given a lethal dose of sodium pentobarbital and perfused intracardially with saline and then 10% formalin. The brains were embedded in celloidin and sectioned in the coronal plane at 25 μm,

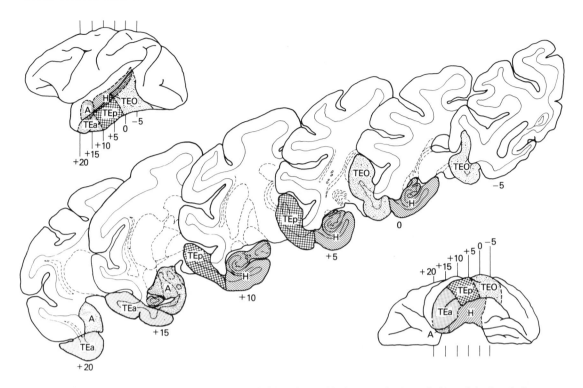

Figure 11.3. Shaded regions indicate intended locations of lesions on the lateral view of the hemisphere (top left), coronal sections (middle), and ventral view (bottom right). Numerals indicate the approximate distance in mm from the interaural plane (0). Abbreviations: A, amygdala (plus periamygdaloid cortex); H, hippocampus (plus parahippocampal gyrus); TEa, anterior portion of cortical area TE; TEp, posterior portion of cortical area TE; TEO, cortical area TEO. Cytoarchitectonic designations are those of Bonin and Bailey (1947). For clarity, the hippocampal formation in the lateral view is pictured slightly dorsal to its actual location.

and every tenth section was stained with thionin. Estimates of tissue damage were derived from planimetric measurements of the damage plotted on standard cross sections.

GROUP AH × TE

All cortical lesions in the right hemisphere were close to those planned. The limbic lesions in the left hemisphere were also generally as intended except for sparing of dorsal amygdaloid tissue, amounting to about 10–15% of the entire complex in cases 2 and 3, and of the caudal 3–4 mm of the hippocampal formation in case 3. In all hippocampectomized hemispheres, however, in this and in the succeeding experiments, there was dense gliosis within the fornix, shrunken mamillary nuclei, and degenerative changes in the lateral dorsal nucleus of the thalamus.

Unintended damage associated with the left amygdalectomy consisted of infarction in both the rostral tip of the tail of the caudate nucleus and the ventral tip of the caudal putamen in cases 1 and 2. Unintended damage associated with the left hippocampectomy consisted of injury to area TE, amounting to 24%, 11%, and 26% in cases 1, 2, and 3, respectively, and to area TEO, amounting to 40%, in case 1. This unintended cortical damage was due both to mechanical injury from lifting the inferior temporal convexity during surgery in order to gain access to the hippocampal formation and to infarcts caused by interruption of the posterior cerebral arterial supply crossing the parahippocampal gyrus. The three deviations from the intended lesions described for case 2 (amygdaloid sparing, striatal infarction, and area TE damage) can be seen in Figure 11.4, AH × TE–2, left hemisphere, levels +15, +10, and +5, respectively.

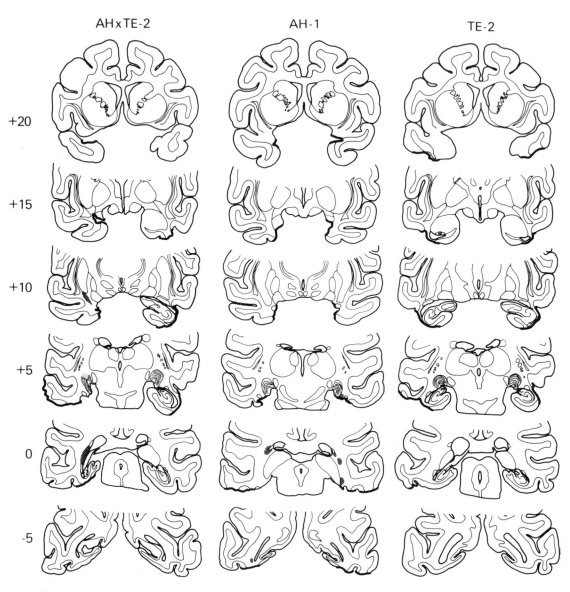

Figure 11.4. Cases from Experiment I. Coronal sections through the lesions of cases AH × TE-2, AH-1, and TE-2, at the levels shown in Figure 11.3. The heavy black line denotes border of lesion, cross-hatching denotes infarction, and shading denotes retrograde degeneration.

A small additional infarct affecting the optic radiations was present in case 2, in the area where the tail of the caudate nucleus begins its descent into the temporal lobe (level 0). This infarct, which is known to be associated with hippocampectomy (though for reasons that are unknown), led to retrograde degeneration in the anterior dorsomedial segment of the lateral geniculate body, a segment representing the lower-right peripheral visual field (level +5).

Deviations from the intended lesions in the two previously reported groups with bilateral lesions of limbic (AH) or visual (TE) tissue, whose scores served as the baseline for those of group AH × TE, are also described here for the purpose of comparison.

GROUP AH

All animals had bilateral sparing of dorsal amygdaloid tissue amounting to about 20%, 8%, and 20% of the entire complex for cases

1, 2, and 3, respectively (Figure 11.4, AH-1, level +15), but none had hippocampal sparing. Cases 2 and 3 sustained unilateral damage to the rostral tip of the tail of the caudate nucleus and the ventral tip of the caudal putamen (similar to that shown for AH × TE-2, level +10). Inadvertent cortical damage, associated with the hippocampectomy, consisted of bilateral injury to area TE, amounting to 10%, 46%, and 10% in cases 1, 2, and 3, respectively, and to area TEO amounting to 12% and 24% in cases 1 and 2, respectively (Figure 11.4, AH-1, levels 0 and −5). Finally, cases 1 and 2 sustained infarcts like that in case AH × TE-2 to the white matter surrounding the dorsal and descending parts of the tail of the caudate nucleus (Figure 11.4, AH-1, level 0), leading, as in that case, to lateral geniculate degeneration in the affected hemispheres (level +5).

GROUP TE

All area TE lesions were as intended (see Figure 11.4, case TE-2). The only exceptions were moderate amounts of unintended damage to the upper bank of the superior temporal sulcus bilaterally in case 1 and unilaterally in case 3.

Except as will be noted in connection with case AH-2, no relationship was apparent between any of the deviations from the intended lesions and test scores.

RESULTS

The scores for the crossed-lesion and comparison groups are presented in Table 11.1 and Figure 11.5. Preoperatively, the animals in group AH × TE required more trials to learn the basic DNMS task than those in the groups tested earlier, but because the task is so easy, the difference is small. Postoperatively, the animals in group AH × TE took as long or longer to relearn the basic task as the two groups of animals with bilaterally symmetrical lesions. Indeed, case AH × TE-3 performed so poorly (70%) at the end of 1,500 trials that it was given an additional 1,000 training trials, 500 with delays decreased from 10 to 5 s and another 500 with a rerun correction procedure in which the original sample remained unbaited on both sample and test re-presentations. The additional training raised the score of case 3 on the basic task to 82%. No explanation for this extreme retardation in relearning is apparent from the animal's lesion. The abnormally high relearning score of case 2 in group AH, on the other hand, is probably attributable to the extensive inadvertent damage that this animal sustained bilaterally to areas TE and TEO.

On the performance test with longer delays and lists, the scores of the animals with crossed lesions were again similar to those of the animals with bilaterally symmetrical AH and TE lesions, the three operated groups having averaged 65%, 60%, and 64%, respectively, or from 30–35% below that of the normal controls (see Figure 11.5).

In short, the overall impairment in group AH × TE, which turned out to be equal in severity to that following bilaterally symmetrical AH or TE lesions, was far greater than anticipated, preventing a direct test of the role of corticolimbic interaction in recognition memory.

Experiment II: Opening up a crossed corticolimbic pathway by sparing area TEa

The design of the crossed lesion in Experiment I was predicated on the assumption that an intact area TE in one hemisphere could directly activate the intact limbic structures in the other through heterotypic connections crossing in the anterior commissure. If the assumption of a heterotypic projection is incorrect, however, or if such connections exist but are too few in number to sustain a functionally effective corticolimbic interaction, then the AH × TE lesion would have prevented such interaction not only within each hemisphere, as planned, but also between the hemispheres. As a consequence, it would have totally disconnected the limbic system from visual input even without commissurotomy.

According to this interpretation of the impairment, utilization of an interhemispheric pathway would require that a crossed corticolimbic lesion leave at least part of area TE intact bilaterally, thereby preserving homotypic connections that are known to cross in the anterior commissure from one area TE to the other (Whitlock and Nauta 1956; Zeki 1973). Such an arrangement is illustrated in Figure 11.6A.

Table 11.1. *DNMS, Experiment I: Effect of crossed AH × TE lesions*[a]

Group	Preop T	Preop (E)	Postop T	Postop (E)	Delays 10	Delays 30	Delays 60	Delays 120	Lists 3	Lists 5	Lists 10	$\overline{X}$[b]
N[c]												
1	100	(26)	0	(0)	91	97	98	96	96	93	91	95
2	80	(28)	0	(0)	98	99	100	98	97	97	94	98
3	40	(19)	0	(0)	99	98	99	98	97	96	92	97
AH × TE[d]												
1	280	(70)	1360	(347)	90	78	76	77	74	63	53	70
2	140	(40)	1500[e]	(408)	85	74	57	63	66	57	56	62
3	240	(87)	1500[e]	(514)	82	71	66	62	66	57	53	63
AH[f]												
1	210	(49)	760	(179)	91	79	65	65	62	64	59	66
2	100	(26)	1500[e]	(429)	81	64	59	63	60	55	61	60
3	80	(22)	700	(203)	90	61	47	52	53	58	44	53
TE[g]												
1	80	(28)	1500[e]	(517)	77	78	75	66	66	62	53	67
2	20	(11)	1500[e]	(461)	88	75	61	64	57	59	57	62
3	120	(40)	1500[e]	(314)	89	64	63	72	63	63	59	64

[a] Scores are trials (and errors) to attain criterion on the basic DNMS task, requiring recognition of a single object after 10 s, final percent correct responses on this basic task, and percent correct responses on each of the six conditions of the performance test. The new experimental group is group AH × TE. The comparison scores for groups N and AH are from Mishkin (1978), and for group TE, from Mishkin and Oubre (1976).
[b] $\overline{X}$ denotes the average score on the performance test (i.e., all delays and lists excluding the 10-s delay).
[c] N is the normal control.
[d] AH × TE is the unilateral amygdalohippocampectomy combined with the contralateral resection of area TE.
[e] Failure.
[f] AH is the bilateral amygdalohippocampectomy.
[g] TE is the bilateral resection of area TE.

Perhaps only in this way could visual signals from the striate cortex in one hemisphere reach the limbic system in the other and thereby preserve the corticolimbic interaction necessary for recognition memory. If a crossed lesion of the type illustrated (Figure 11.6B) did in fact leave recognition memory substantially intact, then the effect of transecting the anterior commissure could be assessed in a later stage.

Before performing this disconnection experiment, however, it was necessary to test first whether a bilaterally symmetrical inferior temporal lesion that preserved the anterior portion of area TE would still yield a recognition impairment comparable in severity to that shown by animals in which area TE had been removed completely. Only if such a test were successful could it be concluded that the new cortical lesion, like the old, blocked the flow of visual information within the hemisphere and could thus be used in a crossed-lesion design. To perform the test, we moved the site of the lesion backward from the rostral two-thirds of inferior temporal cortex (areas TEa and TEp in Figure 11.3) to the caudal two-thirds (areas TEp and TEO in Figure 11.3). The latter site is close to the area originally designated the inferior temporal (IT) cortex in studies of visual learning (Mishkin 1966), and, for convenience, the same designation is used here.

A new group of three experimentally naive rhesus monkeys weighing 4.0 to 5.0 kg were

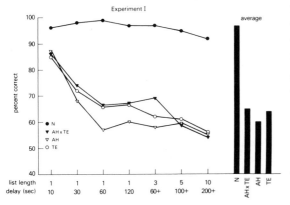

Figure 11.5. Delayed nonmatching-to-sample, Experiment I. Curves indicate average scores at progressively longer delays and list lengths. Bars indicate average scores across the performance test (i.e., all test conditions excluding the 10-s delay). Abbreviations: N, normal control; AH, bilateral amygdalohippocampectomy; TE, bilateral ablation of area TE; AH × TE, unilateral amygdalohippocampectomy combined with contralateral ablation of area TE.

trained preoperatively in the same way as those in the first experiment, given bilaterally symmetrical inferior temporal lesions as will be described, and then retrained. Their performance was compared with that of the group of animals in the first experiment with bilaterally symmetrical lesions of area TE, as well as with a group of identically trained animals from a previous study (Mishkin and Oubre 1976) that were given bilaterally symmetrical lesions of area TEO.

The surgical procedures were the same as before, except that the more posterior placement of the temporal neocortical lesion obviated the need for removal of the zygomatic arch. The cortical removal included the anterior bank of the ascending portion of the inferior occipital sulcus and extended to a line 2 cm rostral and parallel to this sulcus. This removal encompassed area TEO and approximately the posterior half of area TE (TEp).

GROUP IT (TEₚ + TEO)

Examination of the histological material indicated that the lesions were essentially complete. In some hemispheres, removal of area TEO led to infarction of the optic radiations subjacent to the cortex in the depths of the superior temporal sulcus. Such infarction occurred unilaterally in case 2 and bilaterally in case 3, resulting in a small amount of retrograde degeneration in the lateral part of the lateral geniculate nucleus of those hemispheres (see Figure 11.7, IT-3, level +5).

GROUP TEO

All area TEO lesions were complete. As with removal of area IT, however, removal of area TEO led to infarction in the optic radiations in some hemispheres, with resultant minor degeneration in the lateral part of the lateral geniculate nucleus in the affected hemispheres. Such damage occurred bilaterally in cases 2 and 3 (see Figure 11.7, TEO-3, section +5).

RESULTS

All animals in Group IT, like all those in Group TE, failed to reach criterion within the 1,500-trial training limit (Table 11.2). Because the average final score for Group IT was so low, the animals were given additional training as follows. Case 1 received an additional 340 trials, the first 240 with shortened (3–5-s) delays and the last 100 with the original (10-s) delay, raising the performance of this animal from 81% to 90%. Case 2 received 500 additional trials with the shortened delays, but then, because this animal's performance did not improve appreciably, the correction procedure described in Experiment I was introduced for another 500 trials, raising case 2's score from 71% to 80%, a level deemed acceptable for evaluation on the performance test. Case 3, however, failed to achieve even the 80% level with additional training and was not tested further. The additional training thus yielded two animals with an average final score of 85%, matching that of the three animals in group TE.

On the performance test, groups TE and IT obtained similar averages overall (64% and 69%, respectively, see Figure 11.8), but their performance profiles differed. The scores of group TE fell abruptly as soon as the delay was increased and then continued a gradual decline as the lists were lengthened. By contrast, group

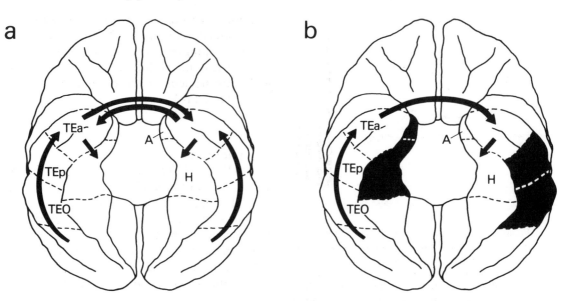

Figure 11.6. (**A**) Revised scheme of corticolimbic visual information flow in the monkey. Here the interaction between area TE in one hemisphere and the limbic system in the other is postulated to be only indirect, being mediated by homotypic connections crossing in the anterior commissure from one area TE to the other. Compare with Figure 11.2A. (**B**) Crossed corticolimbic lesion in Experiment III. The lesion consisted of an amygdalohippocampal ablation in one hemisphere combined with an ablation of IT cortex (i.e., areas TEp + TEO) in the other. Bilateral ablation of IT cortex in Experiment II was found to block memory formation (and, hence, to block intrahemispheric corticolimbic interaction), and the crossed lesion in Experiment III was found to spare memory formation substantially (and, hence, to spare crossed corticolimbic interaction). Thus, the results of Experiments II and III were consistent with the revised scheme shown here and led to evaluation of the effects of anterior commissurotomy. Compare with Figure 11.2B.

IT's scores remained relatively high, exceeding those of group TE under conditions of increasing delay, but then dropped sharply with the lengthened lists (Figure 11.8). A performance profile similar to that of group IT was seen originally in the animals given lesions of area TEO alone. The sharp intensification of impairment on lengthened lists after TEO lesions, illustrated in Figure 11.8, was attributed to the disorder in shape perception that these lesions are thought to induce (Iwai and Mishkin 1968; Yaginuma, Niihara, and Iwai 1982), and to the consequent loss of a visual dimension needed for encoding long lists (Mishkin 1982); the same intensification of deficit in the animals with IT lesions presumably reflects the same disorder and loss. In addition, however, group IT showed a greater impairment overall than group TEO, presumably reflecting a greater disturbance in memory caused by extension of the lesion to include area TEp. Thus, although

the combined removal of areas TEO and TEp did not yield as severe an impairment as the original TE removals on performance at long delays (see Figure 11.8), and therefore presumably did not result in a total disconnection of area TEa from visual input, the impairment and, hence, the disconnection were sufficiently severe to warrant a second crossed-lesion disconnection attempt.

Experiment III: Memory failure after crossed corticolimbic lesions, but only if combined with anterior commissurotomy

In the final experiment, removal of both the amygdala and hippocampus in one hemisphere was combined with removal of the IT cortex in the other. The supposition was that, like the original cortical removal, the relocated cortical removal would largely prevent direct transmission of visual information to the intact

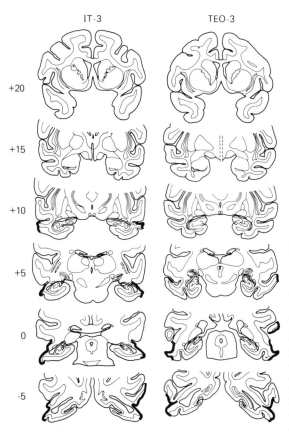

Figure 11.7. Cases from Experiment II. Coronal sections through the lesions of cases IT-3 and TEO-3. Conventions as in Figure 11.4.

limbic structures within that hemisphere. Unlike the original removal, however, the new one should allow information to reach these same intact limbic structures through the homotypic connections of area TEa that cross in the anterior commissure (Figure 11.6B). If so, transection of the anterior commissure in an animal with crossed lesions should disconnect this final corticolimbic pathway.

Six experimentally naive rhesus monkeys weighing 4.0 to 5.0 kg were tested preoperatively as in the previous experiments, after which three were given unilateral amygdalohippocampal removals plus contralateral IT ablations (AH × IT), and the other three were given those same crossed lesions combined with transection of the anterior commissure (AH × IT + AC).

As before, all the lesions were performed in one stage via separate surgical approaches. The AH removal in the left hemisphere was identical to that described in Experiment I (i.e., A + H in Figure 11.3), and the IT removal in the right hemisphere was identical to that described in Experiment II (i.e., TEp + TEO in Figure 11.3). For the commissurotomy, dorsomedial bone and dural flaps were made over the left hemisphere, and a segment of the corpus callosum was then split along the midline in order to expose that portion of the third ventricle, rostral to the mass intermedia, in which the anterior commissure can be seen to cross between the hemispheres. After the anterior commissure was visualized and transected, the dural flap was repositioned but not sewn, the bone flap was replaced and secured to the skull, and the wound was closed.

GROUP AH × IT

Deviations from the intended lesions were as follows. In case AH × IT-3, the left amygdalectomy led to an infarction in both the rostral tip of the tail of the caudate nucleus and the ventral tip of the caudal putamen, and the left hippocampectomy resulted in unintended injury to IT cortex (TEO and TEp), amounting to 15% of the area. These deviations are similar to those illustrated in Figure 11.9 for case AH × IT + AC-1, left hemisphere, levels +10, +5, and 0. In case AH × IT-2, the cortical lesion on the right led to a small infarction in the ventral portion of the optic radiations, with resultant degeneration of the lateral portion of

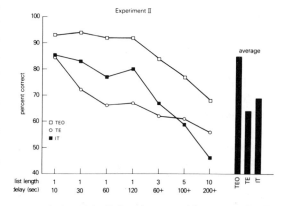

Figure 11.8. Delayed nonmatching-to-sample, Experiment II. Conventions as in Figure 11.5. Abbreviations: IT, bilateral ablation of area IT (i.e., TEp + TEO in Figure 11.3); TEO, bilateral ablation of area TEO; TE, bilateral ablation of area TE (from Experiment I).

Table 11.2. *DNMS, Experiment II: Effect of bilateral IT lesions*[a]

Group	Preop T	(E)	Postop T	(E)	Delays 10	30	60	120	Lists 3	5	10	$\overline{\text{X}}$
IT[b]												
1	60	(31)	1500[e]	(390)	90	83	76	77	77	59	45	70
2	120	(33)	1500[e]	(561)	80	82	77	82	57	59	47	67
3	240	(66)	1500[e]	(464)	77	—	—	—	—	—	—	—
TE[c]												
1	80	(28)	1500[e]	(517)	77	78	75	66	66	62	53	67
2	20	(11)	1500[e]	(461)	88	75	61	64	57	59	57	62
3	120	(40)	1500[e]	(314)	89	64	63	72	63	63	59	64
TEO[d]												
1	160	(36)	20	(5)	93	91	92	94	85	82	76	87
2	140	(49)	40	(28)	92	96	93	89	85	74	65	84
3	80	(22)	160	(35)	93	96	91	93	83	75	64	84

[a] Scores, as in Table 11.1, attained by animals with bilaterally symmetrical lesions of area IT. The comparison scores for group TE (see Experiment I) are from Mishkin and Oubre (1976) and for group TEO, from Mishkin (1982). Following postoperative failure in 1,500 trials, monkeys in group IT were given additional training as follows: case 1, 340 trials; cases 2 and 3, 500 trials (see text).
[b] IT is the bilateral resection of area IT.
[c] TE is the bilateral resection of area TE.
[d] TEO is the bilateral resection of area TEO.
[e] Failure.

the lateral geniculate body (see Figure 11.9, AH × IT-2, right hemisphere, levels −5 and +5, respectively).

GROUP AH × IT + AC

All lesions in cases 2 and 3 of this group were close to those planned. In particular, as illustrated in Figure 11.9, the anterior commissurotomy was complete in these cases, as it was in case 1. In case 1, however, the left limbic removal led to infarction in the ventral part of the tail of the caudate nucleus, and also to IT damage amounting to 10% of the area. In addition, there was sparing of the caudal 2–3 mm of the hippocampal formation. These deviations in the left hemisphere, viz., striatal infarction, IT damage, and hippocampal sparing, are illustrated in Figure 11.9, AH × IT + AC-1, left hemisphere, levels +10, +5, and 0, respectively. In the right hemisphere of this same case, the cortical lesion was incomplete, with moderate sparing (3–6 mm along the rostro-caudal dimension) in the anterior part of area IT. At the same time, this lesion led to an in-

farction in the ventral portion of the optic radiations comparable to that seen in AH × IT-2, resulting in minor degeneration of the lateral portion of the lateral geniculate body. These deviations on the right in case 1, namely, IT sparing, geniculate degeneration, and optic radiation infarction, are shown in Figure 11.9, AH × IT + AC-1, right hemisphere, levels +10, +5, and −5, respectively.

As will be indicated, the deviations from the intended lesions that appeared to be related to test scores were the damage to IT cortex on the left in case AH × IT-3 and the sparing of IT cortex on the right in case AH × IT + AC-1.

RESULTS

The scores for groups AH × IT and AH × IT + AC are presented in Table 11.3 and Figure 11.10. The animals with crossed lesions alone, i.e. with commissures intact, relearned the basic task relatively quickly. The poor performance of case 3 in this group was probably due to the inadvertent damage this animal sustained to area IT on the left. On the perfor-

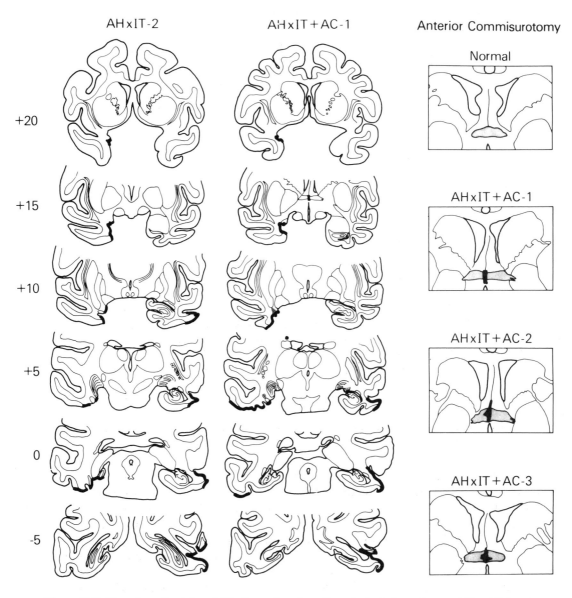

Figure 11.9. Cases from Experiment III. Coronal sections through the lesions of cases AH × IT-2 and AH × IT + AC-1. Conventions as in Figure 11.4. Right-hand column shows anterior commissure at its crossing (stippled) in a normal brain and in the three experimental cases in which it was transected (denoted in black).

mance test, this group attained an average of better than 80% correct responses, a level approximately midway between the scores of the normal controls and the scores of the animals with either bilateral TE, bilateral AH, or AH × TE lesions (see Figure 11.10). Thus, although the crossed AH × IT lesion produced significant impairment in recognition memory, presumably reflecting the considerable damage

to critical structures that this lesion entailed, there was also clearly substantial sparing of recognition memory. The sparing was sufficient to test the effects of adding a commissurotomy.

By contrast to the animals with the crossed lesions alone, two animals in the group with the added anterior commissurotomy failed to reach criterion within the 1,500-trial training limit. The final average for AH × IT + AC-

Table 11.3. *DNMS, Experiment III: Effects of crossed AH × IT lesions, with and without anterior commissurotomy (AC)*[a]

Group	Preop		Postop		Delays				Lists			
	T	(E)	T	(E)	10	30	60	120	3	5	10	X̄
AH × IT[b]												
1	180	(59)	120	(27)	91	97	94	88	83	75	63	83
2	140	(53)	120	(29)	90	92	87	90	75	81	73	83
3	140	(29)	640	(178)	93	84	78	83	81	64	56	75
AH × IT + AC[c]												
1	120	(42)	340	(116)	90	81	77	73	73	63	53	70
2	120	(40)	1500[e]	(341)	81	82	71	66	64	56	49	65
3	200	(45)	1500[e]	(474)	79	63	70	70	65	56	59	64
AH × TE[d]												
1	280	(70)	1360	(347)	90	78	76	77	74	63	53	70
2	140	(40)	1500[e]	(408)	85	74	57	63	66	57	56	62
3	240	(87)	1500[e]	(514)	82	71	66	62	66	57	53	63

[a]Scores, as in Table 11.1, attained by animals with crossed limbic and cortical lesions (groups AH × IT, AH × IT + AC, and AH × TE). Following postoperative failure in 1,500 trials, case 3 of group AH × IT + AC was given 700 additional trials (see text).

[b]AH × IT is the unilateral amygdalohippocampectomy combined with a contralateral resection of area IT.

[c]AH × IT + AC is the unilateral amygdalohippocampectomy combined with a contralateral resection of area IT and transection of the anterior commissure.

[d]AH × TE is the unilateral amygdalohippocampectomy combined with a contralateral resection of area TE (from Experiment I).

[e]Failure.

3 was so low that it was given an additional 700 trials, the first 200 with the original (10-s) delay and the last 500 with both shortened (3–5-s) delays and the rerun correction procedure, which raised the performance of this animal on the basic task from 69% to 79%. The relatively rapid relearning at 10 s shown by the third animal in this group, case AH × IT + AC-1, could well have been due to the moderate sparing in this animal of the anterior portion of area IT on the right. On the performance test, group AH × IT + AC performed at about the same level (66%) as the animals with bilaterally symmetrical lesions of either visual cortex (TE) or limbic structures (AH) (see Figure 11.10). The addition of the anterior commissurotomy thus completed the disconnection of the limbic system from the visual system.

Comment

The results of the final experiment support the proposal that the limbic system's participation in visual memory depends on its receipt of visual input from area TE. Apparently, area TE communicates with the contralateral limbic system primarily, if not exclusively, through interhemispheric corticocortical connections. Consequently, the limbic system of one side can receive input from the visual system of the other only if a portion of area TE is spared bilaterally. When this interhemispheric pathway is the only one left to mediate visuolimbic interaction, then memory formation in vision can be prevented simply by severing the anterior commissure.

The major value of this demonstration is the implication to be drawn from it that the same dependency of limbic function on visual input that was found to exist between the hemispheres also exists within the hemispheres. Because the intrahemispheric corticolimbic connections are nearly inaccessible, a direct test of their function seems prohibitively difficult. Under such circumstances, a crossed-lesion dis-

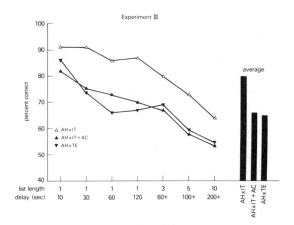

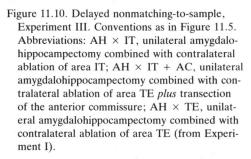

Figure 11.10. Delayed nonmatching-to-sample, Experiment III. Conventions as in Figure 11.5. Abbreviations: AH × IT, unilateral amygdalohippocampectomy combined with contralateral ablation of area IT; AH × IT + AC, unilateral amygdalohippocampectomy combined with contralateral ablation of area TE *plus* transection of the anterior commissure; AH × TE, unilateral amygdalohippocampectomy combined with contralateral ablation of area TE (from Experiment I).

connection experiment appears to offer the best alternative strategy.

If our interpretation of the results of the final experiment is correct, then the results of the initial experiment are accounted for as well. That is, as we proposed for that experiment, complete removal of area TE in one hemisphere combined with ablation of the limbic structures in the other caused a memory failure even without commissurotomy because the crossed lesion alone in this case prevented visuolimbic interaction both within and between the hemispheres simultaneously.

One additional implication of these results deserves comment. Although the need for corticolimbic interaction was demonstrated here only for visual recognition memory, it seems likely that such interaction will turn out to be essential for recognition memory in modalities other than vision, as well as for forms of memory other than recognition. The limbic structures of the temporal lobe have already been found to be critical for tactual as well as for visual memory (Murray and Mishkin 1984), and for a wide variety of associative memories, such as object-reward association (Spiegler and Mishkin 1979, 1981; Phillips and Mishkin

1984), object-place association (Parkinson and Mishkin 1982), and cross-modal association between vision and touch (Murray and Mishkin 1985). Presumably, in each of these forms of memory, just as in visual recognition, the participation of the limbic system will prove to depend on the input it receives from the relevant sensory-processing systems.

But while a functional interaction between sensory and limbic systems may be relatively easy to document further through additional applications of the crossed-lesion disconnection technique, this will still leave unexplained the neural consequences of the interaction. Is the neural product of sensory-limbic interaction the storage of stimulus representations in the sensory-processing systems, as our model proposes, or does the storage occur elsewhere? Indeed, is a storage of stimulus representations even the right initial conception? Clearly, the demonstration that the path to memory requires corticolimbic interaction still leaves us far from our goal.

Acknowledgments

We thank Mr. Leon Dorsey and Mr. Linton Stokes for their invaluable assistance.

References

Bonin, G., and P. Bailey. 1947. *The Neocortex of Macaca mulatta.* University of Illinois Press, Urbana.

Gaffan, D. 1974. Recognition impaired and association intact in the memory of monkeys after transection of the fornix. *J. Comp. Physiol. Psychol.* 86: 1100–9.

Gross, C. G., D. B. Bender, and M. Mishkin. 1977. Contributions of the corpus callosum and the anterior commissure to visual activation of inferior temporal neurons. *Brain Res.* 131: 227–39.

Herzog, A. G., and G. W. Van Hoesen. 1976. Temporal neocortical afferent connections to the amygdala in the rhesus monkey. *Brain Res.* 115: 57–69.

Iwai, E., and M. Mishkin. 1968. Two visual foci in the temporal lobe of monkeys. *In* N. Yoshii and N. A. Buchwald, (eds.) *Neurophysiological Basis of Learning and Behavior.* Osaka University Press, Osaka, Japan, pp. 1–11.

Macko, K. A., C. D. Jarvis, C. Kennedy, M. Miyaoka,

M. Shinohara, L. Sokoloff, and M. Mishkin. 1982. Mapping the primate visual system with 2-^{14}C deoxyglucose. *Science* 218: 394–7.

Mishkin, M. 1958. Visual discrimination impairment after cutting cortical connections between the inferotemporal and striate areas in monkeys. *Am. Psychol.* 13: 414.

–1966. Visual mechanisms beyond the striate cortex. *In* R. Russell (ed.) *Frontiers in Physiological Psychology.* Academic Press, New York, pp. 93–119.

–1978. Memory in monkeys severely impaired by combined but not separate removal of amygdala and hippocampus. *Nature (London)* 273: 297–8.

–1982. A memory system in the monkey. *Phil. Trans. Roy. Soc. London, Ser. B.* 298: 85–95.

Mishkin, M., and J. Delacour. 1975. An analysis of short-term visual memory in the monkey. *J. Exp. Psychol.: Animal Behav. Proc.* 1: 326–34.

Mishkin, M., and J. L. Oubre. 1976. Dissociation of deficits on visual memory tasks after inferior temporal and amygdala lesions in monkeys. *Soc. Neurosci. Abst.* 2: 1127.

Murray, E. A., and M. Mishkin. 1984. Severe tactual as well as visual memory deficits follow combined removal of the amygdala and hippocampus in monkeys. *J. Neurosci.* 4: 2565–80.

–1985. Amygdalectomy impairs crossmodal association in monkeys. *Science* 228: 604–6.

Parkinson, J. K., and M. Mishkin. 1982. A selective mnemonic role for the hippocampus in monkeys: Memory for the location of objects. *Soc. Neurosci. Abst.* 8: 23.

Phillips, R. R., and M. Mishkin. 1984. Further evidence of a severe impairment in associative memory following combined amygdalo-hippocampal lesions in monkeys. *Soc. Neurosci. Abst.* 10: 136.

Rocha-Miranda, C. E., D. B. Bender, C. G. Gross, and M. Mishkin. 1975. Visual activation of neruons in inferotemporal cortex depends on striate cortex and forebrain commissures. *J. Neurophysiol.* 38: 475–91.

Spiegler B. J., and M. Mishkin. 1979. Associative memory severely impaired by combined amygdalo-hippocampal removals. *Soc. Neurosci. Abst.* 5: 323.

–1981. Evidence for sequential participation of inferotemporal cortex and amygdala in the acquisition of stimulus-reward associations. *Behav. Brain Res.* 3: 303–17.

Sperry, R. W. 1958. Physiological plasticity and brain circuit theory. *In* H. F. Harlow and C. N. Woolsey (eds.) *Biological and Biochemical Bases of Behavior.* University of Wisconsin Press, Madison, pp. 401–21.

–1961a. Cerebral organization and behavior. *Science* 133: 1749–57.

–1961b. Some developments in brain lesion studies of learning. *Fed. Proc.* 20: 609–16.

–1967. Split-brain approach to learning problems. *In* G. C. Quarton, T. Melnechuk, and F. O. Schmitt (eds.) *The Neurosciences: A Study Program.* Rockefeller University Press, New York, pp. 714–22.

Turner, B. H., M. Mishkin, and M. E. Knapp. 1980. Organization of the amygdalopetal projections from modality-specific cortical association area in the monkey. *J. Comp. Neurol.* 191: 515–43.

Van Hoesen, G. W., and D. N. Pandya. 1975. Some connections of the entorhinal (area 28) and perirhinal (area 35) cortices of the rhesus monkey. I. Temporal lobe afferents. *Brain Res.* 95: 1–24.

Whitlock, D. G., and W. J. H. Nauta. 1956. Subcortical projections from the temporal neocortex in *Macaca mulatta. J. Comp. Neurol.* 106: 183–212.

Yaginuma, S. Y., T. Niihara, and E. Iwai. 1982. Further evidence on elevated discrimination limens for reduced patterns in monkeys with inferotemporal lesions. *Neuropsychol.* 20: 21–32.

Zeki, S. M. 1973. Comparison of the cortical degeneration in the visual regions of the temporal lobe of the monkey following section of the anterior commissure and the splenium. *J. Comp. Neurol.* 148: 167–76.

Zola-Morgan, S., L. R. Squire, and M. Mishkin. 1982. The neuroanatomy of amnesia: Amygdala-hippocampus versus temporal stem. *Science* 218: 1337–9.

PART III: Cerebral hemispheres and human consciousness

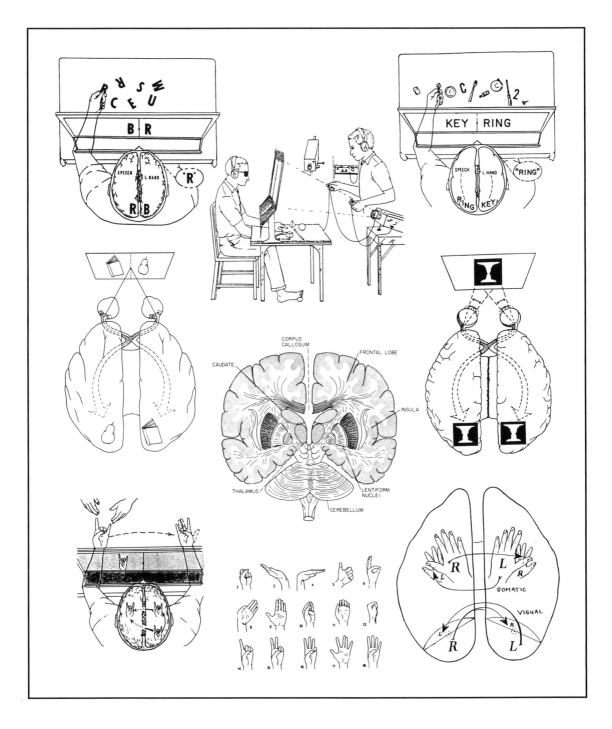

Roger Sperry's Nobel Prize recognized his contribution to understanding of "the organization and functioning of the brain." Special mention was made of his studies with commissurotomy subjects, which demonstrated the powers of consciousness and thinking of the right cerebral hemisphere, previously neglected. Some thought, at the time, that Sperry should have received the prize years before, in recognition of his pathfinding work in neuroembryology. But the imagination of the world – brain scientists, psychologists, neurologists, and lay people – was, naturally, dazzled by the implications of experiments with double consciousness reported by the Caltech group in the 1960s.

The same adventurous "problem-oriented" zeal that led to rapid recognition of the split-brain research with cats and monkeys, quickly gained Roger Sperry, Joseph Bogen, and Michael Gazzaniga fame in the exclusive world of medical neurology and neuropsychology. A definitive description of the commissurotomy syndrome was published in the *Handbook of Clinical Neurology* in 1969. Right up to the present time, the select patient group operated on in Los Angeles by Philip Vogel and Joseph Bogen, and largely studied in Roger Sperry's small laboratory in Caltech, has yielded reports that have extended our comprehension of hemispheric systems for consciousness, thinking, language, and the performance of effective actions. Some highly original attempts have also been made to explore self-knowledge, emotionality, and sociopolitical awareness in subjects with divided neocortex.

Operations of complete commissurotomy, dividing the human brain to prevent spread of epilepsy, and of partial commissure divisions, also undertaken for this purpose or to gain access to tumors, etc., have been performed in many parts of the world. There are reports from other laboratories that confirm and extend the Caltech investigations.

Controversies, about the level of consciousness and language comprehension of the right hemisphere, the significance on reality of divided consciousness, the self-awareness, the basis for coordination of action in the whole body, and so on, have sharpened the terms by which such questions are discussed. No one had been able to encompass such a range of questions as Roger Sperry has asked. We who have accompanied him in the effort recognize this even while we attempt to push questions in new directions, for ourselves.

Joseph Bogen has been a convivial creative member of the team from the start, commissurotomy patients in modern times being a sort of brainchild of his. He has written challenging papers on their mental processes and behavior immediately after the operation, and explored philosophical questions, including indications of duality in ordinary brains, with commissures intact. His vitality and wit are clear in his chapter.

Jerre Levy came to Caltech for her PhD research with an excellent background in psychobiology, biologically rich and psychologically sophisticated. She is to be credited for some of the most ingenious demonstrations of right-hemisphere intelligence and has continued with uninterrupted energy and enthusiasm to lead the field of cognitive neuropsychology in interesting profitable directions. Her chapter discusses evidence for lateralized activation of the neocortex and the importance such a factor of subcortical origin has for explaining both effects of lesions and the individual differences in cognitive function, which are so characteristic of people, and so hard to explain in terms of differences in experience. Brainstem activation stands guard, like Cerebus, deciding what form of experience will enter consciousness and become part of knowledge.

Harold Gordon was the graduate student with interest in how commissurotomy patients appreciated music and odors. Having since measured the visuospatial skills of fighter and helicopter pilots in Israel, he has developed a practical test for obtaining a quick way to measure "hemisphericity" in ordinary men, women, and children – the degree they prefer to use one or other of the hemispheres, each with its characteristic cognitive style. He carries the Sperry mark of a thorough interest in the biology of mental activity and discusses effects of sex hormones on development of lateral preferences and cognitive style as measured by his cognitive laterality battery.

Dahlia Zaidel not only assisted Roger with testing of form perception and memory in the commissurotomy patients over a nine-year period, but also has developed an approach of her own to the structure of memories in the two halves of the human brain. In her chapter, she asks about the way information from vision is handled in two cortices that build up memories in different ways.

Oliver Zangwill and Maria Wyke turn our attention to the illustrious past of neuropsychology, when neurologists were trying to understand the first accurate information about how peoples' awareness and behavior were changed when different pieces of the cortical mantle were injured. Oliver, with Henry Hécaen and Enio DeRenze, pioneered psychological tests that were capable of showing the special visuospatial abilities of the right hemisphere. In this work, they were following Hughlings Jackson. The case histories of this great neurologist help us have a proper perspective, and humility, about our present efforts to give mechanistic interpretation to hemispheric differences in the age of cognitive psychology.

Brenda Milner, Laughlin Taylor, and Marilyn Jones-Gotman discuss findings of Milner and Taylor in a series of tests with commissurotomy patients carried out at Caltech over a number of years in the 1960s and 1970s. Their first experiment was designed to clarify how auditory perception was distributed in left and right temporal lobes for spoken digits presented with dichotic conflict. Then they measured right-hemisphere specialization for tactual form matching with varying delays. Here they also report, for the first time, experiments on the ability of commissurotomy patients to remember arbitrary associations between words that identify items that either are, or are not, easily imaged visually. Commissurotomy patients were remarkably poor at freely recalling associations between words and images. This is important evidence that the corpus callosum and anterior commissure normally help the hemispheres collaborate in focusing consciousness and clarifying memories.

Eran Zaidel discusses the history of another great puzzle – what contribution does a visual right hemisphere make to a linguistic visual task such as reading? Eran's studies of language in the disconnected right hemisphere have helped explain why the hemispheres are different. He has shown that both in adult functioning and in development, they collaborate, performing complementary functions to constitute a more powerful unity. We can only understand the workings of a lesioned brain or one with the commissures sectioned, by grasping that the intact brain has two halves that are mutually involved in all high levels of psychological functioning.

Larry Benowitz and his colleagues at the Harvard Medical School and McLean Hospital bring a fresh, not so "rational," description of right-hemisphere functioning. By examination of emotional processes they bring to light this hemisphere's special capacity for creating and evaluating configurations, estimating their particular state of wholeness. Benowitz carried out experiments on the biochemistry of chick memory at Caltech. He is another Sperry product, not afraid to move from the "biological" to the "mental," and back.

Colwyn Trevarthen has spent much of the past 20 years studying the communications of infants and toddlers, attempting to see human mental biology go through its first steps. But he has not lost the interest in split-brain dynamics he gained from experiments for a PhD at Caltech, on eye–hand coordination and visual learning in chiasm-callosum sectioned monkeys, and from collaboration with Jerre Levy and Sperry on tests of hemispheric functioning with dual stimulation. His chapter attempts to fit ideas about how the hemispheres grow, together but in different ways, into a theory of how knowledge is transmitted from older brains to younger brains. He proposes that new findings on the regulation of learning by subcortical limbic and reticular systems may help bridge the gap between babies and split brains.

Bob Nebes made a crucial contribution to the work on right-hemisphere perception of form and size while he was a graduate student with Sperry. Since then, he has become an expert on the effects of aging on brain activities, the other end of development. He discusses the evidence and the theories concerning the possibility that age affects the hemispheres differently, or at different rates.

Our final chapter is by Roger himself. This paper was first published in 1977, after he had spent ten years working over his ideas on the nature of consciousness and its regulatory role in brain function. We feel it to be an elegant bridge from the laboratory tests of divided consciousness to the more philosophical arguments that draw on a wider stream of evidence. We hope it will convince any sceptics of the scientific soundness of the basis for Roger's bold and original interpretations of the nature of human cognition.

12 Partial hemispheric independence with the neocommissures intact

Joseph E. Bogen
Department of Neurological Surgery
School of Medicine
University of Southern California

The great commissure forms at once a bond of union and a band of separation.

A. L. Wigan, 1844, p. 115

Roger Sperry was awarded the Nobel Prize in 1981 for his work with human split-brain subjects, but the implications of this work have yet to be fully appreciated. The principle of hemispheric specialization, illuminated by him, has been widely recognized, which has stimulated an immense amount of research. But the principle of cerebral duality, first demonstrated in cats and monkeys and then confirmed in humans, has so far had insufficient recognition; the relevant experimental results have been often incidental to other investigations. The main burden of this chapter is to assemble some of these heretofore scattered results in order to encourage a more explicit and systematic study of the potential independence of the hemispheres. This chapter concerns three assertions:

The first is that one cerebral hemisphere is enough, in Wigan's words, "...for the emotion, sentiments and faculties which we call in the aggregate, mind" (Wigan 1844, p. 271). As is well known, the best evidence for that comes from hemispherectomy.

The second assertion is that with two hemispheres, it is possible to have two minds. The best evidence, or at least the most striking (there is quite a lot of other evidence), is from the human split brain, where the two disconnected minds are revealed to be so different (Bogen 1969).

The third assertion is that this duality of mind can be present in the intact brain. I will present some of the evidence and some of the arguments for these three statements – but mainly for the third, because the first two are by now fairly well accepted.

It was about 1820 when an English physician, Arthur Ladbroke Wigan, lost an acquaintance from a relatively sudden death (possibly a heart attack). He went to the postmortem to pay his last respects and, when the head was opened, he and the others present were astonished to see that one hemisphere was completely missing. He was not only astonished, but he also had the wits to recognize that this was meaningful, so he looked around for other cases and he found a few. About 20 years later, he published a book (Wigan 1844) in which he claimed not only that one hemisphere is enough for a mind, but that those of us who have two hemispheres can have two minds. There have been naturally occurring resorptions of a single hemisphere observed since, but the best evidence is from hemispherectomy – first of all in animals. I will not go over all of the experimental observations, having reviewed most of them previously (Bogen 1974). But I would like to quote again what Wenzel, Tschirgi, and Taylor (1962) said about their experience with hemispherectomized kittens. In spite of removal of nearly one-half of the brain, "the behavioral loss is extremely small, or even undetectable."

Perhaps even more impressive than behavioral descriptions are formal quantitative investigations by physiological psychologists. There have been many such studies. One that is especially notable, because of the many years it continued, is the research of Kruper, Patton, and Koskoff (1971). Patton (1961) observed that the hemicerebrectomized monkey can achieve a level of performance on a complex learning task that equals that of the normal animal, although it may take a little longer. Ten years later they said:

> ... showing clear learning deficits when comparing the performance of these animals to the performance of normal monkeys continues to be a compelling challenge (Kruper et al. 1971, p. 175).

Of course, the quality of mind that the residual hemisphere affords depends on the quality of the residual hemisphere and how much damage it has had. If the "mind" includes (at least) the abilities to perceive, discriminate, compare with previously stored information, consider alternative actions, choose among them, and then to act, it is doubtful that any smaller subdivision of a mammalian brain than one hemisphere can support a mind. That is, although these minimal criteria for the "mind" do not distinguish what a hemisphere can do from what the best electronic artefacts can do, it does eliminate any favorite gyrus, cerebral lobe, or cord segment from consideration as the seat of a "mind." By contrast, one hemisphere properly connected to the brainstem *can* support a mind, by these or any other familiar criteria. Not only neuroscientists but by now many laypersons are familiar with these facts. For example, C. E. Marks (a philosopher at the University of Washington in Seattle) wrote that no one nowadays doubts Wigan's original point that one hemisphere is enough for a mind "comfortably characterizable as human" (Marks 1980).

If one hemisphere can be enough for a mind, can two hemispheres be enough for two minds? When they are in separate heads, the answer is clearly "yes." Two people, each with a hemispherectomy, have two minds. But what if the two hemispheres are in the same head?

Most readers already have some familiarity with the split-brain phenomena. Worth emphasizing is that the concept of a duality of mind is not only based on the humans who have had a split-brain operation. The human cases may be more dramatic, but the duality of mind when the brain is split was established before there were any human cases, in hundreds of experiments, by many dozens of investigators, in the cat and monkey (Bogen 1977). This is what Roger Sperry said about the human subjects in 1974:

> Although some authorities have been reluctant to credit the disconnected minor hemisphere even with being conscious, it is our own interpretation – based on a large number and variety of nonverbal tests – that the other hemisphere is indeed a conscious system in its own right – perceiving, thinking, remembering, reasoning, willing, and emoting – all at a characteristically human level, and that both the left and right hemispheres may be conscious simultaneously in different, even mutually conflicting, mental experiences that run along in parallel (Sperry 1974, p. 11).

We come now to the third point. What about two hemispheres inside one head when the two hemispheres are not anatomically disconnected? To what extent does the "duality of mind," easily demonstrable in the split brain, also obtain in the normal brain? This is a principal question affecting most of the inferences, regarding human nature, from the split-brain data. Indeed, hemispheric specialization would be of little more interest than the many other differences in cortical representation of function if it were not for its cooccurrence with a significant degree of hemispheric independence.

To have any duality of mind, hemispherically based, there must be at least some circumstances in which memory traces are unihemispheric and are not communicated to the other hemisphere, even with commissures intact. This question was considered by Doty, Negrão, and Yamaga (1973) when they went so far as to suggest that the corpus callosum may actually act to restrict memory storage to one or the other hemisphere. I shall not take so strong a position here, being content only to claim that the neocommissures cannot effect a complete unification of information processing in the two hemispheres. Nor shall I join Puccetti (1973, 1981) in his view that each of us has two *persons* in one head.

There are two aspects to my claim: first, that *without* the neocommissures, there are nevertheless many effectively unifying mechanisms, and second, that *even with these and the neocommissures,* unification is incomplete, resulting in mental duality, hemispherically based. We consider first some of the extracallosal sources of unification.

Some extracallosal unifying mechanisms

That there must be *some* synchronization (with or without the commissures) is clear enough. Unlike two hemispheres in two different heads, the disconnected hemispheres are (and have been) in the same place at the same time, have the same circulating environment (blood and CSF), and they communicate a great deal subcallosally. This subcallosal sharing includes their possession in common of the "second" (midbrain-dependent) visual system (Trevarthen and Sperry 1973, Weiskrantz et al. 1974). Brainstem connections make for unification in other ways. For example, the duality for cognition demonstrable in the human split brain seems not to be accompanied by as great a disparity of affect (Gazzaniga and LeDoux 1978; Sperry, Zaidel, and Zaidel 1979), perhaps because the two limbic systems are coupled at the hypothalamic level.

An important source of synchronization is the brainstem ascending reticular activating system (ARAS), particularly since generalized arousal via this system can be produced by descending corticofugal influences from one hemisphere (Magoun 1958). Both human hemispheres, whether in the intact or the split condition, are probably asleep and awake simultaneously, just as they are in the split-brain cat (Berlucchi 1966a, 1966b) unless there is a sagittal section of the brainstem (Michel and Roffwarg 1967; Michel 1972). There is no evidence that primate hemispheres (in the same head) can alternate sleeping and waking, as do cetacean hemispheres (Lilly 1962; Serafetinides, Shurley, and Brooks 1972; Mukhametov,

Supin, and Polyakova 1977; Ridgway and Flanigan 1984).

If it were the case that the two hemispheres in normal continuity were sometimes independently awake and asleep, that is, if wakefulness varied independently, then cognition could also vary independently. In the dolphin (whose hemispheres are well connected by a large corpus callosum), this appears to be the case. If the dolphin hemispheres can sometimes be alternately awake (hence, independently thinking) with neocommissures intact, it suggests significant constraints on the synchronizing role, not only of the ARAS, but also that of the corpus callosum.

Before reviewing some of the evidence for partial hemispheric independence in mammals other than cetaceans, we should first take note of other reasons why hemispheric independence should be incomplete in the split brain. The unifying function of the corpus callosum has been unduly emphasized, not only when it is intact (the gist of this chapter) but also when it is absent. That is, the two hemispheres are not altogether independent in the split brain. As noted before, there is a lot of subcortical communication whether or not the neocommissures are cut. In addition, if one hemisphere initiates motion, the other hemisphere receives considerable proprioceptive feedback. What has been less often noted is that the hemispheres share a common blood supply; so it is clear that if one hemisphere causes the secretion of some hormones, the hormones can reach the other hemisphere. This is a means of communication that, although it is less rapid than neuronal communication, is important for mental states. The spinal fluid, of course, is also shared by the two hemispheres and this may be even more important than their common vasculature and more likely as the number of known cerebral peptides continues to increase.

Another noncallosal means of interhemispheric communication is "cross-cueing." Cross-cueing means that one hemisphere initiates a bodily behavior that can provide information to the other hemisphere. One method is "verbal cross-cueing": the speaking left hemisphere names out loud an object being felt in the right hand, resulting in correct retrieval by the left hand of that object after it has been placed in a collection of objects. This is in contrast to the customary failure of cross-retrieval when the split-brain human attempts the same task while remaining silent (Bogen 1984). More intriguing than cross-cueing by the left hemisphere of the right is the reverse. Nonverbal cross-cueing of the left hemisphere by the right takes various forms, as will be described.

Some examples of nonverbal cross-cueing (and of its failure) in the human with complete cerebral commissurotomy

A systematic investigation of nonverbal cross-cueing is as yet a missing brick in the intellectual edifice that Roger Sperry engineered. But nonverbal cross-cueing has been observed incidentally by many people on numerous occasions, and a few examples are appropriate here. As will be readily apparent, any of these "tricks" of cross-cueing could be employed by the normal as well as by the commissurotomized individual.

SUBJECT LB: PROGRESS NOTE
(IN PART) OF SEPTEMBER 18,
1967 (2½ YEARS POSTOP)
During the course of the examination, several objects were placed in his left hand and he was unable to name them. When a paper clip was placed in his hand, he was completely at a loss. He then reached over to take it with his right hand and immediately and correctly named it. (Here the transfer from the left to right hand made sufficient information available to the speaking left hemisphere.)

When a pipe was placed in his left hand, the pipe was turned around and manipulated in various ways and ended up in a correct position. The pipe was then put up to (but not into) his mouth and he then said, "Oh, that's a cigarette." He then was told to feel it with his right hand and immediately after doing so he said, "No, that's a pipe."

When a pair of glasses was put into his left hand, the hand turned it about and then opened the bows and started to put it on his head, at which point his arm was stopped and he was asked to try to name it without trying to do anything further. He was unable to name it. He then flipped the bows closed, which made an audible click. He then quickly said, "Are those your glasses?" (Here the movement of his left hand provided an auditory cue to the left hemisphere.)

A folded handkerchief was put into his left hand; he squeezed it, turned it around and over, and then smoothly reached backwards and slipped it into his left hip pocket. At this point, he said, "Oh, sure, that's a comb." When told he should feel it with his right hand, he did and then shook his head with a chagrined look and said, "A handkerchief." (Here the first left-hand behavior was insufficient to permit accurate identification by the left hemisphere.)

SUBJECT LB: ANOTHER
EXAMPLE OF CROSS-CUEING
Stuart Butler described a situation in which he and Ulf Norrsell were trying to determine if LB's right hemisphere could talk. The idea was to restrict the input to the right hemisphere by using left half-field projection or by putting objects in the left hand that are not apt to provide ipsilateral input, i.e., objects that do not have sharp points, that do not have an obvious temperature, etc. So Butler and Norrsell (1968) were using a wooden sphere, a wooden cube without any sharp edges, and a wooden pyramid. The question was, could LB indicate above chance level, whether he had in his left hand the sphere, or the cube, or the pyramid? Surprisingly, he was identifying them most of the time! He had his hand underneath the screen, so he could not see what was in his hand. Butler and Norrsell couldn't understand how he could recognize them so reliably. They at first thought it might be some kind of subcortical communication. Then they noticed that he was looking around the room. When they put a sphere in his left hand, he would look at the wall clock and he would say, "It's the round one." When they put the cube in his hand, he would look at the door and he would say, "That's the square one." When they put the pyramid in his left hand, he would look up at the ceiling and pause a minute and then say, "It must be that triangular shape." When Butler blindfolded him, instead of letting him look around the room, his verbal reports of what was in his left hand fell to chance.

SUBJECT LB: SELECTION BY GAZE AND CROSS-CUEING

Using chimeric stimuli, Levy, Trevarthen, and Sperry (1972) asked the subjects to point to the picture matching what had just been presented; they observed that either hand could indicate a picture selected by *gaze*. LB was noted on several occasions to use scanning of surroundings and gaze fixation to cue his left hemisphere.

SUBJECT CC: PROGRESS NOTE (IN PART) OF OCTOBER 13, 1973 (8 YEARS POSTOP)

With respect to anomia, the patient's performance is somewhat variable; it is remarkable how he can sometimes identify objects in the left hand on the basis of minimal cues. For example, when a pencil was placed in his left hand, he was rather slow and deliberate about answering, turning the pencil over in his hand and pressing first on the eraser end and then on the pointed end, and then saying, "It's a pencil."

When a dime was placed in his left hand, he rolled it around, rubbed it, and said, "It's a penny." He then said, "Well, isn't it?" When told that he was not correct, he said, "Maybe it's a dime."

When a rubber band was put into his left hand, he first shook his head. However, after rolling it around and then maneuvering it into a position in which it looped over his thumb and opposing fingers so that there was some springy resistance to partial opening of the hand, he said, "a rubber band."

When a pair of glasses was put in his left hand, his fingers rubbed the lenses, closed one bow with a snap, and he then said, "Are these glasses?" When he was told that he should try again, he said, "Well, I don't know." When this same object was then placed into his right hand he immediately said, "Yes, it's a pair of glasses."

When a pipe (still warm) was placed in his left hand, he said, "Is it a cigar?" When he was told that this was incorrect, he shook his head and said, "I don't know." When it was placed in his right hand, he immediately said, "It is a pipe."

When a small paper clip was put into his left hand, he turned it over several times and finally said, "I don't know." When it was placed into his right hand, he immediately said, "It's a clip." He was then asked, "What kind of clip?" and he replied, "To keep papers together."

A small pine cone was placed into the left hand, and he was at a total loss to say what it was. When this same object was placed into the right hand, he said, "It's one of those – I don't know what you call it – it comes from a tree." When he was allowed to see it, he said, "Yes, it is from a tree – what do you call it?" When he was told, "pine cone," he said, "Oh yes, that's what it is."

From this, it is apparent that CC readily recognized and named objects in the right hand, except with the last object (the pine cone), which he could no more readily name in full vision than he could when palpating it in his right hand. In contrast, objects in the left hand were much less readily identified either by verbal description or by naming: any success in this regard apparently depended upon partial information that sometimes led to the correct answer and sometimes to an answer that was related but not correct. The use of pain, from a pencil point, is a clue that has been observed in a number of complete commissurotomy patients. Identification of the rubber band apparently involved some proprioceptive information. The glasses provided a definite auditory clue, and possibly a slight temperature clue. The identification of a pipe as "cigar" is particularly interesting – it is possibly ascribable to an olfactory cue. Alternatively, his speaking left hemisphere may have received some sort of sparse categorical information either from the left hand via uncrossed pathways, or possibly even from the other hemisphere through internal pathways. In any event, it is quite instructive how an individual with an IQ under 70 can use minimal sensory clues to identify objects that are familiar to him.

SUBJECT RM: CROSS-CUEING (MAINLY UNSUCCESSFUL); PROGRESS NOTE (IN PART) OF JULY 13, 1966 (4 MONTHS POSTOP)

He has the usual anomia in the left hand with his eyes covered. When a pencil was placed in his left hand, he held it appropriately but could not name it. It was then put into his right hand, and he said, "a pencil." When a watch was put in his left hand, he said it was a "pencil" even when he was holding the watch up to his left ear. A paper clip was put in his hand, and he could not tell what it was, but when he put it in his right hand, he immediately identified it. A pipe in the left hand was put into his mouth in an appropriate way, but it was called a "pencil" even after the bit was between his teeth. When an ashtray was put in his left hand, he struck the table with it and he immediately told me what it was. When a pair of glasses was put in his hand, he could not name what he was holding until he tried to put them on. A handkerchief was put in his left hand; his left hand immediately put it into his pocket, but he could not say what it was. When he felt it with his right hand, he immediately identified it.

LESS USUAL KINDS OF CROSS-CUEING

Some "tricks" of cross-cueing are quite common across patients (in spite of their only rarely, if ever, meeting one another). Other tricks are more obviously idiosyncratic. Moreover, some tricks are easy to recognize, whereas others are only doubtfully identifiable. Three patients (AA, LB, and CC) have been personally observed by me, each on several occasions, to turn a pencil in the left hand so the sharp point could be pressed into the distal volar surface of a finger. And I have observed five (AA, LB, CC, RY, and RM) loop a rubber band over several fingers to explore its elasticity. (Here there is probably some ipsilateral proprioceptive information from the left hand to the left hemisphere.)

On the other hand, the following are tricks observed only on single occasions:
1. On one occasion, NG was being tested, in full view in the normal way, on the Benton–Van Allen faces test. Part way through the test, she changed her manner of responding. Instead of pointing quickly with her hand (to one of six choices), she would pause before her choices and move her hand only after a motion of her head, which resulted in pointing her chin toward the choice subsequently pointed by hand. When this was recognized and she was asked not to move her head, she resumed the undelayed pointing with her right hand.
2. (Courtesy of E. Zaidel.) On one occasion, LB was being tested by presenting Peabody pictures to one half-field or the other. After a picture of a tree appeared in the left half-field, his hands formed a triangle, and he then said, "teepee."

It is noteworthy that the PhD theses of Roger Sperry's last two graduate students before he retired were concerned with interhemispheric transfer of information for cerebral processes in commissurotomy patients (Cronin-Golomb 1984; Myers 1984).

Other sources of "mental duality"

In addition to the noncommissural communications between the two hemispheres in the split brain, there is another issue needing reemphasis: there are clearly other sources of duality or of ambivalence in the mental state besides having two hemispheres.

All of us are familiar with the distinction between the pyramidal and extrapyramidal motor systems. We know that monkeys can function remarkably well after the pyramids have been transected bilaterally, and this means that extrapyramidal motor control is considerable. All movements are commanded from the spinal cord, but what the spinal cord does can be directed from above in more than one way, and these alternative directives might well be both concurrent and conflicting. So one can see here some opportunity for ambivalence or conflict that requires only one hemisphere.

As another example, there appear to be at least two kinds of memory (in each hemisphere) that are anatomically specifiable: the kind of memory subserved by the hippocampus (Zola-Morgan, Squire, and Mishkin 1982). This difference requires only one hemisphere. There are many kinds of duality that can be checked, and should be checked, in hemispherectomized individuals because, if one saw that kind of duality in them, then there would be no need to suppose that it has anything to do with the duality of the hemispheres. Unfortunately, very little has been done along this line. Indeed, it is astounding that this opportunity is not being pursued to settle convincingly the relevance of hemispheric duality to various kinds of "mental duality."

Having argued that hemispheric integration can occur in the absence of the corpus callosum by a host of other unifying mechanisms, behavioral as well as neuronal and hormonal, I will now consider the complementary claim that even with the commissures intact, there is a significant degree of hemispheric independence. This claim begins with a quantitative argument for duality of mind – that is to say, a significant independence of hemispheric function – and then we shall consider some experimental evidence.

A quantitative anatomy argument for significant hemispheric independence with neocommissures intact

According to both Chauncey Leake (Harvey 1958) and F. H. Garrison (1922), the first time this kind of argument was used in medicine was by William Harvey. Harvey measured the volume of the heart and counted the heart rate. He asserted that the amount of blood that is pumped by the heart in any given time (say, in a day or an hour) could not possibly be produced in such sizable amounts by the lungs. The only reasonable thing to conclude is that the blood circulates. He did not demonstrate the circulation; he just concluded that it *must* be so on this quantitative argument. And it was more than 30 years later (1661) that Malpighi actually demonstrated the capillaries with the microscope.

An argument from quantitative anatomy in the present case is roughly as follows: there are about 800 million nerve fibers in the corpus callosum, whereas within each hemisphere, there are some ten billion nerve cells – each with at least a hundred connections (and many nerve cells, of course, have thousands of connections). This means that the number of connections between the hemispheres are a small fraction of the connections within each hemisphere. That the information generated in one hemisphere can be immediately transferred or made available to the other is hardly credible.

One might suppose that information accumulated by one hemisphere during waking could be transferred later, during sleep; but callosal activity decreases markedly during EEG synchronization and/or REM sleep (Berlucchi 1965). In any event, immediate sensory information in one hemisphere seems fully available to the other only with respect to the midline, since for primary sensory cortices, it is the areas for midline representation that have heavy callosal projections (Myers 1965; Berlucchi 1972; Doty and Negrão 1973; Newsome and Allman 1980; see Chapter 6, this volume).

It might be supposed that hemispheric synchrony with respect to direct sensory experience is unnecessary to avoid mental duality so long as higher-order information (such as that which accompanies learning) is fully shared. But it is often not so shared, according to the evidence to be considered next.

Experimental evidence for significant hemispheric independence with respect to learning

The experimental evidence is of different kinds, mainly having to do with incomplete interhemispheric transfer. While emphasizing the lack of interhemispheric transfer in the split condition, the authors who have reported the split-brain animal experiments have sometimes alluded, albeit briefly, to the fact that in the intact case, there is often (especially in the unsophisticated animal) a lack of transfer. If one trains a monkey to do something with one hand, often he doesn't do it immediately as well with the other hand. After a while, the monkey transfers better, that is, the lack of transfer typically goes away – unlike the anatomically split condition, where the lack of transfer persists.

In a previous review (Bogen and Bogen 1969), we described some evidence for lack of interhemispheric transfer of information in the intact brain, including the cat experiments of Myers (1962). Also mentioned was a lack of transfer of spatial form discrimination from one hand to another during early testing of a difficult task in monkeys (Semmes and Mishkin 1965). Butler and Francis (1973) reinvestigated this often evanescent phenomenon. They arranged for the subjects (baboons) to reach through a tube to manipulate stimuli at the other end, thus restricting movement of proximal joints. The animals learned to rotate the stimuli (to get food) in either a clockwise or counterclockwise direction, depending on the stimulus shape. After the subjects learned the task, the other hand was tested. Two different problems (A and B) were used (three animals learned A first and three learned B first). On the first problem, whether it was A or B, the authors found:

> . . . no animal was able to perform without further training the discrimination learned with the other hand; in all cases the animals required extensive training with the second hand before regaining the proficiency reached with the first one (Butler and Francis 1973, p. 80).

On the second problem (whether B or A), rather than performing at chance as on the first problem, there was often an abundance of errors because of performance in a mirror-image mode. These results could be interpreted as showing the development of a learning set, that is, the animals may actually *learn* to transfer information, with repeated testing (Berlucchi et al. 1978). On the other hand, a lack of intermanual transfer does not rule out interhemispheric communication; it is certainly conceivable that in some cases, information is transmitted but not initially used by the receiving hemisphere, whereas in other situations, the information may not be transmitted from one to the other.

Much earlier, in 1949, Sperry and Clark reported related findings in gobies. (It is worth recalling that the split-brain story started with the question of interocular transfer, i.e., whether learning transferred from one eye to the other; see foreword, this volume.)

In this paper, Sperry and Clarke wrote:

> . . . the results seem to support the conclusion that the brain organization of this teleost fish permits interocular transfer, but at the same time the neural mechanisms involved are not so well developed that good transfer is automatically assured in all instances (Sperry and Clark 1949, p. 278).

In fact, clearcut savings were observed in only five of 16 cases. Lesser degrees of transfer were found in four, whereas transfer was essentially nil in seven. The 11 without good transfer had not simply "forgotten" the task, because retesting of the originally trained hemisphere showed approximately the previous (trained) level of correct responses. Then the untrained eye was again tested in two cases, and excellent transfer was found in one of them.

In considering the previous experiments with fish, we recall that the chiasmal crossing in these animals is essentially complete, so that training one eye is tantamount to training one hemisphere directly and the other only indirectly (if at all). A similar chiasmal crossing is present in the rat and rabbit, which we consider next.

Russell and Morgan (1979) directed the input in the rat to one hemisphere by restricting the input to one eye. (The white rat's chiasm is almost totally crossed – the wild rat has a little bit less crossing, whereas in the human or monkey, it is approximately 50%.) Then they tested the other eye. What they found was that a failure of interocular transfer need not represent some sort of anatomical disconnection. On the contrary, as they said:

> . . . these results suggest that under certain conditions an absence of interhemispheric communication is a characteristic of the intact brain.

Using rabbits, Van Hof (1979) repeatedly found "lateralization of the memory trace," but he cautiously concluded that "it would be premature to regard the rabbit as a 'natural split-brain preparation.'" The rabbit has a corpus callosum, of course, but the engram may not transfer if one sets up the learning situation in a certain way.

Related results have been found in pigeons by a number of investigators, beginning with Beritov and Chichinadze (1937) and recently reviewed by Graves and Goodale (1979), who concluded that the transfer – or lack of it – depended upon the type of problem. Apparently depending upon the experimental conditions, either unilaterality or bilaterality of the engram has been found in newborn chicks (Bell and Gibbs 1977; Benowitz 1974; Greif 1976; Hodge, Gibbs, and Ng 1981).

In this context (monocular training and total chiasmal crossing), it is instructive to consider a case that reinforces a previous point of this chapter: that we could mistakenly over-emphasize the importance of the corpus callosum for interhemispheric communication. Marzi, DiStefano, and Simoni (1979) used Siamese cats, whose optic pathways fully cross, permitting restriction of input to one hemisphere. They found a deficiency of interocular transfer on some more difficult problems, as compared with cats having normal optic chiasmata. The Siamese cats did show essentially complete transfer on simpler problems; *and they did so even with section of the neocommissures*. The authors suggest a role for subcortical connections, which might be more effective in Siamese cats, partially in compensation for their chiasmal peculiarities.

For visual problems, in the experience of most investigators, monkeys usually show transfer as long as the splenium is intact (Hamilton 1977, 1982; Butler 1979; Doty 1983; Doty, Lewine, and Ringo 1984). But even with all commissures intact, lack of transfer has occasionally been evident as a learning deficit on testing of the second hemisphere.

For the purpose of this chapter, it is important that there are certain learning situations giving rise to *certain kinds of information that do not readily transfer in the intact brain*. The likelihood that information will be transferred apparently depends, in part, upon the functional ability of the hemisphere receiving the transfer, particularly if this ability has been reduced by a lesion. Zeki (1967) performed an important experiment to examine this. After making partial lesions in the parastriate cortex, he taught chiasm-sectioned monkeys to do a problem with one eye or the other. When the eye on the side of the lesion was trained first, there was very good transfer. But when the eye on the unlesioned side was trained first, the second eye did not show transfer. He suggested, because the unlesioned side learned with fewer trials, that the interocular transfer in the original circumstance was due to overtraining; a unidirectionality of transfer (for the problems he used) was not found if lesions were placed on both sides.

The influence on interocular transfer of a unilateral juxtastriate lesion was examined in detail by Berlucchi et al. (1979). Their results resembled those of Zeki in that "interhemispheric transfer was clearly present from the injured hemisphere to the intact hemisphere, while it was poor in the opposite direction" (p. 370).

In addition to lack of interocular transfer, another manifestation of hemispheric independence is an inability to cross-compare objects presented to separate eyes; Voneida and Robinson (1970) found this in two chiasm-sectioned cats. These authors were also able to train contradictory habits to separate eyes when the rostral one-third of the callosum was intact and there was still some interocular transfer. Other examples of unilateral engrams include a conditioned salivary response with surgically split tongue of the dog (Abuladze 1963) and a conditioned auditory response in cats (Kaas, Axelrod, and Diamond 1967).

Results with cortical spreading depression (CSD), including a digression on methodological critiques

Next we consider the cortical spreading depression (CSD) experiments. If one puts a few drops of concentrated potassium chloride solution on the cortex of a hemisphere, especially a smooth brain like that of a rat, waves of depression spread over the cortex so that the entire hemisphere becomes temporarily inactivated. Meanwhile, one can train the other hemisphere. Then, after the potassium chloride has been washed away, the rat has two good hemispheres, but only one that has learned the task. If one then inactivates the trained hemisphere with CSD, the untrained hemisphere is found not to know the problem. So, even though the animal was possessed of two hemispheres functioning normally for a while, the learning did not transfer. Bureš, Burešova, and Krivanek (1974) have reviewed this subject in great detail. The main point is that CSD provides an independent kind of information leading to the same conclusion: that there may be lack of interhemispheric transfer with commissures intact.

Experiments using CSD have sometimes been dismissed (Gazzaniga and Le Doux 1978, Denenberg 1983) on the objection that CSD experiments have serious methodologic deficiencies. But, as we shall see, this objection is only narrowly applicable. Before examining this objection, we first recall that *every* technique has its methodologic difficulties and ambiguities; we can consider, as a notable example, the various techniques for cerebral localization.

Cerebral localization (CL) in cases of brain tumor has been extraordinarily productive: many of Hughlings Jacksons' notable conclusions regarding CL were based on tumor cases. Yet it is generally recognized that tumors can be misleading as a result of pressure effects, or because of ongoing diaschsis in the tumors of rapid growth. The phenomenon of tumor "momentum" is well known to neurologists. Indeed, these and related phenomena gave rise to an entire literature on "false localization."

Because of the problems associated with CL in tumor cases, it has often been averred that CL should be based not on tumor cases, but on cases of fixed deficit from thrombotic stroke, preferably cases eventually coming to autopsy, although in recent years, CAT scan localization has significantly complemented autopsy findings. Using stroke cases for CL has a long and illustrious history. But clinicians are aware that the putatively critical infarct is usually accompanied by other infarcts, previously occurring and supposedly "silent," and that these other infarcts contribute in all likelihood to the behavioral deficit consequent to the "critical" infarct. (A well-known example is that when a retrorolandic lesion in the right hemisphere produces a long lasting deficit in face recognition (prosopagnosia), it typically has been preceded by a left hemisphere lesion, often asymptomatic; see Chapter 16, this volume.) Moreover, considerable ambiguity obtains in cases of single thrombotic infarcts, because these usually occur in a brain already affected by arteriosclerosis, with lessened compensatory reserve, or even, as in many cases, with overt manifestations before the stroke.

The ambiguities of CL in the older folks with strokes can be avoided by studying youths wounded in war; this approach has produced not a few well-founded reputations. But missile wounds have boundaries that are rarely well-defined, and their distant effects (for example, by interfering with the blood supply to other brain regions) are largely indeterminate.

And so, should we not rely instead upon certain cases of surgical removal, where the boundaries of the ablation are clean and precisely described? The monumental work at the Montreal Neurological Institute of Milner and her colleagues has utilized just such material. On the other hand, we are not all persuaded of the total reliability of surgeons' reports (especially now that postoperative CAT scans have become so common). Besides, the most reliably precise surgical removals in cases of long-standing epilepsy retain ambiguities attributable to the compensatory changes that inevitably have occurred consequent to the epileptogenic lesions.

Next we can consider hemispherectomy where the anatomic removal is as clean as possible. In such cases, anything in the way of behavior is certainly attributable to the residual hemisphere. But most hemispherectomies have been done for cases of infantile hemiplegia. These, too, have had a long history with much compensatory change in the residual hemisphere between the time of lesion and the time of surgery. Even when the surgery has been done in adults of supposedly normal development, these patients have commonly been tested at some time postsurgery, allowing for reorganization of function.

The confounding effects of compensatory change can be avoided with the "temporary hemispherectomy" of the carotid amytal (Wada) test. But here we have other problems, including that the posterior cerebral artery of the narcotized side often does not feed from the carotid artery. Moreover, carotid branches to the brainstem can seriously affect the behavioral results of the injection.

Does this mean that conclusions from all of the foregoing types of material should be dismissed? Certainly not! The point is that *every* patient population and *every* experimental method has its problems. This is also true of the EEG approach to CL, the use of blood-flow measures, the PET scanner and stimulation mapping, as well as the split brain.

The lesson here is twofold. First, one does not summarily dismiss data having interpretive complications; one takes the time to become familiar with the qualifications and ambiguities, and then relies upon the data with appropriate reservations.

Second, a conclusion indicated by *any* method or material must remain tentative until confirmed by *other* methods having different methodologic problems. When several different approaches point to the same conclusion, we can have increased confidence in the result. It is convergence upon a common conclusion, through a variety of different approaches, which gives us a near certainty in our conviction of complementary hemispheric specialization in the human. Similarly, it is the convergence of a variety of evidence that leaves us in little doubt about the duality of the brain. One kind of evidence for cerebral duality comes from cortical spreading depression (CSD), and we now turn to a closer appraisal of the supposed deficiencies of this approach.

Gazzaniga and Le Doux (1978) and Denenberg (1983) dismissed CSD evidence largely on the basis of a review by Petrinovich (1976). What concerns us in this chapter is whether the methodologic difficulties pointed out by Petrinovich weaken the conclusion that *an engram originally engendered in one hemisphere* (while the other was subjected to CSD) *does not automatically transfer to the other hemisphere* when both are returned to a normal state. In general, for the untrained hemisphere to exhibit the learning on its own, when the originally trained hemisphere is depressed, a number of training trials first are necessary with both hemispheres undepressed. That is, *substantial transfer commonly requires interdepression training (IDT)*. We find on closer examination of the Petrinovich review *not* an objection to this well-known fact, but rather a critique of *other* inferences from CSD studies, in particular, the belief that either the engram is always completely lateralized, or that when it is lateralized, IDT produces transfer with a specific number of trials.

At first glance, Petrinovich's review appears to be summarized in his closing clause: "... it is concluded that the technique (CSD) is of questionable utility in elucidating with any precision mechanisms involved in the formation and transfer of memory traces." But it is the "precision," not the fact of transfer, that is the object of his critique. He specifically singles out for censure the conclusion of Albert that it takes only three minutes for the trained hemisphere to transmit the memory (during IDT),

but it requires two hours for the transmitted memory to consolidate in the untrained hemisphere. The greater part of his review is devoted to the sources of error in three articles by Albert (in *Neuropsychologia* in 1966) and two papers by Mayes (in *Behavioral Biology* in 1973), whose findings were congruent with the findings of Albert. The errors included running animals from light to dark, assuming that washing off KCI quickly restores cortical normality, discarding the results from recalcitrant animals, and the use of inappropriate statistical procedures. Petrinovich does not deny that it is possible to train one hemisphere while keeping the other one untrained with CSD, or that the memory trace or engram subsequently can remain largely lateralized even with both hemispheres functioning. As Petrinovich says in the opening sentence of his discussion, "it is generally agreed that IDT produces transfer, where transfer is defined as the savings observed when the initially depressed cortex is trained undepressed following IDT."

Denenberg (1983), who discounted CSD data, relied not only on Petrinovich, but also on the review by Gaston (1978). But her criticisms are concerned solely with the question of taste aversion, that is, whether CSD experiments can prove the participation of cerebral cortex in a rat learning to avoid certain tastes, learning that possibly can occur without cortex at all. Nowhere does she deny that an originally unilateral engram can remain lateralized in the posttraining undepressed state.

In conclusion, CSD experiments have provided some very clear examples of the failure of intact commissures to effect a synchronization (in the sense of equivalence of information content) of the two cerebral hemispheres.

Hemispheric independence in the intact human

We consider next the human. In the young child, interhemispheric communication might be deficient since myelination of callosal fibers takes ten or more years to reach completion (Yakovlev and Lecours 1967). In fact, deficits in tactile cross-matching have been found in children (Galin et al. 1979). But in the adult, lack of interhemispheric communication has been less directly demonstrable.

It seems reasonable to suppose, as did Butler and Francis (1973), that manual manipulations will show less transfer to the other side, the more distal (in the extremity) are the crucial aspects. This could be expected in humans as well as monkeys, and so it is no surprise that it is for fine digital manipulations or detections that savings seem least. A good example is the learning of Braillelike patterns by sighted adults naive to the task. Although there are usually some savings, it requires further training with the second hand to reach the same level of proficiency as with the first hand. Indeed, when going from left to right in right handers, *just as much* training may be needed for the second hand (Wagner 1977, reproduced in Harris 1980).

The amount of transfer probably depends upon what the second hand is doing while the first is being trained, as shown by Hicks, Frank, and Kinsbourne (1982). They had subjects learn a sequence of key presses on a typewriter with one hand while the second hand was either resting or grasping a table leg; partial transfer occurred to the resting hand, but not to the hand occupied with grasping during the original training.

An ingenious study using dichotic listening to digits and tones was reported by Goodglass and Calderon (1977), and their conclusions were supported in another dichotic study by Sidtis and Bryden (1978). This is not even a situation in which the material is clearly directed to one hemisphere or the other. These results can be summarized by quoting the discussion by Bradshaw and Nettleton (1983) in their excellent review. On page 125 of that book, Bradshaw and Nettleton say:

> These results show that the two hemispheres could concurrently and independently process that component of a complex stimulus for which each is dominant. . . .

Next we come to notable experiments by Landis, Assal, and Perret. The first paper was published in 1979. Their purpose, in the beginning at any rate, was to ask: Is there a right hemisphere superiority for the recognition of facial expression? We know that the right hemisphere is predominant, although not exclusive by any means, for the recognition of faces. The question naturally arises, is the right hemisphere predominant for the recognition of facial *expression?* They did a visual half-field test as follows: they presented centrally a schematic outline of a familiar object, and in one or the other half-field, a photograph of the same thing or of something else and asked, "Are these the same?" For example, a schematic drawing of a corkscrew appeared in the middle at the point of fixation along with a photograph in either the left or right half-field. If it was a photograph of a corkscrew, the subject would push the button; if it was different, no reaction was necessary. They measured the reaction time and repeated the procedure with facial expressions. A schematic diagram of a frontview face appears in the middle, along with a photograph, in either the right or left half-field, of a face in profile with an expression (happy, sad, etc.). Is it the same expression or not? It turned out that the reaction times are *less* in the *left* half-field for the *facial expressions,* whereas the reaction times for objects like the corkscrew are less in the right half-field. Now this is not an altogether surprising finding; it is what most of us would expect. One might also expect that people would be more accurate in recognizing the similarity of objects than in recognizing identity of expressions; and, indeed, the responses were more accurate (96% correct) for the objects than for the expressions (76% correct).

Landis et al. (1979) also noticed that the subjects showed very different levels of awareness of their decisions, often having second thoughts. That is, erroneous object matchings were often followed by rapid recognition of the errors; and accurate object matchings were confirmed. By contrast, when matching expressions, the subjects repeatedly expressed the sense of having made an error when, in fact, the manual response had been accurate. In other words, the subjects seemed to have made many accurate decisions on facial expressions without correctly monitoring their behavior. "However," the author's wrote, "this is an incidental observation which needs to be explored systematically."

There subsequently appeared a paper by Landis, Graves, and Goodglass (1981); the title of the paper asked, "A Split-Brain Phenomenon in Normal Subjects?" The same stimuli were used, but they modified the method of presentation. First, the photographs of objects and faces were presented randomly in one or the other half-field. Also, they made the presentation time sufficiently shorter for the objects, so the subjects were wrong about 25% of the time with both the expressions and the objects. After responding, the subject was expected to report "whenever you think you made a mistake." The principal point here concerns the individual's monitoring of his own behavior. In this second experiment, they were not looking at the reaction times, but wanted to systematically investigate the second thoughts. They found that the monitoring with the object matching was very good, whereas the monitoring for the expression matching was at chance level – *the verbalized corrections did not reflect the person's abilities to make accurate decisions about expressions.* That is to say, when the behavior was presumably controlled by the right hemisphere, second thoughts were not reliable. In the authors' words: "The result for the emotional expression matching task resembles results obtained with split-brain patients."

Hemispheric capabilities have been studied in three principal ways: from studies of patients with lateralized lesions, from studies using lateralized input (as in the half-field studies just described), and from studies using lateralized readout (including both radiographic and electrical methods). The final bit of evidence I will present concerns the last, namely, lateralized readout in the form of tactile evoked potentials. The experiment was done by John Desmedt (1977a, 1977b). He used as a stimulus the flat end of a cylindrical (dowel-shaped) rod. The end of the dowel briefly and repeatedly touched the ball of the palpating finger. If the end of the dowel had a ridge on it, the subject's task was to determine the orientation of the ridge (East–West or North–South). If there was no ridge, the subject did not have to make any spatial orientation judgments. Every time the dowel touches the end of the finger, it evokes a potential recordable from the scalp. And each time, the subject has to decide whether there is a ridge or not, and, if so, how

it is oriented. That keeps him interested, which is quite important because if one wants to do a successful experiment with evoked potentials that involve cognition, it is necessary to keep subjects interested. That Desmedt did so is one reason why his experiment succeeded.

The end surface of the dowel, when it is smooth, elicits a potential that is the same over the two hemispheres. When the end has a ridge, there is a different potential evoked over the right hemisphere, whereas for the left hemisphere, the fact that there is a ridge on the end causes no change. Let me translate the author's conclusion:

> These observations are notable because they show the localization in the right hemisphere of cortical mechanisms put into play by the perception of spatial orientation in normal subjects. They show that the capacities of the right hemisphere inferred from neurological studies of individuals with lateralized lesions do not result from a liberation from control of the left hemisphere. These findings are therefore in favor of the view that there is not a unilateral dominance by the left hemisphere and they are in favor of the notion that each of the two hemispheres possesses different capacities and that the capacities of the right hemispheres can be manifested even when the commissural functions of the corpus callosum are intact (Desmedt 1977a, p. 625).

Since the foregoing was true with *either* hand, it would appear to invoke, in the right-hand testing, a callosal relay rather than direct access (as distinguished by Zaidel 1983). That is, it seems a case of unihemispheric function (with lateralized electrical sign) that is both preceded (for relay of input) and followed (for verbal report) by interhemispheric communications.

Conclusion

The split-brain affords us an anatomically defined circumstance (Bogen, Schultz, and Vogel 1988) in which a single individual can manifest two minds, each with its own discriminative, mnemonic, and volitional capacities. Suppose that we restored the corpus callosum;

would that *reduce* the complexities? To put it differently, if we added 800 million bridging nerve fibers, would a previously complicated situation (that is, mental duality) become more simple? We might even suspect that the mental numerosity of the intact brain is greater than that of the split brain.

If an individual with a hemispherectomy has one mind, and two individuals each with a hemispherectomy have two minds, where between them shall we place people with split brains, who are clearly less double than two individuals with hemispherectomy? And where should we place the intact brain?

If numerosity of mind were a continuum, or even fractionally quantizable, it would be easier to describe the split brain as well as the intact brain. As it is, our current language forces us to jump one way or the other. Between "one mind" and "two minds" to describe *either* the split brain or the intact brain, "two minds" seems closer to being correct.

If the language that we have inherited from the past were changed, we might be able to provide better answers than we have at present. Until we do have a better vocabulary, we are stuck with anthropomorphizing the hemispheres. And we are stuck with the resistance that such usage will elicit in those who (however poorly unified they may be) know that they are better unified than any pair of people with hemispherectomy.

We are on the threshold of a revolution in the way in which we talk about the nature of the mind and about human nature, a revolution in which Roger Sperry's leadership has played a major role. We possess now an abundance of facts that are not adequately comprehended by the concepts that we have inherited from the past. We cannot yet say what new concepts (presumably quantitative) shall serve us best. But we do see that they are needed; we can see, in part, the direction they should take; and we all look forward to the day when the implications of the split-brain research emerge in a form that can help guide human society toward an improved understanding of its own internally conflicted creativity.

Acknowledgments

I am indebted for advice, much of it heeded, from G. M. Bogen, R. W. Doty, D. Galin, C. Hamilton, J. Johnstone, F. Michel, C. Trevarthen, A. van Harreveld, and E. Zaidel. And I am grateful for library assistance from S. Zeind and staff, including P. Logan and V. Caullay of the Huntington Memorial Hospital, and for word processing by Sally Johnstone.

References

Abuladze, K. S. 1963. Functioning of paired organs. *Leningrad: Medgiz 1961* (Russian). Translation by R. Crawford. Macmillan, New York. (Cited by Doty and Negrão 1973.)

Bell, G. A., and M. E. Gibbs. 1977. Unilateral storage of monocular engram in day-old chick. *Brain Res.* 124: 263–70.

Benowitz, L. 1974. Conditions for the bilateral transfer of monocular learning in chicks. *Brain Res.* 65: 204–13.

Beritov, J., and N. Chichinadze. 1937. On the localization of cortical processes evoked by visual stimulation. *Tr. Inst. Fiziol. Beritashvili* 3: 361–4. (Cited by Sperry and Clark 1949.)

Berlucchi, G. 1965. Callosal activity in unrestrained, unanesthetized cats. *Arch. Ital. Biol.* 103: 623–35.

–1966a. Electroencephalographic activity of the isolated hemicerebrum of the cat. *Exp. Neurol.* 15: 220–8.

–1966b. Electroencephalographic studies in "split brain" cats. *Electroencep. Clin. Neurophysiol.* 20: 348–56.

–1972. Anatomical and physiological aspects of visual functions of corpus callosum. *Brain Res.* 37: 371–92.

Berlucchi, G., E. Buchtel, C. A. Marzi, G. G. Mascetti and A. Simoni. 1978. Effects of experience on interocular transfer of pattern discriminations in splitchiasm and split-brain cats. *J. Comp. Physiol. Psychol.* 92: 532–43.

Berlucchi, G., J. M. Sprague, A. Antonini, and A. Simoni. 1979. Learning and interhemispheric transfer of visual pattern discriminations following unilateral suprasylvian lesions in split-chiasm cats. *Exp. Brain Res.* 34: 551–74.

Bogen, J. E. 1969. The other side of the brain. II. An appositional mind. *Bull. L.A. Neurol. Soc.* 34: 135–62.

–1974. Hemispherectomy and the placing reactions in cats. *In* M. Kinsbourne and W. L. Smith (eds.) *Hemisphere Disconnection and Cerebral Function.* Thomas, Springfield (IL).

–1977. Further discussion on split-brains and hemispheric capabilities. *Brit. J. Phil. Sci.* 28: 281–286.

–1984. The callosal syndromes. *In* K. M. Heilman and E. Valenstein (eds.) *Clinical Neuropsychology,* 2nd Ed. Oxford University Press, New York.

Bogen J. E., and G. M. Bogen. 1969. The other side of the brain. III. The corpus callosum and creativity. *Bull. L.A. Neurol. Soc.* 39: 191–220.

Bogen, J. E., D. H. Schultz, and P. J. Vogel. 1988. Completeness of callosotomy shown by magnetic resonance imaging in the long term. *Arch. Neurol.* 45: 1203–5.

Bradshaw, J. L., and N. C. Nettleton. 1983. *Human Cerebral Asymmetry.* Prentice-Hall, Englewood Cliffs (NJ).

Bureš, J., O. Burešova, and J. Krivanek. 1974. *The Mechanism and Application of Leão's Spreading Depression of Electroencephalographic Activity.* Academia Prague, Prague.

Butler, C. R. 1979. Interhemispheric transmission of visual information via the corpus callosum and anterior commissure in the monkey. *In* I. S. Russell, M. W. Van Hof, and G. Berlucchi (eds.) *Structure and Function of Cerebral Commissures.* University Park Press, Baltimore.

Butler, C. R., and A. C. Francis. 1973. Split-brain behavior without splitting. Tactile discriminations in monkeys. *Israel J. Med. Sci.* 9 (Suppl.): 79–84.

Butler, S. R., and U. Norrsell. 1968. Vocalization possibly initiated by the minor hemisphere. *Nature (London)* 220: 793–4.

Cronin-Golomb, A. 1984. *Intrahemispheric Processing and Subcortical Transfer of Non-Verbal Information in Subjects with Complete Forebrain Commissurotomy.* PhD thesis, California Institute of Technology.

Denenberg, V. H. 1983. Micro and macro theories of the brain. *Behav. Brain Sci.* 6: 174–8.

Desmedt, J. E. 1977a. Mise en évidence d'électrogenèses spécifiques de l'hemisphère droit non-dominant chez l'homme intact. *Bull. L'Academie Nationale Médecine* 161: 623–6.

–1977b. Active touch exploration of extrapersonal space elicits specific electrogenesis in the right cerebral hemisphere of intact right-handed man. *Proc. Natl. Acad. Sci. USA* 74: 4037–40.

Doty, R. W. 1983. Some thoughts, and some experiments, on memory. *In* N. Butters and L. Squire (eds.) *The Neuropsychology of Memory.* Guilford Press, New York.

Doty, R. W., J. D. Lewine, and J. L. Ringo. 1984. Mnemonic interaction between and within cerebral hemispheres in macaques. *In* D. L. Alkon and C. D. Woody (eds.) *Neural Mechanisms of Conditioning.* Plenum, New York.

Doty, R. W., and N. Negrão. 1973. Forebrain commissures and vision. *In* R. Jung (ed.) *Handbook of Sensory Physiology VII/3B.* Springer, Berlin.

Doty, R. W., N. Negrão, and K. Yamaga. 1973. The unilateral engram. *Acta Neurobiol. Exp.* 33: 711–28.

Galin, D., J. Johnstone, L. Nakell, and J. Herron. 1979. Development of the capacity for tactile information transfer between hemispheres in normal children. *Science* 204: 1330–32.

Garrison, F. H. 1922. *History of Medicine,* 3rd Ed. Saunders, Philadelphia, p. 243.

Gaston, K. E. 1978. Brain mechanisms of conditioned taste aversion learning: A review of the literature. *Physiol. Psychol.* 6: 340–53.

Gazzaniga, M. S., and J. E. LeDoux. 1978. *The Integrated Mind.* Plenum, New York.

Goodglass, H., and M. Calderon. 1977. Parallel processing of verbal and musical stimuli in right and left hemispheres. *Neuropsychol.* 15: 397–407.

Graves, J. A., and M. A. Goodale. 1979. Do training conditions affect interocular transfer in the pigeon? *In* I. S. Russell, M. W. Van Hof, and G. Berlucchi (eds.) *Structure and Function of Cerebral Commissures.* University Park Press, Baltimore.

Greif, K. F. 1976. Bilateral memory for monocular one-trial passive avoidance in chicks. *Behav. Biol.* 16: 453–62.

Hamilton, C. R. 1977. Investigations of perceptual and mnemonic lateralization in monkeys. *In* S. Harnad, R. W. Doty, L. Goldstein, J. Jaynes, and G. Krauthamer (eds.) *Lateralization in the Nervous System.* Academic Press, New York.

–1982. Mechanisms of interocular equivalence. *In* D. J. Ingle, M. A. Goodale, R. J. W. Mansfield (eds.) *Analyses of Visual Behaviour.* The MIT Press, Cambridge.

Harris, L. J. 1980. Which hand is the "eye" of the blind? – A new look at an old question. *In* J. Herron (ed.) *The Neuropsychology of Left-Handedness.* Academic Press, New York.

Harvey, W. 1958 (originally 1628). *In* C. Leake (trans.) *Anatomical Studies on the Motion of the Heart and Blood.* Thomas, Springfield (IL).

Hicks, R. E., J. M. Frank, and M. Kinsbourne. 1982. The locus of bimanual skill transfer. *J. Gen. Psychol.* 107: 277–81.

Hodge, R. J., M. E. Gibbs, and D. T. Ng. 1981. Engram duplication in the day-old chick. *Behav. Neural Biol.* 31: 283–98.

Kaas, J., S. Axelrod, I. T. Diamond. 1967. An ablation study of the auditory cortex in the cat using binaural tonal patterns. *J. Neurophysiol.* 30: 710–24.

Kruper, D. C., R. A. Patton, and Y. D. Koskoff. 1971. Visual discrimination in hemicerebrectomized monkeys. *Physiol. Behav.* 7: 173–9.

Landis, T., G. Assal, and E. Perret. 1979. Opposite cerebral hemispheric superiorities for visual associative processing of emotional facial expressions and objects. *Nature (London)* 278: 739–40.

Landis, T., R. Graves, and H. Goodglass. 1981. Dissociated awareness of manual performance on two different visual associative tasks: A "split-brain" phenomenon in normal subjects? *Cortex* 17: 435–40.

Levy, J., C. Trevarthen, and R. W. Sperry. 1972. Perception of bilateral chimeric figures following hemispheric deconnexion. *Brain* 95: 61–78.

Lilly, J. C. 1962. Comment on cerebral dominance in the dolphin. *In* V. Mountcastle (ed.) *Interhemispheric Relations and Cerebral Dominance.* Johns Hopkins University Press, Baltimore.

Magoun, H. W. 1958. *The Waking Brain.* Thomas, Springfield (IL) p. 106 ff.

Marks, C. E. 1980. *Commissurotomy, Consciousness, and Unity of Mind.* Bradford Monographs, Montgomery (VT).

Marzi, C. A., M. DiStefano, and A. Simoni. 1979. Pathways of interocular transfer in Siamese cats. *In* I. S. Russell, M. W. Van Hof, and G. Berlucchi (eds.) *Structure and Function of Cerebral Commissures.* University Park Press, Baltimore.

Michel, F. 1972. Sleep and waking in cats with various sagittal sections of the brain. *In* J. Cernaček and F. Podivinsky (eds.) *Cerebral Interhemispheric Relations.* Vydavalestvo Slovenskej Akad., Bratislava, Czechoslovakia.

Michel, F., and Roffwarg, H. P. 1967. Chronic split brainstem preparation: Effect on the sleep–waking cycle. *Experientia* 23: 126–8.

Mukhametov, L. M., A. Y. Supin, and I. G. Polyakova. 1977. Interhemispheric asymmetry of the electroencephalographic sleep patterns in dolphins. *Brain Res.* 134: 581–4.

Myers, J. J. 1984. *Cognitive Transfer from Right to Left Hemisphere after Section of the Forebrain Commissures.* PhD. thesis, California Institute of Technology.

Myers, R. E. 1962. Transmission of visual information within and between the hemispheres: A behavioral study. *In* V. B. Mountcastle (ed.) *Interhemispheric Relations and Cerebral Dominance.* John Hopkins University Press, Baltimore.

−1965. Organization of visual pathways. *In* E. G. Ettlinger (ed.) *Functions of the Corpus Callosum,* Ciba Foundation Study Group No. 20. Little, Brown, Boston, pp. 133–43.

Newsome, W. T., and J. M. Allman. 1980. Interhemispheric connections of visual cortex in the owl monkey, *Aotus trivirgatus,* and the bushbaby, *Galago senegalensis. J. Comp. Neurol.* 194: 209–33.

Patton, R. A. 1961. Hemicerebrectomy and adaptive behavior in the rhesus monkey. *In* H. W. Brosin (ed.) *Experimental Psychiatry.* University of Pittsburgh Press, Pittsburgh.

Petrinovich, L. 1976. Cortical spreading depression and memory transfer: A methodological critique. *Behav. Biol.* 16: 79–84.

Puccetti, R. 1973. Brain bisection and personal identity. *Brit. J. Phil. Sci.* 24: 339–55.

−1981. The case for mental duality: Evidence from split-brain data and other considerations. *Behav. Brain Sci.* 4: 93–123.

Ridgway, S. H., and E. F. Flanigan. 1984. Electrophysiological observations during sleep in the bottlenosed porpoise (*Tursiops truncatus*). Forthcoming.

Russell, I. S., and S. C. Morgan. 1979. Interocular transfer of visual learning in the rat. *In* I. S. Russell, M. W. Van Hof, and G. Berlucchi (eds.) *Structure and Function of Cerebral Commissures.* University Park Press, Baltimore.

Semmes, J., and M. Mishkin. 1965. A search for the cortical substrate of tactual memories. *In* G. Ettlinger (ed.) *Functions of the Corpus Callosum,* Ciba Foundation Study Group No. 20. Little, Brown, Boston.

Serafetinides, E. A., J. T. Shurley, and R. E. Brooks. 1972. Electroencephalogram of the pilot whale, *Globicephala scammoni,* in wakefulness and sleep: Lateralization aspects. *Int. J. Psychobiol.* 2: 129–35.

Sidtis, J. J., and M. P. Bryden. 1978. Asymmetrical perceptions of language and music: Evidence for independent processing strategies. *Neuropsychol.* 16: 627–32.

Sperry, R. W. 1974. Lateral specialization in the surgically separated hemispheres. *In* F. O. Schmitt, and F. G. Worden (eds.) *The Neurosciences: Third Study Program.* The MIT Press, Cambridge, pp. 5–19.

Sperry, R. W., and E. Clark. 1949. Interocular transfer of visual discrimination habits in a teleost fish. *Physiol. Zool.* 22: 372–8.

Sperry, R. W., E. Zaidel, and D. Zaidel. 1979. Self-recognition and social awareness in the deconnected minor hemisphere. *Neuropsychol.* 17: 153–66.

Trevarthen, C. B., and R. W. Sperry, 1973. Perceptual unity of the ambient visual field in human commissurotomy patients. *Brain* 96: 547–70.

Van Hof, M. W. 1979. Interocular transfer and interhemispheric communication in the rabbit. *In* I. S. Russell, M. W. Van Hof, and G. Berlucchi (eds.) *Structure and Function of Cerebral Commissures.* University Park Press, Baltimore.

Voneida, T. J., and J. S. Robinson. 1970. Effect of brain bisection on capacity for cross comparison of patterned visual input. *Exp. Neurol..* 26: 60–71.

Weiskrantz, L., E. K. Warrington, M. D. Sanders, and J. Marshall. 1974. Visual capacity in the hemianopic field following a restricted occipital ablation. *Brain* 97: 709–28.

Wenzel, B. M., R. D. Tschirgi, and J. L. Taylor. 1962. Effects of early postnatal hemidecortication on spatial discrimination in cats. *Exp. Neurol..* 6: 332–9.

Wigan, A. L. 1844. *The duality of the mind: A new view of insanity.* Longman, Brown, Green and Longmans, London.

Yakovlev, P. I., and A. R. Lecours. 1967. The myelogenetic cycles of regional maturation of the brain. *In* A. Minkowski (ed.) *Regional Development of the Brain in Early Life.* Blackwell, Edinburgh.

Zaidel, E. 1983. Disconnection syndrome as a model for laterality effects in the normal brain. *In* J. Hellige (ed.) *Cerebral Hemisphere Asymmetry: Method, Theory and Application.* Praeger, New York.

Zeki, S. M. 1967. Visual deficits related to size of lesion in "prestriate" cortex of optic chiasm sectioned monkeys. *Life Sci.* 6: 1627–38.

Zola-Morgan, S., L. R. Squire, and M. Mishkin. 1982. The neuroanatomy of amnesia: Amygdala-hippocampus versus temporal stem. *Science* 218: 1337–9.

13 Regulation and generation of perception in the asymmetric brain

Jerre Levy
Department of Behavioral Sciences
University of Chicago

There is a certain absurd faith in believing that we can decipher the secrets of this stuff in our heads, especially because, at the current time, we do not even have the foggiest notion regarding the temporal and spatial organizations of matter that make for consciousness. As Sperry (1983) says, "When it comes to even imagining the critical variables in these patterns that correlate with variables that we do know in inner, conscious experience, we are still hopelessly lost" (p. 30). Yet, in spite of this, in spite of the fact that the human brain is the most complex piece of matter in the known universe, and in spite of the absurdity of our faith, enormous progress in understanding has been made in recent decades, and this is due, in no small measure, to Roger Sperry's contributions.

Beyond his purely scientific achievements, Sperry (1983) has offered a new way of viewing the relations between the age-old concerns of philosophers and humanists and those of modern brain science. In this conception, man is truly self-determined, not because he is free of causes, but rather because the spatiotemporal pattern of neural activity that is consciousness encompasses the broadest causal domain in all evolved life, and this is the "top-level regulator" in the causal hierarchy that controls neural activity.

In this chapter, I review and discuss evidence for self-regulatory systems in the human brain as these relate to asymmetric functioning of the two cerebral hemispheres. This issue is closely associated, in my view, with ideas Sperry offered on brain function more than 30 years ago (1952). He emphasized that brains evolved for the regulation of behavior, and that brain activity had this as its ultimate end. Motor activity, instead of being "something to carry out, serve, and satisfy the demands of the higher centers" (Sperry 1952, p. 299), is the end itself, and mental activity is the means to this end. Sperry argued convincingly that adequate stimulus input was radically insufficient for a perception, and that perception occurred when and only when there was a preparation to respond.

He said, "... the preparation for response *is* the perception" (p. 301, his emphasis). This perspective was startling to most students of brain/behavior relations at the time the article was published, and it remains so today. Yet Sperry clearly demonstrated that adequate sensory stimulation was, indeed, insufficient for a perception. Something more was needed, some internal resetting of the brain, some dynamic change in spatiotemporal neural activity that at the same time prepared the organism for action, and that was intrinsic to the brain itself. "The patterning of the perceptual process is determined as much by *the organization of the central mechanisms* as it is by the sensory influx" (Sperry 1952, p. 302, emphasis added).

I shall argue that studies of brain-damaged patients, split-brain patients, and normal individuals give strong support both to Sperry's proposals of more than 30 years ago (Sperry 1952) and to his more recent ideas on human self-determination in consciousness (Sperry 1983). The conceptual models Sperry has presented are, of necessity, broadly outlined and general. Some might contend that they do not allow the derivation of specific experimental predictions. I think that they do, and I believe that the various observations would be difficult to comprehend from any other perspective.

Some historical considerations

THE DOMINANT LEFT HEMISPHERE

Until relatively recent times, neuropsychology was restricted to psychological examination of patients suffering from brain damage. The underlying interpretive assumption of such clinical studies was that if there was a deficiency syndrome in association with a brain lesion, then areas remaining intact must be incompetent for the disordered function, and the damaged area was crucial. At the dawn of neuropsychology, the work of Dax (1865), Broca (1861a, 1861b), and Wernicke (1874) showed that in the vast majority of right-handers, damage to critical regions of the left hemisphere regularly led to language disorders, whereas comparable lesions in the right hemisphere did not. These observations, and many subsequent confirmations, were interpreted to mean that the left hemisphere was dominant in language and that the right hemisphere was linguistically incompetent, either for language production or comprehension.

Since it was a common view that language was synonymous with thought, and since, in any case, symptoms of right-hemisphere damage are not as spectacular as aphasia, the left hemisphere was held to be dominant for all cognitive processes, linguistic and nonlinguistic, and the right hemisphere was seen as a relay station (see Bogen 1969 for review). Yet, Hughlings Jackson (Taylor 1958), as early as 1876, had noted distinctive symptoms resulting from right-hemisphere damage and suggested that the right hemisphere was predominant in "visual ideation" (p. 148), and in subsequent years, similar findings and interpretations appeared.

Weisenberg and McBride (1935) reported that patients with right-side damage showed selective deficits on tasks that were dependent on "the appreciation and manipulation of forms

and spatial relationships" (p. 329). Paterson and Zangwill (1944) described disorders of space perception in patients with right-hemisphere lesions, as did McFie, Piercy, and Zangwill (1950). Hécaen and Angelergues found that right-hemisphere damage, more than left-hemisphere damage, interfered with space perception (1963) and with recognition of faces (1962). In contrast to the prevailing view, these researchers, and others who investigated symptoms of right-hemisphere damage, concluded that both sides of the human brain were highly specialized organs of thought, in which each hemisphere was superior in a set of processes that were complementary to those on the other side.

However, there was great resistance to this dethroning of the left hemisphere, so much so that the fundamental interpretative assumption was abandoned. Alajouanine and Lhermitte (1963) pointed out that symptoms of brain damage not only reflect functional suppression of damaged regions, but also abnormal release of intact regions. They interpreted the symptoms of right-hemisphere damage as being due to pathological activity that was released in the left hemisphere, and they even claimed that right-hemisphere syndromes, rather than revealing any specialized right-hemisphere abilities, demonstrated, instead, the specializations of the *left* hemisphere! These authors never explained why an indirect disruption of left-hemisphere function via a right-hemisphere lesion should produce greater disorders in face recognition than direct left-hemisphere damage.

Nonetheless, the proposal of Alajouanine and Lhermitte left neurological science at an impasse. Once it was offered, it meant that regardless of the nature and severity of symptoms resulting from unilateral lesions, no secure implications could be drawn regarding hemispheric specialization. Symptoms might possibly reflect losses of the specialized processes of the damaged hemisphere, but they could equally likely reflect disordered effects on the specialized processes of the intact hemisphere. On purely logical grounds, there was no way to decide between the two alternatives, and, indeed, by Alajouanine and Lhermitte's (1963) reasoning, language disorders following left-hemisphere lesions might indicate pathological activity in the right hemisphere (an issue they never discussed).

When the classical theory was challenged, a variety of alternatives was possible, and the logical basis for interpreting any functional deficits became much more difficult. In retrospect, based on studies of both split-brain patients and normal people, it is clear that Alajouanine and Lhermitte (1963) were wrong about defects following right-hemisphere damage, but this does not mean that the premise they questioned is correct. This premise, that one can infer locus of function from losses of function, involves two components that have rarely been conceptually separated. First, and most obvious, is the claim that damaged areas are important in the disrupted function. It is also assumed that regions remaining intact are incompetent for the disordered process. Underlying this second claim is the further unstated premise that, by some mysterious mechanism, the brain, whether damaged or not, automatically allocates processing to those regions and systems that are the most competent available anywhere in the brain, so that observable performance becomes a direct indication of the maximum abilities of residual intact areas.

This "automaticity" premise is peculiar on a number of grounds. It posits, though not explicitly, that there is a homunculus who knows precisely all the functions of every system of the brain, not only when the brain is normal, but also when it is damaged. It also knows with perfect accuracy the functions and processes that are called for by a given task or problem. Thus, the homunculus always allocates processing to that brain system that is most competent for the task, and its decisions are always as lucid and logical in the presence of brain damage as in the normal brain. Additionally, it has no preconceived biases that might have been developed through millions of years of evolution and through a lifetime of experience with a complete brain. Prior to a lesion of Wernicke's area of the left hemisphere, the homunculus knew that certain linguistic analyses should be allocated to posterior language-processing regions. Following destruction of these areas, it knows to allocate the processing required for word comprehension to the intact right hemisphere; or if it does not know this immediately, it quickly learns, by trial and error, to make this allocation. Consequently, if patients with left-hemisphere damage do not comprehend words, we can be sure we are seeing the incompetencies of the right hemisphere, not the disordered processing of the damaged left hemisphere. In fact, of course, there is neither an empirical nor logical basis for the foregoing assumptions, and there are both biological and neurological reasons for doubting their validity.

From a biological standpoint, it is difficult to believe that cerebral regulatory systems widespread in the brain would not be biased by anatomy and physiological design to activate those processing organizations that inherently and by experience are normally specialized for particular cognitive operations. Neurologically, it is practically inconceivable that regulatory systems would retain perfect capacities for assessing relative efficiencies of different processing organizations when the brain is damaged. Indeed, the anosognosias consequent to brain damage demonstrate that metacognitive evaluations are frequently disrupted to a serious degree. If a patient with jargon aphasia fails to recognize abnormalities in his speech, there is no reason to suppose that some hidden cerebral system could do so. I know of no reports of patients with total left hemispherectomy who manifest jargon aphasia, and this is an important clue that symptoms of jargon aphasia reflect abnormal processing by a damaged left hemisphere, not characteristics of the intact right hemisphere. And if this is so with respect to jargon aphasia, the neurological implications of other behavioral symptoms of brain damage become far less obvious than has been assumed.

Thus, although Alajouanine and Lhermitte (1963) were wrong in the particular extreme interpretation they offered of right-hemisphere symptoms, they highlighted real conceptual difficulties in moving from observations of deficiency syndromes in brain-damaged patients to conclusions regarding brain organization. Their challenge made it apparent that valid neuropsychological inferences would require converging and consistent evidence from a variety of approaches, including not only studies of patients with cerebral lesions, but also those of split-brain patients and normal individuals. Their emphasis on possible release phenomena brought to attention, also, questions concerning activation effects and general neural regulation.

Brain-damaged and split-brain patients: An inconsistency?

The early studies of split-brain patients by Sperry and his colleagues and students (Sperry, Gazzaniga, and Bogen 1969) demonstrated a remarkable capacity of each isolated hemisphere to perceive, think, and govern behavior, but they also showed, in contrast to earlier opinions, that the right hemisphere could derive associative meaning for both spoken and written words. Indeed, Zaidel (1976a) has found that the isolated right hemisphere possesses an extensive comprehension vocabulary, in spite of its expressive aphasia and its serious deficiencies in syntactical understanding (Hillyard and Gazzaniga 1971, Zaidel 1977), verbal short-term memory (Zaidel 1977), and phonetic analysis (Zaidel 1976b, Levy and Trevarthen 1977).

Additionally, although investigations of aphasic patients with left-hemisphere damage revealed extremely poor performance in associating colors with line drawings of well-known objects (DeRenzi and Spinnler 1967; DeRenzi et al. 1972; Basso, Faglioni, and Spinnler 1976; Cohen and Kelter 1979), the isolated right hemisphere of split-brain patients was shown to perform at least as well as the left on this task, and possibly better (Levy and Trevarthen 1981).

Although some might suggest that the findings from aphasic and split-brain patients are inconsistent regarding the capacities of the right hemisphere, an alternative is that the only inconsistency is in inferences and not in the observations themselves. As discussed, deficiency syndromes associated with unilateral brain damage do not necessarily reveal incompetencies of the intact hemisphere, but might, instead, reflect the disordered mentation of the damaged hemisphere that is still holding control of processing and behavior. If so, this would imply that there are metacontrolling programs in the brain that can allocate processing to and selectively activate specific functional systems of the hemispheres in accordance with inherent or acquired evaluations of task demands. In the following sections, studies of split-brain patients and of normal individuals are reviewed that bear on this issue and on the relation of the selective construction of percepts and behavioral responses.

Behavior, perception, and hemispheric regulation in split-brain patients
PERCEPTUAL CONSTRUCTION
AND MOTOR RESPONSES

Early studies of the California series of split-brain patients suggested the possibility that the left hemisphere might be dominant for executive motor control. Thus, although Sperry et al. (1969) note that voluntary motor responses are not restricted to the left hemisphere, they go on to say that "Except in those special testing situations in which considerable care was taken to evoke leading activity in the minor hemisphere, one had the impression that the separated major hemisphere was in command most of the time" (p. 285).

Yet, by 1971, Levy, Nebes, and Sperry (1971) suggested that "When a hemisphere is intrinsically better equipped to handle some task, it is also easier for that hemisphere to dominate motor pathways. This relationship would suggest that the minor hemisphere would be motor dominant for tasks in which it is superior" (p. 57). The idea that there was an inherent relation between a hemisphere's ability, compared to its partner, and its tendency to dominate processing and behavior is closely associated with, and indeed a prediction from, Sperry's (1952) hypothesis that perception cannot be dissociated from response preparation.

Beginning in 1970, Colwyn Trevarthen and I, with Sperry's guidance and collaboration, designed a series of studies of split-brain patients to investigate hemispheric regulation (Levy, Trevarthen, and Sperry 1972, Levy and Trevarthen 1976, 1977, 1981). Earlier work had confirmed the left hemisphere's predominance in language functions (Sperry et al. 1969) and the right hemisphere's predominance in spatial constructive activities (Bogen and Gazzaniga 1965) and in visuospatial understanding (Levy-Agresti and Sperry 1968), but little was known regarding the conditions under which each hemisphere derived a perception and the mechanisms by which a hemisphere gained control over processing and behavior.

Our method was based on findings that when stimuli are projected in the center of the visual field to split-brain patients, so that each hemisphere receives information only from the contralateral half, there is a perceptual completion in which the perceptual construct is of a whole and complete stimulus (Trevarthen 1974a, 1974b). The tests with commissurotomy patients followed research on visual learning and eye–hand coordination in split-brain monkeys (Trevarthen 1965). The results of simultaneous learning tests with the monkeys indicated that when they were looking at overlapping polarized stimuli, a different one visible to each hemisphere, they could have double awareness. The patterns were received as "left–right chimeras" whenever the monkey with optic chiasma and corpus callosum transected fixated the middle of the compound stimulus on a response screen (Trevarthen 1968). It should be noted here that, beyond the fact that adequate stimulus input is not sufficient for a perception, since an appropriate preparatory set for action is also required, perceptual-completion effects show that inadequate stimulus input does not necessarily imply a similarly depleted perception. Moreover, the completion effect found for single stimuli meeting the vertical meridian on one side operated equally for two-sided chimeric stimuli like those shown in Figure 13.1 (Levy et al. 1972.)

With one half-stimulus joined at the midline to a different half-stimulus to make a "chimera," each hemisphere would receive equivalent, but different, stimulus input, and if two perceptions were gained, they would be in conflict as evidence concerning the object of interest, and the motor responses guided by those percepts would be in conflict. The classical views of cerebral function that Sperry challenged (Sperry 1952) would predict that each hemisphere would derive its own percept, and that double responses, one for each percept, would be given. If, however, perception *is* the preparation to respond, then, except in special circumstances, there should be a single perception linked to a single response under conditions of competitive stimulus input. Further, which hemisphere gains the percept would depend both on the form of motor responses prepared and on the nature of cognitive processes required to recognize the stimulus, since both would determine "the organization of central mechanisms" (Sperry 1952, p. 302).

Our studies overwhelmingly confirmed the predictions of this conceptual model. For all patients examined, and for tasks including the perception of faces, nonsense shapes, pictures of common objects, patterns of Xs and squares, words, word meaning, phonetic images of rhyming pictures, and outline drawings to be matched to colors, patients gave one response on the vast majority of competitive trials. Further, the nonresponding hemisphere gave no evidence that it had any perception at all. Thus, if the right hemisphere responded, there was no indication, by words or facial expression, that the left hemisphere had any argument with the choice made, and, similarly, if the left hemisphere responded, no behavior on the part of the patient suggested a disagreement by the right hemisphere.

When patients were asked to describe the stimulus they saw, the left hemisphere dominated, and the left-hemisphere percept was described, and this was true regardless of the type of stimulus or the task. Obviously, this was expected since the right hemisphere cannot speak. Yet, it could hear the left hemisphere's description, and if this was discordant with some percept it had, then, as had been observed when the left hemisphere confabulates a description of some object that only the right hemisphere knows, one might have expected to see a frown or head shake or some other indication of the right hemisphere's distress at the inaccurate (from its point of view) response.

The foregoing observations strongly indicate that double perceptions did not, in fact, occur in a great majority of trials. When and only when there was a preparation to respond was a perception generated, and without this preparation, no perception was constructed by the nonresponding hemisphere. It could be ar-

TARGET OBJECTS　　CHIMERIC STIMULI

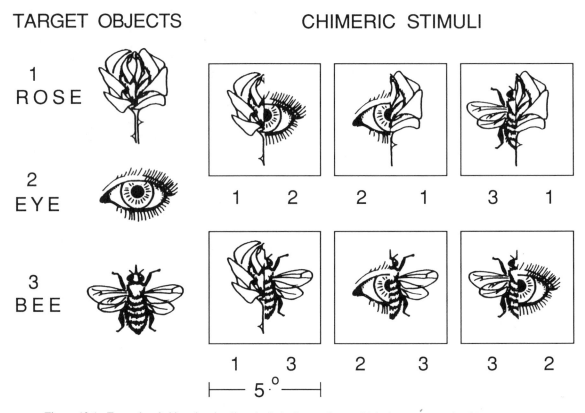

Figure 13.1. Example of chimeric stimuli and whole figures from which they were made. (From Levy, Trevarthen, and Sperry, 1972.)

gued that, for whatever reason, the nonresponding hemisphere simply failed to acquire the necessary sensory information. If so, then it would be impossible to induce a perception, even with an attention-directing procedure. This is discussed next.

UNCONSCIOUS INFORMATION AND THE PERCEPT

There is a phenomenon in psychology called the "what-did-you-say" effect. It is a common experience that we may be engaged in a conversation with A, when B comes up and addresses some comment to us. We know *something* has been said, but we do not know what, and thus ask, "What did you say?" Now the strange thing is, as soon as we ask the question, we know the answer. The auditory input had been stored at a low level and not constructed to the level of a conscious percept since attention had not been directed to it, but our asking the question directs atten-

tion, and as soon as this occurs, the perception is generated.

In a careful and elegant series of experiments, Sperling (1960) investigated this attentional effect by presenting tachistoscopic arrays of from 3 to 12 letters and asking subjects to identify them. There was perfect recall for three-letter and four-letter arrays, but not for larger arrays. For these, only four to five letters could be retrieved, regardless of the size of the array and regardless of whether arrays had been presented for 15, 50, 200, or 500 ms. This made it unlikely that the limit on recall was due to a limit in the amount of information initially extracted. Rather, it seemed that there was a limit on the amount of information that could be taken from a temporary low-level and unconscious storage and turned into a perception.

To examine this, Sperling (1960) presented 12-letter arrays arranged into three rows of four letters each for 50 ms, and *after* the offset of the stimulus, played either a high, middle, or low tone to designate a report of the top, middle, or bottom row, respectively. He found that the proportion of letters recalled greatly increased, indicating that preconscious information could be constructed to a percept if attention was directed toward it.

Thus, it should be that preconscious information in the nonresponding hemisphere of the split-brain patient could be brought to consciousness by an attention-directing procedure. This would then demonstrate that the absence of any indication of a percept under standard conditions could *not* be attributed to a failure of information to penetrate the central nervous system.

In our competitive face-perception task (Levy et al. 1972), there had been a strong right-hemisphere dominance when subjects were required to select a matching face from an array in free vision, and, of course, the left hemisphere dominated when subjects were asked to name or describe the face. For the matching task, therefore, we hypothesized that it was the right hemisphere that was prepared to respond and that thereby gained the perception. To test this, we interrupted the patient on a few trials before a response could occur, removed the array, and asked for a verbal description. We presumed that this procedure would direct attention to information held in the left hemisphere, and, indeed, patients then supplied a description of the face projected to the left hemisphere. When the array was replaced and subjects were asked to pick a matching choice, the face projected to the right hemisphere was picked.

Similarly, when verbal trials were interrupted, and patients were directed to pick a matching face, we presumed that this would direct attention to information in the right hemisphere. Under these conditions patients did, in fact, select a face matching the one projected to the right side of the brain. When they were then asked to describe the face, they described the face projected to the left side of the brain. In brief, preconscious information had evidently been available in the nonresponding hemisphere, and this could be brought to perception by an attention-directing procedure. With instructions that directed attention both ways, both hemispheres would gain a percept,

one because the trial interruption would shift attention to preconsciously stored information, and the other because it had been prepared to respond by a previous and different instruction.

This overt conflict between responses on the interrupted trials resulted in considerable perplexity and confusion on the part of the patients, in quite dramatic contrast to their placid equanimity on noninterrupted trials, when only a single response was given, and when only a single perception was indicated. These data, and similar effects of perceptual retention or erasure obtained with the same subjects when responses of the hemispheres were put in conflict by other procedures (Trevarthen 1974a, 1974b), provide evidence for the close connection between perceptions and responses, but the question still remains as to the factors determining which hemisphere gained control over processing and behavior in a given test. It was not only that the left hemisphere dominated when a verbal response was required, but it also excelled under certain matching conditions, whereas the right hemisphere dominated for other matching tasks. How is such asymmetric hemispheric control regulated?

METACONTROL OF HEMISPHERIC FUNCTION

When subjects were matching stimuli, we found that the right hemisphere was dominant for matching of faces, nonsense shapes, patterns of Xs and squares, pictures of common objects, and even words. In contrast, the left hemisphere dominated when words had to be matched to pictures or when pictures had to be matched for rhyming names. When whole faces or nonsense shapes were projected unilaterally to the left hemisphere, and not in competition with a stimulus in the other field, we found that the left hemisphere's performance was considerably worse than the right hemisphere's had been under competitive conditions with the stimulus chimeras. Similarly, when the rhyming-picture task was given to the right hemisphere alone, we found that it performed at chance.

With only the foregoing observations as a basis, one could propose that, under competitive conditions, the superior hemisphere simply won a speed contest for control over motor pathways that shut out the other hemisphere. In such a case, there would be no need to posit any regulatory system that selectively allocated processing to one side or the other before the response was generated. However, the left hemisphere was essentially perfect at naming pictures of common objects and was actually superior in describing patterns of Xs and squares, as compared to the right hemisphere's ability to match these stimuli. Further, in matching simple words to pictures that they named, the right hemisphere was perfectly competent when it was not in competition with the left. These peculiar discrepancies between competence versus dominance under competitive conditions strongly suggested that the "speed-contest" model was inadequate.

Further insight was gained by examining hemispheric control as a function of task instructions (Levy and Trevarthen 1976). Figure 13.2 shows one of the sets of stimuli we used. On one run of trials, patients were told to select a choice that *looked similar* to the stimulus they saw, and on another run of trials, they were told to pick a choice that would be *used with* or that *went with* the stimulus they saw. The stimuli, choices, and pointing responses remained invariant over instructional conditions.

First, for all four patients tested, there was a highly significant interaction between the instruction given and the hemisphere controlling the response: with visual-similarity instructions, the right hemisphere dominated, and with functional-association instructions, the left hemisphere dominated. Second, although the matching strategy that patients used was sometimes opposite to the instruction given, all except one patient, CC, made relatively more visual matches with visual-similarity instructions and relatively more functional matches with functional-association instructions.

Nevertheless, in spite of the foregoing relations, there were some remarkable dissociations between the strategy of matching used and the hemisphere in control. This is most dramatically highlighted in the case of CC. For 20 out of 22 correct matches with visual-similarity instructions, the right hemisphere controlled responses, and for 19 of these, a visual match was made. For 14 out of 17 correct matches with functional-association instructions, the left hemisphere controlled responses, *but* for all 14, visual and not functional matches were made! Thus, CC had an extremely strong bias to match according to visual similarity, but

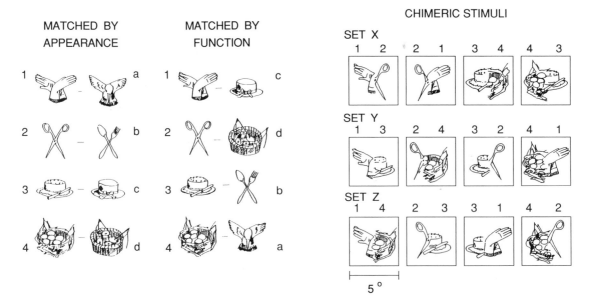

Figure 13.2. One set of chimeric stimuli, whole figures from which they were made, and functional and visual-matching stimuli that were used to explore the effect of task instruction on hemispheric control. (From Levy and Trevarthen 1976.)

nonetheless, opposite hemispheres assumed control in response to instructions to perform visual and functional comparisons.

Such a dissociation means that the control of hemispheric dominance was mediated by a system that, while highly sensitive to task instructions, was quite distinct from that determining the actual processing operations of a hemisphere once it was in control. In that paper, we concluded that hemispheric control "does not depend on the hemisphere's real aptitude but on what it *thinks* it can do" (Levy and Trevarthen, 1976, p. 310, original emphasis). We conceived of this metacontrolling "thinking" system as representing an interaction between higher cortical processes and brainstem "arousal" or "attention-setting" regions. Each hemisphere would process task instructions, evaluate these with respect to its beliefs regarding its cognitive characteristics and competencies, and via corticoreticular pathways would send signals for arousal or appropriate attentional activations. These signals would vary in strength, depending on the outcome of the evaluative process, and brainstem areas would respond accordingly, biasing control, through inherently lateralized component pathways, to either the left or right hemisphere. Under this model, the dominance and competence of a hemisphere would usually be correlated (since beliefs or recollections about and actual effective competencies would be correlated), but the correlation would be imperfect. Dissociations could occur because the underlying mechanisms governing hemispheric arousal are distinct from those involved in task processing itself.

This conception offers a resolution of the finding that patients with left-hemisphere damage often show serious disorders in functions that the isolated right hemisphere of a split-brain patient handles relatively well. When linguistic processes are called for, the metacontrolling system, even in the patient with left-hemisphere damage, would, on occasion, direct control to the left hemisphere. However, once this damaged hemisphere has control of processing, the lesion disrupts cognitive operations and highly abnormal behavior is observed. A similar control by the left hemisphere would

not be unlikely to occur when patients are asked to match line drawings to their typical colors. In this test, features of the depicted object (its shape and color) have been artificially dissociated. The evidence we have suggests that the left hemisphere normally organizes its representations according to a list of describable feature characteristics, whereas right-hemisphere representations tend to integrate and synthesize features into a unified schema or form (see Chapter 19, this volume). If so, the task to associate a drawn object to its color would be "normal" for the left hemisphere and "abnormal" for the right hemisphere, resulting in a bias favoring the left side.

The idea that processing is allocated according to belief systems, that each hemisphere with associated brain systems evaluates itself and directs nerve-impulse traffic according to its evaluation, is precisely the model of cerebral function that Sperry (1983) proposes. It is a model in which those spatiotemporal patterns of neural activity that make up consciousness naturally supersede and regulate lower-level or more peripheral nerve-impulse traffic. The fact that task instructions alone are sufficient to shift control to one hemisphere or the other, even when the controlling hemisphere then fails to follow the instructions, would be difficult to comprehend under any other proposal.

In summary, investigations of both unilaterally brain-damaged patients and split-brain patients point to the conclusion that mental representations are closely bound to preparations for action, and that widely distributed systems in the brain govern the flow of nerve-impulse traffic and the allocation of processing according to belief systems about its competencies for various cognitive tasks. Those beliefs may be wrong, either because a particular task has peculiar characteristics that mislead the evaluative system, or because the brain is damaged or disordered. Thus, in the first case, for example, the right hemisphere may assume control over processing and behavior because general task requirements seem compatible with its functions, whereas specific characteristics of the task are beyond its effective field of operation.

In summarizing their data on competitive

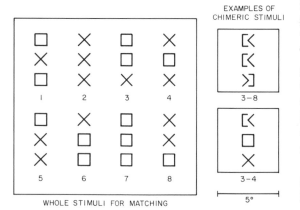

EXAMPLES OF
CHIMERIC STIMULI

3 – 8

3 – 4

|⊢——————⊣|
5°

WHOLE STIMULI FOR MATCHING

Figure 13.3. The stimuli used in the test of perception of vertical triads of "form types," Xs and squares. (From Levy, Trevarthen, and Sperry 1972.)

perception for physical-identity matching, Levy et al. (1972) say, "Where the task needs no more than visual recognition, a visual encoding ensues, mediated by the right hemisphere and based on the form properties of the stimulus as such rather than on separate feature analysis" (p. 75). Thus, the right hemisphere, was dominant in the matching of three-component vertical patterns of Xs and squares (Figure 13.3), yet its actual performance, on this task, was worse than that of the left hemisphere when it was producing descriptions of the patterns. The different triads of Xs and squares had, apparently, no distinctive configurational properties in vision. The type (X or square) and ordering of features in a group of three did not define any global form for the ensemble and possessed no "visual syntax." This is to say that synthesis of features did not generate form, and there were no rules of form that constrained the type and ordering of features. This contrasts with recognition of faces, nonsense shapes, and most visual objects of ordinary experience; these are perceived to have distinctive forms as wholes (Figure 13.1). The right hemisphere's dominance was determined by the general nature of the task (matching for physical identity) and was unaffected by the fact that its specialized programs, although normally superior for tasks of this type, were actually inferior for the unusual stimulus items employed in the former test with Xs and squares.

In the second case, where brain damage

is present, it appears that a similar type of error is made because a brain system has a mistaken "belief" about its own functional competence. The evaluative system bases its decisions on general conclusions about the normal processing abilities and fails to detect or take account of the disruption of function consequent to brain damage. The prevalence of anosognosias with brain damage is easy to explain on this model.

Obviously, the observations so far discussed pertain directly only to various neurological patients or to animals subjected to experimental brain surgery, and it is important to determine whether the inferences derived from these generalize to normal individuals. Studies bearing on this issue are discussed in the following section.

Activation and specialization of the hemispheres in normal people
LATERAL BIASES OF PERCEPTION AND SPECIALIZED PROCESSING

Beginning in the early 1960s, Kimura (1961, 1966, 1967) applied behavioral techniques involving dichotic listening and lateralized tachistoscopic presentation of visual stimuli to investigate hemispheric specialization in normal people. She proposed that under dichotic listening conditions, ipsilateral auditory pathways were blocked so that each hemisphere initially received input only from the contralateral ear. Since each visual half-field projects strictly to the contralateral hemisphere, initial visual input could easily be restricted to a single hemisphere by tachistoscopic methods. Her reasoning was that, in spite of intact commissural pathways, normal people should manifest asymmetries of accuracy or speed in favor of the sensory half-field contralateral to the specialized hemisphere.

This would occur either because each hemisphere would process contralateral information or because there would be a loss of fidelity or speed in the course of commissural transmission from the unspecialized to the specialized hemisphere. Such asymmetries have indeed been found repeatedly in a large number of studies, and consistent with neurological inferences, average asymmetry patterns of left- and right-handers differ (see Bradshaw and Nettleton 1983 for a review). The Kimura explanations of the mechanisms underlying dichotic or tachistoscopic perceptual asymmetries have come to be known as "structural models," the implication being that hemispheric specialization and the anatomy of the commissural pathways are directly responsible for the asymmetries observed, with no intermediate mechanisms.

However, at a conference in 1969, Trevarthen (1972) discussed attentional aspects of hemispheric regulation and noted that when one hemisphere was asymmetrically activated in vertebrate animals, this generated the lateral orientation reflex toward the contralateral side of space. Thus, if a stimulus appears to one side of space, this is initially projected to the contralateral hemisphere, producing a transiently higher arousal of this hemisphere compared to the ipsilateral hemisphere. The asymmetry of arousal triggers, first, a biased attention toward the source of stimulation, and then, actual movements of the eyes, head, and whole body that bring the stimulus into the central behavioral field. He reasoned that in human beings, where each hemisphere is specialized for different functions, asymmetries of hemispheric activation could and would be induced by pure thought, and with the same effects on laterally biased attention and turning as an asymmetric stimulus. On this model, then, a right-ear advantage (REA) or right-visual-field (RVF) advantage on a verbal task would not necessarily depend on restricted hemispheric input, but instead could arise from selective central left-hemisphere activation that biased attention toward the right sensory field.

TASK-SPECIFIC HEMISPHERIC ACTIVATION

Following up on the foregoing ideas, Kinsbourne (1970, 1974a) reviewed neurological evidence that supported the idea that asymmetric hemispheric activation, no matter how produced, did, indeed, induce the lateral orientation reflex. He (Kinsbourne 1972, 1974b) showed that verbal thought induced rightward eye movements and that spatial thought induced leftward eye movements. Studies of electrocortical activity (Morgan, McDonald, and MacDonald 1971; Galin and Ornstein 1972; McKee, Humphrey, and McAdam 1973; Mor-

gan, MacDonald, and Hilgard 1974; Galin and Ellis 1975; Amochaev and Salamy 1979; Spydell, Ford, and Sheer 1979; Ehrlichman and Wiener 1979, 1980) and of cerebral blood flow (Risberg et al. 1975; Gur and Reivich 1980) confirmed that verbal processing was associated with a selective activation of the left hemisphere and that spatial processing was associated with a selective activation of the right hemisphere.

Gilbert and Bakan (1973) were the first to show that right-handed subjects had a leftward perceptual bias when processing face photographs shown in free vision. The left half of photographs was more salient, as indicated by the fact that the majority of right-handers, but not left-handers, judged bisymmetric composites to look more similar to the original face (or its mirror image) when the composite had been made from the half-face to the subject's left. Heller and Levy (1981) observed a perceptual bias toward the left for tachistoscopically presented chimeric faces made from a half-face that was smiling joined to a half-face from the same poser with a neutral expression. However, Levy, Heller, Banich, and Burton (1983a) subsequently showed that this effect was equally strong when face chimeras were shown in free vision. In both the tachistoscopic study (Heller and Levy 1981) and the free-vision study (Levy et al. 1983a), the chimeric face with the smile to the subject's left was perceived as happier than its mirror image.

Bowers and Heilman (1980) found that on a spatial tactile task, performance was superior when stimuli were placed on the left side of space. Thus, it is not only that attention is biased to the left during spatial tasks, but that performance is enhanced for stimuli in the left hemispatial field.

Tweedy, Rinn, and Springer (1980) reported that when two simultaneous syllables were played over loudspeakers, one to the left and one to the right, there was a recognition advantage for syllables played over the right speaker. This effect has also been examined by Morais and Bertelson (1975) and Keller (1977). Recently, Levy and Kueck (1986) found a right hemispatial field advantage for identifying rhyming target words among a large array of distractors when stimulus items were presented in free vision. This was independent of whether subjects scanned items from the left to right or from the right to left.

The foregoing findings strongly support Trevarthen's (1972) proposals and show clearly that each specialized hemisphere is asymmetrically aroused during performance on tasks that call on its specialized functions, an arousal that induces an attentional bias toward the contralateral field. It appears, therefore, that the normal brain, like the commissurotomized brain, directs cerebral activity selectively toward the hemisphere that is differentially specialized for a particular task. It could be maintained, however, that this is not reflective of a metacontrolling system, but instead is merely a reflection of the ongoing processing activities of the hemisphere. In order to establish that hemispheric regulation is based on a separate system from the specialized processing activities of a hemisphere, it would be necessary to demonstrate dissociations between the two.

HEMISPHERIC ACTIVATION VERSUS SPECIALIZED PROCESSING

Investigations of individual differences in hemispheric activation and in perceptual asymmetries provide direct evidence that cognitive specialization and asymmetric activation of hemispheres may have separable effects on perception, which are manifested differently in different circumstances. Normative dichotic and tachistoscopic studies reveal group asymmetry patterns in right-handers that are fully consistent with the neurological literature, but they also show considerable diversity among subjects in both the degree and the direction of perceptual asymmetries. These variations cannot all be attributed to errors of measurement, since, at least in some studies, the individual differences are highly reliable (Heller and Levy 1981; Shankweiler and Studdert-Kennedy 1975).

The source of these diversities is indicated by physiological measurements of brain activity. From data presented by Morgan et al. (1971) of baseline EEG arousal asymmetries in right-handers, calculation shows a test-retest correlation of 0.89. Thus, in a baseline state when subjects are not engaged in any directed

cognitive task, there are highly stable individual differences in characteristic asymmetries of hemispheric arousal. Similarly, Ehrlichman, and Wiener (1979) reported a reliability of 0.74 for baseline EEG arousal asymmetries and a test-retest consistency of 0.88 for the difference in arousal asymmetries for verbal versus spatial processing. As they say, "Subjects maintain their relative positions over sessions" (p. 249), and this is evidently true not only for baseline measures of arousal symmetry, but also for asymmetries that are present during task processing. Further evidence for individual differences among right-handers in task-independent and characteristic asymmetries of hemispheric activity was found by Dabbs and Choo (1980). They measured blood temperature over the left and right ophthalamic arteries, as subjects were lying quietly, as an index of relative blood flow to the two hemispheres, and found a test-retest reliability of 0.69 in the temperature asymmetry.

That these physiological measures of brain activity are true indicators of hemispheric function is confirmed by their associations with verbal and spatial performance. Thus, subjects with an asymmetry of activation in favor of the left hemisphere show enhanced verbal and reduced spatial performance, whereas those with an asymmetry of activation in favor of the right hemisphere show the reversed cognitive pattern (Furst 1976; Glass and Butler 1977; Rebert 1977; Gale, Davies, and Smallbone 1978; Davidson, Taylor, and Saron 1979; Dabbs and Choo 1980; Gur and Reivich 1980). For example, Dabbs and Choo (1980) examined groups of right-handers who showed high verbal and low spatial ability or low verbal and high spatial ability on standardized psychometric instruments. The former had a temperature asymmetry indicating greater left- than right-hemisphere blood flow, and the latter had a temperature asymmetry indicating greater right- than left-hemisphere blood flow. Furst (1976) found that baseline EEG arousal asymmetries predicted spatial performance.

In brief, direct physiological measurements of brain activity show that right-handed subjects differ in the balance of hemispheric activation, that these differences are picked up even during a baseline state when neither hemisphere is engaged in a cognitive task for which it has special aptitude, and that relative verbal and spatial abilities or performance can be predicted by these individual variations. Clearly, then, it is not merely that activation of a hemisphere is a secondary effect of the stimulation of specialized processing activities; it reflects the influence of an independent system that governs the level of activity of the two sides of the brain whether there is a biasing external situation or not.

BEHAVIORAL ASPECTS OF
ASYMMETRIC AROUSAL

The individual differences in hemispheric activity should be matched by comparable differences in bias of lateral eye movements and in perceptual asymmetries, and these behavioral or cognitive consequences of asymmetric hemispheric activity should have the same associations with verbal and spatial performance as the direct physiological measures. Depending on the conditions under which conjugate lateral eye movements are elicited, it is possible to observe some patterns of gaze that are correlated with verbal or spatial processing, as Kinsbourne found (1972, 1974b), or others that are reflective of individual-difference dimensions (Gur, Gur, and Harris 1975). These latter are correlated with individual differences in hemispheric blood flow (Gur and Reivich 1980), and they show strong and predicted associations with verbal and spatial ability (Tucker and Suib 1978).

On standard behavioral measures of laterality, two factors, then, would determine an individual subject's asymmetry of perception. Task-related asymmetric hemispheric processing would tend to bias attention toward the sensory half-field contralateral to the specialized hemisphere, but this effect would be superimposed on an asymmetry of perception arising from the subject's characteristic individual and task-independent profile of asymmetric hemispheric activation. For a group of right-handers, the group-typical asymmetry would indicate hemispheric specialization, which would act in the same direction for the vast majority of subjects, but individual differences among subjects in the balance of hemispheric

activity would generate variations around the mean for the group.

Thus, a subject with an asymmetry of activation in favor of the left hemisphere would perceive more accurately and more quickly in the right sensory field on verbal tasks, since the task-related effect and the individual's balance of brain activity would be acting in the same direction, but the same person would show a reduced or even a reversal of the usual left sensory field advantage on nonverbal tasks, since the task-related and hemisphere activation effects would be in opposite directions. Precisely the reverse would be observed for a subject with an activation asymmetry in favor of the right hemisphere.

A clear example of such effects is provided by Levine, Banich, and Koch-Weser (1984), who gave right-handers tachistoscopic tasks that showed no perceptual asymmetries in favor of either visual field for the group, then divided subjects into those having a left-visual-field (LVF) and right-visual-field (RVF) advantage. Those with a LVF advantage on the nonlateralized task had a large and highly significant LVF advantage on a face-recognition task and no asymmetry on a word-identification task, whereas the RVF subgroup had no asymmetry on the face-recognition task and a large and highly significant RVF advantage on the word-identification task. Also, the greater the LVF advantage for faces, the better was performance with faces, and the greater the RVF advantage for words, the better was performance with words. These relations are expected since activation in favor of the specialized hemisphere would both promote performance and generate large perceptual asymmetries.

Burton and Levy (unpublished) found the same associations between reaction-time asymmetries for recognizing faces and overall speed of performance in right-handed men. The larger the LVF advantage, the faster was overall responding. Levy et al. (1983b) observed that right-handers with a large RVF advantage on a tachistoscopic syllable-identification task had superior performance as compared to those with weak or no visual-field asymmetries.

The various behavioral results discussed before are completely concordant with investigations on individual differences in physiological measures of hemispheric activity and are predictable from them. Nonetheless, it could still be argued that, although mechanisms controlling relative activity in the hemispheres are separable from specialized processing abilities, task-related asymmetries in hemisphere activation are secondary to, rather than prior to, the processing. Can a decision be made between the two alternatives?

HEMISPHERIC ACTIVATION AND
SPECIAL-PROCESSING EFFECTS
ON PERCEPTUAL ASYMMETRY

As noted, Levy et al. (1983b) found that right-handers with a large RVF advantage for syllable identification outperformed those with weak or no visual-field asymmetries (the strong-asymmetry and weak-asymmetry groups, respectively). These groups had been established by separation at the median of visual-field asymmetry scores. The latter group had, in fact, no asymmetry between fields; none of the 16 subjects within it displayed a statistically significant difference in favor of either visual field.

The errors in identifying syllables were examined for each group and each visual field, since, as Levy et al. (1983b) discuss, prior research had indicated that different types of errors are made, depending on whether stimuli are verbally or nonverbally encoded. It was of interest, therefore, to determine whether patterns of errors were asymmetric between visual fields, and whether, if so, the degree or direction of this asymmetry of error patterns differed between the strong-asymmetry and weak-asymmetry groups. The nature of stimulus encoding should be dependent entirely on hemispheric specialization itself. The baseline level of activation of the two hemispheres would affect performance, as discussed, but would not affect the types of processing applied. This, of course, holds only if specialized processing itself is not the inducer of arousal. If it is, then weak-asymmetry subjects should be just as symmetric in error patterns as they are in overall performance.

In fact, a very strong asymmetry of error types emerged. This indicated verbal encoding for the RVF and nonverbal encoding for the LVF, and this asymmetry was just as great for the weak-asymmetry group as for the strong-asymmetry group. The symmetry of overall performance for weak-asymmetry subjects was due to an increase of one type of error in the LVF and of another type of error in the RVF. These subjects applied linguistic processes to RVF syllables and nonlinguistic processes to LVF syllables as much as strong-asymmetry subjects. The lateralized and specialized processes did not, however, produce asymmetries in overall performance that would be indicative of a task-induced asymmetric activation of the brain.

These results show that specialized processing is not the cause of differences in activation between hemispheres. They suggest, instead, that, as for split-brain patients, asymmetries of hemispheric activation are the consequences of brain adjustments prior to execution of processing. The error-type asymmetries demonstrated by Levy et al. (1983b) also show that when a hemisphere is asymmetrically stimulated (as by unilateral projection of a stimulus in the contralateral field), this normally favors its specialized processing strategies. The dissociation between hemispheric control and strategy of processing that was manifested by the commissurotomized subject CC in the experiment discussed earlier represents a pathological exception that probably rarely occurs in the normal brain. Thus, although specialized processing is not the inducer of asymmetric activation, asymmetric stimulation generally is associated with specialized processing strategies. For the normal individual, functional hemispheric asymmetry pertains not only to lateral specializations of cognitive processing that reflect the organizational properties of the hemispheres, but also to regulatory adjustments that govern the activity levels of the two sides. These greatly affect the performance that can be achieved by each hemisphere on a given task.

Two factors, then, affect the manifest ability of a hemisphere. First is hemispheric specialization itself. If hemispheric abilities for a given task are compared when each hemisphere is at its optimal level of activation, differences in competency will appear that are consequences of differences in basic organizations of the two sides of the brain. These affect the speed, accuracy, and strategy of processing. Superimposed on laterally specialized functions are asymmetries of hemispheric activation. Activation differences between the two sides may mean that either the specialized or the unspecialized hemisphere is closer to its optimal activation level. If the specialized hemisphere has the activation advantage, asymmetries of performance will be increased beyond the effects of hemispheric specialization alone. If the unspecialized hemisphere has the activation advantage, asymmetries of performance will be reduced below that expected from hemispheric-specialization effects alone. Although differences in optimal activation levels of the two sides of the brain will affect speed and accuracy of performance, they would not be expected to affect the nature of specialized processing strategies. Both the specialization factor and the activation factor must be considered in any attempt to explain an individual's performance level and asymmetry of perception.

Conclusion

Long before the split-brain revolution, Sperry (1952) was thinking deeply and cogently about the relation between neural organization and mental function. He saw that there was an intimate relation between mental awareness and the adjustment of the highly structured brain in preparation for a response. Independent of the stimulus flux on the receptors, unless and until there was a dynamic adjustment of central neural mechanisms representing an intention to act, there was no perceptual construction and no awareness. He saw, too, that the nature of a perception that was finally achieved was strongly dependent on the central organization of the brain and could not be predicted merely by knowing the physical characteristics of the external stimulus. Thus, there were both static organizational properties of the brain and dynamic regulatory mechanisms that were crucial in determining whether a perception would be generated by a stimulus and, if so, what its properties would be.

These ideas were offered almost two decades before Trevarthen (1972) called attention to the tightly bound association between the lateral orientation reflex and asymmetric hemi-

spheric activation, long before there was any direct evidence that thinking itself could and did entail lateral biases of attention and actual eye movements, long before the elegant microelectrode studies of Mountcastle and his colleagues (Lynch et al. 1975; Lynch et al. 1977; Yin and Mountcastle 1977, 1978) established that attentional biases precede overt motor orientations, and long before split-brain studies and normative investigations of the relations between attention, intentions to act, specialized processes of each hemisphere, perceptions, and behavior. As Sperry's thinking continued to develop (Sperry 1983), he saw a way to bring the effects of human consciousness back into the causal matrix of brain activity and at the top of the hierarchy of central control systems.

It is no accident that Sperry played such a central role in the subsequent research developments, either directly or by molding and directing the thinking of his students and readers. He knew the questions to ask and the pathways to search a decade before the split-brain patients became available for study, and, quite probably, long before that. He was subtle. He taught us, his former students, by his thinking. He secretly placed questions in us and the outlines to their answers, and he did it in secret because he knew that if we could be deluded into believing that it was we who had derived the questions and the paths to their answers, we would try harder and with more enthusiasm. The delusion was a pleasant one, but it could only be maintained briefly.

There were too many insights, too many intuitive leaps that he had, too many "minor" comments that developed into major breakthroughs, too many times when he seemed to argue against "our" ideas, yet gave the game away by a sly grin that he was unable to inhibit. If we were honest with ourselves, we knew. Eventually, that honesty was unavoidable.

Sperry's name is not on every split-brain paper describing the California patients nor does it appear on subsequent papers by his former students. But the questions we ask and our ways of asking them reflect, in a very deep way, his influence. He ended his 1952 paper by saying that the ideas he proposed could "... only be offered tentatively as a possible basis on which to begin to describe the neural events of mental experience" (Sperry 1952, p. 311), and at a Vatican meeting in 1964, he suggested that "consciousness may have real operational value, that it is more than merely an overtone, a by-product, epiphenomenon, or a metaphysical parallel of the objective process" (Sperry 1966, p. 308). It would be the most astonishing coincidence if the subsequent developments, some of which are reviewed in this chapter, were independent of these ideas.

Acknowledgments

The support of The Spencer Foundation is gratefully acknowledged. To Joseph Bogen, much appreciation is due. During my student days, he was generous with his ideas, and he played a major role in my training. To Colwyn Trevarthen, I owe a great deal. In our collaborative efforts, I once accused him of having two right hemispheres, and he accused me of having two left hemispheres. I think we would now modify our charges to say that we are biased in favor of different hemispheres, but it is precisely because of our differing perspectives that I gained so much from our association. As this chapter should make apparent, my debt to Roger Sperry is beyond measure, and it is one that I can never hope to pay. He not only guided and encouraged my research efforts, and not only gave me research opportunities that are available to few, but he communicated his thinking to me and, thus, brought my consciousness into causal contact with his own.

References

Alajouanine, T., and F. Lhermitte. 1963. Some problems concerning the agnosias, apraxias, and aphasia. *In* J. Halpern (ed.) *Problems of Dynamic Neurology.* Hebrew University Hadassah Medical School, Jerusalem.

Amochaev, A., and A. Salamy. 1979. Stability of EEG laterality effects. *Psychophysiol.* 16: 242–6.

Basso, A., P. Faglioni, and H. Spinnler. 1976. Non-verbal colour impairment of aphasics. *Neuropsychol.* 14: 183–93.

Bogen, J. E. 1969. The other side of the brain. II: An appositional mind. *Bull. L.A. Neurol. Soc.* 34: 135–62.

Bogen, J. E., and M. S. Gazzaniga. 1965. Cerebral commissurotomy in man: Minor hemisphere dominance for certain visuospatial functions. *J. Neurosurg.* 23: 394–9.

Bowers, D., and K. M. Heilman. 1980. Pseudoneglect: Effects of hemispace on a tactile line bisection task. *Neurosphychol.* 18: 491–8.

Bradshaw, J. L., and N. C. Nettleton. 1983. *Human Cerebral Asymmetry.* Prentice-Hall, Englewood Cliffs (N.J).

Broca, P. 1861a. Remarques sur le siege de la faculté du langage articulé suives d'une observation d'aphémie. *Bull. Soc. Anat. (Paris)* 6: 330–57.

–1861b. Nouvelle observation d'aphémie produite par une lésion de la moitié postérieure des deuxieme et troisième circonvolutions frontales. *Bull. Soc. Anat. (Paris)* 6: 398–407.

Cohen, R., and S. Kelter. 1979. Cognitive impairment of aphasics in colour-to-picture matching task. *Cortex* 15: 235–45.

Dabbs, J. M., and G. Choo. 1980. Left–right carotid blood flow predicts specialized mental ability. *Neuropsychol.* 18: 711–13.

Davidson, R. J., N. Taylor, and C. Saron. 1979. Hemisphericity and styles of information processing: Individual differences in EEG asymmetry and their relationship to cognitive performance. *Psychophysiol.* 16: 197.

Dax, M. 1865. Lesions de la moitié gauche de l'encéphale coïncident avec l'oubli des signes de la pensée. *Gaz. Hebdomadaire de Med. et de Chirurgie (Paris)* 2: 259–60.

De Renzi, E., P. Faglioni, G. Scotti, and H. Spinnler. 1972. Impairment in associating colour to form, concomitant with aphasia. *Brain* 95: 293–304.

De Renzi, E., and H. Spinnler. 1967. Impaired performance on color tasks in patients with hemispheric damage. *Cortex* 3: 194–217.

Ehrlichman, H., and M. S. Wiener. 1979. Consistency of task-related EEG asymmetries. *Psychophysiol.* 16: 247–52.

–1980. EEG asymmetry during covert mental activity. *Psychophysiol.* 17: 228–35.

Furst, C. J. 1976. EEG asymmetry and visuospatial performance. *Nature (London)* 260: 254–5.

Gale, A., I. Davies, and A. Smallbone. 1978. Changes in the EEG as the subject learns to recall. *Biol. Psychol.* 6: 169–79.

Galin, D., and R. R. Ellis. 1975. Asymmetry in evoked potentials as an index of lateralized cognitive processes: Relation to EEG alpha asymmetry. *Neuropsychol.* 13: 45–50.

Galin, D., and R. Ornstein. 1972. Lateral specialization of cognitive mode: An EEG study. *Psychophysiol.* 9: 412–18.

Gilbert, C., and P. Bakan. 1973. Visual asymmetry in the perception of faces. *Neuropsychol.* 11: 355–62.

Glass, A., and S. R. Butler. 1977. Alpha EEG asymmetry and speed of left hemisphere thinking. *Neurosci. Lett.* 4: 231–5.

Gur, R. C., and M. Reivich. 1980. Cognitive task effects on hemispheric blood flow in humans: Evidence for individual differences in hemispheric activation. *Brain and Lang.* 9: 78–92.

Gur, R. C., R. E. Gur, and L. J. Harris. 1975. Cerebral activation, as measured by subjects' lateral eye movements, is influenced by experimenter location. *Neuropsychol.* 13: 35–44.

Hécaen, H., and R. Angelergues. 1962. Agnosia for faces (prosopagnosia). *AMA Arch. Neurol.* 7: 92–100.

Hécaen, and R. Angelergues. 1963. *La Cécité Psychique. Etude Critique de la Notion d'Agnosie.* Masson et Cie, Paris.

Heller, W., and Levy, J. 1981. Perception and expression of emotion in right-handers and left-handers. *Neuropsychol.* 19: 263–72.

Hillyard, S. A., and M. S. Gazzaniga. 1971. Language and the capacity of the right hemisphere. *Neuropsychol.* 9: 273–80.

Keller, L. A. 1977. Words on the right sound louder than words on the left in free field listening. *Neuropsychol.* 16: 221–3.

Kimura, D. 1961. Cerebral dominance and the perception of verbal stimuli. *Can. J. Psychol.* 15: 166–71.

–1966. Dual functional asymmetry of the brain in visual perception. *Neuropsychol.* 4: 275–85.

–1967. Functional asymmetry of the brain in dichotic listening. *Cortex* 3: 163–78.

Kinsbourne, M. 1970. The cerebral basis of lateral asymmetries in attention. *Acta Psychol.* 33: 193–201.

–1972. Eye and head turning indicates cerebral lateralization. *Science* 176: 539–41.

–1974a. Lateral interactions in the brain. *In* M. Kinsbourne and W. L. Smith (eds.) *Hemispheric Disconnection and Cerebral Function.* Thomas, Springfield (IL).

–1974b. Direction of gaze and distribution of cerebral thought processes. *Neuropsychol.* 12: 279–81.

Levine, S., M. T. Banich, and M. Koch-Weser. 1984. Variation in patterns of lateral asymmetry among dextrals. *Brain and Cog.* 3: 317–34.

Levy, J., W. Heller, M. T. Banich, and L. Burton. 1983a. Asymmetry of perception in free viewing of chimeric faces. *Brain and Cog.* 2: 404–19.

–1983b. Are variations among right-handed individuals in perceptual asymmetries caused by characteristic arousal differences between hemispheres? *J. Exp. Psychol.: Human Percep. Perf.* 9: 329–59.

Levy, J., and L. Kueck. 1986. A right hemispatial field advantage on a verbal free-vision task. *Brain and Lang.* 27: 24–37.

Levy, J., R. Nebes, and R. W. Sperry. 1971. Expressive language in the surgically separated minor hemisphere. *Cortex* 7: 49–58.

Levy, J., and C. Trevarthen. 1976. Metacontrol of hemispheric function in human split-brain patients. *J. Exp. Psychol.: Human Percep. Perf.* 2: 299–312.

–1977. Perceptual, semantic and phonetic aspects of elementary language processes in split-brain patients. *Brain* 100: 105–18.

–1981. Color-matching, color-naming, and color-memory in split-brain patients. *Neuropsychol.* 19: 523–41.

Levy, J., C. Trevarthen, and R. W. Sperry. 1972. Perception of bilateral chimeric figures following hemispheric deconnection. *Brain* 95: 61–78.

Levy-Agresti, J., and R. W. Sperry. 1968. Differential perceptual capacities in major and minor hemispheres. *Proc. Nat. Acad. Sci. USA* 61: 1151.

Lynch, J. C., V. B. Mountcastle, W. H. Talbot, and T. C. T. Yin. 1977. Parietal lobe mechanisms for directed visual attention. *J. Neurophysiol.* 40: 362–89.

Lynch, J. C., T. C. T. Yin, W. H. Talbot, and V. B. Mountcastle. 1975. A cortical source of command signals for visually evoked saccadic movements of the eyes. *Neurosci. Abst.* 1: 59.

McFie, J., M. F. Piercy, and O. L. Zangwill. 1950. Visual-spatial agnosia associated with lesions of the right cerebral hemisphere. *Brain* 73: 167–90.

McKee, G., B. Humphrey, and D. McAdam. 1973. Scaled lateralization of alpha activity during linguistic and musical tasks. *Psychophysiol.* 10: 441–3.

Morais, J., and P. Bertelson. 1975. Spatial position versus ear of entry as determinant of the auditory laterality effects: A stereophonic test. *J. Exp. Psychol.: Human Percep. Perf.* 1: 253–62.

Morgan, A. H., H. MacDonald, and E. R. Hilgard. 1974. EEG alpha: Lateral asymmetry related to task and hynotizability. *Psychophysiol.* 11: 275–82.

Morgan, A. H., P. J. McDonald, and H. MacDonald. 1971. Differences in bilateral alpha activity as a function of experimental task with a note on lateral eye movements and hynotizability. *Neuropsychol.* 9: 459–69.

Paterson, A., and O. L. Zangwill. 1944. Disorders of visual space perception associated with lesions of the right cerebral hemisphere. *Brain* 67: 331–58.

Rebert, C. S. 1977. Functional cerebral asymmetry and performance. I. Reaction time to words and dot patterns as a function of EEG alpha asymmetry. *Behav. Neuropsychiat.* 8: 90–8.

Risberg, J., J. H. Halsey, V. W. Blavenstein, E. M. Wilson, and E. L. Wills. 1975. Bilateral measurements of the rCBF during mental activation in normals and in dysphasic patients. *In* A. M. Harper, W. B. Jennett, J. G. Miller, and J. O. Brown (eds.) *Blood Flow and Metabolism in the Brain.* Churchill Livingstone, London.

Shankweiler, D., and M. Studdert-Kennedy. 1975. A continuum of lateralization for speech perception? *Brain and Lang.* 2: 212–25.

Sperling, G. 1960. The information available in brief visual presentations. *Psychol. Mono.* 74 (No. 11).

Sperry, R. W. 1952. Neurology and the mind-brain problem. *Am. Scientist* 40: 291–312.

–1966. Brain bisection and mechanisms of consciousness. *In* J. C. Eccles (ed.) *Brain and Conscious Experience.* Springer-Verlag, Heidelberg, pp. 298–313.

–1983. *Science and Moral Priority.* Columbia University Press, New York.

Sperry, R. W., M. S. Gazzaniga, and J. E. Bogen. 1969. Interhemispheric relationships: The neocortical commissures; syndromes of hemisphere disconnection. *In* P. J. Vinken and G. W. Bruyn (eds.) *Handbook of Clinical Neurology,* Vol. 4. North-Holland, Amsterdam, pp. 273–290.

Spydell, J. D., M. R. Ford, and D. E. Sheer. 1979. Task dependent cerebral lateralization of the 40 Hertz EEG rhythm. *Psychophysiol.* 16: 347–50.

Taylor, J., (ed.). 1958. *Selected Writings of John Hughlings Jackson,* Vol. II. Basic Books, New York.

Trevarthen, C. 1965. Functional interactions between the cerebral hemispheres of the split-brain monkey. *In* E. G. Ettlinger (ed.) *Functions of the Corpus Callosum.* Ciba Foundation Study Group, No. 20. Churchill Livingstone, London, pp. 24–40.

–1968. Two mechanisms of vision in primates. *Psychol. Forsch.* 31: 299–337.

–1972. Brain bisymmetry and the role of the corpus callosum in behaviour and conscious experience. Paper presented to the *International Colloquium on Cerebral Hemispheric Relations,* Smolenice, Czechoslovakia, 1969. *In* J. Cernacek and F. Podivinsky (eds.) *Cerebral Hemisphere Relations.* Slovak Academy of Science, Bratislava, Czechoslovakia.

–1974a. Analysis of cerebral activities that generate and regulate consciousness in commissurotomy patients. *In* S. J. Dimond and J. G. Beaumont (eds.) *Hemisphere Function in the Human Brain.* Paul Elek (Scientific Books), London, pp. 235–63.

–1974b. Functional relations of disconnected hemispheres with the brainstem and with each other: Monkey and man. *In* M. Kinsbourne and W. L. Smith (eds.) *Hemi-*

spheric Disconnection and Cerebral Function. Thomas, Springfield (IL), pp. 187–207.

Tucker, G. H., and M. R. Suib. 1978. Conjugate lateral eye movement (CLEM) direction and its relationship to performance on verbal and visuospatial tasks. *Neuropsychol.* 16: 251–4.

Tweedy, J. R., W. E. Rinn, and S. P. Springer. 1980. Performance asymmetries in dichotic listening: The role of structural and attentional mechanisms. *Neuropsychol.* 18: 331–8.

Weisenberg, T., and K. McBride. 1935. *Aphasia: A Clinical and Psychological Study.* Commonwealth Fund, New York.

Wernicke, C. 1874. *Der Aphasisische Symptomenkomplex.* Cohn and Weigert, Breslau.

Yin, T. C. T., and V. B. Mountcastle. 1977. Visual input to the visuomotor mechanisms of the monkey's parietal lobe. *Science* 197: 1381–3.

–1978. Mechanisms for neural integration in the parietal lobe for visual attention. *Fed. Proc.* 37: 2251–7.

Zaidel, E. 1976a. Auditory vocabulary of the right hemisphere following brain bisection or hemidecortication. *Cortex* 12: 191–211.

–1976b. Language, dichotic listening, and the disconnected hemispheres. *In* D. O. Walter, L. Rogers, and J. M. Finzi-Fried (eds.) *Conference on Human Brain Function.* Brain Information Service/BRI Publications Office, Los Angeles.

–1977. Unilateral auditory language comprehension on the Token Test following cerebral commissurotomy and hemispherectomy. *Neuropsychol.* 15: 1–18.

14 The neurobiological basis of hemisphericity

Harold W. Gordon
Western Psychiatric Institute and Clinic
University of Pittsburgh

Prologue

It is not immediately obvious how neurospecificity, neurobiology, and neuroembryology might lead to neuropsychology and the understanding of cognitive processes and the mind, but this progression describes the scientific course of Roger Sperry's career. He has performed key experiments in each of these fields, leaving the details for others and moving on to still other key investigations. Pioneer work in specialized cognitive functions of the human brain were the culmination of his experiments with animals, and this work turned out to be the hallmark, by virtue of its recognition in numerous coveted awards topped by the Nobel Prize for Biology and Medicine in October, 1981.

Sperry began investigations of patients who had undergone complete forebrain commissurotomy, for alleviation of intractible epilepsy, at Caltech in the early 1960s; in collaboration with Joseph Bogen, who was also involved with surgery and patient follow-up, and Michael Gazzaniga, who carried out psychological tests for his PhD research (Sperry, Gazzaniga, and Bogen 1969). These early studies sparked a plethora of research programs, scientific and philosophical inquiries, general public interest, and, inevitably, controversy. It was my good fortune to step into Sperry's laboratory near the beginning of work to clarify the separate cognitive abilities attributed to the right and left hemispheres. The studies to be described are some of my efforts to continue these endeavors. After more than 15 years of investigation on the specialized psychological functions of the brain, my work seems to be turning back in the direction of neurobiology and a search for the underlying neurosystems on which these functions are based.

Introduction

Studies at Caltech with the commissurotomy patients confirmed most dramatically not only that the two surgically separated hemispheres had their own volition, thoughts, and ideas (Sperry 1964, 1968), but also that thinking in each hemisphere was qualitatively different (Bogen, DeZure, Tenhouten, and Marsh 1972; Sperry 1974). Prior to surgery, both hemispheres of such individuals had been to the same places, seen the same pictures and scenes, heard the same words and music, and felt the same objects. The dichotomy of cognitive function could not, therefore, be explained by differences in the environment.

The greater contribution of the left hemisphere to speech had been known indirectly for over a century from the speech deficits that followed lesions in that side of the brain. The complete failure of a commissurotomy patient to name or describe objects, scenes, or auditory information arriving only to the right hemisphere, coupled with full verbal disclosure of the same experiences in the left hemisphere (Gazzaniga and Sperry 1967), leaves no doubt that the left hemisphere has the dominant role in verbal expression. Subsequent studies in these and normal subjects have further demonstrated that the right hemisphere may have some role in reception of language and other paralinguistic functions (Zaidel 1978, Gordon 1980a), as well as confirming that the left hemisphere still has the leading responsibility in comprehension of language.

In addition to providing confirmation for the language functions in the left hemisphere, a long series of studies, beginning with the commissurotomy patients in Sperry's laboratory, highlighted a newly emerging set of specialized cognitive functions for which the right cerebral hemisphere has principal control. Although mute and agraphic, the isolated right hemisphere demonstrated a special ability to copy geometrical figures and construct block designs better than the isolated left hemisphere (Bogen 1969). Later work showed the right hemisphere to excel in recognition of shapes, forms, and faces (Nebes 1971, 1972; Levy, Trevarthen, and Sperry 1972; Zaidel and Sperry 1973; Franco and Sperry 1977). While the results on the commissurotomy patients were the most dramatic, similar findings were being reported concurrently in patients with unilateral lesions (De Renzi 1982), and later in normal subjects (Bryden 1982). Converging evidence provides confirmation of the specialized abilities of the right hemisphere.

The advantage of studying commissurotomy patients, of course, is that the performance of the left hemisphere of each individual patient can be compared to his/her own right hemisphere. In patients with unilateral lesions, however, functions attributable to the left or right hemisphere are determined only indirectly, by implication, because only deficits can be observed. In normal subjects, the fact that the hemispheres are still connected through the corpus callosum has always posed the problem of whether differences in visual fields, ears, etc. are due to specialized functions of the left or right hemisphere or deficiencies in interhemispheric transmission. Nevertheless, studies of normal subjects at one extreme and commissurotomy patients at the other, as well as countless other studies on brain-damaged subjects, leave no doubt that there is at least one, and arguably more, cognitive mode of thinking attributable to the left cerebral hemisphere, and another, or others, attributable to the right hemisphere.

Concepts and confusions concerning hemispheric functions

The powerful simplicity of the mental dichotomy claimed for commissurotomy patients incited an inevitable reaction. The concept of *duality* – two functions for two hemispheres – was considered to be an oversimplification. The idea that the right hemisphere could have one kind of function and the left could have another was considered too "perfect." Ironically, critics who focused only on the most striking features of the oft-stated dichotomies, took them at face value and became perpetrators of the simplistic description of a two-sided difference, themselves. In point of fact, the list of functions attributed to the right hemisphere is long and multifaceted. Items include spatial (two-dimensional or three-dimensional) orientation, perception or "imagination" in three dimensions, point localization, form (including facial) recognition, perceptual closure, and certain processing modes in music. The list for the left hemisphere is curiously shorter unless the many different aspects of language are counted separately. Verbal fluency is probably the most "left hemispheric" of the language tasks because the evidence suggests that in the great majority of subjects, the left hemisphere is the only one that produces speech. Other left-hemisphere specialties include phonemic processing in speech perception and generation of syntactical connections. In addition to language, sequential processing or serial ordering is associated with left-hemisphere functioning.

It is clear that problems arise when we try to include the functions of each hemisphere under a single rubric. Thus are born the controversial dichotomies: analytic versus synthetic, verbal and nonverbal, simultaneous and sequential, time-dependent and time-independent, and so on. What must be avoided is the temptation to adopt one or the other of these dichotomies as an absolute rule, thereby forcing an allocation of all cognitive behaviors into one or the other hemisphere.

A second kind of confusion arises from the mistaken belief that a "right-hemisphere" function is something that is *in* the right hemisphere and a "left-hemisphere" function is something that is *in* the left hemisphere. Once again, studies do not suggest this. Rather, data are always relative: the ability of one hemisphere is compared to the ability of the other. Hemispheres are accurately described as being "superior," "dominant," "preferred," or "specialized" for certain functions. But that does not mean that it is the *only* hemisphere that can perform the task; it only means that it may be better at it. The one exception is that the left hemisphere in most adult individuals appears to be the only one capable of verbal production, either through speech or by writing.

What emerges, then, is the concept that there is a cluster of functions that, under normal circumstances, are more strongly represented in the right cerebral hemisphere and another cluster of functions that are more strongly represented in the left hemisphere. Added to this dichotomy of clusters is the most striking conclusion to be drawn from the commissurotomy patients, as indeed it had already been drawn from prior research with commissurotomized animals, namely, that each hemisphere of the brain can function at a high cognitive level on its own, without input from the other side. As Joseph Bogen puts it: "It takes only one hemisphere to have a mind." (See Chapter 12, this volume.)

Neurobiological bases of cognitive function and individual differences

We are led, then, to two lines of enquiry. The first takes its cue from evolutionary concerns and speculation on how natural selection may have produced the structural bases of hemispheric differences in psychological function (Levy 1969). While it is true that modern imaging techniques have demonstrated anatomical differences between hemispheres in recent years (e.g., Galaburda et al. 1978), principles of neurospecificity in the control of nerve connections and function suggest that the qualitative differences between right- and left-hemisphere function are likely to lie ultimately, not in the quantitative features of the anatomy, but rather in the qualitative differences in neurotransmitters, their receptors, and their metabolites. One might look for functional specialization to be under genetic control through regulation of these neurobiological factors. Current and past research on such systems offer promising avenues for understanding the natural organization of cognitive function. One way to observe the effects of genes, hormones

and neurotransmitters on cognitive function is to study patient groups that, by experiments of nature, have abnormal renderings of these features.

Good candidates for study are patients with gonadal dysgenesis, who, for the most part, have a deleted X chromosome and are phenotypically female. The major behavioral characteristic is ineptitude in functions normally attributed to the right hemisphere (Money and Alexander 1966), with normal performance of functions attributed to the left hemisphere (Gordon and Galatzer 1980), and, apparently, symmetrical organization of the two sides of the brain for producing the latter cognitive functions (Netley and Rovet 1983). In addition to a gene deletion in these patients, there is also absence of naturally occurring estrogen and a concomitant elevation of the gonadotropins.

Another case in point, but with an opposite pattern of brain functions, is the developmental dyslexic who appears to have a heritable abnormal dysfunction of cognitive processes attributed to the left hemisphere and a predominance of functions of the kind attributed to the right hemisphere (Gordon 1983; Harness, Epstein, and Gordon 1984), possibly because both hemispheres are organized to form the same (right-hemisphere) type of neurosystem (Witelson 1977). Similar patterns of cognitive asymmetry favoring the functions of the right hemisphere have been reported in parents and siblings of dyslexics (Gordon 1980b), suggesting a dominant genetic link. It is the genetic control of developing neurosystems that is hypothesized to produce the specific cognitive preferences in the dyslexics, and there is anatomical support for this explanation (Galaburda 1983). By the same argument, qualitative differences in the organization of neurosystems may account for individual, group, and even sex differences in cognitive function in normal populations.

The second question emerging from the dichotomy of hemispheric function is more practical. What are the advantages for a person to have a greater ability or proficiency for functions attributed to one cognitive area than for those of another area? Is it desirable, for education or for job allocation, to classify individuals according to hemispheric proficiency as a predictor of success in certain skill areas? Recognition that individuals may fall anywhere along a one-dimensional axis of "left/right" cognitive processing is responsible for popular interest in the notion of separate right- and left-hemisphere function. Courses and workshops have been offered, and books have been written that purport to change a person's position along that axis and to develop the other, hitherto disfavored, side of the brain. It must be admitted that there is, as yet, no scientific validation that these self-help remedies or training exercises are engaging, and strengthening, specialized hemispheric processes in any new or even useful way.

If individual differences in cognitive functions are related to differences in neurosystems, research should focus, rather, on evidence that might help decide if different neurotransmitter systems are the bases of the different cognitive functions that distinguish the two hemispheres. More specifically, it would be important to determine if there is one kind of neurosystem related to all, or a majority, of the functions normally attributed to the left hemisphere, and another, qualitatively different, neurosystem that is related to all or a majority of the functions attributed to the right hemisphere. One way to test this hypothesis is to look at groups of individuals with abnormalities in specific neurosystems to see if they exhibit a consistent increase or decrease of proficiency for functions normally attributed to one hemisphere or the other. The second step is to see if there are differences in cognitive function related to differences in neurosystems across individuals in a mixed population. Additionally, it may be possible to observe shifts in cognitive function in individuals when modifications of neurosystems occur naturally or are produced artificially within them.

The cognitive laterality battery
TESTS TO STUDY HEMISPHERIC FUNCTION (GORDON 1986)

Before any assessment of individual difference or comparison of groups can be made, an instrument of evaluation has to be developed. Clinically oriented neuropsychological tests such as the Halstead–Reitan or the Luria–Nebraska are designed to bring out evidence

for dysfunction in various specified areas of the brain. Since some of the subtests may be selected to identify dysfunction within one of the hemispheres, differences in right/left cognitive deficiencies among certain patient groups can be defined. However, the test batteries are designed to detect brain pathology by observing deficits in a range of special-purpose behavioral tests. Determination of right/left asymmetries are largely based on "soft" motor signs, such as imbalance in gait, reflexes, grip strength, finger-tapping rate, and so on. While useful clinically, these neuropsychological batteries are not suited to assess specialized or "higher" cognitive function of a more normally functioning brain. Furthermore, in individuals where brain damage is not known or suspected, performance would be expected to be near flawless, thereby precluding any assessment of performance asymmetry.

Much of the effort in our laboratory over the past years has been to develop a battery of tests that is capable of assessing a person's abilities in specialized cognitive functions attributed to the left and right hemispheres. The subtests were adapted from those that previously demonstrated hemispheric specialization in patients with forebrain commissurotomy or unilateral lesions, or in normal subjects. If performance on tests attributed to right-hemisphere processing is compared to performance on tests attributed to left-hemisphere processing, an overall cognitive profile of lateral preference may be defined. Early studies showed that patients with unilateral left-hemisphere lesions performed relatively poorly on tests chosen to assess the left hemisphere, whereas patients with right-hemisphere lesions performed poorly on tests chosen to assess the right hemisphere, thereby validating the selection of subtests (Bentin and Gordon 1979). Subsequent studies in the commissurotomy patients demonstrated that the left hemisphere was indeed able to remember sequences better than the right and the right hemisphere was able to better analyze a three-dimensional figure (*1982 Biology Annual Report,* Caltech with E. Zaidel).

Validation of a test battery for lateralized performance is more difficult in normal and unconstrained subjects because the tests are not presented to the right or left hemispheres separately. Instead, factor analyses were carried out in large populations. Two main factors resulted, in which the "right" and "left" groups of subtests loaded separately. While it might be desirable to prove that these right- and left-hemisphere tests separately activate, or are located in, the respective right and left hemispheres, this proof is not necessary. We have hypothesized that different neurosystems form the bases of right and left cognitive functions. A battery of tests designed to assess the level of cognitive functioning is not assessing the location of these functions in the right or left hemispheres. Variation among individuals in the performance of specialized cognitive tasks is distributed along a "right–left" *functional* axis. Performance asymmetry reflects the relative efficiency or dominance of the respective characteristically "right" or "left" neurosystems; these may or may not be located, or more active, in their usual hemisphere.

The fruit of this effort to assess a person's ability in these specialized cognitive functions was the cognitive laterality battery, which has undergone some development (Gordon and Harness 1977; Bentin and Gordon 1979) before reaching its current form and standardization (Gordon 1986). All of the subtests of the cognitive laterality battery have been standardized on normal populations of ages 8 through adult. "Hemisphericity" is measured by the cognitive laterality quotient (CLQ) and defined as the difference between the average performance on tests associated with the right hemisphere and those associated with the left. Since the subtests are standardized, their averages and the average differences are linear combinations of standard scores. Therefore, the population norm would, by definition, have no asymmetry. The distribution of the CLQ scores is normal, so that there are individuals whose performance is predominately better on tests of left-hemisphere function and individuals whose performance is predominately better on tests of right-hemisphere function (Figure 14.1). Groups that are "interesting" are those that differ consistently and significantly from the normal mean of zero (i.e., no asymmetry), giv-

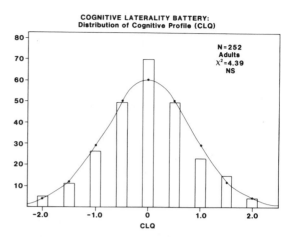

Figure 14.1. Distribution of the cognitive laterality quotient (CLQ), which is the difference between the average performance on tests associated with the right hemisphere and the average performance on tests associated with the left hemisphere. A plot of a normal curve is superimposed on the data.

ing them a cognitive profile – hemisphericity – that favors functions characteristic of either the right hemisphere or of the left.

VISUOSPATIAL TESTS ASSOCIATED
WITH THE RIGHT HEMISPHERE

Localization. A photographic slide containing a small black "x" within a black frame on a white background is flashed on a screen for 3 s. The subject has a similar frame on an answer sheet and must mark with a pencil the exact location of the "x" within it. There are 24 slides arranged in pseudorandom order, counterbalanced such that the same number of "xs" appears in each of the four quadrants. The subject's score is the total error in millimeters accumulated over all trials. (This is the only test in which a high score represents a poor performance.)

Orientation. The stimulus is a slide of 3 three-dimensional S-shaped constructions of 10 stacked cubes (Shepard and Metzler 1971). All three constructions are identical but rotated in space around a vertical axis except that one of the three appears as the mirror image of the other two. The subject is given 15 s to select the two constructions that are alike. There are 24 trials.

A two-dimensional version is also available for young children or low-performing adults. The stimuli are two-dimensional asymmetrical forms ("flags") (Thurstone and Jeffrey 1956) rather than three-dimensional stacked cubes.

Touching blocks (adapted from Mac-Quarrie 1953). The stimulus is a slide of one large cube construction made up of 7–10 stacked rectangular blocks. The blocks are stacked such that anywhere from two to eight blocks may be adjacent to (touching) any one block. For each stimulus slide, five of the rectangular blocks are numbered and the subject is given 45 s to indicate the number of touching blocks for each of the numbered blocks. There are six slides, for a total of 30 items.

Form completion (closure). The stimulus is a slide containing six incomplete silhouette drawings of common objects or scenes appearing white on a blue background. The items were selected from two similar tests (French, Ekstrom, and Price 1962; Thurstone and Jeffrey 1966) and chosen to be as culture-free as possible. The task is to identify and describe, in a word or two, each of the six drawings. Forty-five seconds are allowed for each slide and answers are written on special answer sheets. Four slides are presented, for a total of 24 items.

VERBOSEQUENTIAL TESTS ASSOCIATED WITH THE LEFT HEMISPHERE

Serial sounds. Sequences of four to seven familiar sounds (e.g., baby, bugle, rooster, bird, telephone, etc.) are played from an audio tape. Once the sounds are well-recognized, the subject's task is to write the items in the same sequential order as they were played. The onsets of each sound in the sequence are spaced at 2-s intervals. The subject waits for a start signal at the end of the sequence before writing an answer. Scoring is based on the number of sounds correctly reported in sequence whether or not the whole sequence is correct.

Serial numbers. Sequences of three to nine single-digit numbers are presented at the rate of one per second. At the end of each sequence, the subject is required to write the sequence in the same order as presented. The scoring is the same as for "serial sounds," in which partial credit is given to correct fragments of sequences even if the whole sequence is incorrect.

Word production, letters. The subject is given one minute to write as many words as possible that begin with a given letter of the alphabet. The subject's score is the total of three attempts, each time with a different letter (C, F, L).

Word production, categories. The subject is given one minute to write as many words as possible in a given category (foods, animals). The subject's score is the total of the two categories.

ADMINISTRATION OF THE BATTERY

The cognitive tests are presented on 35-mm slides and audio cassettes. The presentation is automated by use of a sound/sync projector with an internal screen. The audio cassette provides instructions and a cue track that automatically advances the slides according to exact timing. The test apparatus is portable for use in various locations such as in a hospital room. A flip-up mirror in the projector also allows for group testing.

Since the subtests have been standardized on various populations, the average right and left scores may be compared within an experimental population. In this way, relationships among tests – the cognitive profile – may be emphasized rather than overall performance. The cognitive laterality battery has been used with a number of groups in an effort to uncover the neurosystems giving rise to the typical differences between right- and left-hemisphere functions.

Hemispheric asymmetry and psychopathology

One example of individuals believed to have dysfunctional neurosystems without obvious trauma or brain damage are patients with psychopathology, especially those with schizophrenia and those with endogenous depression (Gruzelier and Flor-Henry 1979). Schizophrenics are believed to have an abnormal dopamine system, because dopamine receptor blockers alleviate symptoms, although the nature of the deficit is not known (Rodnight 1982). Depressives are believed to have dysfunction in an amine system, such as the adrenergic neurosystem or the serotonergic neurosystem (Ashcroft 1982).

Not only are neurotransmitter systems differentially affected in these two disorders, but the cognitive deficits of the two kinds of patients appear to be qualitatively different as well. Language disorders are associated with schizophrenia, whereas behavioral deficits indicative of right-hemisphere dysfunction are reported for depressed patients (Yozawitz et al. 1979). However, in this field, much of the evidence is confounded by the diversity of experimental techniques, inconsistencies in patient diagnoses and treatments, and doubt about the validity of various tests. Nonetheless, the data available do seem to point to the existence of an underlying general dichotomy of cognitive processes.

The initial observations of right/left asymmetries in psychopathology were made in patients with epileptic psychoses. Flor-Henry (1969) reported that schizophrenic psychoses were more often associated with left-temporal-lobe epilepsy, and manic-depressive psychoses were associated with right-temporal-lobe epilepsy. Supporting evidence for the hypothesis of left-hemispheric dysfunction in schizophrenics includes language studies that show these patients have many of the features associated with aphasia (Silverberg-Shalev et al. 1981), tachistoscopic studies where right-visual-field inferiorities are found for processing verbal material (Gur 1978), and studies of asymmetrical electrodermal responses (Gruzelier and Venables 1974).

In patients with affective disorders, inferior performances on tests of the right-hemisphere function have been reported (Kronfol et al. 1978). This evidence is supported by the additional finding that while unilateral electroconvulsive therapy (ECT) to either hemisphere effectively reduces depression, the cognitive changes differ, depending on the hemisphere receiving the electric shock. After eight treatments of left ECT, there was a significant decline on a test of word produc-

tion that is attributed to performance by the left hemisphere. After right ECT, judgments of line orientation (attributed to functions of the right hemisphere) improved, whereas performance on other tests stayed the same (Kronfol et al. 1978). These results appear to indicate that ECT to a more normally functioning left hemisphere tends to disrupt activity, whereas ECT to a poorly functioning right hemisphere tends to improve (or "normalize") activity.

In one study using neuropsychological techniques, 114 patients were divided by standard criteria into several diagnostic subgroups, including schizophrenia, mania, hypomania, and depression (both unipolar and bipolar). The subtests of the Halstead–Reitan neuropsychological test battery were analyzed by a stepwise discriminant function that succeeded in separating schizophrenics from both patients with affective disorders and normal controls at a highly significant level (Flor-Henry and Yeudall 1979). But as noted previously, the Halstead–Reitan is a test battery designed to assess brain dysfunction. The cognitive laterality measure, on the other hand, is designed to assess function directly. Asymmetry would be determined by better performance on tests associated with one hemisphere relative to that on tests for the other hemisphere. Accordingly, a pilot study was undertaken in which the cognitive laterality battery was administered to a group of acute schizophrenic and depressed patients. The patients were first diagnosed by an interview given upon admission to the hospital. Testing took place within the next few days before major drug therapy was instituted. Diagnoses were confirmed or modified on the basis of subsequent interviews during the patients' hospital stay.

Results for the acute schizophrenic patients were the most dramatic: 15 out of 15 tested (another 10 were too sick or unwilling to participate) had a profile favoring tests of the right hemisphere, which, in fact, was due to lower than normal functioning on tests of the left hemisphere (Shenkman, Gordon, and Heifetz 1980). For the depressed patients, 60% had the reverse left-hemisphere cognitive profile (Kushnir, Gordon, and Heifetz 1980). Because the diagnosis was made upon admission, there was considerable uncertainty; about one-third of the diagnoses had been changed by the time of discharge. Some patients initially diagnosed as depressed later carried such diagnoses as schizophrenia or neurotic depression. In contrast to those who retained the diagnosis of depression, individuals in the misdiagnosed group performed better on tests of the *right* hemisphere. Furthermore, in a few depressed patients who were tested twice, once during a depressive episode and the second time during a manic phase or during remission, there was a concomitant shift from cognitive performance favoring functions of the left hemisphere toward those favoring functions of the right hemisphere.

The significance of these findings is that they both validate the test battery in its purpose to measure imbalance of hemispheric function and confirm previous findings of studies that had employed other methods. The value of the new approach is that it emphasizes what cognitive functions a patient or subject *can* perform on a relative level, whereas the clinical neuropsychological test batteries usually determine what specific disabilities or deficits are present (i.e., what a patient cannot do). Emphasis on a cognitive profile of ability (rather than disability) encourages a focus on the relationships among tests rather than on levels of performance.

The results with the cognitive laterality battery suggest the cognitive asymmetries in the patients with these psychopathologies may be related to a neurosystemic imbalance associated with the disease condition. As pointed out, depression and schizophrenia are believed to stem from dysfunction in different neurotransmitter systems. This idea is supported because the observed functional asymmetries are not permanent, as might be expected if they were due to fixed anatomical differences in hemispheric organization of cognitive systems. Functional asymmetries have been observed to shift together with the symptomatic improvement following drug therapy. For example, improved performance on tests attributed to the right hemisphere has been observed following administration of lithium in patients with primarily bipolar affective disorders; phenothiazines had less of an effect on cognitive asymmetries in schizophrenics (Small et al.

1973). Other studies have reported changes in left/right asymmetries of the galvanic skin response after administration of chlorpromazine (Gruzelier and Hammond 1978) or propranolol (Gruzelier 1979), and in electrocortical events following chlorpromazine (Serafetinides 1972). The phenothiazines including chlorpromazine effectively block dopamine receptors in controlling schizophrenic psychosis. Tricyclics are the drugs of choice in treating depression. These primarily work on the amine systems, preventing reuptake of the neurotransmitter or sensitizing the receptor. The differences in the treatments for the different psychopathologies reflect differences in the affected neurotransmitter. Of course, there are a number of other drug treatments that alleviate symptoms, yet affect neurosystems by various other mechanisms, not to mention the effect on multiple systems. Qualitatively, however, it appears that the neurotransmitter systems are different or differentially affected for each disease process.

The working hypothesis, based on the presence of different cognitive asymmetries in these patient groups and the subsequent shift in these asymmetries following drug treatment, is that there exists a pharmacologically sensitive neurosystem that is common to both the psychopathological behavior and the asymmetry of each major type of cognitive performance. Since the actions of many drugs in the central nervous system are moderately well-studied, important clues can be derived for understanding the underlying mechanisms producing specialized cognitive functions. By extending the argument, it may be hypothesized that the asymmetries in cognitive function in nonpathological (i.e., normal) individuals are directly or indirectly related to these same neurotransmitter imbalances.

Hormone concentrations and cognitive function

The suggestion that there are correlations between hormone concentrations and right/left cognitive behavior comes from results of studies encompassing patients with chromosomal and endocrinological disorders as well as normal subjects. The most striking and most widely known patient group with deficiencies in cognitive performance are those with gonadal dysgenesis. In particular, these patients have been reported to have deficits in performance IQ (Shaffer 1962), figure drawing (Alexander, Ehrhardt, and Money 1966), orientation (Rovet and Netley 1980), and map reading (Alexander, Walker and Money 1964), whereas the left-hemisphere verbal and sequential functions remain intact (Gordon and Galatzer 1980). Two male groups with supernumerary sex chromosomes, 47,XXY (Klinefelter's syndrome) and 47,XYY, both have cognitive characteristics contrasting with the gonadal dysgenesis. Performance IQs are greater than verbal IQs, implying that right-hemisphere performance is better than left (Pasquiline, Vidal, and Bur 1957; Christensen and Nielsen 1973; Wesner et al. 1973; Zeuthen et al. 1975).

If cognitive asymmetry in patients with chromosomal disorders is mediated by an imbalance of gonadotropins and sex steroid hormones, then a similar cognitive asymmetry would be expected in chromosomally normal individuals with hormone levels abnormal for age, or fluctuating, as during the menstrual cycle. The cognitive laterality battery was administered to a group of 37 individuals (24 males and 13 females) with delayed puberty (Galatzer and Gordon 1982). On the average, performance was better on tests associated with the right hemisphere, worse on tests associated with the left hemisphere, or both. By contrast, performance was better on tests of left-hemisphere function in a group of patients with precocious puberty, where gonadotropins and sex steroids were elevated for chronological age (see Table 14.1). The same left-hemisphere-dominant pattern was also seen in a group of early (but not "precocious") maturers, whereas performance was better on tests associated with right-hemisphere functions in subjects who were late (but not "delayed") maturers (Waber 1976).

Gender differences in cognitive abilities of normal subjects were found for many of the subtests of the cognitive laterality battery. Males were superior in most of the functions attributed to the right cerebral hemisphere, especially orientation, whereas females excelled in the word-production test attributed to the left hemisphere. This does not mean that all functions attributed to the right hemisphere are performed better by males. Notable exceptions are facial perception and recognition of emotion (Ladavas, Umilta, and Ricci-Bitti 1980; Pizzamiglio and Zoccolotti 1981; Pizzamiglio et al. 1983). Conversely, there do not seem to be gender differences in the perception of sequences or serial order usually attributed to the left hemisphere. For those abilities where gender differences do occur, differences in hormone concentrations have been hypothesized as a likely cause (Broverman et al. 1968). Moreover, there have been reports that increased ability in cognitive skills attributed to the left hemisphere are positively related to physical manifestations of androgen levels in males (Klaiber, Broverman, and Kobayashi 1967) and, to some extent, in females (Petersen 1976).

There are also reports of fluctuations in performance of cognitive abilities that coincide with hormonal changes in women during the menstrual cycle. In one study (Wuttke et al. 1975), the fastest and most accurate performance of a test of simple arithmetic calculation (often attributed to the left hemisphere) was in the luteal phase when estradiol and especially progesterone are relatively high. In another study (Ward, Stone, and Sandman 1978), there was a high performance on a dot-detection task (questionably attributable to the left hemi-

Table 14.1. *Cognitive profile of patients with hormonal abnormalities*

Patient	N	P ("left" hemi.)	A ("right" hemi.)	CLQ[a] (A − P)	CPQ[a] (A + P)/2
Constitutional delay of puberty	24	−0.41	0.25	0.64	−0.08
Hypogonadotropic hypogonadism	18	−0.89	−0.05	0.84	−0.48
Precocious puberty	8	−0.22	−0.62	−0.40	−0.55

[a]See definitions in Figure 14.2.

sphere) relative to poor perception of a dot pattern (which is likely to be "right hemispheric") during the same luteal period. There was more equivalence in performances on these tasks during the preovulatory phase and a slight reversal during menstruation when the concentrations of the gonadotropins and sex steroid hormones are at their lowest. The observation that improved performance on tests of left-hemisphere function was related to increased hormone concentrations was supported in another study. Good performance of rapid naming (a left-hemisphere function) and relatively poorer performance on embedded figures (the most "right-hemisphere" test in the battery) occurred during the preovulatory phase, whereas performances were more equivalent during the menstrual phase (Komnenich et al. 1978).

Work in our laboratory (Gordon and Lee 1986) confirms the relationship between hormones and behavior. The cognitive laterality battery was administered to 30 normal young women and 32 normal young men. The four "right" and four "left" subtests of the battery were interspersed in counterbalanced order and presented one at a time. A small sample (8 ml) of blood was withdrawn after each test. Plasma concentrations were obtained for the gonadotropins, FSH and LH, and the appropriate sex steroids: estradiol and progesterone in women and testosterone in men. Gonadotropins are released from the pituitary by stimulation from Luteinizing Releasing Hormone (LRH), whose release is controlled by the hypothalamus. Among other things, the gonadotropins induce the testes in males or ovaries in females and stimulate production of the sex steroids. These concentrations of the sex steroids, in turn, regulate hypothalamic release of LRH.

In males, there was a significant negative correlation between FSH and three of the four tests associated with the right hemisphere (localization: $r = -0.48$, $p < 0.01$; orientation test: $r = -0.35$, $p < 0.05$; blocks: $r = -0.40$, $p < 0.05$). The correlation with the average of all four tests associated with the right hemisphere was strong: $r = -0.52$, $p < 0.01$. The correlation increased in a second session held one week later with the same subjects: localization, $r = -0.53$, $p < 0.01$; blocks, $r = -0.51$, $p < 0.01$; orientation, $r = -0.49$, $p < 0.01$; for the average of four tests, $r = -0.59$, $p < 0.01$. Correlations with LH were less strong and generally positive for all tests, at least in the first session. By contrast, there were virtually no correlations between any cognitive functions and testosterone in men.

The significance of the negative correlations in men between right-hemisphere function and FSH was even more striking in partial correlations where the effects of the other hormones were held statistically constant. Multiple correlational analyses with FSH, LH, and testosterone produced R's ranging from 0.54 to 0.68 among the four tests associated with right-hemisphere function with multiple R's of 0.67 (F = 7.62, $p < 0.01$) and 0.63 (F = 5.25, $p < 0.01$) for the average of the four tests in sessions 1 and 2, respectively. This explains about 39% and 29% of the variance.

tween FSH and visuospatial function was weaker. The correlations were significant ($p < 0.05$) for the orientation test in two successive sessions, but only when the effects of progesterone were controlled. In women, the situation is considerably more complex, possibly due to higher hormone levels as well as consistent shifts of endogenous hormone concentrations.

Additional work indicates that artificial increase of FSH and LH in males (by injection of LRH) has some affect on cognitive processes *within* subjects in the same direction as described *across* subjects. In repeated sessions, subjects injected with LRH significantly improved their fluency score, but failed to improve their score on the orientation test in comparison with themselves when injected with a placebo (Gordon, Lee, and Corbin 1986). These data support the idea that right- and left-hemispheric functions are related to different neurosystems. The data also provide evidence that cognitive function is changeable, depending, in part, on neurobiological factors.

Diurnal or sleep–wake variation in hemispheric functional balance

If the hormone model continues to prove useful in the understanding of neurosystems that underlie cognitive function, it is indeed fortunate, because the study of hormone levels is convenient. Whereas an assay of neurotransmitters is impossible in living subjects, measurement of hormones and even manipulation of some hormone concentrations are relatively benign procedures. However, there is evidence that relates cognitive function to endogenous biorhythms that are not necessarily correlated with the hormone system. This opens the possibility of another system to study.

Throughout an eight-hour test period, it was found that scores on a left-hemisphere task (verbal matching) alternating with a right-hemisphere task (matching of dot patterns) each fluctuated in approximately 90-min cycles between good and poor performances in normal subjects (Klein and Armitage 1979). The important point was that the cycles were 180 degrees out of phase with each other: when the left test was performed well, the right test was performed poorly and vice versa.

Our results in a sleep study support this out-of-phase fluctuation (Gordon, Frooman, and Lavie 1981). The cognitive laterality battery was administered to normal young right-handed males once upon awakening from REM sleep and again upon awakening from NREM sleep, awakenings and test order being counterbalanced across subjects. There was a significant shift in cognitive function: relative performance on right-hemisphere tests was significantly better upon awakening from REM sleep when compared to awakening from NREM sleep. All subtests showed the effect. Left-hemisphere tests were performed better after wakening from the NREM period; right-hemisphere tests were performed better after wakening from the REM period.

These results were replicated in the same laboratory on a group of right-handed women, but were not replicated on left-handers (Lavie, Metania, and Yehuda 1984). In yet another replication by another laboratory, a tactually presented spatial-recognition task was performed better upon wakening from REM sleep than from NREM (Bertini et al. 1983). Once again, the results encourage the view that study of shifts in cognitive behavior during changes in the state of the central nervous system will provide evidence for the neurobiological bases of specialized cognitive behavior.

Cognitive asymmetries and specific disabilities or special talents

As seen in Figure 14.1, scores on the cognitive laterality battery and, in particular, the hemisphericity measure (the cognitive laterality quotient) are distributed normally. Most individuals have little or no asymmetry, some performing slightly better on "right" tests, some performing slightly better on "left" tests. No clear picture of "hemisphericity" (predominance of one hemisphere's functioning) emerges for individuals who have minimal asymmetry. They usually mix their performances, obtaining higher scores on one or two "left" tests and one or two "right" tests. Of greater interest are those individuals found at the right or left extremes of the distribution curve in the absence of obvious causative factors such as unilateral brain damage or chromosomal and hormonal disorders. By studying variation in hormone concentrations, neurotransmitter systems, or other organizational features in the central nervous system and comparing them to cognitive function in these individuals, there is great potential for delineating the underlying neurobiology of specialized cognitive function.

The best illustration of consistent cognitive performance representing the specialized functions of one hemisphere are individuals with specific learning disabilities. This group has puzzled educators, clinicians, and researchers alike because of the striking difference between their intellectual capacities and their inabilities to read and spell. Orton reported a number of years ago that such individuals have abnormally reduced lateral dominance, manifested by a reversed hand preference (or no hand preference) or mixed eye and hand dominance (Orton 1937).

Attention is usually focused on the cognitive inadequacies of these disabled individuals; their strengths are often overlooked. In a study of 108 children referred to a clinic for reading difficulties, 105 performed better on tests associated with right-hemisphere function than on tests associated with left function (Harness, Epstein, and Gordon 1984). This asymmetry did not result just from poor performance on tests of left-hemisphere function; there were unusually good performances on tests of right-hemisphere function. In fact, performance on right-hemisphere tests were just as much above average as tests of left-hemisphere function were below. One explanation is that these individuals were "locked in" to the right-hemisphere mode of thought, which understandably does not work very well for reading skills (Gordon 1983).

These data are not new. They highlight what has often been reported in the literature, but usually without regard to their significance for brain function, except by a few (Rugel 1974, Smith et al. 1977, Kaufman 1979). Children with learning disabilities appear to perform better, often better than average, on tests associated with the right hemisphere as evidenced by their scores on block design and object assembly from the Wechsler Scales (Doehring et al. 1981).

Fortunately, the need for better evaluation techniques is gaining recognition. A new intelligence test, the K-ABC (Kaufman and Kaufman 1983), was purposely designed with regard to specialized functions of the left and right cerebral hemispheres. Scores for each test type (termed "simultaneous" and "sequential") are calculated separately, but a comparison between the two is an integral part of the analysis and evaluation.

Cognitive asymmetries in the learning disabled suggest that these individuals might be an ideal population for studying the underlying causes of cognitive function. The learning disorder has long been thought to have a genetic component, but a workable model of its heritability has not been forthcoming. All that genes can do is tell what proteins are to be synthesized, and so the nature of the supposed "dyslexic" gene is rather obscure (Galaburda 1983). If the cause of specific learning disabilities was based on cognitive asymmetry and such cognitive behavior would be, in turn, based on the development of many different neurosystems, including those that differ in the two sides of the brain, then a genetic model begins to make more sense.

As a first step in determining whether cognitive functions should be dependent variables in a genetic model rather than a particular defect of reading ability, a family study of identified dyslexics was undertaken. The cognitive laterality battery was administered to parents and siblings (and, where possible, second-degree relatives and nonblood-related family members) of children referred to a reading clinic because of difficulties in school. It was found that parents and siblings had the same cognitive profile as the index dyslexics (Gordon 1980b). On the average, performance on tests of left-hemisphere function tended to be below average, and performance on tests attributed to the right hemisphere tended to be above average. Somewhat surprisingly, there were no sex differences in the pattern of the cognitive asymmetry: the magnitude and direction of mothers' cognitive profiles were the same as those of the fathers, sisters, and brothers. The same pattern of asymmetry held for second-degree male relatives (uncles and cousins) as well. No asymmetry was found for second-degree female relatives. Nonrelated family members (spouses) also had no asymmetry, as would be expected (Figure 14.2). The study also included a group of control families chosen because they had at least three male children that were old enough for testing but were otherwise normal, and had no reported reading difficulties. On the average, these subjects had no cognitive asymmetry, that is, they performed like the normal population.

This study indicates that children with learning disabilities (and no evidence of acquired brain damage) may have a cognitive asymmetry that is genetically transmitted. Therefore, cognitive asymmetry favoring right-hemisphere function may be a necessary but not sufficient condition for learning difficulties to occur. It is yet another factor or factors – probably sex-linked because of the predominance of male dyslexics – that determine the presence of serious reading difficulties. It appears that all the family members have a superior ability for tasks associated with the right hemisphere, but they have access to the left-hemisphere processing mode when necessary. The dyslexics appear to be unable to use the left-hemisphere mode and attempt to use the right-hemisphere cognitive mode for performing all tasks, even when it proves to be the less

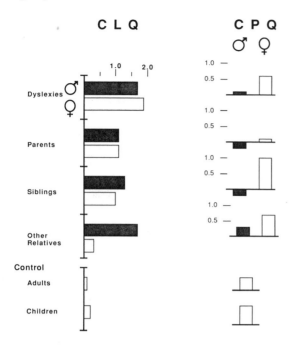

Figure 14.2. The cognitive laterality quotient, CLQ = (performance on "right" tests) – (performance on "left" tests), and the cognitive performance quotient, CPQ = the average performance of all "right" and "left" tests together, for identified dyslexics, their parents and siblings, and other relatives. Adult and children control families are also shown.

efficient strategy, as it is in reading (Gordon 1983).

According to the working hypothesis that specific genetically regulated neurosystems underlie right and left cognitive functions, research might next be directed toward looking for special abnormalities in neurotransmitter systems, or in systems that influence neurotransmitter systems, in the dyslexic population. It should be remembered that attention need not be confined to the right cerebral cortex. A neurosystem that underlies functions normally attributed to the right hemisphere may be predominately found in the right cortex in the "normal" right-handed male, but may have a more widespread distribution in other individuals. For the dyslexic, this system may have an unusual, perhaps bilateral, distribution. With respect to hemispheric organization in dyslexics, an increased bilaterality has already been suggested (Witelson 1977), as has an abnormal developmental history of hormone function (Geschwind and Behan 1982).

There is certainly no requirement that individuals with cognitive asymmetries have some special disability as in the reading disabled. Many individuals have a cognitive profile that favors the right or left hemisphere with no evidence of behavioral or cognitive deficiency. It is not known what distinguishes dysfunctional from nondysfunctional individuals with the same degree of hemispheric preference. But it is likely that individuals favoring primary functions attributed to one hemisphere should be qualitatively different in their abilities and thinking patterns from those favoring functions in the opposite hemisphere. For example, children with an asymmetry in favor of the right hemisphere should still perform less well on achievement tests or verbally loaded school work, even when overall ability (intelligence?) is controlled. Precisely this has been found in three different school populations (Koh 1982; McGranaghan 1983; Gordon 1988).

Fourth- and fifth-grade children were tested in groups in their classrooms with the cognitive laterality battery. Those who performed better on tests of the right-hemisphere function were compared on standard achievement tests to those who performed better on tests of the left-hemisphere function. For reading and language skills but not for arithmetic, the right-hemisphere group was significantly worse than the left-hemisphere group. The difference held when total performance was used as a covariate. That is, the greater success of the left hemisphere group was not because they were smarter. Furthermore, when the "right" and "left" groups were subdivided into above-average and below-average subgroups, the greatest difference was usually found for the above-average subjects (Table 14.2).

The implication from this study is that a general intellectual capacity, or general IQ measure, cannot give a complete account of a person's ability. Achievement testing as well as other intellectual pursuits are also dependent upon the cognitive profile. Gifted children who have a left-hemisphere preference are more likely to enroll in a creative writing class, whereas those with a right-hemisphere preference are likely to enroll in a model-building class (Gordon 1983). In a study where practical relevance was more obvious, it was shown that

Table 14.2. *Achievement scores (national percentiles) of above- and below-average children with "left" and "right" cognitive profiles*

Achievement test		Better on "left" tests	Better on "right" tests	t	p
Vocabulary	Above average	72.5	66.6	2.36	0.02
	Below average	47.6	43.4	1.88	0.07
Reading comprehension	Above average	73.2	66.9	2.74	0.01
	Below average	47.5	42.5	2.20	0.05
Spelling	Above average	78.1	68.1	3.79	0.001
	Below average	58.2	57.2	0.43	NS
Language mechanics	Above average	71.7	70.3	0.55	NS
	Below average	55.8	50.6	1.93	0.06
Language expression	Above average	73.2	67.8	2.14	0.05
	Below average	50.4	45.8	1.93	0.06
Mathematical computation	Above average	72.0	70.5	0.57	NS
	Below average	53.8	55.0	0.49	NS
Mathematical concepts	Above average	72.3	70.4	0.75	NS
	Below average	48.0	47.9	0.06	NS

fighter or combat pilots not only excel in functions attributed to the right hemisphere, but also are significantly better on right-hemisphere tests than pilots who failed to achieve combat status (Gordon, Silverberg-Shalev, and Czernilas 1982) or who left a flight-training program (Gordon and Leighty 1988).

Epilogue

The single "vertical" dimension of intelligence has for too long carried the burden in individual psychometric evaluations. In patients with forebrain commissurotomies, unilateral lesions, and with normal subjects, the converging evidence since the 1960s is that the "horizontal" dimension of hemisphericity is an important component in intellectual endeavors. An unfortunate by-product of this new concept is that popular extrapolations have outstripped scientific validation. Applications of hemispheric differences are undertaken prematurely in countless courses and books purporting to teach how to improve both hemispheres of the brain, how to compensate for a "weak" hemisphere, or how to use a left-hemisphere mode for a right-hemisphere task. So far, none of these attempts have been properly validated by adequate tests or methodology. Proponents of such self-help courses and books hark back to the medicine man of the covered-wagon days or the phrenologist who reads bumps on the skull to determine mental faculties. The courses and books are successful because they satisfy a quest for easy remedies and immediate applicability of science to everyday life.

At the other extreme are the critics who feel right/left dichotomies are not only too simple and overrated, but are also fictitious. If researchers took these dichotomies at face value, the critics would be right. But specialists in the field recognize the dichotomies to be qualitative differences in basic functions of the brain. What complicates the matter further is a failure to find adequate language to describe the specialized brain functions. What may be a semantic disagreement turns into a questioning of the foundations themselves. The scientist who is not a neuropsychologist or a specialist in the field has neither the time nor the basis of experience on which to make a judgment. As a result, scepticism is aroused for the whole field, tarnishing the facts by doubts about the fiction.

Amid the controversy, it is notable that the Nobel Committee recognized the tremendous impact of the discovery of the qualitatively different functions of the brain hemispheres. The Committee also recognized that this discovery will continue to affect everyday life, theoretical scientific constructs, and our own perception of our conscious selves. Roger Sperry's role in the fundamental development of these ideas culminated a lifetime of discoveries in brain organization. Precise analysis of this fundamental mechanism of brain ontogeny will require improved techniques for measuring the distribution of psychological functions between the hemispheres. Findings to date encourage the belief that it will be possible to devise procedures for estimating the great variety of human mentality and the benefits to be derived from this variety. There is much to suggest we can turn full circle on Sperry's work to discover the specificity of brain codes operating in development that instruct a "left hemisphere" to be a left hemisphere and a "right hemisphere" to be a right hemisphere.

References

Alexander, D., A. A. Ehrhardt, and J. Money. 1966. Defective figure drawing, geometric and human, in Turner's Syndrome. *J. Nerv. Ment. Dis.* 142(2): 161–7.

Alexander, D., H. T. Walker, Jr., and J. Money. 1964. Studies in direction sense in Turner's Syndrome. *Arch. Gen. Psychol.* 10: 337–9.

Ashcroft, G. 1982. Biochemistry and pathology of affective psychosis. *In* J. K. Wing and L. Wing (eds.) *Handbook of Psychiatry, Vol. 3.* Cambridge University Press, New York, pp. 160–5.

Bentin, S., and H. W. Gordon. 1979. Assessment of cognitive asymmetries in brain damaged and normal subjects: Validation of a test battery. *J. Neurol. Neurosurg. Psychiat.* 42(8): 715–23.

Bertini, M., C. Violani, P. Zoccolotti, A. Antonelli, and L. DiStefano. 1983. Performance on a unilateral tactile test during waking and upon awakenings from REM and NREM. *Sleep 1982.* 6th European Congress on Sleep Research, Zurich, 1982. Karger, Basel, pp. 383–5.

Bogen, J. E. 1969. The other side of the brain. I. Pysgraphia and dyscopia following cerebral commissurotomy. *Bull. L.A. Neurol. Soc.* 34(2): 73–106.

Bogen, J. E., R. DeZure, W. D. Tenhouten, and J. F. Marsh. 1972. The other side of the brain. IV: The A/P ratio. *Bull. L.A. Neurol. Soc.* 37(2): 49–61.

Broverman, D. M., E. L. Klaiber, Y. Kobayashi, and W. Vogel. 1968. Roles of activation and inhibition in sex differences in cognitive abilities. *Psychol. Rev.* 25(1): 23–50.

Bryden, M. P. 1982. *Laterality. Functional Asymmetry in the Intact Brain.* Academic Press, New York.

Christensen, A. L., and J. Nielsen. 1973. Psychological studies of ten patients with XYY syndrome. *Brit. J. Psychiat.* 123: 219–21.

De Renzi, E. 1982. *Disorders of Space Exploration and Cognition.* Wiley, New York.

Doehring, D. G., R. L. Trites, P. G. Patel, and C. A. M. Fiedorowicz. 1981. *Reading Disabilities.* Academic Press, New York.

Flor-Henry, P. 1969. Psychoses and temporal lobe epilepsy. A controlled investigation. *Epilepsia* 10: 363–95.

Flor-Henry, P., and L. T. Yeudall. 1979. Neuropsychological investigation of schizophrenia and manic-depressive psychoses. *In* J. H. Gruzelier and P. Flor-Henry (eds.) *Hemispheric Asymmetries of Function in Psychopathology.* Elsevier/North-Holland, Amsterdam.

Franco, L., and R. W. Sperry. 1977. Hemisphere lateralization for cognitive processing of geometry. *Neuropsychol.* 15: 107–14.

French, J. W., R. B. Ekstrom, and L. A. Price. 1962. *Kit of Reference Tests for Cognitive Factors.* Educational Testing Service, Princeton.

Galaburda, A. M. 1983. Definition of the anatomical phenotype. *In* C. L. Ludlow and J. A. Cooper (eds.) *Genetic Aspects of Speech and Language Disorders.* Academic Press, New York, pp. 71–84.

Galaburda, A. M., M. Le May, T. L. Kemper, and N. Geschwind. 1978. Right-left asymmetries in the brain. *Science* 199: 852–6.

Galatzer, A., and Gordon, H. W. 1982. Cognitive asymmetries in patients with hormone and genetic abnormalities. Poster at 5th Conference of the International Neuropsychological Society, Deauville, France.

Gazzaniga, M. S., and R. W. Sperry. 1967. Language after section of the cerebral commissure. *Brain* 90: 131–48.

Geschwind, N., and P. Behan. 1982. Left-handeders: Association with immune disease, migraine, and developmental learning disabilities. *Proc. Nat. Acad. Sci. USA* 79: 5097–100.

Gordon, H. W. 1980a. Right hemisphere comprehension of verbs in patients with complete forebrain commissurotomy: Use of the dichotic method and manual performance. *Brain and Lang.* 11: 76–86.

—1980b. Cognitive asymmetries in dyslexic families. *Neuropsychol.* 18: 645–56.

—1983. The learning disabled are cognitively right. *Top. Learn. Learn. Disabil.* 3(1): 29–39.

—1986. The cognitive laterality battery tests: Tests of specialized cognitive functions. *Int. J. Neurosci.* 29(3 & 4): 223–44.

—1988. Specialized cognitive function and school achievement. *Dev. Neuropsychol.* 4(3): 239–57.

Gordon, H. W., B. Frooman, and P. Lavie. 1981. Shift in cognitive asymmetries between wakings from REM and NREM sleep. *Neuropsychol.* 20(1): 99–103.

Gordon, H. W., and A. Galatzer. 1980. Cerebral organization in patients with gonadal dysgenesis. *Psychoneuroendocrinol.* 5(3): 235–44.

Gordon, H. W., and B. Z. Harness. 1977. A test battery for diagnosis and treatment of developmental dyslexia. *DASH. Speech Hear. Disabil.* 8: I–VII.

Gordon, H. W., and P. A. Lee. 1986. A relationship between gonadotropins and visuospatial function. *Neuropsychol.* 24: 563–76.

Gordon, H. W., P. A. Lee, and E. D. Corbin. 1986. Changes in specialized cognitive function following changes in hormone levels. *Cortex* 22(2): 399–415.

Gordon, H. W., and R. Leighty. 1988. Importance of specialized cognitive function in the selection of military pilots. *J. Appl. Psychol.* 73(1): 38–45.

Gordon, H. W., R. Silverberg-Shalev, and J. Czernilas. 1982. Hemispheric asymmetry in fighter and helicopter pilots. *Acta Psychol.* 52: 33–40.

Gruzelier, J. H. 1979. Lateral asymmetries in electrodermal activity and psychosis. *In* J. H. Gruzelier and P. Flor-Henry (eds.) *Hemispheric Asymmetries of Function in Psychopathology.* Elsevier/North-Holland, Amsterdam.

Gruzelier, J. H., and P. Flor-Henry. 1979. *Hemispheric Asymmetries of Function in Psychopathology.* Elsevier/North-Holland, Amsterdam.

Gruzelier, J. H., and N. V. Hammond. 1978. The effect of chlorpromazine upon psychophysiological, endocrine, and information processing measures in schizophrenia. *J. Psychiat. Res.* 14: 167–82.

Gruzelier, J. H., and P. Venables. 1974. Bimodal and lateral asymmetry of skin conductance orienting activity in schizophrenics: Replications and evidence of lateral asymmetry in patients with depression and disorders of personality. *Biol. Psychiat.* 8(1): 56–73.

Gur, R. E. 1978. Left hemisphere dysfunction and left hemisphere overactivation in schizophrenia. *J. Abnormal Psychol.* 87(2): 226–38.

Harness, B. Z., R. Epstein, and H. W. Gordon. 1984. Cognitive profile of children referred to a clinic for learning disabilities. *J. Learn. Disabil.* 17(6): 346–52.

Kaufman, A. S. 1979. Cerebral specialization and intelligence testing. *J. Res. Dev. Educ.* 12(2): 96–107.

Kaufman, A. S., and N. L. Kaufman. 1983. *K-ABC Kaufman Assessment Battery for Children.* American Guidance Service, Circle Pines (MN).

Klaiber, E. L., D. M. Broverman, and Y. Kobayashi. 1967. The automatizative cognitive style, androgens and monamine oxidase. *Psychopharmacol.* 11: 320–36.

Klein, R., and R. Armitage. 1979. Rhythms in human performance. 1½-hour oscillations in cognitive style. *Science* 204: 1326–8.

Koh, Y. H. 1982. *An Analysis of Cognitive Functioning of Korean Middle School Students.* Unpublished doctoral thesis, School of Education, University of Pittsburgh, Pittsburgh.

Komnenich, P., D. M. Lane, R. P. Dickey, and S. C. Stone. 1978. Gonadal hormones and cognitive performance. *Physiol. Psychol.* 6(1): 115–20.

Kronfol, Z., K. deS. Hamsher, K. Digre, and R. Waziri. 1978. Depression and hemispheric functions: Changes associated with unilateral ECT. *Brit. J. Psychiat.* 132: 560–7.

Kushnir, M., H. W. Gordon, and A. Heifetz. 1980. Cognitive asymmetries in bipolar and unipolar depressed patients. Presented at the 8th Annual Meeting of the International Neuropsychological Society, San Francisco.

Ladavas, E., C. Umilta, and P. E. Ricci-Bitti. 1980. Evidence for sex differences in right hemisphere dominance for emotions. *Neuropsychol.* 18: 361–6.

Lavie, P., Y. Metania, and S. Yehuda. 1984. Cognitive asymmetries after wakings from REM and NONREM sleep. *Int. J. Neurosci.* 23(2): 111–16.

Levy, J. 1969. Possible basis for the evolution of lateral specialization of the human brain. *Nature (London)* 224: 614–15.

Levy, J., C. B. Trevarthen, and R. W. Sperry. 1972. Perception of chimeric figures following hemisphere disconnexion. *Brain* 95(1): 61–78.

MacQuarrie, T. W. 1953. *Blocks. MacQuarrie Test for Mechanical Ability.* California Test Bureau, Monterrey.

McGranaghan, K. M. 1983. *The Relationship between Cognitive Profile and Achievement Test Scores for Elementary School Students.* Unpublished master's thesis, School of Education, University of Pittsburgh, Pittsburgh.

Money, J., and D. Alexander. 1966. Turner's syndrome: Further demonstration of the presence of specific cognitive deficiencies. *J. Med. Gen.* 3: 47–8.

Nebes, R. D. 1971. Superiority of the minor hemisphere in commissurotomized man for the perception of the part-whole relations. *Cortex* 7: 333–49.

–1972. Dominance of the minor hemisphere in commissurotomized man on a test of figural unification. *Brain* 95: 633–8.

Netley, C., and J. Rovet. 1983. Relationship among brain organization, maturation rate, and the development of verbal and non-verbal ability. *In* S. J. Segalowitz (ed.) *Language Function and Brain Organization.* Academic Press, New York, pp. 245–66.

Orton, S. T. 1937. *Reading, Writing and Speech Problems in Children.* Norton, New York.

Pasquiline, R. Q., G. Vidal, and G. E. Bur. 1957. Psychopathology of Klinefelter's Syndrome. *Lancet* II: 164–7.

Petersen, A. C. 1976. Physical androgyny and cognitive functioning in adolescence. *Dev. Psychol.* 12(6): 524–33.

Pizzamiglio, L., and P. Zoccolotti. 1981. Sex and cognitive influence on visual hemifield superiority for face and letter recognition. *Cortex* 17: 215–26.

Pizzamiglio, L., P. Zoccolotti, A. Mammucari, and R. Cesaroni. 1983. The independence of face identity and facial expression recognition mechanisms: Relationship to sex and cognitive style. *Brain and Cog.* 2(2): 176–88.

Rodnight, R. 1982. Biochemistry and pathology of schizophrenia. *In* J. K. Wing and L. Wing (eds.) *Handbook of Psychiatry,* Vol. 3. Cambridge University Press, New York, pp. 69–73.

Rovet, J., and C. Netley. 1980. The mental rotation task performance of Turner Syndrome subjects. *Behav. Gen.* 10(5): 437–43.

Rugel, R. P. 1974. WISC subtest scores of disabled readers: A review with respect to Bannatyne's recategorization. *J. Learn. Disabil.* 7(1): 48–65.

Serafetinides, E. A. 1972. Laterality and voltage in the EEG of psychiatric patients. *Diseases Nerv. Syst.* 33: 622–33.

Shaffer, J. W. 1962. A specific cognitive deficit observed in gonadal aplasia (Turner's Syndrome). *J. Clin. Psychol.* 18: 403–6.

Shenkman, A., H. W. Gordon, and A. Heifetz. 1980. Cognitive asymmetries in acute schizophrenics. Presented at the 8th Annual Meeting of the International Neuropsychological Society, San Francisco.

Shepard, R. N., and J. Metzler. 1971. Mental rotation of three-dimensional objects. *Science* 171: 701–3.

Silverberg-Shalev, R., H. W. Gordon, S. Bentin, and A. Aranson. 1981. Selective language deterioration in chronic schizophrenia. *J. Neurol. Neurosurg. Psychiat.* 44(6): 547–51.

Small, I. F., J. G. Small, V. Milstein, and P. Sharpley. 1973. Interhemispheric relationships with somatic therapy. *Diseases Nerv. Syst.* 34: 170–7.

Smith, M. D., J. M. Coleman, P. R. Dokecki, and E. E. Davis. 1977. Recategorized WISC-R scores of learning disabled children. *J. Learn. Disabil.* 10: 437–43.

Sperry, R. W. 1964. Problems outstanding in the evolution of brain function: James Arthur lecture on the evolution of the human Brain. *In* R. Duncan and M. Weston-Smith (eds.) *American Museum of Natural History & The Encyclopedia of Ignorance.* Pergamon Press, Oxford and New York, pp. 423–33.

–1968. Mental unity following surgical disconnection of the cerebral hemispheres. *In The Harvey Lectures, 1966–1967.* Series 62. Academic Press, New York, pp. 293–323.

–1974. Lateral specialization in the surgically separated hemispheres. *In* F. O. Schmitt and F. G. Worden. (eds.) *The Neurosciences: Third Study Program.* The MIT Press, Cambridge, pp. 5–19.

Sperry, R. W., M. S. Gazzaniga, and J. E. Bogen. 1969. Interhemispheric relationships: The neocortical commissures; syndromes of hemisphere disconnection. *In* P. J. Vinken and G. W. Bruyn (eds.) *Handbook of Clinical Neurology,* Vol. 4. North-Holland, Amsterdam, pp. 273–90.

Thurstone, L. L., and T. E. Jeffrey. 1956. *Flags Test.* Industrial Relations Center, Chicago.

Thurstone, L. L., T. G., and T. E. Jeffrey. 1966. *Closure Speed Test.* Industrial Relations Center, Chicago.

Waber, D. 1976. Sex differences in cognition: A function of maturation rate? *Science* 192: 572–4.

Ward, M. M., S. C. Stone, and C. A. Sandman. 1978. Visual perception in women during the menstrual cycle. *Physiol. Behav.* 20: 239–43.

Wesner, C. E., P. Spangler, A. Petrides, D. Baker, and M. A. Telfer. 1973. Prepubertal Klinefelter Syndrome: A report of six cases. *J. Ment. Def. Res.* 17: 237–46.

Witelson, S. F. 1977. Developmental dyslexia: Two right hemispheres and none left. *Science* 195: 309–11.

Wuttke, W., P. Arnold, D. Becker, O. Creutzfeldt, S. Langenstein, and W. Tirsch. 1975. Circulating hormones, EEG and performance in psychological tests of women with and without oral contraceptives. *Psychoneuroendocrinol.* 1: 141–51.

Yozawitz, A., G. Bruder, S. Sutton, L. Sharpe, B. Gurland, J. Fleiss, and L. Costa. 1979. Dichotic perception: Evidence for right hemisphere dysfunction in affective psychosis. *Brit. J. Psychiat.* 135: 224–37.

Zaidel, D., and R. W. Sperry. 1973. Performance on the Raven's Colored Progressive Matrices test by subjects with cerebral commissurotomy. *Cortex* 9: 34–9.

Zaidel, E. 1978. Lexical organization in the right hemisphere. *In* P. Buser and A. Rougeul-Buser (eds.) *Cerebral Correlates of Conscious Experience,* INSERM Symposium No 6. Elsevier/North-Holland, Amsterdam.

Zeuthen, E., M. Nansen, A. L. Christensen, and J. Nielsen. 1975. A psychiatric-psychological study of XYY males found in a general male population. *Acta Psychiat. Scand.* 51: 3–18.

15 Long-term semantic memory in the two cerebral hemispheres

Dahlia W. Zaidel
Department of Psychology
University of California, Los Angeles

It seems a proposition, which will not admit of much dispute, that all of our ideas are nothing but copies of our impressions, or, in other words, that it is impossible for us to think of anything, which we have not antecedently felt, either by our external or internal senses.

David Hume (1748)

Introduction

In this chapter, I will focus initially on work with commissurotomy patients at Caltech that eventually led to my current approach in studying hemispheric specialization – namely, investigation of asymmetries in long-term semantic-cognitive stores.

It seems appropriate in a book honoring Roger Sperry to trace the origin of a new idea. Such a process follows the inquisitive spirit he has always tried to engender in his psychobiology lab at Caltech. My chapter is a tribute to his trust and guidance. He provided facilities and equipment for doing research, consistently tried to instill an appreciation for the beauty of science, and tried to impart lessons on how to make meaningful contributions. The most characteristic feature of his style is an approach to investigation that is unencumbered by elaborate theories or dogmas, an attitude of global curiosity combined with conscientious investigation of every relevant question. Perhaps it was this unique personal style of scientific inquiry, a mixture of simplicity and generality, that caused him to arrive at the idea, in the early 1960s, that the cerebral hemispheres of humans represent two complementary spheres of consciousness (Sperry 1968). Never before had such a conception of the human brain been presented with such clear evidence, and it excited immediate and widespread interest.

What is the nature of long-term semantic memory?

Before the cognitive structure in the brain interprets the significance of such pieces of information, sensory visual input is nothing more than patches of light and color and a jumble of gradients and contours, and auditory sensation is just collections of loudness and pitches. It seems reasonable to assume that a store of abstracted, classified, or categorized experiences from the past interacts with such incoming sensory information to create perception, and that actions or responses reflect what is stored in the mind, as well as information presently exciting the senses.

In information-processing psychology, the theoretical approach adopted in this chapter, long-term semantic memory is considered to be the storehouse of knowledge by which perception and action are organized. Without it, we would not have the ability to write books, make films, perform surgery, paint, or converse. It constitutes the vocabulary of the meaningful world we live in.

At this point, it must be stressed that in my discussion, "semantic" does not refer to linguistic semantics alone. Rather, it refers to the general concept of meaning. As such, it encompasses both linguistic and nonlinguistic knowledge in the brain. Otherwise, it would be impossible to talk about semantic processing in the right hemisphere, a mental system that is only minimally endowed with linguistic capability.

In my analysis of long-term semantic memory, the underlying assumption is that the left and right hemispheres, though they may be exposed to the same external experiences, will lay down different semantic stores or control different retrieval strategies. It is proposed that these hemispheric semantic differences can be examined with the paradigms of information-processing psychology.

In information-processing theory, human memory is viewed as a multiple-component system in which visual information is processed in sequential interrelated stages (see Figure 15.1). Long-term memory (LTM) is the last fixed structural store in the memory system and it links all other fixed components: iconic store, short-term memory, and LTM. For pattern recognition to occur, the material in each of the other two structures in turn requires contact with LTM. The duration of a memory trace in each store is variable: iconic store lasts 250 ms,

short-term memory lasts 20–30 s, and LTM upwards of 30 s to hours or throughout an individual's lifetime (Crowder 1976). Various factors that are in the control of each individual person, such as the context of their experience, their expectations, or attention, may influence the duration of memory. Of these control factors, the context will be given particular attention in subsequent sections of this chapter.

Some psychologists conceive the LTM as providing the interpretive basis for a vast range of everyday functions: crossing the street on a green light, solving conceptual problems, anticipating events, accumulating facts, and so on (Mandler 1967, Norman 1969, Tulving 1972, Klatzky 1975, Rumelhart 1977). Semantic knowledge is an essential component of the LTM built up from past experience, and the LTM may contain the verbal lexicon as well as schematic concepts; in short, it contains all our world knowledge. Meaning or understanding is said to be attained when contact is made between newly perceived information and knowledge stored in LTM.

The constant interaction between the environment and LTM involves the mind in a

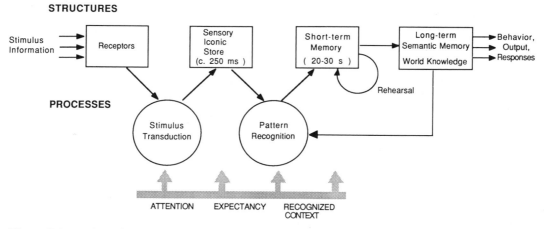

Figure 15.1. A schematic diagram of the information-processing model. Memory is viewed as an interconnected system made of several structural components and control processes. Previously stored knowledge, or long-term memory (LTM), is an important segment of the memory chain that is enriched by some portions and influences others. The structures, though not their content, are more or less fixed, whereas the control processes are subject to the control of the individual (e.g., his or her unique set of experiences leading to specific expectations, or physiological conditions regulating attentional effort, etc.). LTM plays a role in every stage: when perceptual identification demands contact with the repository of stored patterns or when context and expectancy facilitate selection of quick and efficient behavior.

search through coherently organized knowledge and organization of mental functions that make for economy and efficiency in this search. One such organizing construct of the mind is the concept of "schema" described by Norman and Bobrow (1976). Schemata, according to these authors, represent mental structural clusters – of associations, experiences, facts, traditions, or conventions. They are used in pattern recognition of incoming stimuli, in attaining meaning, and, importantly, in guiding the acquisition of new sensory information. During perceptual recognition, an appropriate schema is activated and, as a result of the activation, understanding, recognition, or meaning is achieved.

The British psychologist Sir Frederick Bartlett (1932) is responsible for introducing the concept of schema to the study of memory. Before Bartlett, Sir Henry Head, the British neurologist, attempting to explain the neuropsychological phenomenon of neglect of part of the body, or its converse, the "phantom" limb, used the term schema to describe the concept of a body image that determines our knowledge of the position of our limbs relative to the rest of the body. Bartlett's idea was that newly perceived sensory information is assimilated with reference to a previously stored set of knowledge. More important to the subsequent sections in this chapter is his contention that when new information is perceived, the schemata in a subject's mind into which it becomes organized mentally are not isomorphic with that person's external reality. Consequently, remembering can lead to distorted impressions, the distortions tending in the direction of norms, traditions, or cultural conventions. For example, subjects of Western culture who read Bartlett's best-known stimulus story, "The war of the ghosts," a folktale of North American Indians, made numerous errors in the recall stage. Significantly, the errors were systematic and they revealed consistent adherence to conventions unique to that western culture. In terms of the present discussion, European subjects were unable to remember details from the story because there were no analogous concepts in their culturally fabricated LTM or, put differently, because there was a poor "match" between the details

in the story and the existing schemata in LTM their culture had provided.

That there should be cerebral asymmetries in LTM follows logically from the very evidence for hemispheric specialization in perception and cognition. From studies of patients with unilateral focal lesions as well as those of normal subjects, it has been extensively documented that different thinking processes are controlled by the two cerebral hemispheres and that in most right-handers, certain prominent functions, such as speech, are lateralized mainly to the left, whereas visuospatial abilities are lateralized mainly to the right (Bogen 1969, Levy 1969, Kimura and Durnford 1974, Sperry 1974, Hécaen and Albert 1978). A host of other functions are now believed to be segregated, to some extent, into one or the other hemisphere, and most neuropsychologists today believe in complementarity of function between the two halves of the cerebrum.

In spite of the wealth of knowledge we now possess, however, it is still a mystery how functional integration of the two hemispheres is achieved. Nevertheless, any task that involves mnestic functions, problem-solving strategies, or simple perceptual judgments, whether performed by patients with unilateral localized lesions using free-field testing, or by normal subjects in visual tachistoscopic or dichotic listening experiments, must be presumed to somehow engage or draw upon some aspects of LTM. We can assume, therefore, that consistent asymmetries revealed in tests are attributable, in part, to differences between the two hemispheres in preestablished long-term internal memory stores or in the retrieval strategies that get memories from them. To gain further insights into hemispheric specialization, it is both theoretically and empirically important to explore systematically the possibility that asymmetries in LTM exist, and if so, to determine the nature of LTM in each hemisphere.

A few years ago, following an accidental lead, I decided to investigate just that hypothesis. In the following sections, I will provide a description of the initial insight gained at Roger Sperry's lab from the study of patients in whom the forebrain commissures had been sectioned. This will be followed by a summary of a subsequent study with patients in whom the left or right anterior temporal lobes had been excised. Finally, I will report results obtained recently with normal subjects.

Long-term semantic memory in commissurotomy patients

HOW IT STARTED: A SEARCH
FOR UNDERLYING CAUSES OF
IDEOMOTOR APRAXIA

The idea that led to the study of differential hemispheric LTM was conceived in 1975 with an investigation not concerned with this issue, but rather with the underlying causes for unilateral left-hand ideomotor apraxia that had been observed in five commissurotomy patients (NG, RY, NW, CC, and AA). These patients of P. J. Vogel and J. E. Bogen underwent surgery that effectively disconnected the two cerebral hemispheres. The single-stage complete commissurotomy operation was performed in order to alleviate grand-mal epileptic seizures that could not be controlled with drugs (Bogen, Fisher, and Vogel 1965). Included in the sectioned tissues were the corpus callosum, anterior and hippocampal commissures, and the variable massa intermedia whenever it was visualized. As a consequence of the surgical approach, the column of the right fornix was sectioned in NG and columnar fibers are assumed to have been partially interrupted in the other cases. Extracallosal damage not associated with the surgery is inferred to be present but to vary widely in nature and extent. The behavioral disconnection symptoms are mostly seen only under special lateralized testing conditions (see early reports by Gazzaniga, Bogen, and Sperry 1965; Sperry 1968; Sperry, Gazzaniga, and Bogen 1969).

Ideomotor apraxia is broadly defined as the inability to carry out spoken commands in the absence of sensory or motor deficits. Its presence was tested with short verbal commands such as "put your thumb on your forehead" or "signal for hitchike," these being part of a large series of test items administered to measure motor control and manipulative performance in this population of patients with sectioned forebrain commissures (Zaidel and Sperry 1977).

As part of a continuous effort to delineate functional lateralization and to assess the long-term effects of hemispheric disconnection, trials for ideomotor apraxia were specifically included to test Liepmann's 1905 hypothesis that callosal fibers are required to mediate volitional movements of the left hand following their normal initiation in the left hemisphere (Wilson 1908; Geschwind 1965). Implicit in Liepmann's view is the idea that there is no center for volitional control in the right hemisphere. With callosum-sectioned patients, we felt it should be possible to test this hypothesis directly. To the extent that some ideomotor apraxia was present in the left limbs, Liepmann's proposal was confirmed. However, the deficit was evident in the context of verbal commands and, furthermore, it was variable and never as severe as would be expected if absence of commissural connections had cut the left hand off from all volitional control. Outside the linguistic context, left-hand praxis was normal in all commissurotomy patients tested.

Absence of ideational apraxia and normal ability to copy simple hand postures both provided good evidence for normal praxis in the left hand. Ideational praxis was tested by asking subjects to demonstrate, unilaterally, the use of objects such as a hammer, toothbrush, eraser, etc. Copying of hand postures was tested in free vision by asking subjects to demonstrate the same stationary hand postures as those assumed by the examiner. The postures were all taken from Sperry's previous report (Sperry 1968). Since praxis was, by these tests, unimpaired in the left hand, we suspected that verbal comprehension in the right hemisphere was a major source of the deficit (the dominant language centers being in the left hemisphere). But when we tested the patients under special viewing conditions, we found that they could correctly match a picture confined in the left visual half-field to a spoken command with an accuracy of 80%. Lateralization of a choice array of four action pictures was accomplished through the use of a contact lens occluder (the Z lens), an optical system designed to allow continuous visual presentation of the stimuli to one visual half-field at a time (Zaidel 1975). It requires wearing a specially fitted scleral contact lens on which a light collimator as well as a field occluder are mounted. Only two patients, LB and NG, had been fitted with the lens when this experiment was undertaken. Sperry et al. (1969) reported that these two patients are the best representations of the disconnection syndrome seen in the patients operated by Bogen and Vogel.

In this control test, spoken commands were given in free field and subjects could both monitor their manual response and see the entire multiple-choice array in only one half-field. The two patients were tested in several sessions on a number of tests described in this chapter, in all of which the subject had to match a spoken message with a visual array. The comprehension of instructions by the right hemisphere in these tests was too high to explain the ideomotor apraxia as a consequence of lack of speech comprehension. In view of this finding, and the absence of any impairment in copying hand postures or in ideational apraxia in the left hand, both poor verbal comprehension and poor fine motor control by the right hemisphere were ruled out as principal causes of the observed apraxia of the left hand in commissurotomy patients. The search for other causes continued.

Although there was no previous evidence to support the possibility in commissurotomy patients, there was evidence that body parts themselves might not be easily identified by the right hemisphere, especially when the parts were represented in a linguistic context. According to classical concepts of the anatomical locus of lesion causing autotopagnosia (the acquired inability to identify and name body parts), which points to critical regions in the parietal area of the left hemisphere, we could predict an impairment in recognizing named body parts in the right hemisphere of commissurotomy patients (Selecki and Herron 1965, see Hécaen and Albert 1978 for a review). It seemed worthwhile to investigate this possibility in detail since many items in the ideomotor battery involved commands for touching parts of the body. To test that idea, line drawings of individual body parts and of an entire human figure, with separate front and back views, were prepared. These stimuli were presented to the same two patients (NG and LB) under the same special lateralized viewing conditions described before.

In one set of trials, the two subjects were asked to point to one of four pictures depicting individual parts of the body when the body-part name was spoken aloud by the examiner. In all, there were eighteen trials per subject and the mean correct score was 83% in the LVF and 100% in the RVF. In the other set of trials, drawings of the entire human figure were presented. Again, the examiner named parts and the subjects were required to point to each. Matching responses were 100% in either visual half-field.

In the hope of gaining some additional clues, it was then decided to focus attention on a pictorial representation of the face. Line drawings were prepared of both front and profile views that were presented as described before. The results obtained showed 100% correct identification for the front view in both visual half-fields. In sharp contrast, with the profile view, accuracy was 15% for the right hemisphere while remaining 100% for the left hemisphere.

For the first time in this investigation, error analysis of the profile stimulus hinted at an unusual and unexpected asymmetry in cognitive process. Based on this analysis, I considered that long-term experiential memory (or retrieval from it) in the right hemisphere, with which the perceptual input was presumed to have been processed, may not be identical to the one in the left. Specifically, the errors recorded when commissurotomy patients were pointing with the left hand to stimuli in the LVF revealed a peculiar pattern: they pointed to the ear when they were asked to point to the eye, to the center of the cheek when asked to point to the nose, and to the jaw instead of the lips. Yet, they correctly identified the hair. This result was puzzling in view of the correct identification made of the same parts when they were presented separately or when they were in the front view of the face. Moreover, the right hemisphere has long been associated with superior facial recognition and visuospatial perception when compared to the left (see Warrington and James 1967, Hécaen and Albert 1978). Yet, under the present conditions, with the profile face, performance in the LVF was grossly inaccurate.

How might the hypothesized cognitive differences arise to cause such differences in experiences of the two views of the face? First, in daily interactions, we spend much time looking at people's faces straight-on rather than at their profiles. Hence, we would expect memory units for front views of faces to be stronger than those for side views. Second, in development, faces seem to be in a separate and highly salient class of perceptual experience. Studies with infants (Fantz 1958, 1965) have shown that infants as young as four days prefer pictorial depictions of "real" faces to faces with scrambled features, or to many other simple figures. Thus, sensitivity to a face as a distinct pattern begins early on.

Given this evidence that mental processes in the right hemisphere, and not in the left, were sensitive to the differences in the two views of the face, the following explanation for the previous errors was proposed. First, it was possible that either a different LTM was tapped in each hemisphere or different retrieval strategies were employed. Second, more specifically, storage or retrieval may be specialized for recognition of experimentally familiar perspectives in the right hemisphere.

At this point, it seemed that a cul de sac had been reached in the search for other underlying factors in ideomotor apraxia in the right hemisphere. Clearly, the testing had demonstrated that processing facial features in the context of a front view as well as of individual facial features presented singly was well within the functional control of the right hemisphere. Since in the ideomotor trials, patients had an access to their own bodies or faces, the poor performance on the profile view of a face did not appear in any obvious way to be relevant to the original quest for an explanation of the left hand's inferior performance. Based on the available evidence, then, it was concluded that the behavior of the commissurotomy patients was due to a weak connection between the auditory receiving areas for speech and the motor control centers for the left hand in the right hemisphere (but see Zaidel and Sperry 1977 for a detailed discussion).

EXPLORATION OF A NEW QUESTION: ARE THERE ASYMMETRIES IN LONG-TERM SEMANTIC MEMORY?

Meanwhile, the results with the facial profile led to a new line of investigation and a fresh approach to the study of hemispheric specialization. The working hypothesis in the next series of tests was that information processing in the right hemisphere placed heavy reliance on schemata representing stereotypical or experientially familiar views. An analysis of performance in the recognition of physical features in a configuration that was different from the one in which they normally occur seemed to provide a good test of selective cognitive dependence on common or usual arrays. This would contrast sharply with the view that the right hemisphere specializes in unusual perspective (Warrington and Taylor 1973).

As a start, the heterotopia, "The Rape," painted in the surrealistic tradition in 1945 by Belgian artist Rene Magritte (Torczyner 1979), was chosen for the first stimulus (Figure 15.2). I assumed that a context of a face here is provided by the elliptical outline of a face and adjacent features, e.g., hair, hair-part, neck, etc. Each component in this painting can be recognized easily even though, within the frame of a face, eyes appear to have been transformed into breasts, nose transformed into a navel, and the mouth into the pubic region. The question of interest was whether the components will be recognized in each hemisphere for what they are individually or for the features they appear to have replaced within the face. My hypothesis was that if storage of stereotypes derived from order in the occurrences of external reality is a dominant feature in right-hemisphere mental processes, then a general framing outline, suggesting the stereotype, would prevent recognition of the actual components so that they would not be recognized as such but rather for the components they replaced.

A black-and-white 5×7-inch photograph of the painting was presented to the same two commissurotomy subjects (NG and LB) using the Z-lens optical system. Testing began with the LVF. Names of facial features were read aloud by the examiner and the subject was asked to point to each as it was read. The results were dramatic: both commissurotomy subjects pointed to the breasts when the examiner said "point to the eyes," to the navel when "nose" was said, and to the pubic region when pointing to the mouth was requested. At the same time, the hair and neck were correctly identified;

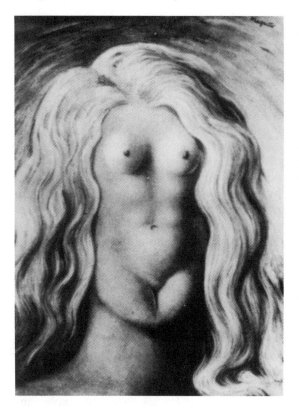

Figure 15.2. The heterotopia, "The Rape," painted by Belgian artist Rene Magritte in 1945. It was shown to two comissurotomy patients under unilateral viewing conditions to reveal hemispheric differences in cognitive processing of stereotypical schemata. In both hemispheres, a facial schema was activated, but the right hemisphere failed to identify the individual body parts, whereas the left did recognize them for what they are. (Reprinted with permission from H. Torczyner, 1979. *Magritte: Ideas and Images*. Abrams, New York.)

forehead and cheeks were identified as the areas above the breasts and on both sides of the navel, respectively.

There was a possibility that perception in the right hemisphere was accurate and the responses reflected an understanding of the symbolic nature of the transformed parts conveyed by the examiner's questions. To find that out, further probing was undertaken as follows: the examiner said, "point to the breasts." Surprisingly, subjects pointed to an area outside the stimulus boundaries but that fell directly below the neck, to a spot where the breasts would normally belong. A request to point to the navel resulted in pointing slightly farther down,

and still farther down from there when "the pubic region" was named. The striking aspect in this performance is that it appeared as if in the right hemisphere, the mental memory trace of a normal woman's figure, rather than the actual stimulus figure, dominated the cognitive process.

Performance in the left hemisphere, by contrast, was accurate throughout. "There are no eyes here," or "if there were eyes, they would be here," were the typical comments made by these two subjects when, immediately following performance with the LVF, they were asked to point to the eyes (with exposure in the RVF). Unlike performance controlled by the right hemisphere, correct identification was provided for the breasts, navel, and pubic region with RVF presentations. Similarly, the hair and neck were correctly identified. Again, these results suggested that whereas in right-hemisphere performance, there appeared cognitive dominance of schemata representing highly common daily images, with a selective emphasis on the frame outlining the contours, performance by the left hemisphere reflected facile ability to separate the contour frame from the components it contains. Subsequent testing in the LVF disclosed the same pattern observed initially on this side.

Perceptual dominance of the contour frame to a point where the contained particulars are not recognized as such was examined further. Instead of the trunk replacing facial features, a line drawing of a heteroclitic (anomalous) face was prepared in which facial features were exchanged with each other. A line drawing of such a surrealistic face (Figure 15.3A) was presented to the two commissurotomy patients with the Z lens. The results were again dramatic. In the LVF, the left hand pointed to the nose and lips when in fact instructed to point to the eyes, and to the eye and ear when asked to point to the nose and lips. Again, hair, neck, forehead, and chin were all correctly identified. One would think that once these were identified, the subject would become sharply aware of the discrepancy in earlier responses. But this did not appear to have occurred.

At the same time, the suggestion that the contours of stereotypical percepts themselves

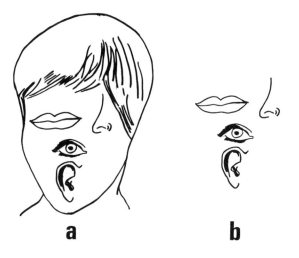

a   **b**

Figure 15.3. (**A**) This stimulus of a heteroclitic face was shown unilaterally to two commissurotomy patients. The right hemisphere failed to recognize the eye, lips, nose, or ear, but gained recognition of the hair and neck. The left hemisphere recognized all the parts. (**B**) When the outline of the facial frame was removed, both hemispheres recognized all the features accurately. This was taken to mean that a schema representing "face" was activated in both hemispheres by the drawn outine of hair, neck, jaw line, but that in the right hemisphere, cognitive processes were dominated by a "preconceived" idea of a face stored in long-term semantic memory and probably activated by the outline.

were the critical elements that interfered with recognition of contained parts had not been directly verified. Accordingly, the outline was erased, leaving only the internal parts (Figure 15.3B). When the new stimulus array was presented in the LVF, each individual part was identified 100% accurately. Thus, in the first part of the experiment, the frame clearly had provided the context for the response and had prevented appropriate cognitive processing of elements inside it. In the RVF, the right hand pointed correctly to the named parts as they were read by the examiner, regardless of the presence or absence of the framing outline.

On the evidence of identical performance by the two hemispheres when the frame was removed, differences in processing of the auditory message – the names of the body parts – cannot explain the hemispheric differences found when the contour frame was present. It would appear, then, that mental processes applied in the right hemisphere to realistic stimuli

may involve a mental "match" with stored concepts that may be characterized by the global contours of a common general percept, e.g., a face. That is not to say that a match with a previously laid store could not take place in the left hemisphere, only that the mental decision there appeared more "tuned in" to the features of the external visual array than the one in the right hemisphere.

One could say that the findings reflect general perceptual or cognitive dominance, within the right hemisphere, of global features over detailed features rather than a dominance in that side for processing of stereotypical or experientially familiar arrays. Whether or not the representation of any enclosure containing parts would result in a comparative neglect of the actual parts in this half of the cerebrum was explored in an additional test.

Several small geometrical figures were drawn inside large geometric shapes such as circle, triangle, or rectangle. These shapes were deemed to have no stereotypical contours relative to the figures they enclosed; they did not represent normal boundaries of familiar arrays. With the experimental conditions used hitherto, the same two subjects, NG and LB, recognized the small geometric figures regardless of the outlined frame, and in either visual field. Thus, the original hypothesis was confirmed: stereotypical frames or percepts play a special role in the storage or retrieval of information from the LTM in the right hemisphere. In view of the results, I continued this intriguing line of investigation with a new population of subjects and employed more complex stimuli than I had done previously.

Performance of patients with unilateral lesions

A new set of stimuli consisting of complex multiple-object scenes was administered to patients who had undergone left (LTL) or right (RTL) temporal lobe removals for the relief of epilepsy (Zaidel and Rausch 1981). In the past, studies of patients who underwent temporal lobe removals have revealed a wealth of data on functional lateralization (see Milner 1975 for a review). Specifically, selective memory impairment has been found for verbal material following surgery on the left side (Milner 1958;

Blakemore and Falconer 1967) and for non-verbal material following surgery on the right side (Kimura 1963, 1969; Milner 1967, 1968).

There are both advantages and disadvantages to testing patients with different etiology from that of the commissurotomy group. The latter are the ideal subjects for studying left–right differences in cognition since the factors of age, education, and sex are all equated in the same individual. Also, conclusions are based on direct evidence of positive hemispheric performance. By contrast, cerebral functional asymmetries found in studies with patients suffering from unilateral lesions are subject to the many uncertainties associated with imperfectly controlled experimental and subject variables and, moreover, conclusions are based on negative inference from deficits in behavior. Nevertheless, although it is more difficult to reach conclusions based on the "noisy preparation" of patients with hemispheric damage, one can partly match the populations for some relevant variables and obtain significant results that transcend interpatient variability. Also, more patients are available for study of the effects of unilateral focal lesions. By contrast, very few individuals have undergone surgical section of the forebrain commissures.

The subjects available for this experiment were patients from the Clinical Neurophysiology Program at UCLA who had undergone unilateral anterior temporal lobectomy at least six months prior to the testing. The surgery included removal of the anterior temporal pole, the uncus, portions of the amygdala, and the pes hippocampi (Crandall, Walter, and Rand 1963). Eight patients had excisions on the left and 11 on the right. Control subjects were 24 normal undergraduate and graduate students and clerical employees at UCLA.

In normal daily experience, objects commonly occur together with other objects of a particular kind. Rarely do we encounter the shapes of things in isolation from a related background. Accordingly, the stimulus scenes used here were pictures depicting two different kinds of semantic organization. These scenes were considered "ecologically valid" means of examining human cognition. Half of the pictures represented organized drawings of common realistic objects in natural groups, while the other half represented unorganized or uncommon arrays of equally realistic and familiar individual objects (see Figures 15.4A and 15.4C).

The neuropsychological literature is replete with hemispheric studies of memory that fail to manipulate this dimension of semantic organization. Cognitive psychologists, on the other hand, have paid much attention to the effects of semantic organization in pictures on memory in normal subjects, but not to possible hemispheric differences in these. Experiments with pictorial scenes have shown that meaningful context facilitates retention and that jumbled pictorial arrays interfere with subsequent recognition (Biederman 1972). Some have reported that pictorial semantic organization is important for good retention, organized stimuli being retained the longest (Mandler and Johnson 1976; Mandler and Parker 1976). Others have concluded that with stimuli depicting either logical organization or unorganized arrays, the degree of component interaction determines the extent of subsequent recognition (Wollen, Weber, and Lowery 1972). In view of these and similar findings, it was hoped that the stimuli administered to patients with left or right temporal lobe excisions would help elucidate hemispheric differences in long-term storage of semantic relationships derived from world knowledge.

I had added to the experimental manipulation with the patients probes for memory of single elements as well as of whole scenes. The question of recognition memory for details versus entire scenes had not been reported previously and it seemed important to assess both in order to obtain a systematic analysis of LTM. Moreover, I was interested in the specific cues that context provides for subsequent retention (Tulving and Thompson 1971; Winograd and Rivers-Bulkeley 1977), and the possible asymmetries that may exist in the use of contextual information by the two hemispheres.

The procedure for testing was as follows. Each subject was presented with a sequence of a set of six pictures (three organized and three unorganized, intermixed within the series) with an exposure duration of five seconds for each picture. Memory for the stimuli was tested in

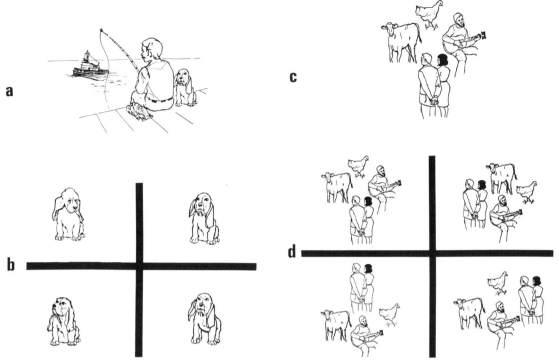

Figure 15.4. Examples of the types of pictorial stimuli and multiple-choice arrays used in a study with patients with left or right temporal lobe excisions. (**A**) An organized scene where the juxtaposition of the elements is "normal" or stereotypical. (**B**) Recognition memory of a single object occurring in the stimulus picture was tested through pointing to the one correct figure that matched the one in the scene. (**C**) An unorganized stimulus scene where the juxtaposition of the component figures is meaningless, although each figure is well known. (**D**) A multiple-choice array used to measure recognition memory of the arrangement of whole stimulus scenes.

a forced-choice recognition paradigm. Immediately following the last stimulus presentation, a distracting task lasting nine minutes was introduced; subjects wrote down as many words as they could beginning with the letter "S," in five minutes; then, in four minutes, they wrote down as many four-letter words as they could that begin with the letter "C". The purpose of this interpolated task was to increase the level of difficulty, since, in this group of patients, memory impairment is typically so subtle that it can go unnoticed in a relatively simple task. Following the completion of the interpolated task, subjects were asked to recognize items from the pictures by pointing to the correct answer in a four-choice array. Both memory for single elements in stimulus scenes and that for entire scenes were measured (see Figures 15.4B and 15.4D). In all there were 12 recog-

nition trials, six for single details and six for entire scenes.

Analysis of the results showed significant main effects of type of probe (details versus whole scenes), but no interaction with type of organization. However, within the group of LTL patients, significantly worse memory for single details was found for the organized than for unorganized pictures. Figure 15.5 gives a graphic presentation of the findings.

Since there was a dissociation between organized and unorganized pictorial arrays within the LTL group, it would seem valid to conclude that there are indeed asymmetries in the semantic memories of the hemispheres. That the dissociation was evident only in the LTL is difficult to reconcile with the hypothesis that real-world schemata are more strongly apprehended in right-hemisphere storage or re-

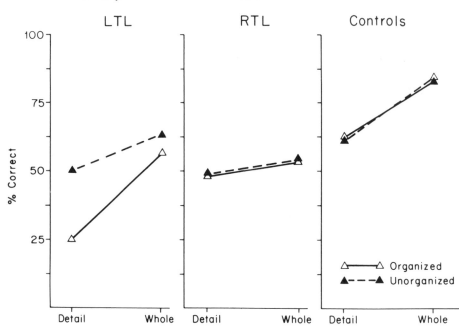

Figure 15.5. A graphic summary of performance by patients with temporal lobe excisions on a successive presentation of the organized and unorganized stimulus pictures as exemplified in Figure 15.4. LTL = left temporal lobe removals, eight patients; RTL = right temporal lobe removals, 11 patients; Controls = normal subjects, 24. Detail = memory for a single figure in the scene; Whole = memory for the entire scene.

trieval (proposed in the section of LTM in commissurotomy patients). If this hypothesis were correct, then there should have been in the RTL group poor memory for organized pictures relative to unorganized ones, the latter stimuli being processed possibly by the intact left hemisphere.

The seeming discrepancy between the findings with patients who have unilateral focal lesions and the hypothesis generated by performance of commissurotomy patients may be the result of pathological inhibitory effects of localized lesions on healthy tissue. It is possible that a surgical lesion in the left temporal lobe inhibited recognition of real-world pictorial schemata, possibly by selectively interfering with the processing of the homologous component in semantic-conceptual structures in the right hemisphere that may be needed for the processing of the organized frames on that side of the brain. If there are such inhibitory processes (cross-callosal?) interfering with processing of schemata in the right hemisphere, they would seem to be asymmetric, i.e., much stronger from left to right than in the opposite direction. Asymmetry of this kind, and the fact

that normal control subjects showed a similar pattern to RTL patients, reflecting the characteristic dominance of the left hemisphere, led to the hypothesis that the patients in the RTL group showed a close approximation to left-hemisphere performance because they were unaffected by inhibitory effects transmitted from the lesion in the right hemisphere (compare Chapter 13, this volume).

Alternatively, the unique performance pattern of the LTL group may signify a different mental process from the one proposed earlier to explain the commissurotomy patients' performance with anomalous faces. The deficit in remembering single objects occurring in organized pictures may be interpreted as follows: considering the factor of context in relation to the experimental procedure, memory for details was tested by requiring recognition of single items without the aid of the original context, whereas recognition of whole scenes involved the presence of the full complement of contextual cues. Contextual changes in probing for effects on memory of elements were first introduced in this experiment during the recognition or retrieval stage of the memory chain.

One aspect of perceiving a change of context must consist of apprehending that new situations deviate from the original context or schema. There was good memory for whole scenes in the LTL group. However, the excision on the left side may have abolished or weakened mechanisms responsible for mentally processing new perspectives comprising stored memory units that are related to a previous perspective. On this interpretation, the distractors in the test for recognition of details of organized scenes, the performance of which showed greatest deficit, could be regarded as introducing novel contexts for those details. The impairment of patients in the LTL group could then be seen as failure to recognize details correctly because of some inhibitory or interference effects in a brain that could not recognize the schema for the new context, i.e., the array of four test stimuli.

Another obvious possibility is that organization of memory for normal stereotypical arrays is dependent upon the parietal lobe (or any other region outside the temporal lobe) in the right hemisphere (Zaidel 1984, 1986, 1988).

An attempt was made, next, to at least partly resolve these puzzles in a study of semantic-memory effects in normal subjects.

Semantic relationships among concepts stored in LTM: Normal subjects

In the previous experiment, complex scenes were used to measure LTM. In the next experiment, the stimuli were, once again, simple figures. Here semantic relationships among specific memory units were probed by analyzing the effects of varying the degree of relatedness of two concepts instantiated by single pictorial figures. I hoped this experiment would provide a graded measure of the relatedness of items in semantic memory in each cerebral hemisphere. The subjects were undergraduate students, all free of neurological signs, and enrolled in introductory psychology courses at UCLA.

Normal subjects have the advantage of directing attention to processes in the organ that we all wish ultimately to understand, namely, the intact brain. They also provide data that are uncontaminated by such complexities as the effects of functional reorganization due to early brain damage, as occurs with the onset of epilepsy in childhood. We cannot rule out this confounding factor in experiments with either temporal-lobe-damaged patients or commissurotomy patients. However, because the forebrain commissures are all intact in normal subjects, testing them can become problematic, their performance being exceedingly difficult to analyze into components. At the same time, we assume that a statistical interaction between the hemisphere factor and the other factors varied experimentally can be taken to indicate direct processing by the hemisphere that received the stimulus first.

The background to the chosen test procedure is as follows. For reasons of economy in processing information in a system of limited capacity, semantic memory is, we presume, highly organized. For the past 15 years, cognitive psychologists have used mental chronometry extensively to gain insights into the nature of this organization. In the process, they have developed excellent tools for studying its structure (Collins and Quillian 1969; Rips, Shoben, and Smith 1973; Guenther, Klatzky, and Putnam 1980). Typically, semantic "distance" and semantic "relatedness" are studied through the use of speeded comparisons between words or concepts, or speeded class membership decisions. Theoretically, memory units that are closely associated have a shorter mental distance between them and a shorter latency of response than unassociated units. The latter have a long "mental distance" separating them and decisions concerning them exhibit a slow reaction time. The implication is that cognitive processes are faster when there is a close relationship in memory between the concepts involved than when there is little association. To illustrate, the latency of response to the statement "a whale is a mammal" may be much longer than the latency of response to the statement "a dog is a mammal" because the concept of "mammal" is stored closer mentally to the concept of a dog (which, like most mammals we know well, has four legs, lives on land, has fur) than to that of a whale (which resembles a fish more than a typical mammal).

In an important series of experiments involving both words and pictures, Rosch

(1975) has shown that latency responses to decisions involving typical instances of natural superordinate categories are, indeed, shorter than those to atypical instances. Rosch determined the level of typicality initially by asking subjects to rate the "degree of representativeness" of specific instances on a seven-point scale. Here latency results can be interpreted to reflect the mental semantic distance between the concept invoked by the name of the category and the concept invoked by the pictorial or verbal representation of the instance.

With this powerful experimental tool, the charting of semantic distances in the left or right cerebral hemispheres offered both theoretical and empirical challenge. I designed my experiment to test the response latencies to decisions involving typical versus atypical instances of natural superordinate categories for stimuli presented in the LVF or RVF of normal subjects (Zaidel 1983, 1985). Norms for typicality ratings were provided in Rosch's (1975) report. Five superordinate categories (furniture, fruit, vehicle, weapon, vegetable) were selected for the testing and instances representing two levels of typicality, high or low, were assigned to each category. Simple line drawings were prepared for each instance as well as for distractors.

Subjects fixated their gaze on a centrally positioned red dot while the figures were flashed at a shutter speed of 150 ms to either side of the fixation point. They had to indicate by pressing a key whether or not the stimuli belonged to the designated category. In this cross-modal matching task, both accuracy and speed were recorded, but only correct responses were included in the data analysis for speed. The error rate was low and did not differ significantly between the two visual half-fields.

There were three main findings relevant to our discussion. (1) The effects of level of typicality were different in each visual half-field and the interaction between these two factors was significant. (2) Whereas responses to highly typical items were fastest in the LVF, responses to atypical items were fastest in the RVF. (3) With stimuli in the LVF, the differences between latencies to high- or low-

level typicality items were significant, whereas with responses to the RVF, no such differences were found.

With each hemisphere performing the membership decision task at an accuracy level well above chance, the latency results suggest asymmetrical hemispheric storage or retrieval of specific semantic relationships. One obvious interpretation of these results is that in right-hemisphere mental processes, there are precise, and possibly few, connections between concepts that lead to a sharp dichotomy between common as opposed to rare instances of category concepts. In the left half of the brain, such a dichotomy is weak or absent, because, possibly, connections or associations are "rich." Alternatively, left-hemisphere semantic memory may be insensitive to the dimension of typicality, whereas semantic memory in the right hemisphere is selectively organized around such a dimension. Given the significantly shorter latency for responses to typical items in the LVF than was the case in the RVF, an extension of the previous interpretation is that during sensory and perceptual analysis of daily events, right-hemisphere cognition may play a special role in the processing of familiar, as distinct from rare, stimuli.

The argument has now come a full circle. I see this last interpretation as reflecting the dominant role of cognitive processing of the right hemisphere for stereotypical schemata, which emerged originally from the study of commissurotomy patients.

What new conceptualization of the two cerebral hemispheres is suggested by the results of the last experiment? The following is one tantalizing possibility. If during daily life, semantic systems in the right hemisphere are selectively dependent on well-rehearsed memory traces, then could these lateralized functions reflect some stability in the interaction of the organism with the environment? Such stability would come at the expense of flexibility or could produce limited adaptability. In contrast, a system where no distinction is made between the stereotypical and the new, as was inferred for the left hemisphere, may represent mental processes that are designed for flexibility, adaptability, and the finding of innovative solutions to new problems. Is it possible that the left hemisphere is, in this sense, more creative than the right?

Concluding remarks

Long-term semantic memory was assumed to be the unifying cognitive process in the sequential analysis of information coming into the brain. By using the theoretical and empirical approaches of information-processing psychology, two experiments were designed to measure functional asymmetries in LTM following initial serendipitous observations on commissurotomy patients. I propose that, taken together, the results suggest differential hemispheric semantic stores or retrieval strategies as well as dichotomous emphases on specific semantic relationships. That asymmetries in LTM were found should not be surprising, given the far-ranging evidence for hemispheric specialization in the brain, but the specific pattern of results could not have been predicted from what was already known about such specialization.

Hemispheric differences in long-term semantic memory are of special importance to our understanding of functional organization in the human brain. First, such differences have to do with different ways of storing natural experience and representing ourselves as the source or part of it. Consequently, the mode of storage/retrieval may determine the different cognitive styles that will have effects extending from problem solving to personality. Second, it is commonly believed by information-processing theorists that comparison with a long-term store of experience is an important component of the activity of perception. Thus, hemispheric differences in long-term semantic memory may in fact underlie the much studied hemispheric differences in perception; they may serve as basis for a whole range of specialized hemispheric cognitive functions that are expressed as these latter differences.

Acknowledgments

I am grateful for the many helpful suggestions on the manuscript by Drs. C. Trevarthen, R. Von Blum, and E. Zaidel. The research was supported by NIH 03372, NIH MH15345, and NIH NS 18973.

References

Bartlett, F. C. 1932. *Remembering*. Cambridge University Press, Cambridge, England.

Biederman, I. 1972, Perceiving real-world scenes. *Science* 177: 77–80.

Blakemore, C. B., and M. Falconer. 1967. The long-term effects of anterior temporal lobectomy on certain cognitive functions. *J. Neurol. Neurosurg. Psychiat.* 30: 364–7.

Bogen, J. E. 1969. The other side of the brain. II: An oppositional mind. *Bull. L.A. Neurol. Soc.* 34: 135–62.

Bogen, J. E., E. D. Fisher, and P. J. Vogel. 1965. Cerebral commissurotomy: A second case report. *J. Am. Med. Assoc.* 194: 1328–9.

Collins, A. M., and M. R. Quillian. 1969. Retrieval time from semantic memory. *J. Verb. Learn. Verb. Behav.* 8: 240–7.

Crandall, P. H., R. D. Walter, and R. W. Rand. 1963. Clinical applications of studies on stereotactically implanted electrodes in temporal lobe epilepsy. *J. Neurosurg.* 21: 827–40.

Crowder, R. G. 1976. *Principles of Learning and Memory*. Lawrence Erlbaum, Hillsdale (NJ).

Fantz, R. L. 1958. Pattern vision in young infants. *Psychol. Rec.* 8: 59–66.

–1965. Visual perception from birth as shown by pattern selectivity. *In* H. E. Whipple (ed.) *New Issues in Infant Development. Ann. N.Y. Acad. Sci.* 18: 793–814.

Gazzaniga, M. S., J. E. Bogen, and R. W. Sperry. 1965. Observations on visual perception after disconnection of the the cerebral hemispheres in man. *Brain* 88: 221–36.

Geschwind, N. 1965. Disconnection syndromes in animals and man. *Brain* 88: 237–94, 585–644.

Guenther, R. K., R. L. Klatzky, and W. Putnam. 1980. Commonalities and differences in semantic decisions about pictures and words. *J. Verb. Learn. Verb. Behav.* 19: 54–74.

Hécaen, H., and M. L. Albert. 1978. *Human Neuropsychology*. Wiley, New York.

Hume, D. 1748. *Enquiries Concerning Human Understanding and Concerning the Principles of Morals*, 3rd Ed. L. A. Selby-Bigge (ed.) 1975. Oxford, Clarendon Press, section vii, Part I, p. 62.

Kimura, D. 1963. Right temporal-lobe damage. *Arch. Neurol.* 8: 264–71.

–1969. Spatial localization in left and right visual fields. *Can. J. Psychol.* 23: 445–58.

Kimura, D., and M. Durnford. 1974. Normal studies on the function of the right hemisphere in vision. *In* S. J.

Dimond and J. G. Beaumont (eds.) *Hemisphere Function in the Human Brain*. Paul Elek, London.

Klatzky, R. L. 1975. *Human Memory: Structures and Processes*. Freeman, San Francisco.

Levy, J. 1969. Possible basis for the evolution of lateral specialization of the human brain. *Nature (London)* 224: 614–15.

Mandler, G. 1967. Organization and memory. *Psychol. Learn. Motiv.* 1: 327–72.

Mandler, J., and N. J. Johnson. 1976. Some of the thousand words a picture is worth. *J. Exp. Psychol.* 2: 529–40.

Mandler, J., and R. Parker. 1976. Memory for descriptive and spatial information in complex scenes. *J. Exp. Psychol.* 2: 529–40.

Milner, B. 1958. Psychological defects produced by temporal-lobe excisions. *Res. Publ. Assoc. Nerv. Ment. Dis.* 36: 244–57.

–1967. Brain mechanisms suggested by studies of temporal lobes. *In* F. L. Darley (ed.) *Brain Mechanisms Underlying Speech and Language*. Grune and Stratton, New York.

–1968. Visual recognition and recall after right temporal-lobe excision in man. *Neuropsychol.* 6: 191–209.

–1975. Psychological aspects of focal epilepsy and its neurosurgical management. *In* D. Purpura, J. Penry, and R. Walters (eds.) *Advances in Neurology*. Raven Press, New York.

Norman, D. A. 1969. *Memory and Attention*, 2nd Ed. Wiley, San Diego.

Norman, D. A., and D. G. Bobrow. 1976. On the role of active memory processes in perception and cognition. *In* C. N. Cofer (ed.) *The Structure of Human Memory*. Freeman, San Francisco.

Rips, L. J., E. J. Shoben, and E. E. Smith. 1973. Semantic distance and the verification of semantic relations. *J. Verb. Learn. Verb. Behav.* 12: 1–20.

Rosch, E. 1975. Cognitive representation of semantic categories. *J. Exp. Psychol.: General.* 104: 192–233.

Rumelhart, D. E. 1977. *Introduction to Human Information Processing*. Wiley, New York.

Selecki, B. R., and J. T. Herron. 1965. Disturbances of the verbal body image: A particular syndrome of sensory aphasia. *J. Nerv. Ment. Diseases* 141: 42–52.

Sperry, R. W. 1968. Hemisphere deconnection and unity in conscious awareness. *Am. Psychol.* 23: 723–33.

–1974. Lateral specialization in the surgically separated hemispheres. *In* F. O. Schmitt and F. G. Worden (eds.) *The Neurosciences: Third Study Program*. The MIT Press, Cambridge, pp. 5–19.

Sperry, R. W., M. S. Gazzaniga, and J. E. Bogen. 1969. Interhemispheric relationships: The neocortical commissures; syndromes of hemisphere disconnection. *In* P. J. Vinken and G. W. Bruyn (eds.) *Handbook of Clinical Neurology*, Vol. 4. North-Holland, Amsterdam, pp. 273–90.

Torczyner, H. 1979. *Magritte: Ideas and Images*. Abrams, New York.

Tulving, E., 1972. Episodic and semantic memory. *In* E. Tulving and W. Donaldson (eds.) *Organization of Memory*. Academic Press, New York.

Tulving, E., and D. M. Thomson. 1971. Retrieval processes in recognition memory: Effects of associative context. *J. Exp. Psychol.* 87: 116–24.

Warrington, E. K., and M. James. 1967. An experimental investigation of facial recognition in patients with unilateral cerebral lesions. *Cortex* 3: 317–26.

Warrington, E. K., and A. M. Taylor. 1973. The contribution of the right parietal lobe to object recognition. *Cortex* 9: 152–64.

Wilson, S. A. K. 1908. A contribution to the study of apraxia, with a review of the literature. *Brain* 54: 164–216.

Winograd, E., and N. T. Rivers-Bulkele. 1977. Effects of changing context on remembering faces. *J. Exp. Psychol.: Human Learn. Mem.* 3: 1–12.

Wollen, K. A., A. Weber, and D. H. Lowery. 1972. Bizarreness versus interaction of mental images as determinants of learning. *Cog. Psychol.* 3: 518–23.

Zaidel, D. W. 1983. Specialized hemispheric retrieval from long-term semantic memory: Convergent evidence from normal and commissurotomy subjects. *Neurosci. Abst.* 9: 527.

–1984. Memory for semantic pictorial organization in patients with posterior hemispheric lesions. *Neurosci. Abst.* 10: 317.

–1985. Hemi-field tachistoscopic presentations and hemispheric specialization in normal subjects. *In* D. F. Benson and E. Zaidel (eds.) *The Dual Brain: Hemispheric Specialization in Humans*. Guildford Press, New York.

–1986. Memory for scenes in stroke patients: Hemispheric processing of semantic organization in pictures. *Brain* 109: 547–60.

–1988. Hemispheric asymmetries in memory for incongruous scenes. *Cortex*, 24: 231–44.

Zaidel, D. W, and R. Rausch. 1981. Effects of semantic organization on the recognition of pictures following temporal lobectomy. *Neuropsychol.* 19: 813–17.

Zaidel, D. W., and R. W. Sperry. 1977. Some long-term motor effects of cerebral commissurotomy in man. *Neuropsychol.* 15: 193–204.

Zaidel, E. 1975. A technique for presenting lateralized visual input with prolonged exposure. *Vis. Res.* 15: 283–9.

16 Hughlings Jackson on the recognition of places, persons, and objects

Oliver L. Zangwill
(d. October 12, 1987)
Formerly of Kings College
Cambridge University
and
Maria A. Wyke
Institute of Psychiatry, London

Introduction

Research with human commissurotomy patients in Sperry's laboratory brought renewed attention to the complex and confusing problem of hemispheric specialization for mental processes. Not only was evidence of dramatic clarity obtained for the regulation of speech by the left hemisphere, but the right hemisphere was revealed in a new light, too. It was shown to possess superior ability for the recognition of objects either seen or felt. Forty years previous to these studies, one of us (O. Z.) was among a small group of psychologists who claimed evidence that unilateral right posterior lesions could lead to visuospatial disorders that had no equivalent in the effects of left-hemisphere damage. But 75 years before that Hughlings Jackson was making a similar claim. In this paper, we wish to examine his evidence for special right-hemisphere abilities.

Whereas Hughlings Jackson had some reservations as regards the localization of psychological functions in the cortex, he never for a moment doubted that in the vast majority of individuals, the functions of speech are largely, if not exclusively, under the control of the left cerebral hemisphere, which, in his terminology, "takes the lead" in the generation and expression of articulate speech. Less widely known, however, is his belief that the right cerebral hemisphere – and more especially its posterior portions – must be assumed to play a no less decisive role in nonverbal intellectual activity, in particular, the visual recognition of places, persons, and objects. The development and implications of this view will be briefly outlined in the present chapter.

The main sources of Jackson's ideas about the functions of the right hemisphere in humans are to be found in an article (Jackson 1868) and, much more importantly, in a full-length thesis (Jackson 1874), which was subsequently reprinted (Head 1915; Taylor 1932). Although this article is somewhat obscure and, in parts, difficult to follow, there can be no doubt that the views expressed are strikingly in advance of their time.

Jackson begins his article on the functions of the cerebral hemispheres with particular reference to speech. While he accepts Broca's contention that the hinder part of the left frontal convolution is the region of the brain most frequently damaged in aphasia, he does not accept Broca's claim that speech is located in "any such small part of the brain" and cites his own famous remark that "to locate the damage that destroys speech and to locate speech are two different things." Although he was aware of exceptional cases in which loss of speech appeared to be due to a right-sided lesion, the significant observation is that damage to the left brain alone can render a man speechless.

Jackson goes on to formulate an important distinction between the two separate systems in the brain, which he believes to have important implications for cerebral lateralization. First, there is what he calls the audioarticulatory system supposedly concerned with the formulation and expression of speech and based on the integrity of the left hemisphere.

Second, there is what Jackson denotes as the retinoocular system, concerned essentially with the recognition of persons, objects and places, i.e., processes that do not depend to any considerable extent upon speech and that owe an outstanding debt to vision. The retinoocular system, which Jackson clearly relates to the activities of the right cerebral hemisphere, finds its most important role in the revival of mental images, which, in his view, clearly constitute the substructure of recognition and recall, as well as having an important role in the comprehension of speech. In developing his ideas on the duality of the brain, however, Jackson takes a somewhat different view. He points out that, according to his analysis of the functions of the cerebral hemispheres, the speechless man has but one side for verbalizing (the damaged left), but two for the revival of images, which no doubt provides him with a degree of intellectual capacity, despite his speechlessness, after a left-hemisphere lesion.

It is most interesting, in view of knowledge gained recently, that Jackson further speculates that the two halves of the brain may differ in anatomical as well as psychological properties. He cites Gratiano as having provided some evidence that the right hemisphere develops more rapidly than the left, and Broca for his suggestion that the convolutions of the occipital lobe are richer on the right side than the left. He expresses himself in agreement with Charlton Bastian, who argued that the posterior lobes of the brain are concerned more especially with those higher intellectual operations that Jackson himself believed to be closely related to the retinoocular system. Now these and kindred speculations about cerebral lateralization have proved groundless, but it has become clear that Jackson's idea of differential lateralization has significance and great interest in contemporary neuropsychology, partly as a result of the work of Roger Sperry and his school with commissurotomy patients.

Jackson on recognition of places

While demonstrating his outstanding originality as a clinical neurologist, it cannot be said that Jackson intended to submit his ideas about the duality of the brain to a convincing experimental test. Nonetheless, he did publish details of his findings with a single case, a patient whose condition appeared to him to provide support for his views concerning the functions of the right cerebral hemisphere. This patient had a large cerebral tumor with left hemiplegia and what Jackson called "imperception." Today the condition would probably be described as visuospatial agnosia. As this appears to have been the first case of its kind to be reported in the literature, a brief account of it may be considered appropriate.

Elisa P. was a lady of 59, whose illness apparently began with an episode of topographical memory loss. She set out to walk in a London park that had been well known to her for many years, but, in spite of the fact that she had lived in her present house for 30 years, she could not find her way to the park nearby and, after making several mistakes, had to ask her way. When she wished to return, she was totally unable to find her way home; fortunately, she was able to gain assistance from a relative who was also in the park.

On arrival home, Elisa seemed at first her usual self, but from that time onwards, she began to deteriorate and would on occasion do odd things, such as putting sugar in the tea several times over and making mistakes in dressing. Five weeks later, her deterioration had become more evident and she developed a left hemiplegia and episodic disorientation for persons. It was found that she could name objects correctly, but made some mistakes in naming coins. She was apparently able to describe some routes in her home town, indicating that her original disorientation for places was not absolute. There was no discoverable anaesthesia on the left side.

The patient died three weeks after the onset of her illness and examination of the brain by Dr. Gowers revealed a large glioma in the posterior part of the right temporal lobe. There was gross involvement of the hippocampus and new growth extending anteriorly in the temporal white matter (temporosphenoidal lobe). The corpus striatum and optic thalamus were unaffected and no abnormality could be found elsewhere in the brain.

Case studies, since Jackson, of loss of temporal memory associated with spatial disorientation for place

Following Jackson's description of topographical memory loss, similar cases were reported from time to time, many of them lacking the element of general confusion that was a prominent feature of the later stages of Elisa P.'s illness. One of the earliest of these included three cases reported in the German literature by Meyer (1900). The lesion is said to have been right-sided in the first case, left-sided in the second, and bilateral in the third. Of these, however, only the first is described in detail; a summary of Meyer's findings has been given by Paterson and Zangwill (1945). Meyer's patient exhibited a most striking difficulty in route finding in his home town, which appears to have been largely, if not wholly, due to a failure of memory apparently limited to long-familiar routes and buildings.

A similar case was reported by Paterson and Zangwill (1945). Their patient, aged 34, was a fully right-handed man who sustained a right-sided penetrating war wound of the brain and, when first admitted, presented a relatively complicated pattern of disability, including a left homonymous hemianopia with superadded neglect of the left side of extrapersonal space and of the left upper extremity (autotopagnosia), apraxia for dressing, and an early general memory defect of the Korsakoff type. There was also a tendency at admission for him to grossly underestimate the passage of time, and test performance revealed marked constructional apraxia.

These disabilities improved considerably during the next few months, leaving a very marked defect in topographical orientation and memory that remained as the most striking disability when the patient was discharged from the hospital and followed up for a further year. While in the hospital, he had shown himself virtually unable to learn his way about or to recognize individuals whom he saw daily. Such orientation as he was still able to achieve was largely due to the recognition of relatively small objects, e.g., an electric light bulb placed close to the patient's bed. On discharge from the hospital, the patient was quite unable to recognize his own house or to name prominent features in his home town of Edinburgh, such as the Scott Monument or the famous hill known as Arthur's Seat, which dominates the town. When pictures of these were pointed out to him, he was unable to name them correctly or to specify their location; nor was he capable of indicating the route from his home to his place of work. In other respects, e.g., in describing events of his early life or his war service, the patient appeared capable of giving accurate information. The memory loss thus appeared to be essentially specific to topographical experience.

Another patient with a striking loss of topographical orientation was studied in great detail by Oldfield over a period of 30 years and an account of this case was given by Whitty and Newcombe (1973) shortly after Oldfield's death. The patient was an electrical engineer who developed a right occipital brain abscess at age 28. Following a prolonged course of surgical treatment, he was found to present a gross defect of spatial orientation and memory that was followed up, mainly by Oldfield himself, over a period of 30 years.

When he first returned home from the hospital, this patient complained of the inability to estimate heights and distances and to take in details of pictures or photographs. He also reported that he had ceased to dream and could picture neither his friends nor the familiar route from his house to his place of work. While in the hospital, he constantly lost his way, but, like Paterson and Zangwill's patient, had learned to recognize small objects that served as landmarks. On reexamination after 10 years, it was established that the patient had been able to return to work, though he still lost his bearings on occasion, particularly at night. He was, however, still unable to work from a map, or plan, or to give directions to a stranger. It was, therefore, evident that despite good recovery, some residue of the early disabilities remained.

On reexamination after 30 years, the patient still complained of some difficulty in the recognition of buildings and streets unless some distinguishing detail was in evidence. He also reported that he met them every day; faces, in particular, were soon forgotten and he was also liable to confuse characters he watched on television or at the cinema. It was thus evident that despite considerable recovery and good occupational and social adjustment over 30 years, the patient still suffered a disabling handicap.

More recently, De Renzi, Faglioni, and Villa (1977) have described a patient with a marked topographical amnesia. This was a case of a 62-year-old housewife who was admitted to hospital with a left hemiparesis and aphasia, both of which resolved within eight days, leaving only a mild dysarthria. She was discharged after 15 days with a diagnosis of having a cerebrovascular accident. The patient subsequently showed a profound loss of spatial orientation both at home, where she had lived for many years, and in keeping her bearings in the town whenever she went out alone. On readmission to the hospital after several months, she was found to have a mild dysarthria and a left homonymous hemianopia, with macular sparing. The patient easily became lost within the building, and, when shown a simple route in the garden of the clinic, invariably lost her way. At the same time, this patient showed no written or oral speech disorder and no difficulty in recognizing objects or pictures. She was, however, incapable of learning a simple visual maze. The brain scan revealed a moderate uptake of isotope in the right temporal region.

Comparative incidence of right- and left-hemisphere lesions in loss of topographical memory

The question of whether loss of topographical memory is associated with right- or left-sided lesions has been asked by Critchley (1953) and by Hécaen and Angelergues (1963), though their findings are hardly comparable. Critchley lists 17 cases, mostly under the care of consultant physicians, who appear to have presented the syndrome of topographical memory loss, though, in several cases, the evidence is distinctly slight. Hécaen and Angelergues have made a more systematic study of the comparative incidence of the various forms of agnosia as defined clinically and classified by the two authors. We shall confine ourselves here to cases that appear to meet the requirements of a diagnosis of topgraphical memory loss associated with impaired spatial orientation. De-

fects of topgraphical memory were recorded in 15 out of their 398 patients.

Critchley's 17 cases comprise two with right-sided lesions, seven with left-sided lesions, and eight with bilateral lesions. Not all cases, however, are reported as verified. Of Hécaen and Angelergues's 15 cases, nine had right-sided lesions, two left-sided, and four bilateral. In the case of De Renzi et al. (1977) cited before, it was clear that despite the initial aphasia, the patient's severe and apparently persistent topographical amnesia for familiar places was the outcome of damage to the right cerebral hemisphere.

It seems, therefore, that with careful examination, a distinct majority of patients with defective recognition of place have right (i.e. minor hemisphere) lesions. The two latter reports and those of Paterson and Zangwill and of Oldfield appear to confirm the view of Jackson that there is a relationship between defective recognition of familiar places in the environment and lesions of the right cerebral hemisphere.

Jackson on the recognition of persons

Although, so far as the authors are aware, Jackson did not himself make any reference to failure of recognition of individual human faces by vision, the disorder now known as prosopagnosia, there can be no doubt that he regarded the recognition of persons as indisputably within the special functional province of the right cerebral hemisphere. He was probably aware of the work of Wilbrandt (1897), who first described what was then known as mind blindness, which Wilbrandt regarded as a focal cerebral syndrome. It is, therefore, appropriate to inquire whether there is evidence – as Jackson claimed – that awareness of persons no less than of places depends, predominantly, on the activity of the right cerebral hemisphere.

The syndrome of agnosia for faces (prosopagnosia) was apparently first described by Bodamer (1947), whose work has been well reviewed by Critchley (1953), but the most informative account of its clinical manifestations is probably that published in English by Hécaen and Angelergues (1962) on the basis of 22 personally studied cases as well as a number of previously published case reports. These authors present a convincing account of the clinical picture of prosopagnosia, pointing out, for example, that whereas the patient with this condition may describe more or less adequately the appearance of the face of someone well known, e.g., a member of the family, the patient is nonetheless incapable of recognizing the individual concerned unless he should speak to him, whereupon he recognizes him instantly but only transiently. He may likewise recognize his wife by her dress, should he happen to remember what she is wearing, though consistently fails to recognize her from her visual appearance. Hécaen and Angelergues also note that some patients with prosopagnosia fail to recognize their own faces in a mirror.

In considering the clinical associations with prosopagnosia, Hécaen and Angelergues report that visual-field deficits (especially left-sided) are among the most common symptoms. Other features not uncommonly found are constructional apraxia, difficulties in dressing, and vestibular or directional disturbances and metamorphosia. On the other hand, aphasic disorders were very seldom observed. Hécaen and Angelergues stress that the condition itself appears to be a relatively rare occurrence; it appeared in only 22 of their 382 patients with retrolandic lesions personally studied by the authors. They also directed attention to the "decisive role" (16 of their patients) of the minor hemisphere in determining the presence of prosopagnosia, thus strengthening the apparent relationship between the recognition of faces and places and the unilateral disorder of the right cerebral hemisphere.

Of the more recent studies of prosopagnosia to appear in the literature, a paper by Meadows (1974) on the anatomical basis of prosopagnosia merits particular attention. Meadows devotes some preliminary discussion to the complex and sophisticated achievement involved in normal facial recognition, which he evidently considers to have no other counterpart in human experience. He argues that facial recognition requires one to discriminate in detail and remember very minor differences by predominantly nonverbal means. At the same time, he has little doubt that learning to discriminate faces is essentially an acquired rather than an inborn skill, thereby subscribing to the point of view put forward by Hebb (1949). Recent research with infants, on the other hand, would seem to support the view that perception of faces and learning to identify individuals is based on a strong inborn predisposition (see Chapter 20, this volume).

Meadows suggests that prosopagnosia may perhaps represent a localized form of amnesic syndrome. This interpretation, first proposed by Hécaen (Hécaen and Angelergues 1962) and supported by others (e.g., Tzavaras, Hécaen, and Le Bras 1970; Whiteley and Warrington 1977; Geschwind 1979), has also gained some support from Milner's observation that delayed recognition of faces is impaired, though not to the extent seen in prosopagnosia, after right temporal lobectomy (Milner 1968). Meadows, like Hécaen before him, likewise touches on the frequency with which topographical amnesia is related to prosopagnosia. At the same time, however, there is evidence from cases of war wounds of the brain that these two deficits may be dissociable; thus, a study by Newcombe and Russell (1969) has suggested that whereas a maze-learning task is appreciably impaired by right parietal lesions, defect on the facial-discrimination task is more clearly impaired with right temporal lesions. Meadows is, therefore, led to propose that prosopagnosia might depend upon a lesion intermediate between a posterior area required for facial recognition and a more anterior temporal area that might operate in motor learning, with possible limbic connections relevant when there is damage to topographical memory. Although highly speculative, these suggestions do, at least, point to possible relationships between the recognition of faces and places.

Laterality of hemisphere lesion and prosopagnosia

Regarding the anatomical basis in the aetiology of prosopagnosia, we seem to confront a major incompatibility between the evidence of clinical and psychological studies (see Ellis 1983), which indicate with consistency the important role of the right hemisphere in perceptual recognition of faces, and the postmortem anatomical studies, which appear to indicate mainly bilateral lesions. Five out of the eight cases discussed by Meadows had bilateral lesions. The cases in question were seven patients reviewed by Meadows himself and the case described by Rubens and Benson (1971) whose postmortem report (Benson, Segarra, and Albert 1974) revealed the presence of bilateral lesions.

Meadows stressed that a right occipitotemporal lesion was present in all cases of prosopagnosia that have so far come to necropsy. He also pointed out that this correlates with the exceptionally high incidence of upper quadrantic field defects in these patients. For these reasons, Meadows regarded it as quite proper to discuss what he called "the problem of the right hemisphere lesion," and he doubted that bilateral lesions are essential for the presence of prosopagnosia. Such a view would seem to concur with the findings of the split-brain research, which shows that the right hemisphere dominates the visual-matching responses of split-brain patients when they are presented simultaneously with pictures of unfamiliar faces in the right and left visual fields (Levy, Trevarthen, and Sperry 1972).

There is no evidence that prosopagnosia can result from an isolated left hemisphere lesion. For a definitive appraisal of the views of Jackson, who strongly supported a right-hemisphere specialization for facial recognition, we need more detailed anatomical data. This issue may soon be clarified by further extensive investigation of patients with prosopagnosia in whom the site of the lesion has been clearly established by modern methods of brain imaging. Damasio (Damasio, Damasio, and Van Hoesen 1982; Damasio 1985) has marshalled evidence that, while the right hemisphere may "take the lead" in facial recognition, both hemispheres must be damaged to produce the peculiar defect of memory of which prosopagnosia is one manifestation (see Chapter 15, this volume)

Visual agnosia and the recognition of objects

We may now turn to the recognition of objects or "things" that, along with persons and places, Jackson believed to be represented in the right cerebral hemisphere. Although he makes few explicit references to the perception of objects, it seems highly likely that he was fully aware of the prestigious experiments of Munk (1877), who described the effects of ablation of the occipital lobes in dogs. Munk reported that his findings indicated that, whereas the operated animals appeared to be indifferent to food and persons or places well known to them, they were nonetheless far from blind, though they might become blind as a result of a second and more extensive operation. He concluded that the original operation had left the animals capable of seeing without recognizing – a condition that was first designated *Seelenblindheit* (mind blindness) and later "visual object agnosia," by which name it is generally known today.

Not surprisingly, visual agnosia soon attracted the attention of clinical neurologists, more particularly in Germany. While relatively rare, the condition appeared to duplicate the findings of Munk in so far as the patients were, like the operated dogs, held to see, though not to recognize, objects in common use with which they were presented. Among them was a case reported by Stauffenberg in 1914 and summarized by Head (1926). As a classic representative of "mind blindness," this case may be briefly reported.

A 61-year-old woman had a series of cardiovascular lesions and was found to present a left hemiplegia and left hemianopia along with a transient dysphasia. Her main disability, however, was a persistent failure to recognize either persons or common objects, such as a key or a sponge, in spite of the fact that her powers of vision were said to have largely recovered and her intellectual capacities were considered to be substantially intact. At the time of her death in 1912, she was still incapable of reliably naming, or otherwise indicating, the nature of objects or colors with which she was confronted. Necropsy revealed an extensive softening of both occipital lobes. All appropriate paths on the right side and most of those on the left were affected; the right temporal lobe was completely destroyed and there was considerable degeneration of the splenium and the anterior commissure.

Other early studies have been summarized by Critchley (1953) and although several have proved distinctly controversial, the reality of the condition cannot certainly be gainsaid. It should be mentioned that A. B. Rubens (1979) and Ratcliff and Newcombe (1982) have recently contributed full and up-to-date accounts of visual agnosia.

Lissauer on "mind blindness," and two contrasting cases of visual agnosia

Lissauer (1889) proposed an important distinction between what he believed to be two distinct forms of mind blindness; these he termed *apperceptive* and *associative,* respectively. The former he regarded as a failure of recognition due to distortion or defective processing of visually perceived objects, whereas the latter is due to failure to link information that has been accurately perceived with appropriate meaning and relationship to previous experience. In short, the patient with apperceptive visual agnosia is unable to match or copy a picture presented to him, whereas the patient with associative agnosia fails to recognize objects or pictures in spite of adequate visual capacity. At the same time, such a patient is able to copy accurately an object or picture even if unable to appreciate its name or nature. Although this dichotomy has given rise to much criticism, it has held its place in clinical neurology for almost 100 years and finds ready application in psychological discussion today, under the heading of "episodic memory." Two comparatively recent cases of visual agnosia with contrasting patterns of visual disability (Benson and Greenberg 1969; Rubens and Benson 1971) lend support to Lissauer's conception.

The first patient was admitted to hospital suffering from accidental carbon monoxide poisoning and was at first considered blind, but when admitted to hospital seven months after the onset of the illness, it was found that he could navigate corridors successfully in his wheelchair. He could also name colors and follow moving visual stimuli, but was unable to identify familiar objects by vision alone, although visual acuity determined indirectly was normal. The patient was unable to read or recognize faces, names, or visual symbols to confrontation. Detailed psychophysical testing was undertaken by Efron (1968). The patient was able to distinguish light intensity, object size, color, and direction, but he could not differentiate between simple forms, e.g., a circle and a square. Eye-movement control was appreciably disturbed. The patient maintained that he had ceased to dream since his illness, and, although rapid eye movements were observed during sleep, when awakened, the patient denied dreaming.

In spite of the fact that most of this patient's symptoms referred to visual deficits, the authors considered it appropriate to describe his condition as "visual form apperception." They were satisfied that this present case clearly falls under Lissauer's category of apperceptive visual agnosia, although only in the broadest sense could the defect of perception be considered an elementary visual disorder.

The second case conforms to the description of associative visual agnosia.

The patient was a 47-year-old right-handed physician with a history of alcoholism and an episode of confusion and disorientation, following which he was found to have a dense right homonymous hemianopia with macular sparing. He was able to name neither objects presented visually nor pictures of objects or faces, nor colors or printed words. Drawings of geometrical forms were satisfactory and he could copy line drawings of objects though often misnamed what he had drawn. He frequently misnamed colors and was unable to recognize members of his family, the hospital staff, or even his own face in the mirror. Thus, there was clearly a severe prosopagnosia in addition to his difficulty in recognizing objects; topographical orientation, on the other hand, appeared to be substantially unimpaired. In addition, this patient exhibited several other patterns of disability, among them alexia without agraphia, color agnosia, and impaired verbal learning. He was discharged from the hospital after four months, by which time his memory for everyday events was normal and reading much improved. Naming of colors remained slow, but, as a rule, correct, and misidentification of objects was now rare. On the other hand, prosopagnosia remained severe.

The patient died three years after the onset of his agnosia and the brain was made available for neuropathological study. The findings are reported by Benson, Segarra, and Albert (1974).

Gross examination revealed several abnormalities, among which were: (1) a change in the appearance of the left posterior cerebral artery, which, on section, had the appearance of a solid cord with no demonstrable lumen; (2) a deeply depressed vascular lesion on the undersurface of the left temporooccipital lobe that continued as a narrow strip running almost the entire length of the fusiform gyrus; (3) no lesion was visible on the surface of the right occipital lobe, but a concave deformity of the undersurface suggested a loss of bulk in the posterior part of the hemisphere.

Brain sections showed the following: (1) Small infarcts in both the right and left globus pallidus. (2) Sections at the level of the pulvinar showed a lesion of the left temporal lobe that involved a well-healed infarct involving the white matter of the parahippocampal cortex and the anterior third of the fusiform lobe. This lesion expanded as it extended posteriorly and finally extended to the pial surface of the lingual gyrus. (3) Sections of the right hemisphere posteriorly revealed an elongated cystic lesion occupying the white matter of the fusiform gyrus. (4) Sections through the corpus callosum revealed necrosis that involved the lower half of the splenium. (5) The occipital lesions appeared to interrupt several fiber systems; on the left side, the inferior longitudinal fasciculus connecting the fusiform gyrus to the temporal lobe structures was involved. The optic radiation and hippocampal connections were severed by the extent of the hippocampal infarct. The lesion on the right side was less extensive, but almost symmetrical; the optic radiations escaped but several occipitotemporal connections were affected. (6) The corpus callosum was damaged, probably producing complete interruption of the interhemispheric connections between right and left visual areas. The calcarine cortex was intact bilaterally, though on the left virtually isolated, whereas on the right side, only the major outflow pathways to the central lobe were interrupted. All possible visual interhemispheric connections were deemed to be destroyed, though no mention was made of the condition of the anterior commissure.

Visual object agnosia and unilateral lesions

Although the lesion in many of the early cases of visual object agnosia has been indisputably bilateral, the question of whether or not this syndrome can ever result from a purely unilateral lesion is of considerable interest and has led to some differences of view. Gowers (1888) took the view that "we do not know whether complete mind blindness can be produced from a lesion in one hemisphere or whether disease of both hemispheres is necessary for production of the symptom." Oppenheim (1911), on the other hand, argued that if the paths from the right occipital lobe and those from the left calcarine area to the left occipital cortex are destroyed at the same time, unilateral hemianopia together with mind blindness will result. Mingazzini (1922) claimed that "on the basis of numerous clinical observations, at times a disease focuses in one occipital lobe, usually the left, and is enough to cause signs of mind blindness." Potzl (1928) likewise held that left-sided brain lesions at the base of the occipital lobe are particularly liable to occur in cases of mind blindness, but only when, besides cortical disturbances of variable degree and extent, much of the white matter is destroyed and the splenium of the corpus callosum is severely affected. A less impressionistic judgment had to wait, however, until Nielsen (1937) made a more thorough inquiry into the evidence regarding the incidence of unilateral visual-object agnosia.

Nielsen selected thirteen cases of visual-object agnosia, originally reported from 1875 to 1922, according to the following principles:

1. The record of the case not only must state that visual agnosia for objects was present, but must offer evidence for scrutiny and independent diagnosis.
2. Only one occipital lobe must have been affected.
3. Failure of recognition of objects had not been due to general cerebral involvement.

4. The agnosia had been more than trivial. If the patient recovered before death or if diaschisis had been the cause of the syndrome, the case was not included.
5. The syndrome must have been verified.

These cases were classified in three groups:

1. Cases of visual-object agnosia due to compression of one occipital lobe (two cases).
2. Cases of visual-object agnosia due to superficial softening of one occipital lobe (two cases).
3. Cases of large deep lesions of one occipital lobe (nine cases).

In this small series of patients who suffered from visual-object agnosia allegedly associated with lesions of one or other cerebral hemisphere, 10 sustained lesions of a single cerebral hemisphere, right or left. They are summarized in Table 16.1.

Many of the 13 patients showed certain other deficits in addition to visual-object agnosia. Apart from visual-field defects, the most interesting of these are failure of color recognition, alexia without agraphia, and topographical amnesia. As we have already seen, certain of these deficits, likewise in evidence in Rubens and Benson's case, were present in the older cases considered before. On the other hand, even among the cases with left-sided lesions, aphasia was seldom recorded.

Four patients had right-sided lesions compared with six whose lesions were left-sided. In three cases, which were carefully reviewed by the present writers, the lesions were considered in all probability to have been bilateral.

Conclusions

Can we draw any clear conclusions from this study as regards the standing of Jackson's conception of cerebral lateralization and, in particular, his idea of right-hemisphere functions? It is true that our material is very limited and is to be regarded as illustrative rather than as a formal analysis of the lateralization of cortical function. Nonetheless, the following tentative conclusions may serve to guide the design and conduct of future more substantial clinical studies relating to agnosia and kindred disorders.

1. Defects in topographical memory and in failure of spatial orientation in highly familiar surroundings appear to be recorded with a fair degree of frequency in association with lesions of the right cerebral hemisphere, most commonly involving the mesial cortex. Such defects do, however, occur from time to time as a result of comparable lesions of the dominant cerebral hemisphere. Neither the severity nor the duration of the disability appears to bear a clear relation to the side of the lesion.

2. Whereas prosopagnosia, which appears to be appreciably less common than topographical memory loss, is likewise observed more commonly after lesions of the right rather than the left hemisphere, recent studies verified at necropsy strongly suggest that involvement of the left, i.e., dominant, hemisphere may play a role in the genesis of this condition. The possible role of bilateral lesions in prosopagnosia still remains to be determined.

3. Visual-object agnosia appears to be appreciably less common than other forms of spatial loss or prosopagnosia. It also appears to be associated more frequently with left and bilateral lesions than either of these two other forms of visual agnosia, as well as being associated beyond any doubt whatsoever with lesions involving the occipital lobes of either one or both hemispheres. In cases of unilateral lesion, however, it is doubtful whether this disability is related in a causal manner to factors of cerebral dominance, such as those that operate in relation to language.

Jackson was undoubtedly right in stressing the importance of the right hemisphere in relation to intellectual activity, but there is reason to believe that, in some respects, he exaggerated its role in the perception of persons and things. In spite of this caveat, we should estimate his contribution to our understanding of cerebral organization to be in no way less important than that of Paul Broca. Sperry's research on commissurotomy patients has helped energize the search for special cognitive and memory capacities of the right hemisphere that Jackson pioneered.

Table 16.1. *Lateralization of lesion in 13 cases of unilateral cerebral lesions associated with defective recognition of objects*

Case	Group	Lesion side	Pathology	Remarks	Verification
1. Wandenberg	I	Right	Head injury: parasagittal meningioma.	Apraxia for dressing. Failed to recognize houses or find his way about.	Necropsy
2. McEwen	I	Left	Cerebellar abscess affecting posterior portion of both the temporal and occipital lobes.	Good postoperative recovery.	Operation
3. Luciani & Seppilli	II	Bilateral	Cortical softening affecting both temporal lobes but only left occipital lobe.	Jargon aphasia.	Necropsy
4. Pousepp	II	Left	Toxaemia of pregnancy.	No hemianopia. Alexia without agraphia. Visual constructive disability.	Necropsy
5. Henschen	III	Right	Tumor right occipital lobe. Degeneration of splenium. Left hemisphere normal.	Left-handed. Left homonymous hemianopia. Agraphia. Speech unaffected. Acalculia.	Necropsy
6. Lissauer	III	? Bilateral	Softening of left occipital lobe. Continuation of splenium to right side degenerated.	Alexia. Apraxia for dressing. Impaired spatial orientation. Color recognition impaired. Alexia without agraphia.	Necropsy
7. Lountz	III	Right	Softening of internal two-thirds of right occipital lobe.	Handedness not stated. Left hemiparesis.	Necropsy
8. Jackson	III	Right	Glioma involving entire right temporooccipital region and lying close to medial border of right hemisphere destroying fibers of splenium.	Loss of topographical orientation. Some difficulty in recognizing coins and perhaps also places. Left homonymous hemianopia.	Necropsy
9. Rabus	III	Left	Large cyst involving much of the left hemisphere. Calcarine cortex on both sides separate from the convex surface of left occipital lobe.	Apraxia. Tactile agnosia in right hand.	Necropsy

Table 16.1. (*cont.*)

Case	Group	Lesion side	Pathology	Remarks	Verification
10. Müller	III	? Bilteral	Large tumor in left occipital lobe involving splenium of corpus callosum. Tumor compressed right occipital lobe extending across the midline.	Some apraxia. Complete right homonymous hemianopia with constriction of the left field.	Necropsy
11. Jack	III	Left	Large tumor of left temporal lobe and extensive softening of left occipital lobe.	Marked defect in topographical orientation and memory. Agraphia. Alexia.	Necropsy
12. Giannuli	III	Left	Cyst on left occipital lobe destroying second and third occipital convolutions.	Disorientation in own house. Ideokinetic apraxia.	Necropsy
13. Nodet	III	Left	Subcortical softening of left occipital lobe and destruction of the splenium.	Failed to name colors. Right homonymous hemianopia. Could read letters but not words.	Necropsy

Source: After Nielsen (1937).

References

Benson, A. J., J. Segarra, and M. L. Albert. 1974. Visual agnosia – Prosopagnosia: A clinicopathological correlation. *Arch. Neurol.* 30: 307–10.

Benson, D. F., and J. P. Greenberg. 1969. Visual form agnosia. *Arch. Neurol.* 20: 82–90.

Bodamer, J. 1947. The prosop-agnosic (Die Agnosie des Physio-Gnomiee rhennens). *Arch. Psychiat. Nouv.* 179: 653.

Critchley, M. 1953. *The Parietal Lobes*. Arnold, London.

Damasio, A. R. 1985. Prosopagnosia. *Trends in Neurosci.* 8: 132–5.

Damasio, A. R., H. Damasio, and G. W. Van Hoesen. 1982. Prosopagnosia: Anatomical basis and behavioral mechanisms. *Neurol.* 32: 331–41.

DeRenzi, E., P. Faglioni, and P. Villa. 1977. Spatial memory and hemispheric locus of lesion. *J. Neurol. Neurosurg. Psychiat.* 40: 495–505.

Efron, R. 1968. *What is Perception?* (Boston Studies in the Philosophy of Science, Vol. 4). Humanities Press, New York.

Ellis, A. W. 1983. *Normality and Pathology in Cognitive Functions*. Academic Press, London.

Geschwind, N. 1979. Specialization of the human brain. *Sci. Am.* 241: 158–68.

Gowers, W. R. 1888. *A Manual of Diseases of the Nervous System*. Churchill, London.

Head, H. 1915. Hughlings Jackson on aphasia and kindred affections of speech. *Brain* 38: 1–190.

Hebb, D. 1949. *The Organization of Behavior*. Wiley, New York.

Hécaen, H., and R. Angelergues. 1962. Agnosia for faces (prosopagnosia). *Arch. Neurol.* 7: 92–100.

–1963. *La Cécité Psychique: Etude Critique de la Notion D'Agnosie*. Masson et Cie, Paris.

Jackson, H. 1868. Language and thought – The duality of mental processes. *Med. Times Gaz.* 1: 526–8.

–1874. The duality of the brain. *Med. Press Circ.* 1: 19, 41, 63.

Levy, J., C. Trevarthen, and R. W. Sperry. 1972. Perception of bilateral chimeric figures following hemispheric disconnection. *Brain* 95: 61–78.

Lissauer, H. 1889. Ein Fall von Seelenblindheit nebst einem Beitrag zur Theorie derseben. *Arch. f. Psychiat. Nerv.* 22: 222–70.

Meadows, J. C. 1974. The anatomical basis of prosopagnosia. *J. Neurol. Neurosurg. Psychiat.* 37: 489–501.

Meyer, I. O. 1900. Ein und doppelseitige Homonyme Hemianopsie mit Orientierungs Storungen. *Monatschr. Psychiat. Neurol.* 8: 440–56.

Milner, B. 1968. Visual recognition and recall after right temporal lobe excision in man. *Neuropsychol.* 6: 191–209.

Mingazzini, G. 1922. *Der Balken.* Springer, Berlin, p. 184.

Munk, H. 1877. Zur physiologie der Grosshirnrinde. (Verh. Physiol. Ges., Berlin). *Dtsch. Med. Wschr.* Jahr 3, Nr. 13: 153–4.

Newcombe, F., and W. R. Russell. 1969. Dissociated visual perceptual and spatial deficits in focal lesions of the right hemisphere. *J. Neurol. Neurosurg. Psychiat.* 32: 73–81.

Nielsen, J. M. 1937. Unilateral cerebral dominance as related to mind blindness. *Arch. Neurol. Psychiat.* 38: 108–35.

Oppenheim, H. 1911. *Text Book of Nervous Diseases,* 2 Vols. (A. Bruce trans.) Foulis, London.

Potzl, O. 1928. *Die Optisch – Agnostischen Storungen* Deuticke, Leipzig.

Paterson, A., and O. L. Zangwill. 1945. Disorders of visual space perception associated with lesions of the right cerebral hemisphere. *Brain* 67: 331–58.

Ratcliff, G., and F. Newcombe. 1982. Object recognition: Some deductions from the clinical evidence. *In* A. W. Ellis (ed.) *Normality and Pathology in Cognitive Function* Academic Press, London and New York.

Rubens, A. B. 1979. Agnosia. *In* K. N. Heilman and E. Valenstein (eds.) *Clinical Neuropsychology.* Oxford University Press, London and New York.

Rubens, A. B., and D. F. Benson. 1971. Associative visual agnosia. *Arch. Neurol.* 24: 305–16.

Taylor, J. 1932. *Selected Writings of John Hughlings Jackson,* Vol. II. Hodder and Stoughton, London.

Tzavaras, A., H. Hécaen, and H. LeBras. 1970. Le Problème de la Spécifité de la Reconnaissance du Visage Humaine lors des Lesions Hémisphériques Unilateral. *Neuropsychol.* 8: 403–16.

Whiteley, A. M., and E. K. Warrington. 1977. Prosopagnosia: A clinical, psychological and anatomical study of three patients. *J. Neurol. Neurosurg. Psychiat.* 40: 395–403.

Whitty, C. W. M., and F. Newcombe. 1973. R. C. Oldfield's study of visual and topographic disturbances in a right occipito-parietal lesion of thirty years duration. *Neuropsychol.* 11: 471–5.

Wilbrandt, H. 1897. *Die Seelenblindheit als Herderscheinung.* Bergmann, Weisbaden.

17 Lessons from cerebral commissurotomy: Auditory attention, haptic memory, and visual images in verbal associative-learning[*]

Brenda Milner
Laughlin Taylor
and
Marilyn Jones-Gotman
McGill University

The most direct and compelling evidence of dual functional asymmetry in the human brain comes from the observations of Roger Sperry on a small group of patients in whom the main interhemispheric commissures had been transected as a therapy for medically intractable epilepsy (Bogen and Vogel 1962; Bogen, Fisher, and Vogel 1965). In these patients, Sperry and his colleagues have been able, by appropriate techniques, to confine sensory input and motor output to one cerebral hemisphere and thus bring out the contrasting specializations of the two sides (Sperry, Gazzaniga, and Bogen 1969), as well as demonstrating within one person the coexistence of two relatively independent streams of conscious awareness (Sperry 1968, 1974; Levy, Trevarthen, and Sperry 1972).

We have had the privilege of studying this group of patients on several occasions; in each case, the experiments were designed to answer specific questions arising from our ongoing research on the human temporal lobes. In this retrospective account of three studies, we describe our findings and examine their implications in the light of subsequent work.

Dichotic-listening tests of hemispheric differences

In our first study (Milner, Taylor, and Sperry 1968), we were able to demonstrate a critical role played by the callosal pathway in the performance of a verbal dichotic-listening task (Broadbent 1954; Kimura 1961). One ma-

jor consequence of hemispheric disconnection is that the patients can only give a verbal report on sensory information that has been channeled to the language-dominant left hemisphere (Gazzaniga and Sperry 1967). For example, such patients cannot name or describe objects flashed in the left visual field, but name only those flashed on the right, because each field projects solely to the contralateral hemisphere. Nor can they name objects palpated by the left hand, although manipulating them appropriately. In audition, however, the anatomical situation is quite different, with each ear represented bilaterally at every stage of the afferent pathway, from the cochlear nucleus to the auditory cortex of the temporal lobe, and, therefore, sound input cannot be restricted to one cerebral hemisphere. Yet, by presenting different verbal stimuli simultaneously to the two ears, as in Kimura's dichotic-digits task, it is possible to show a complete or near-complete suppression by the left or speaking hemisphere of input from the ipsilateral ear (Milner et al. 1968; Sparks and Geschwind 1968; Musick and Reeves 1986).

Our first testing of the commissurotomy patients took place from six months to four years postoperatively, at which time five of the

---

[*]In a series of visits to Pasadena over a 10-year period, Milner and Taylor had the opportunity to carry out several studies with the commissurotomy patients in Sperry's laboratory at Caltech. This chapter reviews these findings and reports in full an experiment on image-mediated learning that is an extension of M. Jones-Gotman's research with other patient groups.

seven patients obtained near-zero scores for the left ear in the dichotic condition, whereas the remaining two patients (LB and NG) reported about one-third fewer digits for the left ear than for the right. In contrast, no patient had any difficulty in reporting digits from the left ear under monaural conditions, thereby showing that the ipsilateral pathway was viable. These results cannot be attributed to extracallosal damage in the right hemisphere (either preexisting or occurring as a complication of the surgical intervention), as Lassonde, Bryden, and Demers (in press) have argued, because CC, the one patient with a well-lateralized focal left-hemisphere lesion, together with a surgical approach over the left hemisphere, also showed a complete extinction of verbal input to the left ear in the presence of competing input from the right.

An instructive finding, in our study, was the magnitude of the left-ear suppression, in view of the much less striking loss on the left ear seen in patients tested from two to three weeks after a right temporal lobectomy that included excision of the primary auditory cortex of Heschl's gyrus. This difference was interpreted (Milner 1974) as consistent with an earlier physiological study in the monkey (Pribram, Rosner, and Rosenblith 1954), which had suggested an extension of auditory cortex into the parietal lobe. Subsequent evidence from cortical evoked-potential recording in awake patients (Celesia 1976), and in the owl monkey (Immig et al. 1977), where responses were elicited from the superior bank of the Sylvian fissure, has strengthened this interpretation, as has a more recent cytoarchitectonic study of the human brain (Galaburda and Sanides 1980), which indicated the presence of auditory-related cortex in the parietal operculum and inferior parietal lobule.

We were able to retest all seven patients, two years later, and observed a marked improvement in the left-ear score (from 0 to 67%) in patient NW, previously tested six months after commissurotomy, but the scores of the other six patients were essentially unchanged. No patient came close to the normal level of left-ear performance in the dichotic condition and two patients (including CC) continued to show complete extinction of verbal input to the left ear four years after the commissurotomy.

Taken as a whole, the dichotic-listening studies carried out in patients with section of the corpus callosum testify to the dominance of the contralateral auditory pathway over the ipsilateral, as Kimura (1961) had proposed; they also point to the importance of the transcallosal input in the normal performance of such tasks. It is also evident that there are marked individual differences in the extent to which the ipsilateral pathway can be used to compensate for loss of input from the opposite hemisphere.

In our original study, we had hoped to demonstrate the converse phenomenon of right-ear suppression (Kimura 1964) if simple melodies of three or four notes were presented to the patients dichotically with the instruction to sing or hum the melodies they heard. Instead, it proved impossible to obtain a consistent readout from the right hemisphere, except in the case of CC, who hummed only the melodies that had been presented to the left ear, although he had shown a complete suppression of that ear on the verbal dichotic task. For the other five patients tested, the results were quite disorderly, as though the right hemisphere could not compete effectively for control of the vocal musculature, even though speech was not involved.

Delayed matching-to-sample tests of haptic shape perception: Right-hemisphere superiority; memory loss

On our next visit to California, we were more successful in tapping the specialized capacities of the right hemisphere. The aim of the study was to show that the disconnected right cerebral hemisphere, though mute, could perform a delayed matching-to-sample task more efficiently than the amnesic patient HM; in this patient, the uncus and amygdala, together with the bulk of the hippocampus and parahippocampal gyrus, had been removed bilaterally to control epileptic seizures, but the corpus callosum was intact (Scoville and Milner 1957). This study had some theoretical importance, because Sidman, Stoddard, and Mohr (1968) had claimed that HM's poor performance on

Examiner

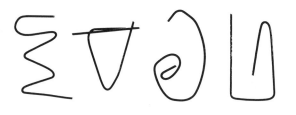

Subject

Figure 17.1 The four wire figures used to test tactile pattern matching, in the orientation in which they are presented to the subject. In the delayed-matching procedure, a sample figure from the set of four is given to the subject to palpate for 10 s. It is then replaced among the other figures to form a horizontal array, as shown here. At the end of the intratrial delay, the subject uses the same hand to find the sample again by blind touch. The order of the figures in the array is changed at random from trial to trial. (From Milner and Taylor 1972.)

the delayed matching of ellipses was due to his failure to code the stimuli verbally. We were convinced from other behavioral evidence that this was not so, but it seemed that a more telling proof would be to show that the isolated right hemisphere could bridge longer intratrial delays than HM.

Up till then, HM's delayed matching had been assessed only in the visual and auditory modalities (Prisko 1963, Sidman et al. 1968), where he typically showed normal matching at zero delay, with performance falling to chance after an intratrial interval of 30 s. In order to have a procedure more appropriate for use with the commissurotomy patients (where it is important to be able to confine input to one hemisphere), a tactual pattern-matching task was devised and was administered to HM on two occasions, three months apart.

The test material consisted of four irregular patterns, each constructed out of a 10-in piece of wire, bent into the desired flat shape (Figure 17.1). These items were taken from a larger series devised by Corkin (1964, 1978) and were chosen to be easily discriminable from one another by touch but not easily named.

During testing, the subject placed one hand inside a cardboard frame, which was covered by an opaque curtain that hid the test material from view. A terry-cloth towel was stretched over the base of the frame to reduce possible auditory cues. In the delayed-matching task, the subject rested his hand on the towel throughout the intratrial interval, keeping the hand that was not being tested outside the frame at all times.

The procedure followed with HM was similar to that used with the commissurotomy patients (Milner and Taylor 1972) and which will be described. Because, in the latter case, our main purpose was to assess the memory capacities of the right hemisphere, the left hand was always tested first, and, therefore, the initial testing of HM was also limited to the left hand.

On this task, which involved unfamiliar abstract figures, subjects were first allowed to manipulate each of the figures in turn for 10 s. They were then tested for their ability to match to sample at zero delay. At the beginning of each trial, the four figures were placed on the towel in a horizontal array (Figure 17.1). The subject was then given one of them to palpate for not more than 10 s. The sample figure was then returned to the array and the subject searched for it immediately, using the same hand as before. Subjects were required to feel each of the figures in the array before selecting the one they thought matched the sample and returning it to the examiner.

Each block of four trials constituted a single testing unit, and the order of presentation of the figures varied at random from one block of trials to the next, as did the distribution of shapes within the array. Thus, successful matching had to be on the basis of pattern recognition, not serial order or spatial arrangement. After each trial, subjects were told whether or not they had chosen correctly, but if they had made an error, they were not allowed to correct it.

Testing at zero delay was continued until a single block of four trials had been completed without error. An intratrial delay of 15 s was then introduced, during which the subject sat quietly until signaled to search for the matching

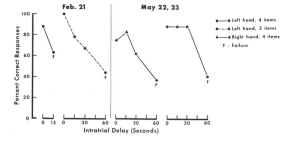

Figure 17.2. Tactile pattern-matching performance of amnesic patient HM, as a function of intratrial interval and number of memoranda. Errors are plotted as a percentage of total trials needed to reach criterion. F signifies failure to complete one errorless block of four trials within the limits of testing.

figure in the array. Again, testing was continued until all four trials within a single block had been successfully completed. If criterion was not reached within five blocks of trials, the zero-delay baseline was reestablished before continuing with the 15-s interval. If errors were still being made after another five blocks of trials, testing was discontinued. If, instead, the subject succeeded at 15 s, the interval was extended to 30 s, then to 60 s, and finally to 120 s. No more than five blocks of trials were allowed at any of these intervals, and in each case, the subject was required to complete one errorless block before the interval could be extended.

On a tactual task of this kind, the zero-delay condition is not a true zero (as it can be in vision), because the figures have to be explored seriatim, and thus several seconds may elapse before a choice is made. This may well increase the difficulty of the task initially for an amnesic patient. HM was, therefore, tested over more trials than the commissurotomy patients, since it seemed particularly important in his case to establish a stable baseline against which his performance after an intratrial delay could be judged.

Figure 17.2 summarizes the results obtained and indicates the order in which the various tests were carried out. In the initial session with the left hand, HM had difficulty maintaining a stable baseline when working with four patterns, and he failed to reach criterion when a 15-s delay was introduced. When the number of wire figures was reduced to three, he made

no errors in the baseline condition, but performance deteriorated with increasing intratrial interval and he was unable to match the figures correctly after a delay of 60 s.

When testing was resumed three months later, HM was able to achieve accurate baseline performance with either hand after a few initial errors, but once again his performance deteriorated every time the intratrial interval was lengthened and he failed with both hands at the 60-s interval. At this stage, every time the intratrial delay was eliminated, errorless performance ensued, but matching broke down again as soon as the 60-s interval was reintroduced. Thus, HM's results for touch are similar to those obtained for delayed matching in other modalities and point to a rapid forgetting of information that cannot readily be verbalized.

In the course of examining HM, we encountered an instance of procedural learning occurring in the absence of any conscious recollection of the testing experience. After HM had spent an entire morning performing the delayed-matching task with his left hand, we returned from lunch and asked him, as he sat once more before the covered frame that concealed the wire figures, if he remembered what he had done that morning. When he could not tell us, we explained that he had had to place one hand under the curtain and feel some wire shapes. At this point, we asked him to try to remember which hand he had used. He hesitated, and then said:

> I was just having a little argument with myself. I was going to say "My right hand," because I am right-handed, but then I noticed my left hand coming up to the table, so I suppose it must have been my left.

This observation not only highlights the contrast between the two kinds of learning (one lost and the other preserved in HM), but also provides a good example of his insightful use of extraneous cues.

When the wire-figures task was administered to seven patients with complete section of the cerebral commissures (Milner and Taylor 1972), the performance of the right hemisphere was found to be far superior to that of HM, with four patients succeeding with the left hand at delays of 120 s (the longest interval sampled) and only one patient (NG, with a performance IQ of 69) doing less well than HM, whose performance IQ was 125. The commissurotomy patients initially had difficulty in matching the patterns, but once this was accomplished, increasing the delay rarely disrupted performance for long. In contrast, when working with the right hand and left cerebral hemisphere, five patients failed to reach criterion at zero delay, despite the introduction of a correction technique in the later trials; yet only AA had sensory defects on the right hand that could account for the failure in pattern recognition (Corkin, Milner, and Rasmussen 1970; Milner and Taylor 1970). For every patient except LB (whose performance with both hands broke down at the 120-s delay), the results for the left hand were superior to those for the right.

These results for the callosotomy patients, though demonstrating a striking superiority of the right hemisphere over the left in tactual pattern matching, raise the question of why their overall performance, even with the right hemisphere, should be so bad. Patients with temporal or frontal unilateral cortical excisions but with intact commissures made virtually no errors either on baseline testing or at any of the intratrial delays, and many of them complained that the task was too easy to be challenging. It thus seems clear that efficient performance of the task requires the conjoint action of the two hemispheres.

Subsequent work by Zaidel and Sperry (1974) has demonstrated a more general memory impairment after cerebral commissurotomy, as revealed by abnormally low scores on a variety of standard learning and memory tests. This led them to conclude that the "processes mediating the initial encoding of engrams and the retrieval and readout of contralateral engram elements depend upon the functioning of the interhemispheric commissures." The work reported in what follows provides further support for this view (see also Chapters 11 and 15, this volume).

Image-mediated verbal learning after cerebral commissurotomy

Our final experiment, first reported in detail here, concerned the use of visual im-

agery to facilitate performance on a verbal associative-learning task. It is well established that concrete words are easier to recall than abstract words of equal frequency in the language, and this is thought to be largely due to their greater power to evoke images (Paivio, Yuille, and Madigan 1968). In work with normal subjects, this image-evoking power has been exploited by instructions to use images as mediators of links between words, and under these conditions, a considerably higher level of recall is achieved (Bugelski, Kidd, and Segmens 1968; Paivio et al. 1968; Paivio 1969; Bower 1970; Elliott 1973). Imagery mnemonics have also been found to improve the verbal-learning performance of some aphasic patients (Patten 1972), and of patients with verbal memory deficits consequent to left temporal lobectomy (Jones 1974), although in this case, scores still remain below the normal level.

In our own earlier work (Jones-Gotman and Milner 1978), patients with right nondominant temporal-lobe lesions showed a slight but significant reduction of the ability to benefit from imagery on a difficult associative-learning task involving 60 pairs of concrete words, although they performed normally on a still more demanding task involving abstract words to be linked by sentence mediation. It thus seemed likely that commissurotomized patients, deprived of input from the right hemisphere to the left, would be handicapped on a verbal-learning task that embodied an imagery mnemonic. In making this prediction, we were also influenced by the mass of evidence showing that the right hemisphere makes a more important contribution than the left to the perception and retention of complex visual patterns (for reviews, see Milner, 1974, 1980). Nevertheless, our prediction was not confirmed. Instead, we found that the commissurotomy group, though performing poorly overall on our learning task, derived as much benefit as other patient groups from instructions to use imagery.

METHOD

Subjects. In all, eight commissurotomy patients were tested, six (AA, LB, CC, NG, NW, RY) with presumed complete section of the interhemispheric commissures (Bogen, Fisher and Vogel 1965; Bogen 1969), and two

(NF, DM) with partial section, sparing the splenium of the corpus callosum (Gordon, Bogen, and Sperry 1971). Because the performance of the latter two patients on the associative learning task did not differ from that of the patients with the complete section, the results were pooled across all eight patients. The patients were tested from four to nine years after the commissurotomy.

The performance of this group was compared with that of a subset of 11 patients from Jones's original study (1974), chosen to match the commissurotomy patients as closely as possible with respect to age and IQ. Each of these patients had undergone a unilateral cortical excision for the relief of epilepsy (one left frontal, two left temporal, one left frontotemporal, two right frontal, one right frontocentral, two right temporal, and two right frontotemporal). As with the commissurotomy patients, the epileptogenic lesions were static and atrophic, dating from birth or early life. Nine patients were tested two weeks postoperatively, the remaining two in followup examination, one or more years later. Table 17.1 summarizes the age and IQ distribution for the two groups.

In addition, it was decided to compare the performance of LB, the most intelligent of the commissurotomy patients, with that of a group of seven patients with cortical excisions (one right frontal, six right temporal) matched to LB specifically with respect to age, sex, and intelligence (see Table 17.2). Three patients were tested two weeks postoperatively, the other four from one and one-half to nine years after surgery.

Materials and procedure. The test material consisted of three equivalent lists of 10 word pairs, seven concrete and three abstract. The concrete pairs were composed of words rated high in image-evoking properties and the abstract pairs were composed of words rated low (Paivio et al. 1968). Although all words were in common use, no two members of a pair sounded alike or belonged to the same semantic category; they were thus relatively difficult to associate.

A set of colored drawings was prepared for use with the concrete pairs of list II, showing the two items represented by each pair of words in interaction. The abstract pairs of that list were just written out in large colored letters (Figure 17.3).

The procedure followed is outlined in Table 17.3. For comparability with Jones's study, training was limited to three trials per list, followed by a delayed recall test for each list, two hours later, the interval being occupied with unrelated nonverbal tasks. Each list was read aloud the first time at the rate of one pair every 10 s, followed immediately by a cued recall test, in which the first word of each pair was given and the subject had 20 s in which to respond with the word that had been paired with it. A correction method was used throughout, and the order of presentation was different for every learning trial and every recall test. For trials 2 and 3, the presentation rate was increased to one pair every 5 s.

No mnemonic was prescribed for list I, which thus provided a baseline estimate of the subject's ability to learn verbal paired associates by rote. The following instructions were given before presentation of list II:

I am now going to read you another list, very much like the first one, but this time

Table 17.1. *Image-mediated learning: Age, IQ, and verbal learning scores for 8 commissurotomy patients and 11 patients with cortical excisions*

Patient group		Age (yr)	Wechsler IQ	Wechsler paired words
Commissure section (5M, 3F)	Mean	31.8	84.4	8.1
	Range	21 – 49	72 – 106	5.0 – 10.5
Cortical excision (10M, 1F)	Mean	24.8	92.0	12.3
	Range	15 – 46	79 – 114	6.0 – 19.0

Table 17.2. *Image-mediated learning: Age, IQ, and verbal learning scores for LB and formatched cortical control group of seven male patients tested after right temporal or frontal lobectomy*

Patients		Age (yr)	Wechsler IQ	Wechsler paired words
LB		22	106	10.5
Cortical control group	Mean	22.3	106.7	15.2
	Range	16 – 33	90 – 115	12 – 20

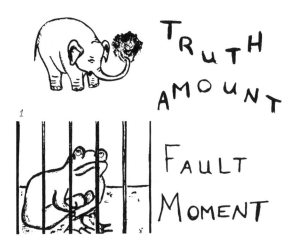

Figure 17.3. Examples of illustrations provided on trial 1 for use with the word-pairs of list II. Left, concrete words: bouquet-elephant; jail-frog. Right, abstract words: truth-amount; fault-moment. Originals in color. (After Jones 1974.)

Table 17.3. *Procedure for image-mediated verbal associative-learning task*

		No. of trials	
List	Condition	Learning	Delayed recall (2-h)
I	Baseline: No images provided	3	1
II	Training: Imagery instructions plus pictures	3	1
III	Test: Generate own images	3	1

when I read the pairs I shall show you a memory trick that I want you to use to help you remember. I want you to imagine the objects named by the two words of each pair in some sort of interaction together, and to see this as a picture in your mind. In order to show you exactly what I mean, I shall describe an image for you after I read each pair, and at the same time I shall show you a drawing of each image I describe, to illustrate what I mean by actual pictures in your mind.

List II was then read aloud to the subject, and after each pair, an image was described briefly while the corresponding drawing was shown. For example, the word-pair "bouquet-elephant" would be read, followed by presentation of the drawing (Figure 17.3, upper left) and the verbal description: "You might imagine an elephant holding a bouquet." The abstract word-pairs were shown in a similar manner, with the explanation that, because these words were difficult to picture, they had simply been written out. Before the second and third readings of the list (trials 2 and 3), subjects were merely told to imagine again the pictures that had been shown on trial 1.

With list III, subjects were instructed to make up their own images: "to try to imagine the objects named by the two words of each pair, in interaction, and to see that as a vivid picture in the mind." On trials 2 and 3, they were told to imagine again the same pictures they had formed the first time the list was read.

Normal control subjects tested on all three lists without imagery instructions showed no improvement from list I to list III on either concrete or abstract words (Jones 1974); the

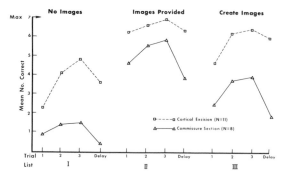

Figure 17.4. Concrete word-pairs: learning curves across three trials, and mean two-hour delayed-recall scores for eight commissurotomy patients and for 11 patients with unilateral cortical excisions.

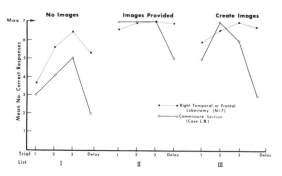

Figure 17.5. Concrete word-pairs: learning curves across three trials, and two-hour delayed-recall scores for cerebral commissurotomy patient LB, and corresponding mean recall scores for a matched group of seven patients with right frontal or right temporal lobectomy.

lists thus appear to have been well matched and any improvement over baseline in the present experiment can be attributed to the imagery instructions.

RESULTS

Concrete words. The performance of the eight patients with commissure section was first compared with that of the control group of 11 patients tested after an unilateral cortical excision for epilepsy.

Figure 17.4 shows the learning curves and two-hour delayed-recall scores of the two groups for the three conditions of testing. A three-way analysis of variance (list x trial x group) with repeated measures yielded a significant main effect of list (F = 56.4, p < 0.001), but no list x group interaction. Both groups were able to benefit from the instructions to use imagery, with performance better on list II (where the images were provided) than on list III (where the subjects had to create their own), but with performance on list III still superior to that on list 1. There was also a significant trial x group interaction (F = 4.66, p < 0.01), because the commissurotomy group was inferior to the cortical-excision group on trial 3 and on delayed recall, and that on lists II and III, the commissurotomy patients showed significant forgetting from trial 3 to the delayed-recall test and the control group did not.

It could be argued that the more rapid forgetting shown by the callosotomy patients

was because they had not reached the same level of learning as the control group before the two-hour delay. We, therefore, examined separately the performance of LB, the only patient with callosal section to reach criterion within the three learning trials. Figure 17.5 shows LB's recall scores as compared with the mean scores of the seven male patients with right temporal or right frontal lobectomy (Jones 1974) matched to him as far as possible for age and IQ. Despite LB's efficient learning under imagery conditions, he showed a clear loss on delayed recall, whereas the control group had near-perfect recall.

Abstract words. In Figure 17.6, the lower graphs show the performance on abstract words of the eight commissurotomy patients and the control group of 11 patients with cortical excisions. Analysis of variance in this case revealed significant effects of group (F = 18.5, p < 0.001), and of trial (F = 15.4, p < 0.001) but not of list, the degree of learning being the same under all three conditions. For both groups, performance on trials 2 and 3 was superior to that on trial 1, but trials 2 and 3 did not differ from each other. The delayed-recall trial did not differ from trial 1, showing no residual beneficial effect of training for either group at this stage.

The upper graphs in Figure 17.6 show the performance of LB, as compared with the mean

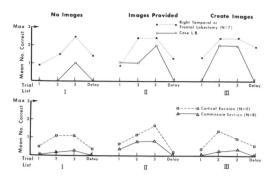

Figure 17.6. Abstract word-pairs: learning curves and two-hour delayed-recall scores. (*Top*) Results for LB and for means of matched cortical-excision group. (*Bottom*) Results for commissurotomy group and for control group of patients with unilateral cortical excisions.

of the matched group of patients with right frontal- or right temporal-lobe excisions. We again see LB's rapid decline in performance after the two-hour delay, whereas the control group showed relatively little loss. Thus, despite the fact that LB was learning a verbal task, the same rapid forgetting is apparent as was seen in the concrete imagery part of the task.

COMMENT

The two main findings in this study were, first, the generally low level of performance achieved by the cerebral commissurotomy group, and, second, the fact that these patients were nevertheless able to derive the same amount of benefit from the use of an imagery mnemonic as the patients whose commissures were intact. These findings have since been replicated with a different control group consisting of unoperated patients subject to frequent epileptic seizures and also matched to the commissurotomy patients as far as possible with respect to age and IQ. Again, both groups benefited equally from the imagery instructions, and, again, the performance of the commissurotomy group was inferior to that of the control group on both concrete and abstract words and under all three testing conditions. In the discussion that follows, these two findings will be considered separately.

The finding that the disconnected left hemisphere responds normally to imagery instructions was contrary to our prediction, but, in retrospect, it seems that that prediction was based on a failure to analyze the requirements of our learning task. The use of an imagery mnemonic imposes no constraints as to the accuracy or wealth of detail in the image evoked, but only that it function as an adequate mediator between words. There is no evidence that the evocation of such images is critically dependent upon the right hemisphere (Ehrlichman and Barrett 1983) and indeed there is some evidence to suggest that the ability to evoke visual images may depend more on the left posterior cortex than the right (Farah 1984, Farah et al. 1985).

The slow learning and poor delayed recall shown by the commissurotomy patients in the present study add to the evidence of impaired memory in this patient group (Zaidel and Sperry 1974). This impairment is shown most strikingly on tests of free recall and, in this respect, accords well with our observations on patients undergoing memory tests after intracarotid injection of sodium amytal into one cerebral hemisphere (Milner, Branch, and Rasmussen 1962; Milner 1978).

In the preoperative assessment of patients with temporal-lobe epilepsy, the carotid-amytal technique has proved to be a valid screening device, enabling one to test memory in patients temporarily deprived of most of one hemisphere by the action of the drug, and thus to uncover possible risk to memory in a planned temporal lobectomy. When we began this research, we did not expect to encounter any striking failures of recall after injection on the same side as the patient's lesion. This was because the test material was simple and had been chosen to permit the use of both verbal and visual coding. Instead, in this case also, our predictions proved wrong and we have become increasingly aware of the frequent total failure of recall for objects, pictures, and sentences presented after the injection (and thus to one hemisphere only), even in patients who have no difficulty in recalling similar material from the preinjection baseline test, and no impairment of recognition. These recall failures are equally frequent after injection into the dominant and into the nondominant hemisphere. These observations have led us to consider that the only valid criterion of amnesia for material presented while the drug was active is a failure to recognize the material after recovery from the effects of the drug.

Further evidence along the same lines comes from a recent study by Lesser et al. (1986). These authors showed that patients were later able to recognize objects that had been shown to them during the first minutes after injection into the left hemisphere, while the patients were not only mute, but also confused and partially inattentive, with complete contralateral hemiplegia, and before the EEG disturbance over the contralateral hemisphere had cleared. Again, the patients could not recall the objects later, but could recognize them from a longer series. Comparable injections into the right nondominant hemisphere did not provoke the same initial confusion, but a similar failure of recall was seen for objects, pictures, and words presented soon after the injection, with good recognition of the same material, provided the injection was to the side of the temporal-lobe lesion.

In the light of these findings, the postinjection impairment of free recall for material presented to the nondominant hemisphere, with subsequent recognition by palpating with the left hand, cannot be interpreted as implying that the right hemisphere keeps its secrets to itself (Risse and Gazzaniga 1978), and by extension that the left hemisphere does also (Bogen 1986). We certainly agree that a mute hemisphere can encode a nonverbal representation of an object, but the subsequent failure of verbal recall for that object does not tell one anything about the failure of interhemispheric transfer, since we have seen that a similarly severe deficit in free recall, with recognition intact, follows injection into the mute hemisphere, and that this occurs for both verbal and nonverbal material (Milner 1978; Lesser et al. 1986).

These carotid-amytal findings provide further evidence of an impairment in free recall for material presented to a single hemisphere, but they do not explain it. Ellenberg and Sperry (1980) have suggested that "the cerebral commissures force the two hemispheres to work together and maintain attentional unity in the intact brain." If this is so, then it is possible that the breakdown of this focused attentional system contributes significantly to the recall difficulties seen after cerebral commissurotomy (see Chapter 13, this volume).

Acknowledgments

We are indebted to Roger Sperry for the opportunity to study the patients with cerebral commissurotomy, and to Joseph E. Bogen for making their clinical histories available to us. The work was supported in part by the United States Public Health Service, through NIMH grant MH–07332 to Dr. Sperry, and in part by the Medical Research Council of Canada, through grant MT–2624 to Brenda Milner.

References

Bogen, J. E. 1969. The other side of the brain. I. Dysgraphia and dyscopia following cerebral commissurotomy. *Bull. L.A. Neurol. Soc.* 34: 73–105.

–1986. One brain, two brains, or both? *In* F. Leporé, M. Ptito, and H. H. Jasper (eds.) *Two Hemispheres – One Brain: Functions of the Corpus Callosum.*, Vol. 17: *Neurology and Biology.* Alan Liss, New York, pp. 21–34.

Bogen, J. E., E. D. Fisher, and P. J. Vogel. 1965. Cerebral commissurotomy: A second case report. *J. Am. Med. Assoc.* 194: 1328–9.

Bogen, J. E., and P. J. Vogel. 1962. Cerebral commissurotomy in man: Preliminary case report. *Bull. L.A. Neurol. Soc.* 27: 169.

Bower, G. H. 1970. Imagery as a relational organizer in associative learning and memory. *J. Verb. Learn. Verb. Behav.* 9: 529–33.

Broadbent, D. E. 1954. The role of auditory localization in attention and memory. *J. Exp. Psychol.* 47: 191–6.

Bugelski, B. R., E. Kidd, and J. Segmens. 1968. Imagery versus repetition encoding in short- and long-term memory. *J. Exp. Psychol.* 100: 270–6.

Celesia, G. G. 1976. Organization of the auditory cortical areas in man. *Brain* 99: 403–14.

Corkin, S. 1964. *Somesthetic Function after Focal Cerebral Damage in Man.* Unpublished PhD thesis, McGill University, Montreal.

–1978. The role of different cerebral structures in somesthetic function. *In* E. C. Carterette and H. P. Friedman (eds.) *Handbook of Perception*, Vol. 6B. Academic Press, New York, pp. 105–55.

Corkin, S., B. Milner, and T. Rasmussen. 1970. Somatosensory thresholds: Contrasting effects of postcentral gyrus and posterior parietal-lobe excisions. *Arch. Neurol.* 23: 41–58.

Ellenberg, L., and R. W. Sperry. 1980. Lateralized division of attention in the commissurotomized and intact brain. *Neuropsychol.* 12: 411–18.

Elliott, L. 1973. Imagery versus repetition encoding in short- and long-term memory. *J. Exp. Psychol.* 100: 270–6.

Erlichman, H., and J. Barrett. 1983. Right hemisphere specialization for mental imagery: A review of the evidence. *Brain and Cog.* 2: 55–76.

Farah, M. J. 1984. The neurological basis of mental images: A componential analysis. *Cognition* 18: 245–72.

Farah, M. J., M. S. Gazzaniga, J. D. Holtzman, and S. M. Kosslyn. 1985. A left hemisphere bias for visual mental imagery? *Neuropsychol.* 23: 115–18.

Galaburda, A., and F. Sanides. 1980. Cytoarchitectonic organization of the human auditory cortex. *J. Comp. Neurol.* 190: 597–610.

Gazzaniga, M. S., and R. W. Sperry. 1967. Language after section of the cerebral commissures. *Brain* 90: 131–48.

Gordon, H. W., J. E. Bogen, and R. W. Sperry. 1971. Absence of deconnexion syndrome in two patients with partial section of the neocommissures. *Brain* 94: 327–36.

Immig, T. J., M. A. Ruggero, L. M. Kitzes, E. Javel, and J. F. Brugge. 1977. Organization of auditory cortex in the owl monkey (*Atus trivirgatus*). *J. Comp. Neurol.* 171: 111–28.

Jones, M. K. 1974. Imagery as a mnemonic aid after left temporal lobectomy: Contrast between material-specific and generalized memory disorders. *Neuropsychol.* 12: 21–30.

Jones-Gotman, M., and B. Milner. 1978. Right temporal-lobe contribution to image-mediated verbal learning. *Neuropsychol.* 16: 61–71.

Kimura, D. 1961. Some effects of temporal-lobe damage on auditory perception. *Can. J. Psychol.* 15: 156–65.

–1964. Left-right differences in the perception of melodies. *Quart. J. Exp. Psychol.* 16: 355–8.

Lassonde, M., M. P. Bryden, and P. Demers. In press. The corpus callosum and cerebral speech lateralization.

Lesser, R. P., D. S. Dinner, H. Lüders, and H. H. Morris. 1986. Memory for objects presented soon after intracarotid amobarbital sodium injections in patients with medically intractable complex partial seizures. *Neurol.* 36: 895–9.

Levy, J., C. Trevarthen, and R. W. Sperry. 1972. Perception of bilateral chimeric figures following hemispheric deconnection. *Brain* 95: 61–78.

Milner, B. 1974. Hemispheric specialization: Scope and limits. *In* F. O. Schmidt and F. G. Worden (eds.) *The Neurosciences: Third Study Program.* The MIT Press, Cambridge, pp. 5–19.

–1978. Clues to the cerebral organization of memory. *In* P. A. Buser and A. Rougeul-Buser (eds.) *Cerebral Correlates of Conscious Experience,* INSERM Symposium No. 6. Elsevier/North-Holland, Amsterdam, pp. 139–53.

–1980. Complementary functional specializations of the human cerebral hemispheres. *In* R. Levi-Montalcini, (ed.) *Nerve Cells, Transmitters and Behavior.* Pontificiae Academiae Scripta Varia, Vatican City, pp. 601–25.

Milner, B., C. Branch, and T. Rasmussen. 1962. Study of short-term memory after intracarotid injection of Sodium Amytal. *Trans. Am. Neurol. Assoc.* 87: 224–6.

Milner, B., and L. Taylor. 1970. Somesthetic thresholds after commissural section in man. *Neurol.* 20: 378.

–1972. Right-hemisphere superiority in tactile pattern-recognition after cerebral commissurotomy: Evidence for nonverbal memory. *Neuropsychol.* 10: 1–15.

Milner, B., L. Taylor, and R. W. Sperry. 1968. Lateralized suppression of dichotically presented digits after commissural section in man. *Science* 161: 184–6.

Musick, F. E., and A. Reeves. 1986. Effects of partial and complete corpus callosotomy on central auditory function. *In* F. Leporé, M. Ptito, and H. H. Jasper (eds.) *Two Hemispheres – One Brain: Functions of the Corpus Callosum,* Vol. 17: *Neurology and Biology.* Alan Liss, New York. pp. 423–33.

Paivio, A. 1969. Mental imagery in associative learning and memory. *Psychol. Rev.* 76: 241–63.

Paivio, A., J. C. Yuille, and S. A. Madigan. 1968. Concreteness, imagery, and meaningfulness values for 925 nouns. *J. Exp. Psychol. Monogr. Suppl.* 76(2): 1–25.

Patten, B. M. 1972. The ancient art of memory. *Arch. Neurol.* 26: 25–31.

Pribram, K. H., B. S. Rosner, and W. A. Rosenblith. 1954. Electrical respones to acoustic clicks in monkeys: Extent of neocortex activated. *J. Neurophysiol.* 17: 336–44.

Prisko, L.-H. 1963. *Short-Term Memory in Focal Cerebral Damage.* Unpublished PhD thesis, McGill University, Montreal.

Risse, G. L., and M. S. Gazzaniga. 1978. Well-kept secrets of the right hemisphere: A carotid amytal study of restricted memory transfer. *Neurol.* 28: 950–2.

Scoville, W. B. and B. Milner. 1957. Loss of recent memory after bilateral hippocampal lesions. *J. Neurol. Neurosurg. Psychiat.* 20: 11–21.

Sidman, M., L. D. Stoddard, and J. P. Mohr. 1968. Some additional quantitative observations of immediate memory in a patient with bilateral hippocampal lesions. *Neuropsychol.* 6: 245–54.

Sparks, R., and N. Geschwind. 1968. Dichotic listening in man after section of neocortical commissures. *Cortex* 4: 3–16.

Sperry, R. W. 1968. Hemisphere deconnection and unity of conscious awareness. *Am. Psychol.* 23: 723–33.

–1974. Lateral specialization in the surgically separated hemispheres. *In* F. O. Schmidt and F. G. Worden (eds.) *The Neurosciences: Third Study Program.* The MIT Press, Cambridge, pp. 5–19.

Sperry, R. W., M. S. Gazzaniga, and J. E. Bogen. 1969. Interhemispheric relationships: The neocortical commissures; syndromes of hemisphere disconnection. *In* P. J. Vinken and G. W. Bruyn (eds.) *Handbook of Clinical Neurology,* Vol. 4. North-Holland, Amsterdam, pp. 273–90.

Zaidel, D., and R. W. Sperry. 1974. Memory impairment after commissurotomy in man. *Brain* 97: 263–72.

18 The saga of right-hemisphere reading[*]

Eran Zaidel
Department of Psychology
University of California, Los Angeles

Prologue: At Caltech

In March 1967, about to graduate from Columbia College, I had to decide which graduate school to attend. I was interested in human language and cognition and had a long experience with computers, so that artificial intelligence seemed like a natural choice for a research career. At first, my preference was for the Computer Science Department in Carnegie Mellon University. But the brochure that just arrived from the Information Science Department at Caltech featured palm trees, and the school earned a high "overall academic excellence index" as part of my complex evaluation algorithm. I went to Pasadena. For the next three years, the work with my advisor, Fred Thompson, was extremely interesting, focusing on mathematical linguistics. Unfortunately, Thompson was primarily interested in computer "language" and "cognition" and he did not believe that the computer can simulate human cognition.

Caltech did not have a Psychology Department. Over in Humanities and Social Sciences, Louis Breger did psychoanalytically motivated dream research; in Information Science, Derek Fender used contact lenses for stabilized retinal images to study human visual perception; and across the campus, 300 yards away, Roger Sperry was studying hemispheric specialization in split-brain patients. My wife, Dahlia W. Zaidel, had been working in his lab since 1967, and the research there seemed exciting and full of opportunities for a skeptical formalist.

One sunny afternoon in the Fall of 1970, I went to Roger Sperry's office and proposed a new technique for presenting visual information to one visual half-field (VHF) at a time while permitting continuous hemispheric ocular scanning. Sperry was skeptical. Others have tried different electronic approaches to restrict vision and failed, he said. Nevertheless, he provided funding for developing the technique and space in his psychobiology lab. For the next nine months, I struggled with the optical design and with the precision machinists in the Chemistry Instrument Shop. Only later, when comparing notes with my wife and other fellow and former students, did I realize that Sperry's skepticism was his usual "survival test" for commitment. The question was, does the student have enough commitment to persevere in spite of doubts? Does he have enough insight to follow his own hunches? Sperry never responded to those students who kept asking what experiments to run, but he always provided insightful critical analysis when required and reminded us to keep the big picture in mind, to ask the critical question, run the critical experiment. He said, if the man in the street will not understand the significance of your results, then the experiment is not worth doing. One may argue whether this is a sufficient general criterion, but there is no doubt that the "man-in-the-street" rule is a powerful antidote to being lost in the technicalities of one's own

[*]This chapter was written in 1984. An update on the status of right-hemisphere reading is available in Zaidel (in press) and in Zaidel et al. (in press).

field, to losing sight of the overall goals of the research program. We absorbed the rule by osmosis during a period of apprenticeship.

I survived, and the application of the contact-lens technique to the language abilities of the two hemispheres of the commissurotomy patients in Sperry's laboratory gave me the opportunity I was seeking for my PhD research. Not everyone flourished in this laissez-faire environment. Some students, younger, or perhaps less desperate, did not enjoy the "survival test." I was not the only one of Sperry's students to have made a move. We were a motley crew. Half of us were transfers from other departments or "special admits." Not everywhere are such transfers possible. Caltech is a small school; it prides itself on flexibility and encourages interdisciplinary research. For my part, I will always be grateful for the opportunity to make the move that gained me entry to the science of human neuropsychology.

The classical tradition

The clinical neurological account of acquired reading disorders consequent to brain damage has changed incredibly little in the past century. Its main outline was set by Jules Déjerine in the 1880s, when he presented clinical-anatomical evidence for two types of acquired alexia: alexia with agraphia (Déjerine 1891) and alexia without agraphia (Déjerine 1892). Alexia without agraphia, pure word blindness with a preserved ability to write, was said to result from a lesion in the visual (occipital) cortex of the language-dominant hemisphere, coupled with a lesion in the splenium of the corpus callosum. Déjerine believed that the left angular gyrus, anterior to the visual cortex on that side, served as the exclusive center for verbal–visual images and thus subserved reading, and that the occipital lesion (in the white matter) destroyed the fibers connecting the calcarine region of the visual cortex to the angular gyrus. Nonetheless, Déjerine did not ascribe any role to the splenial lesion in the pathogenesis of alexia.

Albert (1979) points out that both Brissaud, in 1900, and Redlich, in 1895, noted that two lesions, one involving the left primary visual area, and the other involving the corpus callosum, might prevent the transfer of visual

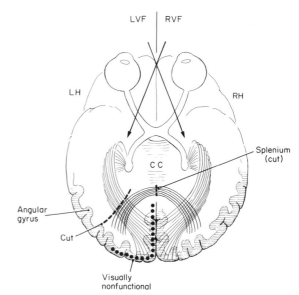

Figure 18.1. Schematic diagram of the disconnecting lesions that give rise to a pure alexia.

information. But according to Albert, it was Quensel, in 1931, who stressed the necessity of the callosal lesion, and emphasized the "disconnection" aspect of the syndrome.

In this 50-year-old theory, which was revived and championed by Geschwind in 1965, the lesion in the left visual area prevents visual stimuli entering the left hemisphere (LH) from reaching the left angular gyrus, which is necessary for reading, while visual stimuli that enter the intact right hemisphere (RH) are prevented from reaching the left angular gyrus because the splenium of the corpus callosum has been destroyed. The cause of pure alexia is, therefore, a combination of lesions in the dominant occipital lobe and in the splenium of the corpus callosum (Figure 18.1).

It turns out, in fact, that neither the splenial lesion nor right homonymous hemianopsia is necessary for the syndrome of pure alexia. The angular gyrus is said to receive dorsal and ventral inputs from the splenium of the corpus callosum as well as medial and lateral inputs from the visual cortex. Thus, small lesions in the occipital lobe may disconnect afferent pathways from the left calcarine cortex, leaving both calcarine areas intact. In particular, lesions in the white matter beneath the angular gyrus (subangular alexia) can undercut and isolate it from visual information originating in both left and right visual cortices, and if the lesion spares the optic radiations, no right hemianopsia should occur.

Frequently, pure alexics can name some objects, letters or digits. How does this preserved naming square with the alleged visual disconnection? Geschwind (1965) suggested that such stimuli can evoke nonvisual sensory associations in the RH and that this representation may cross the corpus callosum through the intact and more anterior portion. Colors, lacking tactile associations, would not be named.

F. Michel (personal communication) distinguishes two forms of the syndrome. According to him, the first is due to a large softening involving the temporal lobe. Symptoms include right homonymous hemianopsia, a memory loss and word-finding difficulties. Patients can usually name objects, sometimes with semantic errors, and can often read digits and letters but cannot name colors. The second form of pure alexia is due to bleeding into the visual radiation and inferior longitudinal fasciculus and extending to the occipital horn; there are frequent cases without hemianopsia, there is little memory disturbance, and there is usually good reading of digits and letters, good color naming, and good object naming. Recovery from alexia is more likely in the second form than in the first. Both forms are consistent with the disconnection account and they explain why neither right homonymous hemianopsian nor a splenial lesion are necessary.

Alternative explanations of alexia without agraphia in terms of visual agnosia were offered as early as 1889 (by Lissauer, see Albert 1979) and persist to this day (Albert 1979). But all agree that the disorder can be observed with lesions restricted to the LH. In fact, an acquired reading disorder is considered a more reliable lateralizing sign for a (dominant) LH lesion than is speech deficit (Benson 1979). Thus, the clinical neurologic tradition denied that the RH can read at all! This goes beyond merely claiming LH superiority; it posits a LH specialization for reading at least as exclusive as for speech.

The dramatic conflict

When Sperry, Gazzaniga, and Bogen (1969) summarized the first phase of split-brain work, they confirmed classical clinical neurological views about LH specialization for expressive language in general and for speech in particular. The disconnected RH seemed essentially mute. It was easy to demonstrate the language disconnection syndrome by "left-hand or LVF anomia" in the presence of good RH perception. While these observations challenged directly the observations of Akelaitis in the late thirties and early forties (Akelaitis 1944), they conformed well to the classical descriptions of disconnection syndromes by the "diagram makers" and localizationists. But, quite early in the California series, there also emerged evidence for some receptive language capacity in the RH, especially auditory comprehension (Sperry and Gazzaniga 1967). This was in direct opposition to established neurological tradition, and, indeed, led Bogen to withdraw his name from the first papers summarizing the findings (Gazzaniga and Sperry 1967, Sperry and Gazzaniga 1967). For Sperry, the conflict created a "problem" whose explication was bound to lead to a scientific advance. For him, a modicum of verbal RH comprehension was consistent with the presence in the RH of a complete and potentially independent, cognitive system.

When I started experiments in Sperry's lab in the Spring of 1970, I was interested in using commissurotomy patients to understand the structure of human language and its relation to thought. RH language provided a partially developed model of natural language that might be more transparent to experimental analysis. At the same time, the RH provided a model of thought unconstrained by language. Using the new contact-lens technique, I embarked on three consecutive series of experiments extended over a period of nine years.

The first series used developmental analysis to characterize the language profile of the disconnected RH in terms of an hypothesized stage in first language acquisition. These experiments were motivated by the question of the ontogenesis of hemispheric specialization for language. The second approach compared RH language to the classical aphasiological profiles from standardized aphasia tests. Here the motivation was to try to resolve the apparent conflict between findings of clinical aphasiology and the view of RH language emerging from the disconnection syndrome. The answer had important clinical implications for a RH role in recovery of language functions in aphasia. The third approach sought to characterize the differences between the LH and RH language systems in terms of an information-processing/psycholinguistic analysis of lexical organization. The next question was whether the observed hemispheric differences extended to the normal brain (Zaidel 1985).

DEVELOPMENTAL ANALYSIS

When we examine an equivalent mental-age profile for RH competence on a series of standardized language-comprehension tests, ranging from auditory discrimination and phonological encoding to lexical phonetics, auditory and visual vocabulary, phrase comprehension, and syntax (cf. Zaidel 1978; Zaidel and Peters 1981), it is clear that RH comprehension does not correspond to any one stage in normal language acquisition. In particular, the disconnected RH did not stop acquiring language uniformly at age 5 (or 13, for that matter). The RH did acquire some reading, but the visual vocabulary of the disconnected RH remained smaller than its auditory vocabulary. In linguistic terms, the RH appeared to have developed a rich lexical semantic and conceptual system, a limited syntactic system, and an impoverished phonological system (Zaidel 1978).

APHASIOLOGICAL ANALYSIS

The language profile of the disconnected RH does not correspond to any classical aphasic type. No classical syndrome has the following pattern: little or no speech and very little writing, substantial comprehension of single words, which is better for auditory than visually presented stimuli, and poor comprehension of sentences. But is the reading profile of the RH like that of any acquired alexia? The RH is not word blind; it has neither literal nor verbal alexia (Kertesz 1979). It may be regarded as having a form of aphasic alexia, perhaps of the type associated with an anterior speech deficit, or, perhaps, like "sentence alexia" (Kertesz 1979). But "sentence alexia" is prominent in all of the

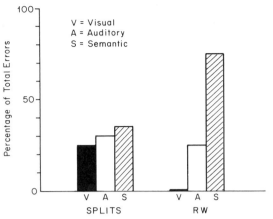

Figure 18.2. Predominance of semantic errors in matching words to pictures by commissurotomy patients LB and NG, and by deep dyslexic patient RW. (Subtest B.3 of Schuell's Minnesota Test for Differential Diagnosis of Aphasia with visual, auditory, and semantic decoys; Schuell, 1965.)

classical aphasic syndromes (Kertesz 1979). Thus, there is no one alexia syndrome that parallels the reading profile of the RH of a commissurotomy patient.

A notable feature of RH reading, accompanying auditory comprehension of single words, is a predilection for semantic errors when the multiple-choice responses contain decoys that are closely related in meaning or context to the target. This pattern is illustrated in Figure 18.2. It may reflect a "looser," more associative lexical/semantic or conceptual organization in the RH than in the LH. Alternatively, these semantic errors may reflect a direct route from the modality-specific patterndriven lexical representation to a central amodal representation of meaning, without the benefits of multimodal representations, or of richer rule-governed phonological constraints. Moreover, the semantic organization of the visual and auditory lexicons of the RH may well be different. Indeed, the same semantic categories (objects, colors, actions, geometric shapes, and numbers) show a different ordering of preservation in the visual and auditory lexicons of the disconnected RHs. For example, the disconnected RHs comprehend spoken object names best, but comprehend written object names worst (Zaidel 1982).

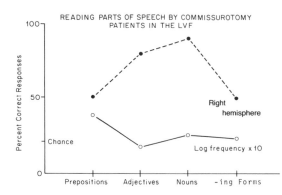

Figure 18.3. Effect of part-of-speech on reading single words in the LVF of commissurotomy patients LB and NG.

It is easy to demonstrate that the disconnected RH can comprehend the meanings of abstract words. Here the correct answer in the multiple-choice picture array is simply chosen to instantiate the abstract concept. For example, the drawing of Minerva holding the scales can identify the concept "justice." We found that frequency of occurrence of spoken words in language use rather than their rated abstraction predicts their availability to either hemisphere, and that the RH has a higher frequency threshold for retrieving the meaning of words (Zaidel 1976). But when word frequency is controlled, reading tests suggest that the disconnected RH reads concrete nouns better than function words (Zaidel 1983a; Figure 18.3). A similar dissociation is frequently observed in a variety of aphasic syndromes (cf. Patterson and Besner 1984).

INFORMATION-PROCESSING ANALYSIS

A lexical item can be represented by its spoken or acoustic form, its printed or orthographic form, or, in the case of many words, by its referent, say depicted by a picture. Any child who has learned to read phonetically can easily recognize or identify any one representation of a lexical item (spoken word, written or printed word, picture of referent) given another. But this is not true of the RH. The disconnected RH can match either a spoken or a printed word with a picture, but its auditory vocabulary is larger. We do not know how much writing the RH has, but this seems severely limited (cf. Levy, Nebes, and Sperry

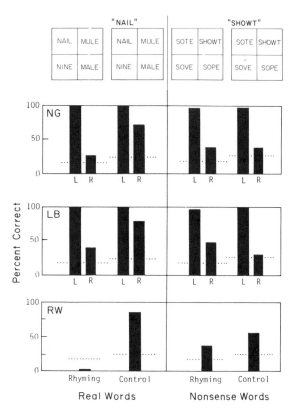

Figure 18.4. Performance of commissurotomy patients LB and NG and of deep dyslexic patient RW on rhyming and control tests using real and nonsense words. The control tests require the subject to point to a word in response to its auditory form. L = LH and R = RH.

1971). Although the RH has virtually no speech, it, surprisingly, may have some limited ability to evoke the phonological or acoustic representation of the name of the concept, as assessed by the ability to match pictures with homonymous names, without being able to name them aloud (Zaidel and Peters 1981). The RH can apparently also evoke the orthographic representation from the acoustic representation, as determined by tests requiring it to match spoken names with written multiple choices. This phoneme–grapheme conversion route may operate indirectly via intermediate, say semantic, representations.

At the same time, the evidence suggests that the disconnected RHs do not have grapheme–phoneme conversion rules; they are unable to match the written forms of either meaningful or nonsense words for rhyming

(Figure 18.4). Thus, RH reading seems to access meaning directly from the orthography, without intermediate phonetic recoding. Such reading is nonetheless invariant across numerous perceptual changes, including handwriting style and case. Therefore, the internal "orthographic" representation of lexical items in the RH must be relatively abstract and normalized, rather than iconic.

GENERALIZABILITY: LEXICAL DECISION AND SEMANTIC FACILITATION

The foregoing conclusions about the RH reading profile were based largely on the patterns observed with LVF testing, using the contact-lens method for hemispheric occular scanning in two commissurotomy patients, LB and NG, who had been fitted with lenses. Do the results generalize to every commissurotomy patient? In order to extend our conclusions concerning the scope of RH reading to other commissurotomy patients of the California series, we used a hemifield tachistoscopic lexical decision and semantic facilitation paradigm that can be administered easily to commissurotomy patients, aphasics, and normal subjects alike.

The task required the subjects to decide whether or not briefly and randomly lateralized target character strings spelled out meaningful English words (lexical decision). Commissurotomy patients responded with the hand homolateral to the input VF by pressing a centrally placed button only if the target was a word. Half of the target strings were orthographically regular, pronounceable nonsense words; the other half were meaningful, concrete, and frequent words from four to six letters long. In a variant of the task, targets were preceded by randomly lateralized word primes. Of the primes paired with target words, half were semantically associated with the targets (as determined by free word association norms) and half were not. Another variant of the task included auditory rather than printed primes, spoken by the examiner. Six commissurotomy patients received the task: five had complete cerebral commissurotomy including the corpus callosum, anterior commissure, and hippocampal commissure (LB, NG, RY, AA, and NW), and one had partial section, sparing the splen-

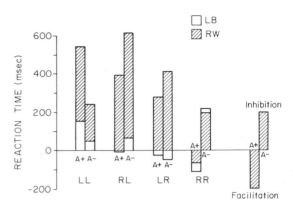

Figure 18.5. Latency difference between lexical decision of targets with primes and lexical decision of targets alone. Ideally, semantically associated primes (A+) should create facilitation and unassociated primes (A−) should create inhibition. LL = prime presented in the left visual hemifield (LVF), target in LVF; LR = prime in LVF, target in RVF; etc. In the case of targets alone, ignore the prime VF.

ium (NF). Latency and accuracy were used as dependent measures of performance.

Lexical decision of targets alone disclosed bilateral competence. All patients except NG could make lexical decisions of targets in both VFs. Most patients showed more accurate LH decisions (RVF targets and right-hand responses). But of those patients whose accuracy was above chance bilaterally, most were equally fast with both hemispheres. Partial-commissurotomy patient NF showed the same pattern as the complete commissurotomy patients. Thus, though different in accuracy and processing style, both hemispheres of commissurotomy patients can decide whether or not a word is meaningful.

Only one patient (LB) showed significant facilitation, i.e., shorter reaction times for decisions of targets with associated than unassociated primes, and then only in the LH (Figure 18.5). However, both hemispheres of LB showed similar facilitation by auditory primes. Thus, lexical decision by both hemispheres involves semantic access. This also suggests that semantic access in auditory comprehension is superior to semantic access in reading comprehension in either hemisphere.

Is competence for lexical decision indicative of competence for conscious lexical/semantic access in reading? Two commissurotomy patients, LB and NG, participated subsequently in a reading experiment using the same target words. Here, instead of lexical decision, the task required the subject to view the briefly lateralized target and then to point to the correct picture from a multiple-choice quartet exposed in free vision. Results for both hemispheres yielded higher estimates of tachistoscopic vocabulary size in the reading than in the lexical decision task (Zaidel 1983b). In turn, the results on the tachistoscopic reading test were then compared with results on the same test when both target words and multiple-choice pictures were lateralized for free ocular scanning, using the contact lens. Again, the tachistoscopic data underestimated the vocabulary size obtained with hemispheric scanning. Thus, the lateralized tachistoscopic lexical decision paradigm seems to provide a conservative estimate of the reading ability of the disconnected RH.

All five patients with complete commissurotomy tested in the California series, then, show evidence for RH reading comprehension of single words. But do these conclusions generalize to the normal brain, or do they reflect abnormal language development in the RH due to early epileptogenic lesions in the language area of the LH? We will attempt to answer this question more directly by experiments probing the competence of the normal RH on the same lexical decision and semantic faciliation paradigms. At this point, we may note that there is no neurological evidence (EEG, seizure pattern, neurosurgical accounts, etc.) in these patients for a LH lesion of a size that would lead to compensatory language development in the RH. Moreover, there is no evidence in any of these patients for any gross linguistic deficit in the LH, now or during their developmental histories (Zaidel 1983a).

Gazzaniga (1983) argues that the normal RH has no language since patients in the Wilson series tested by him usually show no RH language competence. Furthermore, he finds that when the RH does develop language, this could be of any level of competence with no unique profile. The data presented in support of these arguments are not compelling (Zaidel 1983c; Myers 1984). Patients in the Wilson series typically have intact anterior commissures through which information from one hemisphere may transfer to the other as occurs in monkeys (Sullivan and Hamilton 1973), and some of the patients have large LH lesions. Under these circumstances, estimates of RH language competence are especially uncertain (Myers 1984). The argument arising from conflicting claims for commissurotomy patients may be resolved if it can be demonstrated that the RH has language in the normal brain and in adult aphasics, as will be discussed.

DOES THE DISCONNECTED LH
HAVE A LANGUAGE DEFICIT?

Using a variety of clinical tests, we have verified repeatedly that the disconnected LH has no clinically detectable language deficit. In particular, there is no gross LH impairment in the comprehension of spoken or written words, or in the other domains where the RH has a selective relative competence. Why then are any linguistic abilities developed in the RH? Three alternative answers can be put forth. First, these rudimentary linguistic abilities, particularly in lexical semantics, may be necessary for adequate independent RH orientation to the environment during communication. Second, the RH may be important in acquiring certain linguistic skills, such as reading, where it offers an "ideographic" alternative to phonetic reading (cf. Zaidel 1979a). Third, these RH abilities may be prerequisites to other functions that it contributes to support the LH during normal communication. Candidate functions are (1) the modulation of affective prosody and intonation during receptive and expressive sentence processing (cf. Ross 1981), (2) thematic analysis in discourse and affective orientation to narrative (cf. Meyers 1984), (3) implementation of pragmatic strategies (Foldi, Cicone, and Gardner 1983), and (4) recognition of recurring patterns in speed reading (Zaidel 1979a). If any of these skills is really dependent on the integrity of the RH, then the disconnected LH should show corresponding deficits.

We have not observed such deficits using the usual gross clinical measures, but we did not test specifically for subtle or high-order deficits.[†] It is possible that subcallosal interhemispheric transfer still mediates at least some of these supporting functions in the split brain, but it is unlikely to do so for the full range of any of these skills (such as phonological and syntactic aspects of prosody). More testing is needed to resolve these issues.

While it is difficult to exhibit any gross linguistic deficits in the disconnected LH, it is nonetheless surprisingly easy to demonstrate both left- and right-hemisphere deficits in the split brain on a variety of allegedly related cognitive functions, such as those making up the Illinois Test of Psycholinguistic Abilities (Zaidel 1979b). Here the free-vision profiles of six commissurotomy patients are subnormal and erratic and they do not correspond to a normal profile at any age. While these "psycholinguistic abilities" may require interhemispheric interaction in the mature brain and may even underlie the acquisition of some linguistic structures in children, they apparently have little to do with mature language functioning.

To summarize, the disconnected RH has a unique reading profile. It has no grapheme–phoneme conversion, it reads concrete nouns better than function words, and it cannot tell apart close associates from actual meanings of real words. Reading mechanisms in the disconnected LH, on the other hand, show none of these patterns. In particular, the LH can read phonetically, i.e., it can translate orthography into sound.

Interlude: A change of scene; At UCLA

In September 1979, I moved my books and files from quiet Pasadena to bustling West-

---

†More recently, we have documented severe and persistent deficits in the ability of split-brain patients to comprehend extended reading discourse. We have also tested them on a battery of loosely termed parapragmatic functions found to be impaired following unilateral right-hemisphere damage (Gardner and Brownell 1986). The patients showed consistent and severe deficits on three subtests during normal administration: (1) interpreting the affect expressed by prosody in spoken sentences (prosody), (2) associating spoken expressions with pictorial representation of their metaphoric rather than literal meanings (pictorial metaphor), and (3) comprehension of spoken discourse tested by retelling of a heard story (narrative retelling) (Zaidel, Spence, and Kasher, in preparation). On the assumption that the disconnected left hemisphere controls the verbal interaction with the examiner during free-field testing in these patients, it follows that these left hemispheres do have some parapragmatic deficits.

wood. Larger and more impersonal than Caltech, UCLA had a huge Department of Psychology. Moreover, I found people actively interested in hemispheric specialization not only in the departments of neurology, neurosurgery, psychiatry, radiology, anatomy, and physiology, at the medical school to the South, but also in computer science, linguistics, philosophy, education, and sociology, further to the North.

UCLA is a commuter school; many offices and labs quickly empty after 5 P.M. I still remember the "good old days," when, as a graduate student in Sperry's lab, I would cross the street from home to lab and start serious work at 10 P.M. Chuck Hamilton was always there to develop a constructive scientific dialogue in an amazingly short time (we usually talked simultaneously). Larry Benowitz would be there to examine what it all meant in the context of wider perspectives, such as psychoanalysis or socialism, and Hal Gordon was always ready for a strong personal argument, whatever the topic. But it was Dahlia who taught me how to discriminate left from right and introduced me to the excitement of experimental neuropsychology. I miss the intense intellectual encounters that started in the laboratory and continued across the street in the student-run coffee house surrounded by loud music and mountains of science-fiction paperbacks and comic books. Sperry was never at the lab at night, but his spirit was wandering around, dominating the conversations.

At UCLA, I embarked on a new research program to seek convergent evidence from the split-brain data, from hemisphere-damaged patients, and from normal subjects. This required interaction between cognitive psychology and neuroscience, linguistics and psychology, bringing together cognition and affect. UCLA was the ideal place to work at the interface. When I felt homesick, I went back to test the commissurotomy patients at Caltech, where I retained a part-time affiliation as a visiting associate in biology.

Working through

The normal brain remains the ultimate focus for any account of hemispheric specialization. Such focus is motivated by two implicit underlying assumptions. The first is the "transparency" hypothesis, which holds that lesion-induced cognitive deficit exposes or "makes transparent" normal cognition. Using a computer analogy, we may say that aphasia, agnosia, apraxia, and amnesia are the result of lawful losses of distinguishable "software modules" from the complex anatomically arranged cognitive program of the brain. Changes in anatomy (structure) dictate predictable changes in function. The second, related, assumption is the "simulation" hypothesis. It says that it is possible in principle to simulate deficit conditions in the normal brain under appropriate load and stress. For example, laterality (dichotic listening or hemifield tachistoscopic) experiments can be said to simulate callosal section with measures of speed or accuracy of information processing (Filbey and Gazzaniga 1969).

What is the evidence for RH reading in the normal brain? Answers to this question have a long and interesting history. As early as 1933, S. I. Franz believed in the simulation hypothesis and recognized the usefulness of the hemifield tachistoscopic paradigm as a method of probing hemispheric specialization for normal reading (Franz 1933). From numerous aphasia studies, including his own, Franz knew that the LH is specialized for reading in dextrals. For his experiment, Franz used a surprisingly modern design: target exposure was set at 100 ms using a gravity tachistoscope; a central stimulus had to be identified in addition to the lateralized letters to ensure fixation; and responses consisted of named identification of the stimulus words or letters (cf. Zaidel 1983b). The dependent measure was accuracy rather than reaction time. But for stimuli, Franz used four-letter words split apart by 10° (degrees of visual angle) across the horizontal meridian. Thus, the two letters making up the first half of the target were flashed 5° to the left of fixation, and the two letters making up the second half of the word were flashed 5° to the right of fixation. He found an unexpected left-visual-field advantage (LVFA) (Franz and Kilduff 1933) and concluded pessimistically that hemispheric control can shift as a function of psychological task parameters (Franz 1933). Clearly, Franz's experiment confounded the reading habit (in English) for scanning from left to right with hemispheric specialization. Twenty years

later, Mishkin and Forgays (1952) deliberately tested the influence of reading scanning habit but failed to detect a general left-hemisphere specialization for reading perhaps because they inappropriately chose Yiddish instead of Hebrew as a right-to-left scanning language (Zaidel 1983b).

One fundamental concept missing from the earlier experiments was the distinction between tasks that can be performed by either hemisphere alone ("direct-access" tasks) and those that can only be processed in one hemisphere and may require callosal transfer prior to processing ("callosal relay" tasks). Without a principled set of behavioral criteria for identifying the two models, it is impossible to interpret a right-visual-field advantage (RVFA) in a linguistic experiment (Zaidel, 1983b). One common criterion for direct access is an interaction between some linguistic stimulus dimension (say concreteness of targets in a lexical decision task) with visual field of presentation when other dimensions (such as length, visual complexity, etc.) are the same (the "processing dissociation" criterion). Another useful criterion is the observation of a mild RVFA that is the same in both the split and normal brain, suggesting that each hemisphere can perform the task and that no callosal transfer is involved (Zaidel 1983b).

DIRECT ACCESS FOR LEXICAL DECISION IN THE NORMAL BRAIN

The student who came into my office one afternoon in the fall of 1980 said he was looking for a topic and an advisor to supervise an honors thesis in psychology. After a short discussion, it became clear that Allen Radant was interested in the problem of anxiety. He hypothesized that level of anxiety is inversely proportional to callosal connectivity. I suggested interhemispheric semantic facilitation in lexical decision as a paradigm for measuring the effect of anxiety and the project was under way. With a minimum of instruction, Radant designed the decision and facilitation task that we subsequently administered to the commissurotomy patients.

Subjects were required to fill out the Spielberger State and Trait Anxiety Questionnaire (Spielberger, Gorsuch, and Lushene 1970). Results showed bigger facilitation in the LVF then in the RVF, suggesting a direct-access model. And, there was an inverse correlation between state anxiety and inter-hemispheric facilitation, especially from the left to the right hemisphere (prime in RVF, target in LVF), consistent with increased RH activation under increasing anxiety or stress (Radant 1981).

Radant's experiment used 100-ms primes, a 500-ms ISI (to maximize semantic facilitation), and about 50-ms targets (titrated individually to achieve a fixed performance level of about 85%). Other people in the lab continued the experiment and extended the results over the next two years. Lexical decision of primes preceding targets was compared with lexical decision of targets alone. It is believed that semantically related primes facilitate the decision of their paired targets, relative to decision of these targets alone, whereas unrelated primes actually inhibit decision (slow it down) relative to targets alone (Posner 1978). We found out that both facilitation and inhibition occur predominantly in the LVF under the conditions of our experiment. This suggests, among other things, that automatic activation of lexical semantics is stronger in the RH than in the LH. The results also indicate a "processing dissociation" indicative of direct access.

Thus, we now have convergent evidence that lexical decision is a direct-access task. Both commissurotomy patients and normal subjects exhibit a mild RVFA and both groups show evidence for bilateral processing competence.

Concerning semantic facilitation, it is interesting to note that the normal RH shows facilitation, whereas the disconnected RH does not. This could reflect a simple population difference in RH language ability, but it more likely reflects a greater RH contribution to lexical semantic access in the normal RH than in the disconnected RH. It is as if the normal LH facilitates normal RH processing of linguistic processing though cross-callosal interaction. If this is so, the disconnected RH *underrepresents* the linguistic competence of the normal RH.

OTHER HEMIFIELD TACHISTOSCOPIC
EVIDENCE FOR LEXICAL ANALYSIS
IN THE NORMAL BRAIN

The word-superiority effect. One rarely quoted paper supporting the absence of pho-netic recoding in normal RH reading was drawn to my attention by Jerre Levy. In 1975, Krueger reported that better letter recognition in words than in nonwords (the word-superiority effect) was found in the RVF but not in the LVF of normal subjects, both for horizontal and vertical strings. On the interpretation (disputed by some) that the word-superiority effect is due to the information provided by a phonological code (cf. Johnstone 1981), this direct-access task (by processing dissociation) suggests an absence of phonological recoding during RH reading and, in turn, an absence of grapheme–phoneme conversion there.

The nonword pseudohomophone effect. In a lexical decision, task words are generally recognized faster than nonwords, and nonwords that are homophones of real words are recognized slowest, presumably because the valid phonological code is evoked automatically and conflicts with the invalid orthography. Cohen and Freeman (1978) found that such phonologically induced inhibition occurs in the RVF but not in the LVF of normal subjects. This direct-access task again supports the conclusion reached for the disconnected RH that RH reading does not involve intermediate phonological representation, i.e., that RH reading is "ideographic." Cohen and Freeman's results were not replicated by Barry (1981) and more data are needed to resolve this issue.

The concreteness effect. We have been able to demonstrate that the disconnected RH comprehends abstract spoken target words such as "justice" or "grief" when the multiple-choice pictures are concrete instantiations of the targets. In a post hoc analysis of the effect of concreteness on hemispheric differences in comprehension, I found only an overwhelming bilateral word-frequency effect (Zaidel 1976). We did not attempt to analyze the effect of word concreteness as a function of other lexical dimensions such as frequency or imageability, especially in reading. The stimuli in Radant's lexical decision task, which shows bilateral competence, were all chosen to be relatively high in concreteness, imageability, and frequency.

Numerous hemifield tachistoscopic experiments with normal subjects claim to have demonstrated selective RH comprehension of concrete nouns. Such a result would constitute strong evidence for direct access in lexical analysis. Unfortunately, none of these studies applied procedures for deciding whether the task is indeed of direct access or callosal relay. Patterson and Besner (1984) review 16 hemifield tachistoscopic studies of the concreteness effect and argue that the bulk of evidence does not support the hypothesis of selective RH reading of concrete words. But their arguments are not altogether compelling (Zaidel and Schweiger 1984). Many of the cited studies involve naming, which makes it harder to obtain the direct-access effect since the obligatory speech component is presumably always mediated by the LH. Others involve lexical decision whose relationship to semantic access during reading remains obscure since it seems to involve a metalinguistic analysis and, apparently, some postlexical-access components (Koriat 1981). Day (1979) used a lexical decision task and still found a concreteness effect. More importantly, Day (1977) has evidence for direct access in a semantic categorization task, but he does not report separately the effects of concreteness on VF. In sum, we believe that the hypothesis of RH predilection for reading concrete words remains viable.[‡]

Resolution: A second look at right-hemisphere reading in aphasics

It would seem that accounts of RH reading in disconnected and normal brains are in agreement. But the conflict with aphasic data persists. Why do aphasics with lesions restricted exclusively to the LH not show residual reading (let alone auditory comprehension) compatible with at least the reading competence of the dis-

connected RH? Some observers take the aphasiological data as primary and uncomplicated and dismiss the paradox of "ideographic" reading in the disconnected RH as an aberration, an abnormal state to be explained away (cf. Whitaker and Ojemann 1977). Instead, we take the position that disconnection and aphasiological data are equally primary and that neither is simple.

There are several possible explanations of the conflict. First, it may be that as a recent evolutionary development, RH reading is labile and subject to large interindividual differences. Then those uncommon aphasics with pure word blindness due to a localized LH lesion would reflect individuals at one extreme end of the continuum with no RH reading. It is also the case that the syndrome of pure word blindness is usually diagnosed by gross clinical criteria, which do not always allow for nonspeech responses, such as pointing to multiple-choice pictures. But F. Michel has data (personal communication) suggesting that patients suffering from alexia without agraphia, who fail to read words aloud, also fail to show reading comprehension by pointing to multiple-choice pictures (cf. also Patterson and Kay 1982).

Some suggest that RH reading is only released under certain circumstances, depending on the etiology, size, location, and nature of the aphasiogenic lesion in the LH (e.g., Lansdell 1969, Milner 1974). For example, a common argument is that only massive lesions in the LH, encompassing much of the "speech area," will transfer control over language processing to the RH (Milner 1974). Implicit in this view is some form of the "pathological inhibition" argument, according to which latent RH reading is masked by LH control and inhibition. The pathological inhibition argument has been criticized recently by Patterson and Besner (1984) as being merely a description rather than an explanation. We disagree (Zaidel and Schweiger 1984, Bogen 1974). Their dismissal of the concept of LH inhibition of RH language competence is premature. The following arguments may be offered in support of the inhibition hypothesis.

Just as normal interhemispheric interaction may be controlled by a central integrating

---

[‡]Since the writing of this chapter, we have amassed overwhelming evidence for independent lexical analysis in the two normal hemispheres. We have demonstrated independent right-hemisphere contribution to semantic, orthographic, morphologic, even phonological and grammatical variables. We also found independent lexical congruity effects in the two normal hemispheres, including automatic facilitory and inhibitory semantic and orthographic "strooplike" effects, and congruity effects in symbolic comparative judgment tasks, in addition to the associative priming results mentioned above (Zaidel et al. 1988).

mechanism, perhaps involving the brainstem, so the RH contribution to normal language processing would be regulated by some linguistic control mechanism. When language functions are lost following a LH lesion, higher-order monitoring, evaluating, or metalinguistic control functions may also be impaired to a larger or smaller extent. When the linguistic monitoring functions are not impaired, the RH may contribute specific processing components missing from the LH, or it may be available to help the LH when the latter is incompetent, overloaded, or fatigued. We believe this is the case in deep dyslexia (Zaidel and Schweiger 1984; see the section after next). When the monitoring function is impaired, it may lead to distorted, overoptimistic estimates of LH competence and failure to relinquish control to the RH. Alternatively, the mechanism that regulates the RH contribution to language processing in the LH may itself be impaired, especially if it is "localized" in the LH, leading to an apparent pathological cross-callosal inhibition. We believe that this is partly what happens in alexia without agraphia (pure alexia) (Zaidel and Schweiger 1984).

ALEXIA WITHOUT AGRAPHIA

Recently, Landis, Regard, and Serrat (1980) studied the existence of a range of task parameters that yields inhibition and a range that, in turn, releases RH reading. They showed that a patient with alexia without agraphia caused by a tumor could not read words at speeds that allowed him to name some individual letters, but could correctly point to objects in response to brief tachistoscopic words at higher speeds that did not allow him to name individual letters and led him to deny that he had seen anything. Moreover, he subsequently lost this reading-by-pointing ability when he improved enough to be able to name more individual letters of the flashed object names. Although inferences from tumor cases are often problematic, the implication here is that as long as the task parameters are within the reduced "competence" of the LH, control is still assigned to the LH. Only when the task parameters exclude *all* LH competence, does RH reading become functional. This is likely to occur when the residual LH reading strategy is incompatible with RH strategy (as in letter-by-letter reading) and when, in addition, the LH strategy cannot cope with a given stimulus. Thus, it should be possible in principle to demonstrate RH reading in pure alexia as long as we can manipulate the task parameters (such as presentation time) out of the range of LH competence while remaining within the range of RH competence.

A CASE OF DEEP DYSLEXIA

In April 1982, Avraham Schweiger, then an NIMH postdoctoral fellow in my lab, first saw RW, a 38-year-old woman with aphasia due to presumed occlusion of the left middle cerebral artery following an automobile accident eight months prior to testing. At that time, RW had residual hemiparesis and no visual-field defects. Her expressive speech was minimal, consisting largely of concrete nouns. Her comprehension was moderately good. She had a Western Aphasia Battery aphasia quotient of 31.1, consistent with the symptoms of Broca's aphasia. On the Token Test, she had a pass–fail score of 19 correct out of 31 (61.3%) and a weighted score of 94 out of 117 (80%) (Schweiger et al. in press).

In reading aloud, RW made numerous semantic errors in all classes of words. A similar pattern occurred in writing to dictation. She also made predominantly semantic errors in reading comprehension by pointing to multiple-choice pictures (Figure 18.2). Reading of function words was almost impossible for her, whereas verbs and abstract nouns were somewhat easier, and concrete nouns the easiest. RW could not match either meaningful or nonsense words for rhyming (Figure 18.4), even though she could frequently match pictures for identity of names (the Homonym Test, Zaidel and Peters 1981). RW was diagnosed as deep dyslexic and deep dysgraphic (cf. Marshall and Newcombe 1973).

The syndrome of acquired deep dyslexia (Coltheart, Patterson, and Marshall 1980) recognizes several "obligatory" and "optional" symptoms in reading. The necessary features are semantic errors in reading aloud, better reading of concrete nouns than of abstract function words, and no grapheme–phoneme conversion. (Some believe that the concreteness and part-of-speech effects are independent.) Some patients also have semantic errors in "reading comprehension" assessed by pointing to multiple-choice pictures, one of which is semantically related to the targets. Since the same three symptoms occur in RH reading by commissurotomy patients, it is natural to hypothesize that the RH of the deep dyslexic is used for lexical semantic access during reading (Coltheart 1980). Does a systematic comparison between the reading profile of RW and those of the disconnected RH hemispheres justify this "right-hemisphere hypothesis"?

Figures 18.3 and 18.4 show that the disconnected RHs of patients LB and NG, discussed previously, and RW all satisfy two of the three symptoms of deep dyslexia. But the reading competence of RW far exceeds that of the disconnected RHs. Thus, in order to survive, the right-hemisphere hypothesis must be weakened. In the weaker version, the RH of a deep dyslexia is said to be used for lexical/semantic access only when the (impaired) reading mechanism of the damaged LH cannot cope with the stimulus, or when it is slower than the "ideographic reader" in the RH. Even when the RH is used for lexical/semantic access, the phonological and articulatory mechanism of the LH are still necessary to name the word aloud. Thus, in this view, all of speaking and most of reading in deep dyslexics, particularly for longer phrases and sentences, are still subserved by the damaged LH.

But do we have any direct evidence that lexical access in the RH of a deep dyslexic is superior to lexical access in the LH and thus that it can provide an alternative mechanism when LH competence is poor? Just such data come from the lexical decision and semantic facilitation task of Radant. This task was administered in the usual manner to RW, who has intact fields. She responded with the nonhemiplegic left hand. In order to exclude the possibility of more subtle agnosic deficits in the RVF, a control counting task was administered as well. The same targets were presented as before, but in this task, RW was required to press the button if the target string was more than four letters long, whether a word or not. The results showed that RW was equally accurate for lexical decision in both VFs (more than 80% correct), but that LVF latency was significantly lower and had a smaller standard deviation than the RVF. By contrast, there was excellent performance in the control test in both visual half-fields (99% correct) and there was no significant difference in latency. The same control test showed no visual-field advantage in normal subjects (Schweiger et al. in press).

Like commissurotomy patients, RW had evidence for facilitation of lexical decision by semantically related primes only in the LH. Thus, RW shows evidence for direct access in lexical decision together with a strong RH superiority, which is not due to a general perceptual deficit in the RVF. This pattern is consistent with occasional reliance on the RH for lexical semantic access during reading aloud, as required by the weak version of the right-hemisphere hypothesis.

We saw that when RW made lexical decisions of targets that were flashed for 150 ms, she showed evidence of direct access and of RH superiority. We reasoned further that as a linguistic task becomes increasingly difficult, it should recruit progressively greater RH participation and control. Six months after the lexical decision task, the same targets were presented for 90 ms, this time to be read aloud, in an attempt to maximize the number of reading errors. Of a total of 51 correct readings aloud, 28 (55%) occurred in the RVF (LH). By sharp contrast, of a total of 22 blatant semantic errors, 16 (73%) occurred in the LVF (RH)! Both derivational errors (8) and visual errors (19) were predominantly in the RVF (5 and 11, respectively). The double dissociation between correct reading aloud and semantic errors as a function of VF of target is statistically significant ($\chi^2 = 4.4$, $p < 0.05$) and it supports the hypothesis of RH takeover of lexical access when LH access fails. Assuming direct access, it would seem that control is released to the RH on a trial-by-trial basis. However, such release may only be possible when LH competence is challenged.

Conclusion: A happy ending?

A systematic comparison of reading in aphasics, the disconnected RHs, and the normal RHs now converges on the view that the RH is competent for "ideographic" lexical/semantic access, that it can be used as a backup system in aphasia, and that, for some reading-related processes, it is actually superior to the LH in the normal brain. We interpret the apparent conflict between reading competence in the disconnected RHs and that in some aphasics as reflecting variability, limitation, and deficiency in the assignment of control to the intact RH when the language mechanism in the LH is impaired. Such control is more likely to be assigned in deep dyslexia than in pure alexia.

Thus, the theoretical importance of the reading profile of the disconnected RH is that it specifies limit conditions on RH interaction with the LH during reading, i.e., that it serves as a model for interhemispheric interactions. Limited data on RH reading can be misleading. Reading in the disconnected RH does not provide an accurate estimate of the reading competence in the normal RH. The deep dyslexia demonstrates an aphasic syndrome with reading competence superior to the disconnected RH; the pure alexic demonstrates a syndrome with reading competence inferior to the disconnected RH; and the normal RH seems superior in reading to the disconnected RH. Each approach to brain functions is tentative and methodologically insecure; each source of information gives only a partial view of the system. Only convergent evidence from these different cases can give us a coherent picture of language organization in the brain.

Epilogue

As scientists, we often ask ourselves when is an unexpected observation an aberration, an error to be attributed to random noise and ignored, and when is it a clue to a new insight? When one is in the throes of day-to-day science without the benefit of hindsight, the answer is not always clear. Few scientists feel secure facing such ambiguity in data and even fewer are gifted enough to resolve it. Sperry searched out paradoxes. In two separate and notable cases, one focusing on neural plasticity, the other on hemispheric specialization, he re-

solved apparent paradoxes with critical experiments. He is a master in designing dramatic experiments unencumbered by special cases and a complex theoretical machinery. Once the basic distinctions are made and time comes for mopping up and elaboration, he advised us, it is time to move on to new problems.

The question of RH language has not yet reached that stage; its solution can still be conceptualized in simple terms. If we are correct that RH language is unique and available both to the aphasic and normal brain, then converging evidence will soon amass in support of this view. A dramatic demonstration of this view in the Sperry mold would consist in experimentally improving an aphasic's language through release of RH competence. Then it will be time to move on to the next big question: How does interhemispheric integration occur? Even better, the next step would be to check this out with Sperry. He does seem to know the royal road to the scientific unconscious.

Acknowledgments

Thanks to Joseph Bogen, Colwyn Trevarthen, and Dahlia Zaidel for comments on the manuscript. This work was supported by NIH grant NS 20187 and by an NIMH RSDA MH 00179.

References

Akelaitis, A. J. 1944. A study of gnosis, praxis and language following section of the corpus collosum and anterior commissure. *J. Neurosurg.* 1: 94–102.

Albert, M. L. 1979. Alexia. *In* K. M. Heilman and E. Valenstein (eds.) *Clinical Neuropsychology.* Oxford University Press, New York, pp. 59–91.

Barry, C. 1981. Hemispheric asymmetry in lexical access and phonological encoding. *Neuropsychol.* 19: 473–8.

Benson, D. F. 1979. *Aphasia, Alexia, and Agraphia.* Churchill Livingston, New York.

Bogen, J. E. 1974. Dysfunction from defacilitation. Letter to the Editor. *Arch. Neurol.* 32: 421–2.

Cohen, G., and R. Freeman. 1978. Individual differences in reading strategies in relation to cerebral asymmetry. *In* J. Requin (ed.) *Attention and Performance, VII.* Lawrence Erlbaum, Hillsdale (NJ), pp. 411–26.

Coltheart, M. 1980. Deep dyslexia: A right hemisphere hypothesis. *In* M. Coltheart, K. Patterson, and J. Marshall (eds.) *Deep Dyslexia.* Routledge and Kegan Paul, London, pp. 326–80.

Coltheart, M., K. Patterson, and J. C. Marshall (eds.). 1980. *Deep Dyslexia.* Routledge and Kegan Paul. London.

Day, J. 1977. Right hemisphere language processing in normal right handers. *J. Exp. Psychol.: Human Percep. Perf.* 3: 518–28.

–1979. Visual half-field word recognition as a function of syntactic class and imageability. *Neuropsychol.* 17: 515–19.

Déjerine, J. 1891. Sur un cas de cécité verbale avec agraphie, suivi d'autopsie, *Mém. Soc. Biol.* 3: 197–201.

–1892. Contribution a l'étude anatomo-pathologique et clinique des différentes variétés de cécité verbale. *Compt. Rend. Soc. Biol.* 44: 61–90.

Filbey, R. A., and M. S. Gazzaniga. 1969. Splitting the normal brain with reaction time. *Psychon. Sci.* 17: 335–6.

Foldi, N. S., M. Cicone, and H. Gardner. 1983. Pragmatic aspects of communication in brain-damaged patients. *In* S. J. Segalowitz (ed.) *Language Functions and Brain Organization.* Academic Press, New York, pp. 51–86.

Franz, S. I. 1933. The inadequacy of the concept of unilateral cerebral dominance in learning. *J. Exp. Psychol.* 16: 73–5.

Franz, S. I., and S. Kilduff. 1933. Cerebral dominance as shown by segmental visual learning. *Stud. Cereb. Func., II.* 1: 79–90.

Gardner, H., and H. Brownell. 1986. *Right Hemisphere Communication Battery.* Psychology Service, VAMC, Boston.

Gazzaniga, M. S. 1983. Right hemisphere language following brain bisection: A 20-year perspective. *Am. Psychol.* 38: 525–37

Gazzaniga, M. S., and R. W. Sperry 1967. Language after section of the verbal commissures. *Brain* 90: 131–48.

Geschwind, N. 1965. Disconnexion syndromes in animals and man. *Brain* 88: 237–94, 585–644.

Johnstone, J. C. 1981. Effects of advance precuing of alternatives on the perception of letters alone and in words. *J. Exp. Psychol.: Human Percep. Perf.* 7: 560–72.

Kertesz, A. 1979. *Aphasia and Associated Disorders: Taxonomy, Localization and Recovery.* Grune and Stratton, New York.

Koriat, A. 1981. Semantic facilitation in lexical decision as a function of prime-target association. *Mem. Cog.* 9: 587–98.

Krueger, L. E. 1975. The word-superiority effect: Is its locus visual spatial or verbal? *Bull. Psychonom. Soc.* 6: 465–8.

Landis, T., M. Regard, and A. Serrat. 1980. Iconic reading in a case of alexia without agraphia caused by a brain tumour: A tachistoscopic study. *Brain and Lang.* 11: 45–53.

Lansdell, H. 1969. Verbal and nonverbal factors in right hemisphere speech. *J. Comp. Physiol. Psychol.* 69: 734–8.

Levy, J., R. Nebes, and R. W. Sperry. 1971. Expressive language in the surgically separated minor hemisphere. *Cortex* 7: 49–58.

Marshall, J. C., and F. Newcombe. 1973. Patterns of paralexia: A psycholinguistic approach. *J. Psycholing. Res.* 2: 175–99.

Meyers, P. S. 1984. Right hemisphere impairment. *In* A. Holland (ed.) *Language Disorders in Adults.* College Hill, San Diego, pp. 315–20.

Milner, B. 1974. Hemispheric specialization: Scope and limits. *In* F. O. Schmitt and F. G. Worden (eds.) *The Neurosciences: Third Study Program.* The MIT Press, Cambridge, pp. 698–717.

Mishkin, M., and D. G. Forgays. 1952. Word recognition as a function of retinal locus. *J. Exp. Psychol.* 43: 43–8.

Myers, J. J. 1984. Right hemisphere language: Science or fiction? *Am. Psychol.* 39: 315–20.

Patterson, K., and D. Besner. 1984. Is the right hemisphere literate? *Cog. Neuropsychol.* 1: 315–41.

Patterson, K., and J. Kay. 1982. Letter-by-letter reading: Psychological descriptions of a neurological syndrome. *Quart. J. Exp. Psychol.* 34A: 411–41.

Posner, M. I. 1978. *Chronometric Explorations of Mind.* Lawrence Erlbaum, Hillsdale (NJ).

Radant, A. 1981. *Facilitation in a Lexical Decision Task: Effects of Visual Field, Sex, Handedness and Anxiety.* Honors undergraduate thesis, Department of Psychology, UCLA.

Ross, E. D. 1981. The aprosodias. *Arch. Neurol.* 38: 561–9.

Schuell, H. 1965. *The Minnesota Test for Differential Diagnosis of Aphasia.* University of Minnesota Press, Minneapolis.

Schweiger, A., E. Zaidel, T. Field, and B. Dobkin. In press. Right hemisphere contribution to lexical access in an aphasic with deep dyslexia. *Brain and Lang.*

Sperry, R. W., and M. S. Gazzaniga. 1967. Language following surgical disconnection of the hemispheres. *In* F. L. Darley (ed.) *Brain Mechanisms Underlying Speech and Language.* Grune and Stratton, New York, pp. 108–21.

Sperry, R. W., M. S. Gazzaniga, and J. E. Bogen. 1969. Interhemispheric relationships: The neocortical commissures; syndromes of hemispheric disconnection. *In* P. J. Vinken and G. Bruyn (eds.) *Handbook of Clinical Neurology,* Vol. 4. North-Holland, Amsterdam, pp. 273–90.

Spielberger, C. D., R. L. Gorsuch, and R. E. Lushene. 1970. *State Trait Anxiety Inventory Manual.* Consulting Psychologists Press, Palo Alto (CA).

Sullivan, M. V., and C. R. Hamilton. 1973. Memory establishment via the anterior commissure of monkeys. *Physiol. Behav.* 11: 873–9.

Whitaker, H. A., and G. A. Ojemann. 1977. Lateralization of higher cortical functions. A critique. *In* S. J. Dimond and D. A. Blizard (eds.) *Evolution and Lateralization of the Brain.* New York Academy of Sciences, New York, pp. 459–73.

Zaidel, E. 1976. Auditory vocabulary of the right hemisphere following brain bisection or hemidecortication. *Cortex* 12: 191–211.

–1978. Lexical organization in the right hemisphere. *In* P. A. Buser and A. Rougeul-Buser (eds.) *Cerebral Correlates of Conscious Experience*. Elsevier, Amsterdam, pp. 177–97.

–1979a. The split and half brain as models of congenital language disability. *In* C. L. Ludlow and M. E. Doran-Quine (eds.) *The Neurological Bases of Language Disorders in Children: Methods and Directions for Research*. National Institute for Neurological and Communicative Diseases and Stroke, Monograph 22. U.S. Government Printing Office, Washington, D.C., pp. 55–89.

–1979b. Performance on the ITPA following cerebral commissurotomy and hemispherectomy. *Neuropsychol.* 17: 259–80.

–1982. Reading in the disconnected right hemisphere: An aphasiological perspective. *In* Y. Zotterman (ed.) *Dyslexia: Neuronal, Cognitive and Linguistic Aspects*. Wenner-Gren Symposium Series, Vol. 35. Pergamon, Oxford, pp. 67–91.

–1983a. On multiple representations of the lexicon in the brain: The case of the two hemispheres, *In* M. Studdert-Kennedy (ed.) *Psychobiology of Language*. The MIT Press, Cambridge, pp. 105–125.

–1983b. Disconnection syndrome as a model for laterality effects in the normal brain. *In* J. Hellige (ed.) *Cerebral Hemisphere Asymmetry: Method, Theory and Application*. Praeger, New York, pp. 95–151.

–1983c. A response to Gazzaniga: Language in the right hemisphere, convergent perspectives. *Am. Psychol.* 38: 542–6.

–1985. Language in the right hemisphere. *In* D. F. Benson and E. Zaidel (eds.) *The Dual Brain*. Guildford, New York, pp. 205–31.

Zaidel, E. In press. Hemispheric independence and interaction in word recognition. *In* C. von Euler, I. Lundberg, and G. Lennerstrand (eds.) *Brain and Reading*. Hampshire, Macmillan.

Zaidel, E., J. Clarke, and B. Suyenobu. In press. Hemispheric independence: A paradigm case for cognitive neuroscience. *In* A. Scheibel and A. Wechsler (eds.) *Neurobiological Foundations of Higher Cognitive Function*. Guilford Press, New York.

Zaidel, E., and A. M. Peters. 1981. Phonological encoding and ideographic reading by the disconnected right hemisphere: Two case studies. *Brain and Lang.* 14: 205–34.

Zaidel, E., and A. Schweiger. 1984. On wrong hypotheses about the right hemisphere: Commentary on K. Patterson and D. Besner. Is the right hemisphere literate? *Cog. Neuropsychol.* 1: 351–64.

Zaidel, E., H. White, E. Sakurai, and W. Banks. 1988. Hemispheric locus of lexical congruity effects: Neuropsychological reinterpretation of psycholinguistic results. *In* C. Chiarello (ed.) *Right Hemisphere Contributions to Lexical Semantics*. Springer, New York, pp. 71–88.

19 The role of the right cerebral hemisphere in evaluating configurations

**Larry I. Benowitz, Seth Finkelstein
David N. Levine** and **Kenneth Moya**
Departments of Psychiatry and Neurology
Harvard Medical School; McLean Hospital;
Massachusetts General Hospital; and
Spaulding Rehabilitation Hospital

Introduction

Following the classical discoveries of the nineteenth century that verbal language was controlled in specialized systems of the left cerebral hemisphere in most people, the general view developed that the left hemisphere was responsible for all higher psychological processes. The right side was called the "minor" or "nondominant" hemisphere, and was thought to contribute little beyond sensory and motor processes. This idea persisted despite Hughlings Jackson's suggestion (Jackson 1932) that the right hemisphere played a special role in perceptual functions, and in spite of a number of observations from the 1930s on of deficits that were associated primarily with right-hemisphere damage (Brain 1941; Patterson and Zangwill 1944; Hécaen, de Ajuriaguerra, and Massonnet 1951; McFie, Piercy, and Zangwill 1960; Hécaen 1962).

The late 1960s and early 1970s witnessed a turnaround in how human brain organization was conceptualized. The view of the left hemisphere as the seat of the intellect and of consciousness was replaced as it became apparent that both sides of the human brain were specialized and superior in some functions, that the specializations of each side were complementary to those on the other side, and that normal brain function depends on an integration between the right and left hemispheres. This perspective, which is so central to current neuropsychological thinking, was, in large part, a consequence of the studies of Roger Sperry (1974) on hemispheric function in split-brain

patients. Sperry, with his students and his colleagues, showed that the right hemisphere, as well as the left, was a thinking, feeling, perceiving, and conscious organ, and that in some domains, its capacities were superior to those of the left side of the brain.

Studies of both brain-damaged patients and of normal individuals have been in full agreement with the split-brain investigations in showing that the left hemisphere's superiority for language is complemented by a superiority of the right hemisphere for visuospatial processes. Moreover, a number of recent studies of selected neurological patients, in whom chronic changes in personality and cognition can be studied with relatively few methodological restrictions, indicate that the specializations of the right hemisphere extend well beyond its involvement in visuospatial tasks. Through these studies, it is becoming increasingly apparent that damage to the right hemisphere affects such fundamental aspects of behavior as social communication, the ability to evaluate the significance of one's experiences, and even certain higher-order aspects of language.

A patient recently seen at the Massachusetts Rehabilitation Hospital offers a fairly typical illustration of right brain damage. JW, a 64-year-old man who suffered an embolic stroke in the territory of the anterior and middle cerebral arteries, was shown by CT radiography to have sustained a large right frontoparietal infarct. The patient had previously been in good health and had worked for many

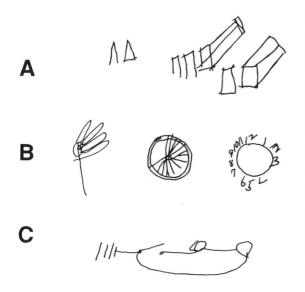

A

B

C

Figure 19.1. Drawings by patient JW two months after a right frontoparietal CVA. (**A**) Multiple attempts to copy a triangle and a cube. (**B**) A flower drawn from memory and attempts to fill in the spokes of a wheel and numbers on a clock face. Note the left-sided neglect in the flower and wheel. (**C**) Circuit diagram completed without including the voltage source; patient was certain it was correct when he reexamined it.

years as an electrician. When examined two months after the stroke, he was alert and oriented to time, place, and person. Language was intact, though speech was somewhat aprosodic and staccato. JW was cooperative about being tested, but at times, he seemed inappropriately familiar and even mildly insulting to his examiners. He was largely unaware of his extensive left-sided sensory and motor losses, and would occasionally attempt to stand up and walk. On one occasion, he described his main problem to be an inability to put on his socks, and only after lengthy questioning did he mention the weakness in his left shoulder. When pressed he would say that the "doctors told me I had a stroke," though he seemed to have little direct awareness of the change in his state. Nevertheless, he was undisturbed about remaining in the hospital for another two months, occasionally offering vague alternative explanations for being there.

Constructional apraxia and left-sided neglect were apparent in his drawings (Figure 19.1). A triangle was drawn without a base, the first two attempts at drawing a cube were incomplete squares, only the petals on the right side of a flower were drawn, and only the spokes on the right side of a bicycle wheel; the numbers of a clock face were filled in fairly well. In the patient's area of expertise, he drew a circuit diagram with a power source, a switch, and two bulbs in series, then completed it by connecting the bulbs to the switch. When questioned whether the lights could work without the power on the left side of his diagram, he redrew the wire, but was undisturbed about his error. Photographs of well-known political figures and actors were all recognized, but on the Profile of Nonverbal Sensitivity (PONS) test, which is to be described, he scored poorly in identifying facial expressions.

The disorganization seen in this patient's drawings was paralleled in the way he recounted his experiences. On one occasion, he told us that the week before he had felt cold at night and had phoned his wife to bring in a blanket. When we reacted with surprise that he did not just ring for a nurse, he casually changed his story and said that he did, and, actually, the heat had been off for the entire week and that everyone else in the hospital was in the same boat. He said that he took all this calmly because he used to work for the housing authority and knew that it often took a week or more for new equipment to come in. In attempting to verify this story, we discovered that the heat had never gone off (the week before had been the coldest of the winter), and that the patient had been estranged from his wife for years.

This patient illustrates a number of the well-known characteristics of right-brain damage, including constructional apraxia (Piercy, Hécaen, and de Ajuriaguerra 1960), left-sided neglect, and unconcern (Denny-Brown, Meyer, and Horenstein 1952), along with a number of other behavioral changes that will be the topics of the following sections.

Nonverbal communication in patients with right-hemisphere lesions

The occasional lapses in social appropriateness and the emotionless manner of speaking noted in patient JW are not uncommon after right brain damage (Gardner 1975;

Tucker, Watson, and Heilman 1977; Ross and Rush 1981). To examine whether such changes might also be associated with an imperception of social cues from the expressive behaviors of other people (Izard 1971; Buck et al. 1972; Ekman, Friesen, and Ellsworth 1972), we have been giving unilaterally brain-damaged patients the Profile of Nonverbal Sensitivity (PONS), a scale that assesses competence in decoding emotional content in communication through facial expressions, body gestures, and vocal intonation (Rosenthal et al. 1979a and 1979b). The PONS has been validated as a reliable measure of social sensitivity, and has been given to thousands of people of various ages, cultures, and educational backgrounds, providing extensive normative data against which the performance of neurological subjects could be compared. The full test is a film consisting of 220 two-second video and/or audio segments. These present the face, body, or vocal intonation pattern of an actress portraying emotional situations. Subjects choose between two alternative descriptions of the scene that are read to them.

In our first study (Benowitz 1980; Benowitz et al. 1983), right brain-damaged subjects were found to average nearly two standard deviations below normal on the PONS test. Two of these subjects had verbal IQs, measured after their strokes, of 135 and 148, yet both scored more than three standard deviations below normal on the PONS test. Such findings emphasize the dissociation between verbal ability, on the one hand, and sensitivity to nonverbal cues on the other. A comparison group of mild-to-moderately aphasic left brain-damaged subjects scored significantly better, averaging within one-half standard deviation of normal on their overall test performance.

Facial emotions generally provide highly salient information in nonverbal communication (Izard 1971; Buck et al. 1972; Ekman et al. 1972), and it was in this area that right brain-damaged subjects showed the greatest deficit. All but one patient in this group scored in the fourth percentile or lower in recognizing emotions from a film of facial expressions; the left brain-damaged patients who were tested all performed normally. Surprisingly, most of the right brain-damaged patients who were unable

to judge facial expressions were well within the normal range in evaluating gestures of hands and body ($+0.8$ standard deviations of the normal mean score).

An additional group of unilaterally brain-damaged patients, not previously reported, included five patients who had suffered infarcts of the right temporoparietal cortex within three months of testing (all verified by CT scan; average age of 65; two female; all right-handed); all five of these subjects scored in the fifth percentile or lower in judging facial emotions. Yet, only one of these patients had difficulty in recognizing familiar faces of actors and political figures. Five other patients, similar in age and right-handed, but with other types of right-hemisphere damage (two frontoparietal, two deep frontal plus capsular damage, and one with a recent central plus an old temporoparietal infarct), averaged somewhat better in judging emotions from facial expressions (tenth percentile) and were normal in evaluating the PONS body gestures (average forty-second percentile) and in recognizing familiar faces.

Figure 19.2 summarizes the performance of all of the unilaterally brain-damaged subjects to whom we have given the PONS test. Right brain-damaged subjects whose lesions included the temporal cortex (N = 11) averaged 2.3 standard deviations (SD) below normal in judging emotions from facial expressions (i.e., in the bottom first percentile), but only 1.1 SD below normal in judging body gestures; these subjects were not impaired, on the average, in evaluating intonational qualities of the voice. Subjects with right-sided lesions that spared the temporal cortex (N = 6) did better in judging facial emotions, but showed a relative impairment in evaluating tonal qualities of the voice. The left brain-damaged subjects shown in Figure 19.2 were unimpaired on all channels of the PONS test.

Using the "split-retina" lens system developed by Zaidel (1977), we also had the opportunity, at Caltech, to present video portions of the PONS test to each cerebral hemisphere separately in commissurotomy patients who had all neocortical commissures divided. Signaling with the fingers of the contralateral hand to indicate the choices of each hemisphere, one "split-brain" subject (LB) scored normally (fif-

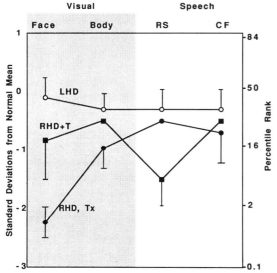

Figure 19.2. Summary of patients tested on the Profile of Nonverbal Sensitivity (Rosenthal et al. 1979a, 1979b). Scores on different channels of nonverbal communication are given in terms of percentile ranking and standard deviations from the mean of the normal population. Video channels include facial expressions and body gestures. Audio channels include random splices (RS) and content-filtered (CF) speech. LHD = left-hemisphere-damaged subjects (N = 6); RHD + T = right-hemisphere-damaged subjects with the temporal lobe intact (N = 6); RHD − Tx = right-hemisphere-damaged subjects with the temporal lobe damaged (N = 11).

tieth percentile) in identifying facial expressions viewed by his right hemisphere, but at a near-chance level when choosing items seen by the left (language) hemisphere. Three other split-brain subjects (RY, NG, AA), also tested in Sperry's lab at Caltech, scored in the fourth percentile or lower when verbally identifying emotions from faces viewed freely, presumably reflecting the inability of the left hemisphere in this domain (Benowitz et al. 1983).

Several other studies have described similar deficits in evaluating emotions from photographs of faces after right, but not left, hemisphere lesions (Cicone, Wapner, and Gardner 1980; DeKosky et al. 1980; Kolb and Taylor 1981). In two of these studies (Cicone et al. 1980; DeKosky et al. 1980), deficits in judging facial expressions were found to be dissociable from the ability to identify individual faces, as we have also observed. Moreover, in normal subjects, localized stimulation of the

right posterior middle temporal gyrus arrests identification of emotions expressed on the face without impairing the ability to distinguish individual faces (Ojemann et al. 1980). Evidence for right-hemispheric superiority in evaluating facial expressions also comes from studies in normal subjects, using either chimeric "split-emotion" faces (Campbell 1978, Heller and Levy 1981) or whole faces expressing emotion presented tachistoscopically to each hemifield (Suberi and McKeever 1977, Ley and Bryden 1979). In all of these, a left visual hemifield, and thus a right-hemisphere, superiority for recognition of facial expressions has been found. These latter studies also suggest a greater right-hemisphere involvement in evaluating emotions as compared to recognizing individual faces.

Other studies indicate that the right hemisphere may dominate not only in recognition of emotion, but also in emotional expression by facial movements. In right-handers, both positive (Heller and Levy 1981) and negative (Sackeim, Gur, and Saucy 1978) emotions appear to be expressed more intensely on the left side of the face than the right (i.e., contralateral to the right hemisphere), both in spontaneous and posed situations (Moskovitch and Olds 1981; Borod, Caron, and Koff 1981). Consistent evidence from unilaterally brain-damaged patients indicates that facial expressions in response to emotive stimuli are diminished after right-, but not left-, hemisphere lesions (Buck and Duffy 1980).

A lesser involvement of the right hemisphere in judging body gestures as compared to facial expressions was regularly observed in our patients. Perhaps body gestures involve more sequences of discrete movements and fewer holistic or simultaneous configurations than facial expressions, and may therefore be more languagelike and hence left hemispheric. In conformance with this interpretation is the finding that both expression and perception of body movements are impaired after left-hemisphere lesions (Goodglass and Kaplan 1963, Gainotti and Lemmo 1976); however, another study also discusses diminution of gestures expressive of emotions in relation to right-hemisphere damage (Ross and Mesulam 1979).

Impairments in discriminating and encoding vocal intonations have been reported after right temporoparietal damage (Heilman, Scholes, and Watson 1974; Tucker et al. 1977). Whether these abilities are lateralized to the right hemisphere, however, is unclear since similar impairments have been reported after left-sided lesions as well (Schlanger, Schlanger, and Gerstman 1976). Dichotic listening studies in normal subjects have likewise given varying results on laterality for processing prosodic qualities of speech, showing a right-hemisphere superiority in cases where tonal and melodic qualities are separated from linguistic context (Carmon and Nachshon 1973; Blumstein and Cooper 1974; Bryden, Ley, and Sugarman 1982), but not when the two are integrated (Zurif 1972). In our studies, right-left differences in evaluating tonal qualities of the voice were generally not as striking as were the differences in judging facial expressions; however, several of the patients with right frontoparietal damage were impaired in evaluating tonal qualities of the voice, in agreement with the findings of Heilman and others (Heilman et al. 1974, Tucker et al. 1977).

Emotional behavior, emotional state, and self-evaluation

As recently discussed by Ross and Rush (1981), components of emotional behavior that might potentially be dissociated from one another in brain-damaged patients include the verbal-cognitive set (i.e., the words used to describe one's state), affect (facial expressions, body posture and prosody of speech), and "vegetative" behavior (appetite, sexual drive, sleep, motivational level); mood (inner state) is usually inferred from the other three. Damage to the right hemisphere, as described before, can alter the expression of affect, as well as its perception in other persons.

Patients such as the one described at the beginning of this chapter frequently show changes in their verbal-cognitive set, often being strikingly indifferent in the way they talk about their disabilities. In a classic description of this phenomenon, Denny-Brown, Meyer, and Horenstein (1952) described a woman who, after a right-hemisphere stroke, denied her left hemiparesis, was unconcerned over details about which she had previously been metic-

ulous, showed poor planning for the future, and did not comprehend the significance of her deficit. In a large group of unilaterally brain-damaged subjects, Gainotti (1972) found those with right-hemisphere lesions to have a higher incidence of fatuous joking, indifference toward family feelings and failures, anosognosia (denial of illness), and minimization of deficits. Those with left-sided lesions, in contrast, showed more swearing, anxiety, crying, and unwillingness to be evaluated. In agreement with this, Gasparrini et al. (1978) reported that left-brain damaged patients, independent of aphasia, showed evidence of depression on the Minnesota Multiphasic Personality Inventory, with a profile suggesting a major affective disorder; right brain-damaged patients, in general, did not show such responses. A series of studies by Robinson and co-workers suggests that the depression associated with left-sided lesions is independent of aphasia and other functional disabilities, being correlated instead with the proximity of the lesion to the left frontal pole (Robinson and Benson 1981).

Another dimension of emotional behavior that we have been studying after unilateral brain damage is neuroendocrine and vegetative functioning (Finkelstein et al. 1982). In addition to evaluating such conventional symptoms of depression as crying, psychomotor state, subjective mood, motivation, self-esteem, guilt, appetite, and sleep disorders, we also examined the response to a single-dose dexamethasone suppression test (DST), a measure of neuroendocrine dysfunction that has been related to "endogenous" depression (Carroll, Feinberg, and Greden 1981).

Patients with cortical strokes lateralized to the left (N = 13) or right (N = 12) hemisphere, along with a group of 13 controls matched for age, length of hospitalization, and other medical problems, were evaluated using criteria from the Hamilton Depression Scale and Research Diagnostic Criteria, and nurses' ratings were also obtained. Abnormally high serum-cortisol levels after dexamethasone were found in 52% of the stroke patients, as compared to 8% of controls. No difference was observed in the prevalence of abnormally high DST results after left or right hemisphere lesions. Moderate-to-severe disturbances of sleep and/or appetite were also equally common regardless of the side of lesion, occurring in 54% of left and 50% of right brain-damaged patients. The one dimension that differed between the groups, however, was their overt and verbalized signs of mood disturbance; whereas 69% of left brain-damaged patients were rated as being moderately-to-severely depressed, only 25% of the right brain-damaged group were dysphoric, and none severely so. These findings suggest that while cortical strokes in either hemisphere may lead to a disequilibrium in sleep, appetite, and neuroendocrine functions, mood in right brain-damaged subjects is not always consonant with these disorders; some of these patients are frankly indifferent to their state.

A similar dissociation of depressive symptoms has been noted by Ross and Rush (1981), who describe a young patient with a large infarction in the right superior temporoparietal region and a small left anterofrontal lesion. This patient showed a positive DST response, was irritable, uncooperative, unsociable, anorexic, insomniac, and abrasive toward her children. Nevertheless, she was emotionally unreactive to her left-sided motor and sensory losses and denied all signs of depression, including the dysphoria, anorexia, and insomnia. These authors have proposed that the right temporoparietal region may play a critical role in formulating the verbal-cognitive representation of emotion.

An even more basic involvement of this brain region in emotional behavior is suggested by the lowered arousal threshold seen in patients with right temporoparietal damage. These subjects have a low galvanic skin reaction, even to stimuli on the ipsilateral side of the body, an effect that is not seen after left-brain damage (Heilman, Schwartz, and Watson 1978). In tests of simple reaction time, right brain-damaged patients take much longer than left brain-damaged controls to press a button in response to an auditory or visual stimulus with their nonparetic hand (DeRenzi and Faglioni 1965). Howes and Boller (1975) have shown that such changes in reaction time are not a function of lesion size, but depend upon the inclusion of either the right temporoparietal cortex or basal ganglia in the lesion.

Experimental studies in normal subjects support the contention that the right hemisphere may be preferentially involved in evaluating the emotional qualities of stimuli, and may help to explain some of the spontaneous behavioral changes seen after right brain damage. Normal subjects have been reported to show an increased incidence of leftward orientation of gaze when presented with emotive, but not neutral, material (Schwartz, Davidson, and Maer 1975), a greater degree of cardiac acceleration when a negatively emotional film is partially lateralized to the right hemisphere using a split-retina contact-lens system (Dimond and Farrington 1977), and an increase in EEG desynchronization selectively over the right parietal cortex while viewing or imagining emotional scenes (Davidson et al. 1979). Differential responses over the frontal cortex dependent upon the polarity of stimuli have also been reported, with increased left-sided activation during positive, and increased right-sided activation during negative episodes (Davidson et al. 1979; Tucker, Stenslie, and Roth, 1981). The possibility that the left hemisphere may in fact dominate in generating positive emotions has been suggested by others (Perria, Rosadini, and Rossi 1961; Dimond and Farrington 1977; Sackeim et al. 1982), but most studies in the literature suggest a dominant role of the right hemisphere in reacting to emotive material regardless of the polarity of affect.

Thought and language

Returning once more to patient JW described at the beginning of this chapter, while syntax, phonology, and word usage were intact, evidence of a thought disorder was suggested both in his poor visuospatial constructions and in confusions in his verbal narrative. In the circuit diagram drawn by this patient, all of the appropriate elements were included, but the figure was completed without including the power source on the left, resulting in an illogical overall form. Such an error, usually considered a manifestation of constructional apraxia, might also be viewed as reflecting a disruption of mental schemata, in which the capacity to evaluate relational properties is impaired. In the verbal sphere, a similar description might apply to JW's story, in which he said he phoned his wife for a blanket when the hospital's heating system failed. Here, again, individual elements of the story seemed plausible enough, but the concatenation was a sheer confabulation.

Another man, seen two months after a massive right-hemisphere CVA, denied his hemiplegia and hemisensory losses, explaining that he had been chosen to participate in a joint Canadian–American rehabilitation project due to poor general health. A woman with a right-hemisphere infarct resulting from an intracerebral bleed was in pain from a toothache when we saw her. She maintained that we were the dentists she sent for even after we repeatedly told her who we were. She also related a story about slipping on ice to explain the brain surgery that she had undergone, although, in fact, this surgery had occurred in the spring, to evacuate a hematoma. Both patients displayed profound constructional apraxia.

Fisher (1982) has recently described a series of patients with lesions in the right parieto-occipital region who, in addition to left-sided neglect and constructional apraxia, were disoriented as to place. One patient acknowledged that he was in the Massachusetts General Hospital, but on different occasions claimed it was the "extension" in California, London, Paris, Baghdad, Tokyo, or elsewhere. As we have also found, such a patient seldom "said he did not know or was not sure. He had little insight into his errors. He failed to use clues from events and circumstances around him" (Fisher 1982). Hécaen (1962, p. 217, note 1) has also commented on the high prevalence (36%) of confusion and dementia in association with right-sided lesions.

We have begun to investigate whether the bizarre ways in which right brain-damaged patients often recount their experiences, on the one hand, and constructional apraxia, on the other, might be functionally related to one another, both possibly stemming from an underlying inability to mentally construct or evaluate relationships among individual elements in the context of an overall schema. To investigate this hypothesis, we developed a parallel set of tests for story comprehension and constructional abilities, with a scoring protocol that allowed us to evaluate representation of individual details, inference of relationships among elements, and appreciation of overall form in both the spatial and verbal domains; we also recorded instances of confabulation, errors of reference, and perseveration, along with left-sided neglect in the drawings.

Sample drawings and recollected stories for three right brain-damaged subjects are shown in Figure 19.3 and in Table 19.1. At first glance, the two domains explored in these studies would seem to require rather different abilities, each comprised of diverse and probably independent perceptual, motor, and cognitive elements. Nevertheless, parallels between story recall and the drawing ability are apparent in the samples in terms of accuracy in details, appreciation of the overall "form," and unwarranted intrusions.

In the 18 right brain-damaged subjects included in our study, the correlations between story comprehension deficits and constructional apraxia were striking (Moya, et al. 1986).

As noted by the underlining in Table 19.2, all aspects of story comprehension correlated with analogous visuospatial abilities. Accuracy in reproducing details in the figures (e.g., copying a Rey–Osterreith Diagram, or drawing a clock from memory), in maintaining proper relationships among elements, and the overall form of the figures were all found to be correlated with the ability to recall the details of a story and to answer questions about relationships among story elements. On the negative side, the appearance of intrusions in drawings correlated with intrusions in recounting stories, while perseverative errors in the two domains also covaried. Among all aspects of story comprehension, it was the ability to infer relationships among story elements, probably the most abstract level of performance examined, that showed the highest degree of covariation with visuospatial abilities. These findings lend support to the possibility of a common right-hemispheric mechanism underlying both visuospatial abilities and the ability to construct story schemata.

Impairments in story recall after right-hemisphere lesions (Wechsler 1973; Wapner, Hamby, and Gardner 1981) and commissurotomy (Zaidel and Sperry 1974) have also been described by others, and contrast with the pres-

	Copy Rey Diagram	Copy Cube	Draw Clock	Draw Flower

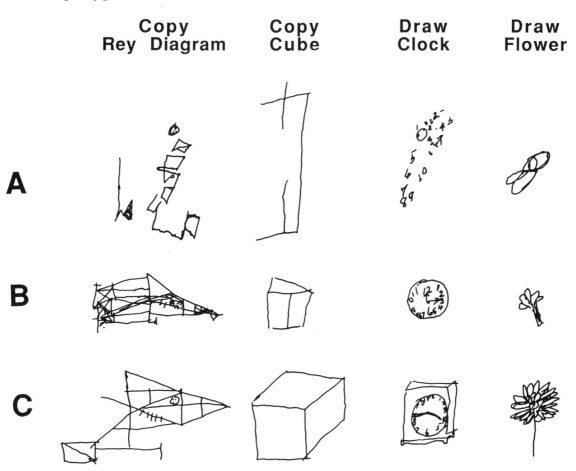

Figure 19.3. Drawings of three right-handed subjects, all of whom suffered strokes in the distribution of the right middle cerebral artery (temporoparietal + central regions). Subjects were asked to copy a Rey–Osterreith figure and a cube and to draw a clock and flower from memory. (Subject A: 74 years, male, 1½ months after stroke, former proofreader; B: 77 years, male, 1 month after stroke, former merchant; C: 50 years, female, 8 months after stroke, former secretary.) Sample stories recollected by these subjects are given in Table 19.1.

ervation of more basic verbal skills in these people (Weinstein 1962, Matarazzo 1979). In our study, we also found story-comprehension deficits to be unrelated to basic language skills, simple arithmetic ability, and forward digit span. Wechsler (1973) has reported that right brain-damaged subjects perform as poorly as aphasic left brain-damaged subjects on story recall, but unlike the latter group, they fail to show improvements in performance when the stories are made emotional. In split-brain patients, story recall and other verbal memory deficits are considerably greater than would be expected given the subjects' IQs, a finding that Zaidel and Sperry (1974) attribute to a contribution of the right hemisphere in the encoding of memory for even some language-based material (see Chapter 15, this volume).

Other language-related deficits described in right brain-damaged patients include impairments in solving simple verbal problems based upon antonymic adjectives (Caramazza et al. 1976), in judging the connotation of words (Gardner and Denes 1973), and in evaluating humorous material (Gardner et al. 1975, Brownell et al. 1983), metaphors (Winner and Gardner 1977), and emotional scenes (Cicone et al. 1980). Patients in these studies have been

Table 19.1. *Sample story recall of right brain-damaged subjects*[a]

	Story 2. At 6:00 P.M. last night, rush hour traffic leaving Boston through the Callahan Tunnel was backed up about two miles. The reason was that two of the automatic toll machines stopped working. Four employees rushed to the scene and in about a half hour the machines were working properly. However, it wasn't until 7:15 P.M. that traffic was flowing normally again. This had been the fifth traffic tie-up of the month.	Story 4. John drove out of town on a stormy day. Rain clouds obscured the city's skyline, which was on his left-hand side. The river, which was on his right, began rising and soon overflowed on to the road. In his sideview mirror John noticed a car skidding towards him. As he swerved to avoid it his heart leapt as he saw only a guard rail separating him from the river.
Patient		
A	The traffic tie up. The traffic leaving the city, it was, of course that wasn't in the story, but I did hear that the traffic tie-up was due to ice on the side, in the road way. The time of the tie-up was fifteen minutes or something like that.	(It was) about John leaving in his car. He saw a road on his left and he turned and he skidded, missing a car, I think the other car was coming up on his right, or it was on the same road.
B	Traffic leaving Boston at 4:00 P.M. was kind of tied up, 'cause two of the machines at the toll booths weren't working properly. I think it was four men came to repair the machines, and they got them working properly. And traffic resumed its normal pace. And there was a tie up before that – traffic, because of the failure of the machines at the booths, the toll booths.	John (was) in his car, heading north, the skyline was obscured. His car swerved, and then there (was) nothing between him and the car but the guard rail. And the river was rising.
C	During the rush hour at 7 P.M. traffic through the Callahan tunnel out of Boston was backed up about two miles. The reason was that two of the automatic toll booths were jammed so people couldn't get through. Two employees came to check it out and fix it. But it took quite a while as it was about 7:15 before traffic was flowing normally.	John left the city during a heavy storm. To his left the city was obscured by clouds. To his right the river was flowing rampantly, which soon began to spill over its banks onto the road. In or through his rear view mirror, he . . . side view mirror, he noticed a car swerving towards him.

[a] Stories were read slowly to patients. Immediate recall on two of the five stories is shown for the same three subjects described in the legend for Figure 19.3.

characterized as occasionally confabulating explanations of the test materials, at times making wild unjustified inferences about the situations depicted (Gardner et al. 1975), accepting absurd literal translations of metaphors (Winner and Gardner 1977), or confusing particular emotions even with their polar opposites (Cicone et al. 1980). On story-recall tasks, Wapner et al. (1981) describe right brain-damaged patients as being impaired in assessing characters' motivations, in appreciating fictitious story boundaries, in extracting a moral from a story, or in integrating individual elements into a coherent narrative. The patients frequently confabulate or rationalize foreign elements of a story and inject personal references, while seldom being aware of the inappropriateness of their responses. In interpreting these observations, the authors suggested that "bereft of a structure into which to place the element, unaware of (or insensitive to) the rules which govern discourse in an area, the patient must make

Table 19.2. *Correlation between story comprehension and visuospatial abilities after right-hemisphere damage*

Visuospatial items	Story-recall items						
	Details	Logical relationships	Form	Intrusions	Perseverations	Substitutions	Confabulations
Details	0.54[a]	0.67[c]	0.54[a]	−0.34	−0.30	−0.32	−0.14
Relationships	0.59[b]	0.68[c]	0.41	−0.29	−0.14	−0.26	−0.12
Form	0.60[b]	0.68[c]	0.53[a]	−0.58[b]	−0.06	−0.36	−0.28
Intrusions	−0.33	−0.51[a]	−0.31	0.55[b]	0.20	0.34	0.01
Perseverations	−0.27	−0.50[a]	−0.41	0.27	0.57[b]	−0.02	0.14
Neglect	0.34	−0.50[a]	−0.28	0.57[b]	−0.07	−0.44	−0.21

[a] $p < 0.025$.
[b] $p < 0.010$.
[c] $p < 0.005$.

an assessment based only on the element itself. . . . These deficits can also be viewed as an inability to evaluate the gestalt or form of the linguistic entity, or as a disruption of schemata."

The notion of a schematic organization of memory was first proposed by Bartlett (1932), who presented experimental evidence that the recall both of spatial designs and of narrative material represents a mental reconstruction of the interrelationships among the principal features, such as organizational or functional features, determined by the subjects' prior experiences with like configurations. The schematic organization of memory for narrative material has been investigated further in recent years (e.g., Rumelhart 1975, Mandler and Johnson 1977, Thorndyke 1977), with a number of studies showing that the components of stories that are best recalled by normal subjects reflect the context (e.g., setting) and the basic outline of the event structure. An extension of these ideas views schemata as the units of perceiving and conscious thought processes (Neisser 1976), continuously being modified by the subject's expectations and ongoing sensory input.

On Rorschach tests, right brain-damaged patients' performance is marked by a free undisciplined expansiveness (Hall, Hall, and Lavoie 1968). In contrast to left brain-damaged patients, who are cautious, self-critical, concrete, and restricted in their interpretations, subjects with right-sided lesions show little perplexity, are not self-critical, and inappropriately combine individual elements to construct preposterous or bizarre, rather than genuinely imaginative, interpretations (Hall et al. 1968).

Conclusions

In the foregoing sections, we have reviewed evidence that the right cerebral hemisphere plays a role in perceiving emotions expressed on the face, in appreciating the significance of one's state, and in apprehending relational properties and overall form, even for linguistic material.

The Rorschach testing of Hall et. al (1968) provides an interesting insight into the "cognitive style" of the right hemisphere, sug-

gesting that it normally participates in evaluating individual elements of an array in the context of the overall form and in critically evaluating the resulting constructs. The confabulations occasionally produced by right brain-damaged patients in recounting their histories, recalling stories, explaining jokes, or accounting for their hospitalization or their geographical location all seem to be consistent with the uncritical, undisciplined, expansive style seen in the Rorschach studies. These patients' inability to give an overview or extract a moral from a story, to assess humourous material, to appreciate fully the significance of their disabilities, or to assess properly social situations would all seem to reflect a breakdown in normal contextual evaluation or conative awareness. Even constructional apraxia might be seen along these lines. Here, too, right brain-damaged subjects fail to appreciate the relationship of component objects or elements to the overall form or task, and, in so doing, are seldom aware of their impairments and are rarely affronted or upset when corrected. Perhaps constructional apraxia, one of the "core" cognitive deficits in right brain-damaged patients, should not be viewed in isolation from the other behavioral changes described in this chapter, but might be seen instead as the most accessible and mildest form of a disorder in mental organization and evaluation, which, with greater degrees of impairment, becomes manifest in many other spheres of intelligence and behavior.

Our main conclusion is as follows. In addition to the classical deficits in visuospatial abilities, people with right-hemisphere damage show impairments in social communication, in evaluating the significance of their disabilities, and in appreciating story schemata, word connotations, humor, and logical relations. The constellation of deficits we have found suggests a general involvement of the right hemisphere in the ability to critically evaluate the interrelationships among elements with respect to an overall schema. The loss of such a faculty may underlie the constructional deficits as well as many of the other behavioral changes that are seen after right cerebral lesions.

Much of the present interest in the role of the right hemisphere in psychological function can be traced directly to Sperry's seminal split-brain investigations. They stimulated an entirely new outlook on how the human brain is organized, led to a reevaluation of the earlier clinical studies of patients with right-hemisphere damage, and generated hypotheses leading to new research. One consequence of this revolution has been the realization that the right side of the brain makes a major specialized contribution to our intelligence and behavior – it can no longer be regarded as a "minor" hemisphere.

Acknowledgments

We gratefully acknowledge the support of the Alfred P. Sloan Foundation to Dr. Benowitz and the American Heart Association to Dr. Finklestein. We wish to thank Drs. Jerre Levy, David Bear, and Ross J. Baldessarini for helpful comments on the manuscript.

References

Bartlett, F. C. 1932. *Remembering*. Cambridge University Press. Cambridge.

Benowitz, L. I. 1980. Cerebral lateralization in the perception of nonverbal emotional cues. *McLean Hosp. J.* 5: 146–67.

Benowitz, L. I., D. M. Bear, R. Rosenthal, M.-M. Mesulam, E. Zaidel, and R. W. Sperry. 1983. Hemispheric specialization in nonverbal communication. *Cortex* 19: 5–11.

Blumstein, S., and W. E. Cooper. 1974. Hemispheric processing of intonation contours. *Cortex* 10: 146–58.

Borod, J. C., H. S. Caron, and E. Koff. 1981. Asymmetry of facial expression related to handedness, footedness, and eyedness: A quantitative study. *Cortex* 17: 381–90.

Brain, R. 1941. Visual disorientation with special reference to the lesions of the right cerebral hemisphere. *Brain* 64: 244–72.

Brownell, H. H., D. Michel, J. Powelson, and H. Gardner. 1983. Surprise but not coherence: Sensitivity to verbal humor in right hemisphere patients. *Brain Lang.* 18: 20–7.

Bryden, M. P., R. G. Ley, and J. H. Sugarman. 1982. A left-ear advantage for identifying the emotional quality of tonal sequences. *Neuropsychol.* 20: 83–7.

Buck, R., and R. J. Duffy. 1980. Nonverbal communication of affect in brain-damaged patients. *Cortex* 16: 351–62.

Buck, R. W., V. J. Savin, R. E. Miller, and W. F. Caul. 1972. Communication of affect through facial expressions in humans. *J. Person. Soc. Psychol.* 23: 362–71.

Campbell, R. 1978. Asymmetries in interpreting and expressing a posed facial expression. *Cortex* 14: 327–42.

Carmon, A., and I. Nachshon. 1973. Ear asymmetry in perception of emotional non-verbal stimuli. *Acta Psychol.* 37: 351–57.

Caramazza, S., J. Gordon, E. G. Zurif, and D. DeLuca. 1976. Right-hemispheric damage and verbal problem solving behavior. *Brain Lang.* 3: 41–6.

Carroll, B. J., M. Feinberg, and J. F. Greden. 1981. A specific laboratory test for the diagnosis of melancholia. *Arch. Gen. Psychiat.* 38: 41–5.

Cicone, M., W. Wapner, and H. Gardner. 1980. Sensitivity to emotional expressions and situations in organic patients. *Cortex* 16: 145–58.

Davidson, R. J., G. E. Schwartz, C. Saron, J. Bennett, and D. J. Goleman. 1979. Frontal vs. parietal EEG asymmetry during positive and negative affect. *Psychophysiol.* 16: 202–3.

DeKosky, S. T., K. M. Heilman, D. Bowers, and E. Valenstein. 1980. Recognition and discrimination of emotional faces and pictures. *Brain Lang.* 9: 206–14.

Denny-Brown, D., J. S. Meyer, and S. Horenstein. 1952. The significance of perceptual rivalry resulting from parietal lesion. *Brain* 75: 433–71.

DeRenzi, E., and P. Faglioni. 1965. The comparative efficiency of intelligence and vigilance tests in detecting hemispheric cerebral damage. *Cortex* 1: 410–33.

Dimond, S. J., and L. Farrington. 1977. Emotional response to films shown to the right or left hemisphere of the brain measured by heart rate. *Acta Psychol.* (*AMST*) 41: 255–60.

Ekman, P., W. Friesen, and P. Ellsworth. 1972. *Emotion in the Human Face: Guidelines for Research and an Integration of Findings*. Pergamon Press, New York.

Finkelstein, S., L. I. Benowitz, R. J. Baldessarini, G. W. Arana, D. N. Levine, R. Woo, D. M. Bear, K. Moya, and A. Stoll. 1982. Mood, vegetative disturbance and dexamethasone suppression test after stroke. *Ann. Neurol.* 12: 463–8.

Fisher, C. M. 1982. Disorientation for place. *Arch. Neurol.* 39: 33–6.

Gainotti, G. 1972. Emotional behavior and hemispheric side of the lesion. *Cortex* 8: 41–55.

Gainotti, G., and M. A. Lemmo. 1976. Comprehension of symbolic gestures in aphasia. *Brain Lang.* 3: 451–60.

Gardner, H. 1975. *The Shattered Mind*. Knopf, New York.

Gardner, H., and G. Denes. 1973. Connotative judgments by aphasic patients on a pictorial adaptation of the semantic differential. *Cortex* 9: 183–96.

Gardner, H., P. K. Ling, L. Flamm, and J. Silverman. 1975. Comprehension and appreciation of humorous material following brain damage. *Brain* 98: 399–412.

Gasparrini, W. G., P. Satz, K. M. Heilman, and F. L. Coolidge. 1978. Hemispheric asymmetries of affective processing as determined by the Minnesota Multiphasic Personality Inventory. *J. Neurol. Neurosurg. Psychiat.* 41: 470–3.

Goodglass, H., and E. Kaplan. 1963. Disturbance of gesture and pantomime in aphasia. *Brain* 86: 703–20.

Hall, M. M., G. C. Hall, and P. Lavoie. 1968. Ideation in patients with unilateral or bilateral midline brain lesions. *J. Abnormal Psychol.* 73: 526–31.

Hécaen, H. 1962. Clinical symptomatology in right and left hemispheric lesions. *In* V. B. Mountcastle (ed.) *Interhemispheric Relations and Cerebral Dominance.* The Johns Hopkins Press, Baltimore. pp. 215–43.

Hécaen, H., J. de Ajuriaguerra, and J. Massonnet. 1951. Les troubles visuo-constructifs par lesion parieto-occipitale droite. Role des perturbations vestibulaires. *Encephale* 1: 122–79.

Heilman, K. M., R. Scholes, and R. T. Watson. 1974. Auditory affective agnosia. *J. Neurol. Neurosurg. Psychiat.* 38: 69–72.

Heilman, K. M., H. D. Schwartz, and R. T. Watson. 1978. Hypoarousal in patients with the neglect syndrome and emotional indifference. *Neurol.* 28: 229–32.

Heller, W., and J. E. Levy. 1981. Perception and expression of emotion in right-handers and left-handers. *Neuropsychol.* 19: 263–72.

Howes, D., and F. Boller. 1975. Simple reaction time: Evidence for focal impairment from lesions of the right hemisphere. *Brain* 98: 317–32.

Izard, C. E. 1971. *The Face of Emotion.* Appleton-Century-Crofts, New York.

Jackson, J. H. 1932. *Selected Writings,* J. Taylor (ed.). Hodder and Stoughton, London.

Kolb, B., and L. Taylor. 1981. Affective behavior in patients with localized cortical excisions: Role of lesion site and side. *Science* 214: 89–91.

Ley, R. G., and M. P. Bryden. 1979. Hemispheric differences in processing emotions and faces. *Brain Lang.* 7: 127–38.

Mandler, J. M., and N. S. Johnson. 1977. Remembrance of things parsed: Story structure and recall. *Cog. Psychol.* 9: 111–51.

Matarazzo, J. D. 1979. *Wechsler's Measurement and Appraisal of Adult Intelligence,* 5th Ed. Oxford University Press, New York.

McFie, J., M. F. Piercy, and O. L. Zangwill. 1960. Visual-constructive disabilities associated with lesions of the right cerebral hemisphere. *Brain* 73: 167–90.

Moskovitch, M., and J. Olds. 1981. Asymmetries in spontaneous facial expressions and their possible relation to hemispheric specialization. *Neuropsychol.* 20: 71–81.

Moya, K. L., L. I. Benowitz, D. N. Levine, and S. P. Finkelstein. 1986. Covariant defects in visuospatial abilities and recall of verbal narrative after right hemisphere stroke. *Cortex* 22: 381–97.

Neisser, U. 1976. *Cognition and Reality.* Freeman, San Francisco.

Ojemann, G., I. Fried, C. Mateer, R. Wohns, and P. Fedio. 1980. Organization of visuospatial functions in human non-dominant cortex: Evidence from electrical stimulation. *Neurosci. Abst.* 6: 418.

Patterson, A., and O. L. Zangwill. 1944. Disorders of visual space perception associated with lesions of the right cerebral hemisphere. *Brain* 67: 331–58.

Perria, L., G. Rosadini, and G. F. Rossi. 1961. Determination of side of cerebral dominance with amobarbital. *Arch. Neurol.* 4: 173–81.

Piercy, M., H. Hécaen, and J. de Ajuriaguerra. 1960. Constructional apraxia associated with unilateral cerebral lesions: Left- and right-sided cases compared. *Brain* 83: 225–42.

Robinson, R. G., and D. F. Benson. 1981. Depression in aphasic patients: Frequency, severity and clinical-pathological correlations. *Brain Lang.* 14: 282–91.

Rosenthal, R., J. A. Hall, D. Archer, M. R. DiMatteo, and P. Rogers. 1979. The PONS test: Measuring sensitivity to nonverbal cues. *In* S. Weitz (ed.) *Nonverbal Communication.* Oxford University Press, New York, pp. 357–70.

Rosenthal, R., J. A. Hall, M. R. DiMatteo, P. L. Rogers, and D. Archer. 1979. *Sensitivity to Nonverbal Communication: The PONS Test.* The Johns Hopkins Press, Baltimore.

Ross, E. D., and M.-M. Mesulam. 1979. Dominant language functions of the right hemisphere? *Arch. Neurol.* 36: 144–8.

Ross, E. D., and A. J. Rush. 1981. Diagnosis and neuroanatomical correlates of depression in brain-damaged patients. *Arch. Gen. Psychiat.* 38: 1344–54.

Rumelhart, D. E. 1975. Notes on a schema for stories. *In* D. G. Bobrow and A. Collins (eds.) *Representation and Understanding: Studies in Cognitive Science.* Academic Press, New York.

Sackeim, H. A., M. S. Greenberg, A. L. Weiman, R. C. Gur, J. P. Hungerbuhler, and N. Geschwind. 1982. Hemispheric asymmetry in the expression of positive and negative emotions. *Arch. Neurol.* 39: 210–18.

Sackeim, H. A., R. C. Gur, and M. D. Saucy. 1978. Emotions are expressed more intensely on the left side of the face. *Science* 202: 434–6.

Schlanger, B. B., P. Schlanger, and L. J. Gerstman. 1976. The perception of emotionally-toned sentences by right-hemispheric damaged and aphasic subjects. *Brain Lang.* 3: 396–403.

Schwartz, G. E., R. J. Davidson, and F. Maer. 1975. Right hemisphere lateralization for emotion in the human brain: Interactions with cognition. *Science* 190: 286–8.

Sperry, R. W. 1974. Lateral specialization in the surgically separated hemispheres. *In* F. O. Schmitt and F. G. Worden (eds.) *The Neurosciences: Third Study Program.* The MIT Press, Cambridge, pp. 5–19.

Suberi, M., and W. F. McKeever. 1977. Differential right hemispheric memory storage of emotional and non-emotional faces. *Neuropsychol.* 15: 757–68.

Thorndyke, P. 1977. Cognitive structures in comprehension and memory of narrative discourse. *Cog. Psychol.* 9: 77–110.

Tucker, D., C. E. Stenslie, and R. S. Roth. 1981. Right frontal lobe activation and right hemisphere performance decrement during a depressed mood. *Arch. Gen. Psychiat.* 38: 169–74.

Tucker, D. M., R. T. Watson, and K. M. Heilman. 1977. Discrimination and evocation of affectively intoned speech in patients with right parietal disease. *Neurol.* 27: 947–50.

Wapner, W., S. Hamby, and H. Gardner. 1981. The role of the right hemisphere in the apprehension of complex linguistic material. *Brain Lang.* 14: 15–33.

Wechsler, A. F. 1973. The effect of organic brain disease on recall of emotionally charged versus neutral narrative texts. *Neurol.* 23: 130–5.

Weinstein, S. 1962. Differences in effects of brain wounds implicating right and left hemispheres: Differential effects on certain intellectual and complex perceptual functions. *In* V. B. Mountcastle (ed.) *Interhemispheric Relations and Cerebral Dominance.* The Johns Hopkins Press, Baltimore; pp. 159–76.

Winner, E., and H. Gardner. 1977. The comprehension of metaphor in brain-damaged patients. *Brain* 100: 717–29.

Zaidel, D., and R. W. Sperry. 1974. Memory impairment after commissurotomy in man. *Brain* 97: 263–72.

Zaidel, E. 1977. Concepts of cerebral dominance in the split-brain. *In* P. Bouser and A. Rogeul-Buser (eds.) *Cerebral Correlates of Conscious Experience.* Elsevier, Amsterdam.

Zurif, E. B. 1972. Auditory lateralization: Prosodic and syntactical factors. *Brain Lang.* 1: 391–404.

20 Growth and education of the hemispheres

Colwyn Trevarthen
Department of Psychology
University of Edinburgh

If he or she is to thrive in a human world, every newborn child will have to learn how to be intelligent according to the set of meanings peculiar to one culture. Cultural learning, which is beyond any other species, takes place in a brain that is the largest in proportion to body weight, the most elaborate in anatomy, and the one with most neocortex. It is a brain that is already very elaborate soon after birth, but that reaches full maturity with exceptional slowness – some cells and circuits of the cortex and brain core do not complete differentiation until middle life or old age (Yakovlev and Lecours 1967). Finally, the human brain is characterized by functional asymmetry, a highly variable hemispheric difference for just those cognitive functions that are essential for the cognitions and skills of a responsible adult in the culture. (Dimond 1972; Corballis and Beale 1976; Sperry 1982, 1983; Bradshaw and Nettleton 1983; Trevarthen 1984a; Witelson 1987; Witelson and Kigar 1987).

In our attempt to understand how cultural transmission depends on brain anatomy, Roger Sperry's research has unique importance. His developmental studies support the concept of a genetic regulation of the growth of nerve circuity even for the highest mental functions. The research with commissurotomy patients leads from his early ideas about the regulation of perception by action to a new theory of complementary systems of consciousness that "cause" human knowledge and human values (Sperry 1983; Nobel Prize Conversations 1985).

Since the first of Sperry's psychological tests with commissurotomy patients (Sperry 1967, 1974; Sperry, Gazzaniga, and Bogen 1969), hemispheric functional asymmetries have been the target for a burgeoning research effort (Bradshaw and Nettleton 1983; Corballis, 1983; Trevarthen 1984a). One important finding has been that we humans have brains with marked individuality. Different persons' brains lean toward proficiency in different tasks, their different mental aptitudes relating to traditional fields of knowledge, skill, and belief, and to distinct roles in society. Recent data strengthen the view that psychological individuality (which is not reduceable to differences in quantity, speed, or strength of general intelligence) owes as much to inherited factors in the growth of major component systems in the brain, to stable personality characteristics, as to differences in experience (e.g., Harshman and Hampson 1987; Loehlin, Willerman, and Horn 1988). Variation in activation of the hemispheres may explain a considerable part of individual differences in mental functions (see Chapters 13 and 14, this volume).

In this chapter, I explore how growth of the brain, and of its hemispheric asymmetry, can be related to learning in society. I review such evidence as we have on what governs the way functions in left and right hemispheres transform during growth of a child's brain, while he or she is learning to live in intelligent cooperation with other persons and their brains.

Transmission of culture by brain growth: A new approach

The classic view in modern psychology has been that genetic regulation of brain growth will provide only general preparation for the learning of symbols and practices of adult society. A child's brain must be hugely impressionable if language and the rest of arbitrary traditional knowledge are picked up from experience and by conditioning in society. Why the brain should be asymmetric for a complex skill like language is, in this view, a mystery. It does not seem to be trained to have that asymmetry.

It has been found that the cerebral hemispheres are different in midfetal stages (Strauss, Kosaka, and Wada 1983; Witelson and Kigar 1987), and findings in infant psychology confirm that there is elaborate preparation in brain growth for cultural learning (Trevarthen 1983, 1987a, 1987b; Trevarthen and Logotheti 1987). It appears that growth regulations having effect from the fetal period equip a child with a set of motives evolved for acquiring cultural knowledge through communicating. The crucial process appears to reside in a mechanism that requires older brains to engage with mental states of awareness, interest, intention, and emotion in receptive younger brains. Brain asymmetry, affecting learned cultural skills, may be an adaptation for this brain-to-brain engagement. Arbitrary and historic ideas and customs would not be passed on unless there were some such mechanism.

Regional differences in cortical functions of adults, including the balance of different hemispheric contributions, are being traced to differences appearing first in modulatory reticular nuclei on left and right of the core of the brain (see what follows). The modulatory systems develop in embryo stages before the cortex starts to differentiate. Genetic control of individual differences in cerebral development, including differences in laterality of psychological function, may, therefore, be initiated by way of the wide ramifications of relatively few reticular neurones that project a variety of regulatory instructions to cell bodies throughout the cortex (McGeer, Eccles, and McGeer 1978;

Scheibel 1984; Hökfelt 1987). Core regulatory neurone activities set the conditions for responses of cortical cells to stimuli from the world outside the body (Trevarthen 1987d). They also control how new nerve network associations grow and how mechanisms for perceiving goals and for acting on them are coupled in development and learning (Singer 1987).

This theory of how brain development is controlled from inside the brain itself, reinforced by new concepts of how learning is motivated by activity of reticular and limbic neurones (see Chapter 11, this volume, and Goldman-Rakic 1987), offers the possibility that transmission of concepts and skills from one generation to the next is facilitated by direct coordination between the motivations generated in a child and the feelings of adults, who already have mastered those concepts and skills, and who can interpret or evaluate the world for the child. If this is so, we will have to revise the traditional theory of how biological matter gains social abilities.

The new theory would explain transmission of culture in terms of a specific and highly active epigenetic program for brain growth that needs brain–brain interaction. Adaptation of a given brain to a particular social world depends, not on reinforcement by physiological rules for maintaining vital states of the body (primary drives), but on a motivated search by the young for certain target experiences; experiences that are capable of yielding information needed to solve specific problems that have been set by the young instinctively behaving in a particular way. One such innate way of behaving is expressing mental or motivational states to others, and getting into contact with their mental states. The genetically regulated strategy of brain development in a child will be, therefore, one that generates motives to engage with signs of complementary and constructive motives in other human beings.

In the first year of an infant's life, close attachments form between a baby and his or her primary caretaker, and the brain-linking person-to-person communication process is set up in a companionship framed by emotions (Trevarthen 1980, 1984c). Infancy is the phase in which circuits of the cerebral cortex undergo their greatest transformations, when the functional systems are blocked for accurate perception of one world by several sense modalities acting together, and for the precise performance of effective acts that move a complex multisegmented body in coordination (Trevarthen 1985a). These integrative brain developments occur in the context of an intimate affectionate relationship between infant and mother, or other caretaker. In tracing how an infant changes into a speaking toddler who has great curiosity about conventions in social life, we can observe brain function transforming and watch the emergence of cultural awareness within friendships maintained by emotions. We can identify the motives that drive the process (Trevarthen 1982, Trevarthen and Logotheti 1989).

Cortical growth in utero

The cerebral hemispheres start as bulges on the end of the brain in midembryo, one month after conception, their thin walls made up of undifferentiated cells. Neurons form in basal ganglia and limbic parts in the next few weeks, appearing in the neocortex at about eight weeks. This marks the beginning of the fetal period, in which the cerebral hemispheres and the cerebellum develop the basic arrangement of their complex tissues (Trevarthen 1985a). Their growth is conditioned by events in earlier stages.

In the brainstem and spinal cord of a human embryo, nerve circuits comparable to those of an adult lower vertebrate, such as the salamander of Herrick's classical study (Herrick 1948), grow between four and eight weeks (Windle 1970). Motor axons grow from the ventral cord at four weeks, then the dorsal input of the cord by bipolar sensory neurones grows at four and one-half weeks. Selective connections between sensory axons and dendrites of motor cells in the spinal cord, forming the basis for spinal locomotor and autonomic reflexes, are guided, in this midembryo phase, by spontaneous activity of reticular interneurones (Baker 1985), and this appears to be a principle of morphogenetic regulation that is repeated over and over in other parts of developing brains. Motor cell groups attain a pri-

mary organization and exhibit spontaneous activity before sensory input from the surface of the body reaches them; then interneurones of the reticular core of the brain assist in coupling sensorimotor links (Hamburger 1973, Oppenheim and Reitzel 1975, Oppenheim 1984). The chemical communication system of reticular interneurones, capable of influencing gene action in differentiating nerve cells everywhere in the brain, appears to be active even before synaptic relations have been established (Oppenheim, 1984).

Evidently, the interneurones, assisted by glia cells, mediate in genetic control of sensorimotor links. When far-reaching connections grow into the forebrain from reticular nuclei and hypothalamus in the brainstem, axons penetrate the developing striatum and the primordial hippocampus and pyriform cortex (palaeopalium) before the neocortex begins to differentiate (Windle 1970; Björklund and Stenevi 1979; Dunnett, Björklund, and Stenevi 1983). The diverse neurotransmitter systems of brain-core neurones, which later regulate motivation and emotion in the adult, thus appear, in the late embryo, as probable regulators of morphogensis in the hemispheres (McGeer, Eccles, and McGeer 1978; Scheibel 1984; Hökfelt 1987; Singer 1987; Wied 1987). They are evidently a source of trophic substances and intracellular messengers that govern survival, migration, and differentiation of cortical neurones from before the time that cortical synaptic networks form (see Chapter 1, this volume).

Undifferentiated neurones multiply in the lateral cerebral wall and then appear in the roof and the medial wall above the hippocampus. They are in the frontal and occipital poles by nine and one-half weeks. In the next two months (10–18 weeks), there is peak rate of multiplication of neocortical nerve cells migrating from the germinal tissue (ependyma) around the cavities of the cerebral hemispheres (Dobbing 1981). Nearly all the cortical neurones for the whole life of the individual are produced in this "neuronal growth spurt," four to five months before birth. The immature neurones creep in waves along supporting glia cells that connect inner and outer membranes of the hemisphere wall, and they congregate in a stratum called the "cortical plate," late ar-

→ primary cortical areas maturing first

rivals infiltrating between earlier arrivals so that the youngest cells accumulate toward the outside of the plate (Sidman and Rakic 1973). These younger cells will later constitute the intracortical associative system of higher mental functions, the older deeper layers being destined to form close links with subcortical systems.

Migration, survival, and differentiation of cortical cells in the fetus depends, we can be sure, upon both local factors and influences projected into the cortex from the brainstem core. Thalamic afferents and projections from ventromedial reticular nuclei and hypothalamus arrive while the cortical cells are still migrating (Marin-Padilla 1970, Morest 1970, Sidman and Rakic 1973). Neither thalamic nor cortical cells are mature at this stage. Cortical dendrite trees and synaptic systems start to differentiate in late fetal stages and complete in the first postnatal year or two, primary sensory areas attaining maturity first (Conel 1939–1963, Huttenlocher 1979, Huttenlocher et al. 1982, Rakic et al. 1986, Goldman-Rakic 1987).

Tissue asymmetries can be seen in the human cortex before cortical cells differentiate (Strauss, Kosaka, and Wada 1983). The migration and selective survival of cells round the Sylvian sulcus, where important asymmetries appear (Witelson and Kigar 1987), is presumably also subject to influences projected upward from the brainstem core, hypothalamus, and limbic system, subhemispheric and palaeocortical parts of the brain known to have asymmetries in mammals (Nordeen and Yahr 1982; Sherman, Galaburda, and Geschwind 1982; Strauss, Kosaka, and Wada 1983; Gerendai 1987). Many asymmetries are now reported for the cortex of rats (Diamond 1987).

Brain development is reciprocally linked with differentiation of the gonads and the appearance of secondary sexual features of the body (MacKinnon and Greenstein 1985), and sex differences in both brain anatomy and in the gonads appear to stem from differences in the organization of neurohumoral systems of the brain stem (Geschwind and Galaburda 1985, Wierman and Crowley 1985). Removal of the gonads at birth produces effects on cortical growth in rats, changing hemispheric asymmetry (Gerendai 1987). In monkeys, there are sex differences in growth of the temporal neocortex involved in habit formation, due to high levels of testosterone in newborn males, which slows cortical maturation (Hagger, Bachevalier, and Bercu 1986). Hormonal control of sexual differentiation in behavior is related to the biochemical mechanism by which gene expression is controlled in the central nervous system itself. Thus, for example, peptides, first known as important hormones outside the brain, are now perceived to be abundant intracerebral transmitters that act in intricate combinations within the regulatory circuits of the CNS (Iverson 1987, Wied 1987). There is a feedback loop between neurones of the hypothalamus and medioventral reticular formation and the endocrine system of gonads and adrenals that regulate reproductive activities and development of the body and its secondary sexual features. This connection, which is of importance in the postnatal growth of the mental abilities in children, is first evident in the early fetal stages (MacKinnon and Greenstein 1985).

Three steps by which cells become connected in the central nervous system

In 1965, Sperry summarized his chemoaffinity theory of how genes regulate growth of nerve circuits by tagging nerve cells for connectivity (Sperry 1965). His famous surgical experiments on how regeneration of nerves is regulated in lower vertebrates led to the proposal that the pathways responsible for instinctive sensorimotor coordinations, as in orienting to capture food outside the body, achieve their layout by selective cell-to-cell attachments. Each growing axon branch flourishes a superabundance of exploratory filaments from the growth cones at its tips and these are guided between cells of brain and body by a chemoaffinity matching mechanism. The axon-filaments were imagined to follow chemical labels on target cell surfaces that had been produced in orthogonal gradients by gene action (see the foreword and Chapters 1–5, this volume). Sperry allowed that learning could make additional selections from a set of templates for matching to stimulus features, defining categories for form, color, etc., but these features, too, would be formulated a priori, by a chemical coding in sensory projections, with sufficient distinctness to provide for all possible useful discriminations. In early papers, produced while he was working with Paul Weiss, Sperry accepted Weiss's view that the surface features of the body (skin, muscles, retina, etc.) might impress a coding on nerves (Sperry 1940). Later he decided that the neurones of the CNS could themselves be specified chemically to determine connective affinities, and he presented experimental evidence to support this theory (Sperry 1963, 1965; see Chapters 1 and 2, this volume).

Nearly half a century of research supports Sperry's chemoaffinity explanation for the basic route finding and somatotopic layout of sensory projections, central interneuronal mappings, and neuromuscular systems in embryos, even though the molecular mechanism of nerve-cell affinities is still unknown. However, it is also the case that extensive refinements of perceptual and motor projections, and elaborate new combinations of sensory and motor processes, are acquired by self-selection of functional nerve connections. Moreover, the principles of cooperative interaction between neurones allow them to respond to stimuli. This is how the brain learns.

Sperry's mechanism of innate chemoaffinity gradients is now generally thought to be complemented by a principle that Hebb proposed to explain formation of cortical neurone assemblies in learning (Hebb 1949). Convergent effects transmitted from different active axon terminals to postsynaptic cells can, Hebb proposed, change the network cooperatively, according to how action potentials and secreted transmitter chemicals become distributed in space and time within the nerve network and interact (Singer 1987; von der Malsburg and Singer 1988).

In the epigenetics of the developing nervous system, cell multiplications, cell migrations and extension of cell projections, while constrained by chemical guidance factors under regulation by genes, all result in an exuberant mingling of elements produced in extravagant excess. Subsequently, more refined functional cell groups and cell-to-cell transmission lines are selected by eliminating the great majority of elements, or closing off contacts (Mark 1974;

Changeux, Heidmann, and Patter 1984; Changeux, 1985). Quantitative matching of cell systems is achieved by competitions of neurones in newly connected systems for growth substances, unsupported cells dying (Oppenheim 1984; see Chapter 1, this volume). As the neurones become functional in a nerve net, the cells, axons, or effective synaptic connections that are retained are those that synchronize and cooperate in excitation of a cell on which they converge, the postsynaptic cell with its receptor sites for neurotransmitters acting as an integrator and selector. The coincidence and spatial registration of action potentials assist in deciding which transmission lines will prosper, while others that do not cooperate are lost.

Selection processes in this second phase of brain development, by deletion of unfavored contacts, are driven by impulse activity of the cells and exchange of messenger substances. This begins *in utero* by spontaneous discharge of the neurones and transmission of growth substances down axons, i.e., without the benefit of excitation from stimuli of environmental origin (Malsburg and Singer 1988). Thus, when the environment does start to have a decisive voice in the selection process, by patterning sensory excitation in receptors, its input infiltrates an already active and highly structured nervous system. Shaping of the brain by the pattern of stimuli is conditioned by the prior genetic coding of acceptable circuits, *à la* Sperry, prenatal and "self-patterning" of the nerve network.

Recently, a third principle of nerve-net formation has been found that allows for a late regulation of cooperative assemblies of neurones, and this process ensures that the retained assemblies will embody additional "life value," according to rules acquired in evolution and laid down earlier in development, but different from the ones guiding formation of the basic nerve net. A second voice is given to gene regulation of nerve-circuit formation, different from the cell-surface coding Sperry proposed, and adding an important qualification of Hebb's hypothesis for accretion of cell assemblies. A system of neurones in the core of the brain, prewired in the embryo, is capable of vetting the effects of stimulation in creation of cooperative cell assemblies. It confers prior information, validated by evolution, about what the environment should afford, giving appropriate a priori values for experiences.

Singer and his colleagues (Singer and Rauschecker 1982; Singer, Tretter, and Yinon 1982; Singer 1987) have shown that the brainstem reticular formation "gates" the responses of cortical neurones in kittens to convergent information from the two eyes. Collaborating with the oculomotor system of the brainstem, which aims, converges, and focuses the eyes on objects of interest (Hein et al. 1979, Imbert 1985), an ascending noradrenergic reticular influence selects which cells will retain simultaneously active binocular inputs. This builds up (selects) binocular cells in a mechanism for stereo acuity and depth perception by a process that is driven, not only by stimuli, but also by the coordinated, internally generated, interest and attention of the young animal. Such a system would be capable, in later phases of development, of selectively enhancing, and retaining in a discriminatory or "semantic" memory, certain classificatory or category-defining cell assemblies. These assemblies would correspond with stimuli that come immediately after the brain has commanded orientation of receptors to aid recognition of an object, the object being picked out from the field round the animal because it is "felt" to have a particular life value or motivation attached to it; e.g., it is in an object already taken to be "good" or "bad" to eat. The internally generated "interest" effectively "rewards" or "punishes" the receptive networks.

In summary, then, Sperry's chemoaffinity mechanism can explain the basic mapping between cell arrays that portray the spatial organization of the body and its congruent field of action – the bilaterally symmetrical, anteroposteriorly and dorsoventrally polarized "behavior field" (Trevarthen 1974). It can indicate how mechanisms are formed for coorienting and bringing together different parts of the body (i.e., converging the eyes; bringing hand to mouth to transport something from visual pericorporal space into the body; guiding locomotion to achieve selective mobility in a spatial array of gaps, surfaces, and goals; etc.). An additional mechanism, such as Singer's, is needed to explain how neural connections of

learning, Hebbian synapses, are made to conform to innate adaptive evaluations. How such connections become capable of identifying goal objects in terms of their invariant stimulus indices, their "constancies," and their properties and values with respect to dependable and inherent vital needs to which the organism must be attentive, and about which it must generate positive or negative feelings.

Now we can see more easily how pathways of communication formed among cells of the developing brainstem could direct gene transcription in target cells in the cortex and so determine the formation, consolidation, or loss of effective interneuronal contacts. Core regulator neurones can exercise a decisive influence over the process whereby cortical cells join in cooperative assemblies.

Messages governing nerve-net formation are not always conveyed by other neurones. They include, also, products of nonneural glia cells, as well as hormones circulating in cerebrospinal fluid and in blood vessels, hormones produced by the brain itself or by endocrine glands, including the gonads. Nevertheless, it is interneurones of specialized form that produce the most differentiated trophic and regulator substances, and that transmit them along their axons with refined precision. These neurones form a small fraction of the brain's population in number (about 5%), but they manufacture different potent chemical messenger substances and they distribute their disproportionally elaborate projections to many distant parts of the brain (Scheibel 1984, Nauta and Feirtag 1986, Hökfelt 1987, Iverson 1987). Their products can excite local or widely separated aggregates of cells that thereby become synchronized in their state of activity and receptivity. We note, moreover, that asymmetries have been reported for neurotransmitters in subcortical structures of the human brain (Oke et al. 1978; Glick et al. 1987; see what follows).

The neurobiology and genetic significance of motives

In the adult brain, regulator neurones of the reticular core form the anatomical space/time frame of behavior. They constitute the coupled system of spontaneously active oscillators, or clocks, that give the essential beat for motor coordination and for communication between individuals. They also regulate the focus of attention and the rhythm and balance of different cognitive states of alertness, readiness to act, flexibility of orientation or scanning, and the allocation of information processing (Trevarthen 1987d). Finally, they are capable of initiating different levels or moods of activity – restless, forceful, cautious, purposeful, casting about, etc. – at the same time as they control the initiation, coordination, and sequencing of motor activity. All these "programming" elements in cerebral activity can be generated independently of input or output, though they are formed to organize the cooperative effects of stimulation in sense organs and of muscle contractions in motor systems. The general term "motivation" is used to describe activity of central origin that sets the state of information pickup, and an underlying form, pace, and direction of activity in relation to which sensory afference becomes informative. The distinct organized forms of motivation built into the brain for particular purposes may be called *motives* (Trevarthen 1982).

The existence of adaptive motives in behavior is evident, and their value to animal life is obvious. They are replicated in offspring faithfully, and can be used to identify a species. Indeed, motive systems in brains help control evolution itself. Brains have greatly accelerated the rate of evolution of distinct animal forms and their organs (Wilson 1985). Instincts in brains determine how genes will be multiplied and dispersed in living populations. Different animal bodies have evolved in response to different ways of behaving directed by different motives in the brains. The "higher" animals enrich their motives by learning specific reactions to identified environmental conditions, but in no way does this mean they replace inherited motives by learning. Indeed, their motives are inherently richer and more elaborately coordinated than in "lower" forms. In development, motives, changing according to a gene-regulated program, assist in the cooperative self-organizing principles of brain growth, so that learning in the life of the individual will build increasingly effective perception of the environment and increasingly selective and effective action.

Intrinsic regulation of brain growth and the social transmission of knowledge

Subcortical neurones, by way of their motor and neurochemical effects, pattern brain development, the ongoing flow of behavior and consciousness, and the building of memories. Limbic structures of the hemispheres, reciprocally connected to the hypothalamus and brainstem reticular nuclei, enter into memory formation in the neocortex and are essential for transfer of learning between modalities as well as the retrieval of associations from memory (Mishkin 1982; Murray and Mishkin 1985; Mishkin and Phillips, Chapter 11, this volume).

Against this background, the origin of functional asymmetries in the forebrain, as of other regional differences in brain functioning, must be sought in neocortical epigenetics – from the stage of multiplication of cells in the germ layer, and their migration away from it, through patterning of regulatory mechanisms that project up from the brainstem to the cortex as its cell networks are forming. In general, brainstem reticular systems project to the cortex ipsilaterally, so differences between left and right halves of the reticular system are reflected in parallel differential effects in left and right hemispheres.

Hemispheric asymmetries, of interest because they concern late maturing functions of great significance in human cultural intelligence, it is here proposed, come about as a consequence of asymmetric transfusion of trophic and regulator molecules from brainstem to the cortex throughout brain development. Subsequently, sensory information, given cohesion by recurring patterns in the physics of the external world, is crucial for the selection of cooperative assemblies of neurones that will perform the cognitive operations of perception, memory, and voluntary motor coordination. Outgrowth of transcortical associative links, including those through the corpus callosum, is essential to this later phase of the process. But, even in these late stages of brain development, the selective influence of subcortical gating processes, operating through attention and motivation, will remain effective.

The neurochemical regulators of brains in higher animals have evolved to control and respond to social influences. In social mammals, brain development comes under control of signals that direct the motives of all individuals in a social group, with particularly strong effects on the young. Primates have young that are born, at great cost in nutrient energy from the mother, with big but immature brains, ready for an intensive "education" while their cerebral cortices are being completed (Armstrong 1985). In humans, this strategy is elaborated for the transmission of culture (Lancaster 1986). Human cerebral hemispheres gain their anatomical and functional definition by a process of education, immature brains and mature brains entering into a long program of communication that is directed by a transforming complex of emotions. Children pass through stages of attachment to adult caretakers, who change their expressions and responses to meet the needs of the young and to give them appropriate guidance and instruction so they learn what culture offers. The instruction must fit what Vygotsky called the child's "zone of proximal development" (Rogoff and Wertsch 1984).

Support for this theory of culture genesis by regulated growth of brains in social communication comes from the neurobiology of emotions. Recent discoveries concerning the neurochemistry of emotional states and their effects on brain function and brain growth link up with findings concerning the role that emotions play in regulating cognitive developments in infancy (Tucker 1986). Important evidence comes from the patterns of asymmetry in brain chemistry (Oke et al. 1978), in emotional function (Gainotti 1987), and in infant communication behavior, all confirming the idea that intrinsic cerebral factors guide the associative processes of cognitive development and learning (Fox and Davidson 1984; Tucker and Williamson 1984; Tucker and Frederick 1987; see Chapters 14 and 18, this volume). Finally, as we shall see, emotional and communication disorders in infant mental growth give evidence for a

genetic determination of critical factors in brain chemistry that may help explain cerebral asymmetries, as well as many other characteristic differentiations of brain function.

Cultural intelligence in infants and toddlers

Fifty years ago, infants were thought to be reflex organisms that build up coordination by trial and error and by conditioned reinforcement of new sensorimotor connections. Consciousness, rationality, skillful action, emotional responses, and morality were all thought to be built up by associative learning, the learning of language being given a central role in the internalization of symbolic terms for thought and for representation of causal relations in reality.

Modern developmental cognitive psychology was created by Piaget (1970). He emphasized that mental schemata, on which intelligence bases its predictions about consequences of action, are built from the spontaneous motor activity of children who test feedback in playful sensorimotor "circular reactions." He taught that after schemata for the movements of body parts are coordinated through exercise of primary reflexes, and mutual assimilation of sensorimotor "means–ends" schemes, the infant, about one year old, builds a concept of an ideal external object that is capable of acquiring properties that exist independently of the infant's given act of orientation or manipulation. Thought about persistent reality and causality is built up in the child's mind by coordination of schemata for two or more objects, and by representation of reversible operations by which the child learns to combine or separate objects and to make them interact in different ways. Emotions, according to Piaget, are part of the child's "energetics" – they regulate cognitive operations by controlling the expenditure of behavioral and mental energy (Piaget 1962, Piaget and Inhelder 1969).

After building up mental schemata for reality and its transformations, the child gains, through imitation, according to Piaget (1962) a basic representation of other people and their actions. Only then, after these schemata for the interests of other minds have been built, is symbolic and linguistic awareness possible. That is how Piaget explains why humans wait nearly two years before they speak. They need to develop a coherent cognitive system through practice of sensorimotor coordinations, and adapt to society, before they can articulate with the different point of view and different focus of experience in another person. He described young children as "egocentric," meaning they were incapable of taking account of another's viewpoint.

Piaget portrays the development of intelligence through an invariant sequence of stages. Cognitive and rational structures are made by a self-regulated process of experimentation through action that sets its own pace and course while assimilating environmental information.

A different view of infant intelligence has come from study of early spontaneous reactions to persons, rather than problem solving (Trevarthen and Logotheti 1987). It has been shown that before a baby gains postural stability, manipulation, and locomotion, he or she has refined awareness of other persons and their emotions. Infants express elaborate emotions, and they are ready to enter from birth into an engagement of feeling with another (Trevarthen 1984c, 1985b; Murray and Trevarthen 1985; Figure 20.1). The effects of this engagement on the child's mental activity are profoundly important for the early development of perception, perceptuomotor coordination, and cognitive processes. To a degree unequalled in any other primate, human newborns start to learn by communicating. Subsequent developments show that the regulation of learning by emotion in communication is of primary importance for the whole strategy of human mental growth. The foundations for communication by emotional expression are innate, as is the course of their development. New motives for communication emerge in a predictable age-related progression, setting changing goals for learning (Trevarthen 1982, 1986b).

A theory of the innate foundations for cultural intelligence has come from study of these developmental changes (Trevarthen 1987c; Trevarthen and Logotheti 1987, 1989). It proposes that human offspring enter into a

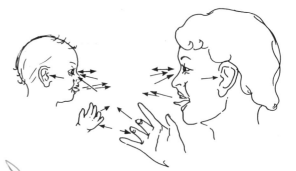

Figure 20.1. Mothers and infants, both, can regulate complex emotional engagements by means of expressions of eyes, face, voice, and hands. Infants under three months respond selectively to expressions of the mother's eyes, face, voice, and hands, one at a time or in coordination. For example, infants can seek eye contact; react to, and imitate, facial expressions of happiness, sadness, and anger; respond sensitively to, and imitate, changes in voice setting and intonation; imitate hand movements seen; and respond to touching by the mother's hand. And they react quickly to mood changes signaled in all these parts together. Mothers also use the same channels, separately or in coordination. After three months, infants pay increasing attention to the actions performed by mothers' hands and are more aware of sounds made by their own manipulation of objects or by other persons moving objects.

sharing of motives with older mentors and then extend their cooperative play to peers. In the process, ideas about conventions of behavior and of symbolic meanings come to dominate the child's consciousness and learning. Language is seen, not as the sole means for communication of conventional ideas, but as the most powerful expression and vehicle for the system of meanings (collective semantics). Words help to define the purposes by which cooperation is achieved. Children learn to understand speech, and to speak, read and write, as a refinement of an inherent interest they already have in sharing experiences, tasks and feelings in conventional form (Hubley and Trevarthen 1979; Trevarthen 1987c). This interest is clearly expressed in the imaginative and "prerepresentational" (symbolic and role-taking) play that appears before speech (Piaget 1962; Trevarthen and Logotheti 1987, 1989).

The regular stages observed in the emergence of language, when put in the full context of all kinds of cooperative behavior, give evidence for a particular intersubjective strategy of brain development. The transformation of skill in communicating and cooperating can be related to general developments, and learning, in perception, motor coordination, and cognition; but the strategy of development seems most coherent when viewed as a growth in specific interpersonal or intersubjective functions. That is to say, the regulation of developments inside the child's brain appears to be centered in core motivating systems active in the child and open to the expressions of mental activity in other persons (Trevarthen 1983, 1985b, 1987b).

In the earliest communicative engagements, human babies show rudiments of conversational expressiveness that foreshadow later development of symbolic expression (Studdert-Kennedy 1983, 1987; Trevarthen and Marwick 1986, Trevarthen and Logotheti 1987). A second human species-specific feature emerges later, toward the end of the first year, while the human child is still unable to walk. This involves an active engagement with a partner to share in some arbitrary manipulation of the environment – it is genuinely "protosymbolic." The child shows willingness to coordinate interest with another in manipulation of objects, giving deliberate attention to the others' interests and purposes so as to learn a new way of employing or combining objects (Trevarthen and Hubley 1978; Hubley and Trevarthen 1979; Trevarthen and Logotheti 1987). Simultaneously with this development, the infant makes the first signals of "protolanguage" – a set of vocalizations or hand signs, learned in communication with a known and trusted companion, and used consistently to perform communicative "acts of meaning" (Halliday 1975; Trevarthen 1987c). A one-year-old who is interacting with familiars will share eye contact combined with vocal, facial, and gestural expression to involve another in a joint manipulative task. This kind of play leads directly into the symbolic and role-playing imagination of a toddler who is eager to act in conventional ways, taking objects for their "proper" use, assuming imitated postures and roles for the appreciation of others (Trevarthen and Logotheti 1987, 1989).

Joint task performance, coordinated so-cial display, posturing, and sociodramatic expression all occur, of course, in ape societies and in the play of juvenile apes. The difference is that play of apes or monkeys is not open to variation by learning of new conventional applications to anything approaching the same extent as is normal for a human infant.

Lateral asymmetries in early expressive communication and in perception of expressions

In the earliest expressions of the two-month-old infant seeking protoconversational interaction, or of the one-year-old starting to communicate about joint task performance or cultural world awareness, there are spontaneous lateral asymmetries (Studdert-Kennedy 1983, 1987; Trevarthen 1986a). The asymmetries seem strongest for the most typically human activities, including antecedents of speech and gesture.

By the end of the first month, a full-term infant can join in a "protoconversation," looking at the mother intently, with a "knit brow and jaw drop" expression of concentrated attention, then smiling in recognition of the mother's imitative sounds of pleasure and her smile. In a few seconds, the baby becomes "serious" and either makes a cooing vocalization, or moves lip or tongue in what looks like rudimentary speech, and is called "prespeech" (Trevarthen 1979, 1985b, 1986b). Accompanying these facial/oral expressions are hand movements. Wrist and finger movements are often precisely synchronized with the lip and tongue movements to form an integrated act of expression or "utterance" (Trevarthen 1986a). These behaviors give evidence for a coordination, within the infant, between gaze, vocalization, and hand gestures (Trevarthen 1984b), and also for a central emotional process that tunes itself to the expressions of the mother's emotion (Trevarthen 1985b, 1986b). The two persons enter into a "couple" of feeling, moving in unison or in alternation, and acting in complementary address-and-reply or question-and-answer modes (Stern 1985; Trevarthen 1986b).

Face-to-face protoconversations can be sustained by means of TV images linking, by sight and sound alone, a mother and a two-month-old baby who can be in separate rooms (Murray and Trevarthen 1985; Trevarthen 1985b, 1986b). It is important to note that such exchanges are well-organized, in timing and affective modulation, before the baby shows much interest in visual, auditory, and tactual exploration of physical surroundings, and before effective grasping and manipulation are possible (Trevarthen 1984b). The latter skills are strengthened with the differentiation of the cortical systems of vision, and the stabilization of gravity-defying posture and mobility of the trunk, head and arms, in the third and fourth month. The mechanism in the striate cortex for visual hyperacuity and binocular stereoacuity evidently does not develop until the fifth month (Held 1985), indicating that protoconversations are controlled with little benefit from more elaborate neocortical processes and the information that they will eventually process.

Precocious though they are, with a probable anatomical substrate in subcortical and limbic mechanisms, protoconversations already reveal the existence of a number of asymmetrical or lateralized processes in the infant's brains. A majority of two-month-old infants, when being expressive in engagement with a supportive and responsive person, are more active with their right hands (Figure 20.2) and they turn their eyes toward the right (Trevarthen 1985b). They also show asymmetries of facial expression (Strauss et al. 1983; Studdert-Kennedy 1983, 1987; Trevarthen 1985b; Tucker and Frederick 1987) that resemble those reported for adults (Chaurasia and Goswami 1975; Sackheim and Gur 1978; Graves, Goodglass, and Landis 1982; Moscovich and Olds 1982; Wolf and Goodale, 1987; Figure 20.3). This suggests infants have greater activity, when attempting an utterance, in coordinative or regulatory systems located in the left side of their brains and at a level below the hemispheres. One possible contributor to this is the corpus striatum, which has a dopamine asymmetry that correlates with handedness (Glick et al. 1987). Asymmetries have also been demonstrated in electrical activity of the frontal lobes of infants about 10 months of age in response to face expressions of happiness (Davidson and Fox 1982).

It has been suggested that early asym-

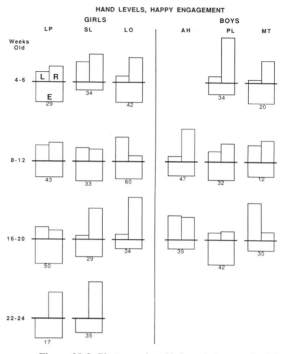

Figure 20.2. Photographs of infants in happy playful communication with their mothers revealed that the infants' hands were sometimes held at different levels when the baby was being expressive (Trevarthen 1986a). In a majority of cases the right hand (R) was held higher than the left (L). In many photographs, the levels of the two hands were equal (E). The histograms show that girls' gestures were right-handed at four to six weeks, but not at 8 to 12 weeks. Right-handedness returned after 16 weeks. Boys appeared to remain right-handed into the third month, and two of three boys showed a loss of right-handedness up to five months. This pilot study suggests that asymmetry of gestures is present at one to two months in boys and girls and tends to disappear in the period from three to six months and earlier in girls. The numbers of photographs used for each subject at each age, first selected without reference to hand positions, are indicated under the histograms. The areas of the rectangle represent the proportion of photographs for each positioning of the hands.

metries in infant behavior are the consequence of a one-sidedness in arousal or attention, which, in turn, is triggered by asymmetric sensory or motor systems or one-sided orienting reflexes (Turkewitz 1977, Michel 1981). However, complementary asymmetries in different kinds of behavior show that this theory of a single peripherally driven unmotivated asymmetry is inadequate (Kinsbourne and Hiscock

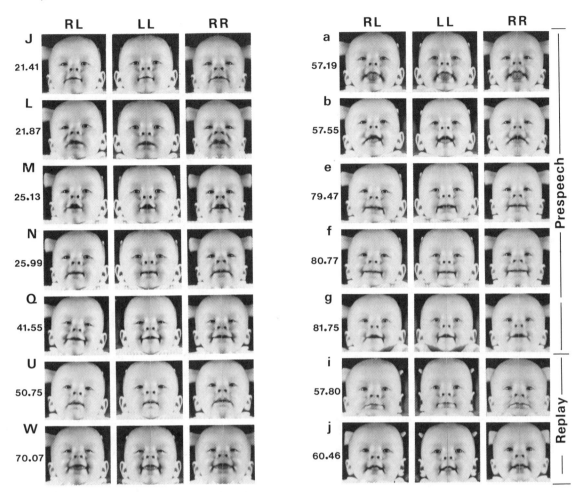

Figure 20.3. Photographs of TV images of an eight-week-old infant girl communicating with her mother's televised image (Trevarthen 1985b) show asymmetries in expressive movements. Full-face pictures, from the television screen (RL), are paired with double left (LL) and double right (RR) prints. Photographs are labeled according to a microanalysis previously published (Trevarthen 1985b). The time, in seconds, from the start of the analyzed sequence of communication is indicated by each photo. J to W sample moments in the engagement. After making eye contact, the baby smiles (J), with upper lip curled more on the right. The baby starts to coo, but moves only on the right (L); the full coo is also more curled up on the right (M). Asymmetries are also clear as the lips close (N). Smiles (Q and W) are stronger on the right, but a resting attentive face (U) is more symmetric. Movements from two prespeech sequences (a and b; e to g) show small asymmetries in tongue and lip movements. Note that the grimacelike movement in e and f starts larger on the left. Pictures i and j are taken from a sequence where the videotape of the mother was replayed to the baby, which caused distress. Time indications are taken from the tape of the mother. The infant is making attempts to communicate but these attempts are tense and challenging. In both photographs, the upper lips curl up more on the right, but i is more tightly closed on the left. Note that LL photos are "fatter" than RR photos when the infant is turning her head slightly to the right (L, M, N; e and f). This is particularly clear for the climax of the coo (M). The infant appears to turn slightly left when grimacing in i.

1983, Trevarthen 1986a). Newborns are sensitive to the human voice and they show evidence of prenatal learning of features of their mother's voice, preferring hers, from birth, to other female voices. Most tend to turn right when sleeping and they react more quickly to stimuli on the right. Dichotic listening tests indicate that a left-ear (right-hemisphere) advantage for musical sounds develops by two months, but a right-ear advantage for speech does not develop until later (Shucard, Shucard, and Thomas 1984; Mehler 1985). Young infants already have larger cortical evoked responses to speech from stimulation of the right ear. However, they also show stronger cortical responses to left-ear stimulation with musical notes, vocal prosody, and other "environmental" sounds, and music causes selective blockage of the infant precursors of the α rhythm in the right hemisphere (see Trevarthen 1984a, Mehler 1985, Shucard et al. 1984). The electrophysiological evidence thus supports the conclusion that infants perceive human vocalizatons by two different hemispheric systems from birth. The asymmetric activities recorded from the scalp of newborns will be projected up from deep subcortical asymmetries, rather than resulting from anatomicofunctional differences restricted to the cortex. Auditory input will be shunted to left or right hemisphere by mechanisms of the brainstem. Cortical areas concerned with speech are among the slowest to mature. They are certainly in a very different condition in the newborn from that in an adult brain.

Shucard et al. (1984) report interesting sex differences in the emergence of asymmetries in auditory evoked responses. At three months, speech and music both cause larger effects in the right hemisphere of males and the left hemisphere of females. At six months, the males have changed little, but the females show larger left-hemisphere responses to speech and larger right-hemisphere responses to music, as in adults. Evidently, the females are ahead of males at six months in this, as in other signs of hemispheric specialization (Held, Shimojo, and Gwiazda 1984; Trevarthen 1986a; Humphrey and Humphrey 1987). At six months, infants with strongest right-hand preferences for grasping, male and female, were the most advanced in hemispheric asymmetry for auditory effects (Shucard et al. 1984).

Experimental disruption of the infant's contact with the mother causes negative emotional reactions that show different lateralization from the positive expressions. In general, self-touching increases in distress (Murray and Trevarthen 1985), and this is usually done more by the left hand of one-to-six-month-olds (Trevarthen 1986a; Figure 20.4).

In infants three to five months of age, expressive hand movements are not so clearly lateralized as earlier or later (Figure 20.2). In this period, infants neither maintain eye contact with their mothers for long nor engage in protoconversational games. They prefer to explore surroundings, having acquired strong muscular support for the head and trunk, and thus a base for visual exploration that is both more stable and more mobile (Trevarthen 1984b). At four months, control of arm extension toward objects also improves, and it rapidly leads to effective prehension and development of controlled manipulation (Hofsten 1983, Trevarthen 1984b).

Asymmetries in use of the hands reappear after six months, most infants making reaching movements to pick up or extract objects with their right hands while tending to stabilize themselves, or objects, with the left hand (Seth 1973; Bresson et al. 1977; Ramsay, Campos, and Fenson 1979; Ramsay 1980; Trevarthen 1986a). Between three and six months, there may be a preference to reach out with the left hand (Gesell and Ames 1947, Seth 1973, Young 1977). Asymmetries also appear when the baby intercepts moving objects (von Hofsten and Lindhagen 1979, von Hofsten 1984). While it may express a postural asymmetry inherited from lower primates (MacNeilage, Studdert-Kennedy, and Lindblom 1987), right-handedness in prehension and manipulation of six-month-olds may also be coupled in a central mechanism that generates all expressive communication; Ramsay (1984) reports that the individual differences in the age at which a clear hand preference emerges correlate with the ages at which different babies start babbling. A right-hemisphere (left-visual-field) advantage has been reported for recognition of familiar faces by infants four to nine months, who

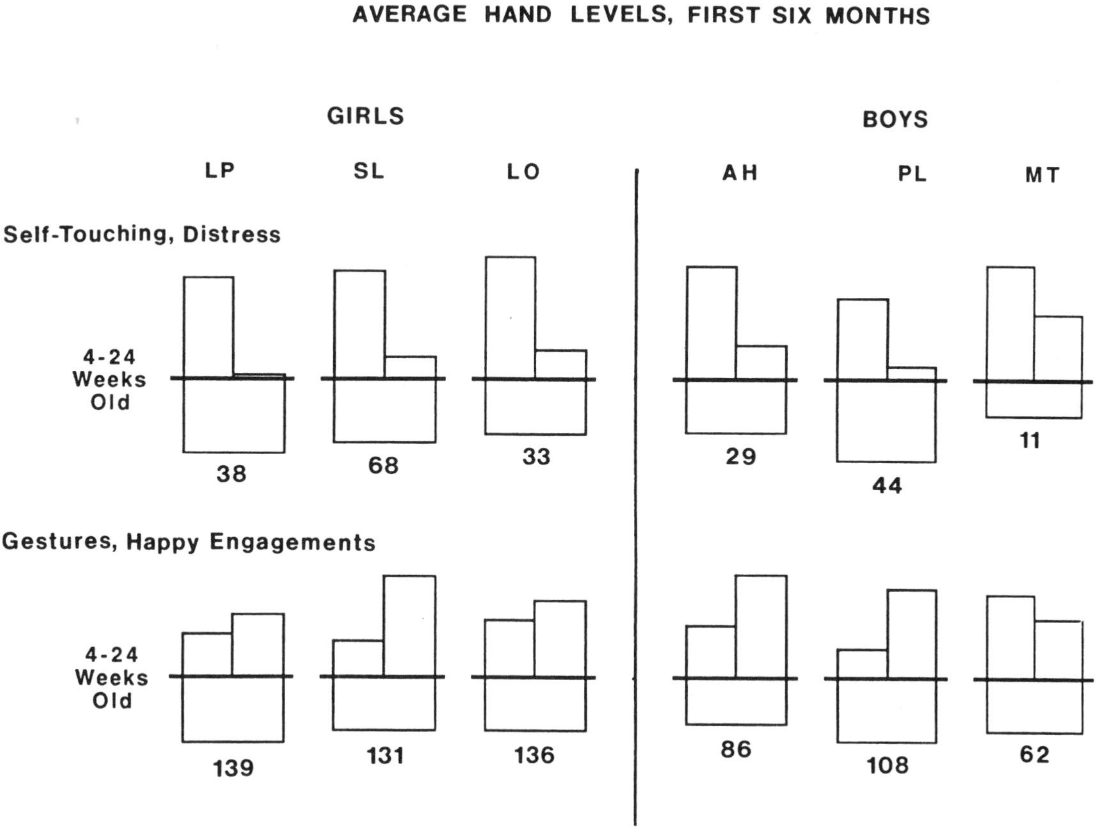

Figure 20.4. In the first six months, infants showed complementary asymmetries in hand positions, depending on their mood or state of communication (Trevarthen 1986a). In distress, when confronted by the mother keeping her face immobile or by a stranger, the babies tended to touch their clothes more with the left hand, which was also, in most cases, higher that the right. When in happy engagement with responsive mother, they were more likely to have the right hand raised higher. Conventions as in Figure 20.2.

distinguish them from unfamiliar faces (Schonen, Gild de Diaz, and Mathivet 1986).

Genetic disorders of brain growth that block development of symbolic intelligence

A rare condition called Rett's syndrome (Rett 1966) proves the power of intrinsic regulators of brain development over growth of cognition and the capacity to learn (Hagberg et al. 1983; Nomura, Segawa and Hasegawa 1984; Kerr and Stephenson 1985). This permanent infancy, or speechless mental handicap, known only in females, is associated with an X-chromosome fault that is evidently fatal in males in embryo (Comings 1986). At around nine months, a baby, who at six months was thought to be normal, shows signs of distracted attention, weak posture, and poor coordination of limb movements. The girl may advance through protolanguage and learn a few words, but by 18 months, she will be retarded and deeply disturbed in motivation and emotions. She will show autistic withdrawal from people, and fits of agitation, with screaming, lose voluntary use of her arms and hands, and make stereotyped patting or stroking movements, rubbing the hands together and bringing them, with athetoid twisting, to the mouth. Object prehension will cease, as will all deliberate gestures of communication.

By two, the autistic and agitated emotional features pass, leaving a condition of profound mental handicap that remains stable through three or four decades. Far from being avoidant, the girls, who can utter only undifferentiated calls and laughter, now seek eye contact and give quick social recognition, smiling or laughing in response to an approaching face, especially if it is accompanied by friendly cheerful speech and encouraging hand contact. Almost all Rett's syndrome girls have delicate attractive features and their gentle movements, seeming alertness, and positive orientation to people elicit strong efforts at communication from parents and siblings. Nevertheless, behind this expressiveness, their cognitive powers are minimal and they show little evidence of learning and no comprehension of language. Voluntary hand movements remain virtually absent; only crude hitting or grasping movements may be made to salient targets, often at moments when the child's efforts are being supported by a closely shadowing pattern of communication, as is practiced in music therapy. These movements of the Rett's child are not accompanied by deliberate visual orientation to the target. There is no speech, only infrequent cries and, in some cases, screaming. Most of the girls grind their teeth, which become displaced, and they exhibit poor control of lips and tongue, which often move in outbursts of activity that resemble prespeech of young infants, in synchrony with the periodic flailing, writhing, and clasping movements of the arms and hands. Inadequate oral control leads to dribbling.

Endocrine development and sexual maturation in Rett's girls appear unremarkable, and their brains appear surprisingly normal in standard neuropathological examination, though measures of head circumference are subnormal by 6 to 12 months, and below the 2% level of the normal population by two to four years, the brain growing little thereafter (Kerr and Stephenson 1985). Histochemistry of the brain has, so far, yielded no evidence of abnormality, except for suggestions of low pigmentation on the *substantia nigra* and *locus ceruleus*. The cause of catastrophic arrest of brain maturation, apparently cutting off neocortical development completely, is thus unknown, but available evidence points to a non-Mendelian gene fault expressed somewhere in the core of the brain, among neurones whose activity is essential to the formation of effective cortical networks (Kerr 1987).

Comparison between Rett's syndrome and autism is instructive. According to Kanner's original description (Kanner 1943), autism begins in the first two and one-half years. Cognitive and language development are interfered with following a disturbance of motivation affecting human contact. Notwithstanding a persistent conviction that the key fault is to be found in sensory or cognitive mechanisms, there is clear evidence for a primary emotional or motivational defect (Richer 1978), and it seems likely that widespread brain dysfunction results from faults in paramedian limbic and frontal parts, and in parts of the cerebellum (Damasio and Maurer 1978; Bauman and Kemper 1985). Autistic symptoms are produced in six-month-old monkeys by amygdala and hippocampus lesions made shortly after birth (Merjanian et al. 1986).

Autistic children do not orient normally to persons. Most avoid eye contact and they do not smile. Facial or vocal expressions of emotion are poorly perceived. Peculiarities of language, which is retarded, include confusion of personal reference. There is evidence for reduced left-hemisphere involvement in language in autistic children (Dawson et al. 1986). Intense narrowly focused concentration on manipulation and sensory exploration of objects, and fascination with music, drawing, or verbal games directed to the self are features of autistic children, including intelligent or "gifted" ones. In contrast to Rett's syndrome, autism is extremely varied and about four times more common in males. Where Rett's syndrome is essentially a genetic disease, autism appears to have multiple and variable etiology. Virus infection in early intrauterine stages is one likely factor. There is, however, a high incidence of Fragile X-chromosome disorder (Brown et al. 1986; Fisch et al. 1986; Hagerman et al. 1986a, 1986b).

In both autism and Rett's syndrome, a failure in deep affective communication is coupled to arrest or slowing of cognitive and linguistic development. Girls with Rett's syndrome can play with a partner at the level of a three to six-month-old, engaging in subtle exchanges of feelings, but they are incapable of imitative gestures or babbling, and they cannot manipulate objects. They show fluctuating awareness and motivation, having "absences" or blank periods. Episodes of hyperventilation may be linked to emotional panic or confused fear, and the complex motor stereotypes tend to increase when the girls are frightened or stressed. They can be patterned by music or the prosody of a story read slowly with dramatic emphasis. Autistic children also go into strange ecstatic states, in which they "float off," reaching out their arms, looking upward, and smiling in a vague "beatific" way. Thus, in spite of marked differences, the two conditions seem to share patterns of intrinsic fluctuation in motivation for experience, associated with poor communication with other human beings.

Rett's girls and autistic children, like a majority of profoundly mentally handicapped children, respond positively to a basal level of human expression; in almost every case, their alertness and motivation can be captured by music and movement therapy. This is evidence for retention of a fundamental, probably subcortical, system for coordination of motives with other persons, probably homologous with that which regulates play between a mother and a young infant. It remains to be determined how far restitution of a more complete communication and an increased measure of cognitive ability can be fostered by means of such techniques of emotional "transfusion."

These two diseases, in which cognitive development is powerfully impeded or distorted by a fault in brainstem motivating systems, lend support to the hypothesis that differential cognitive growth in the hemispheres of normal children may be regulated by asymmetric factors originating from beneath the cortex in the brainstem. Furthermore, multiple genetic factors, including a number in X chromosomes, may have the role of varying the patterns of hemispheric development to produce individual differences in patterning of cognitive competence (see also Grigsby, Kemper, and Hagerman 1987, who report an association between Gerstmann syndrome and Fragile X). Lateral asymmetries in behavior of Rett's girls or autistic children have yet to receive systematic study.

"Inner expression" is made coherent by asymmetric cerebral motives for communication from the start

In adults, the brain mechanism for communication is asymmetric as a whole; speech and hearing, hand signs and seeing, and writing and reading are all under dominant control by the left hemisphere. Language coordinates all organs of expression, including the hands in spontaneous movements that accompany conversational speech and express aspects of thinking in the message. The thinking of language gives times, spatial coordination, and conceptual integrity to movements of different body parts at a deep level (McNeill 1987). Furthermore, most people are right-handed for an endless variety of socially useful skills, not all of which are linguistic. There is evidence that, for oral and manual movements, all rapid serial motor coordination (motor sequencing) is lateralized to the left hemisphere (Kimura 1982). This may be based on a postural asymmetry inherited from monkeys (MacNeilage et al. 1987), but motor asymmetry is certainly associated with lateralized perception mechanisms (including the asymmetric auditory association cortex of the *planum temporale*).

Development of language shows the same unity, and asymmetry of intrinsic coordination, from the beginning and through all its stages. Research on the learning of sign language by deaf and hearing-impaired children indicates that, provided there is helpful and explicit input from the human environment to encourage the alternative to speech, similar stages of babbling, one-word, two-word syntax, and acquisition of morphology, inflexions, and anaphora occur in the mastery of language by hand-signing as by speech, and at the same ages. Thus, in the first three years, the child advances like a normal hearing and speaking child, through one word, sentence, and coherent discourse stages. Between three and six, the child, while already understanding syntax (how nominals are established and verbs made to agree), gains proficiency in signing these grammatical distinctions correctly, as a speaking child does.

In spite of the very different sensory and motor processes involved in using hand signs or speech, parallel advance is made through an order of communicative and grammatical skills, provided that a natural affectively positive environment of communication in the medium is given, beginning with a clarified "motherese" (Volterra 1981, 1986; Newport and Meier 1985; Bellugi et al. 1988). Moreover, similar errors of expression are made at the same ages in speech and signing. Remarkably, the same progression also appears when deaf, hearing-impaired, or hearing children are given early instruction in reading, an apparently more artificial form of communication that, nevertheless, can start as a natural language at the middle of the second year (Söderbergh 1981). That is, as soon as a child can be expected to speak, or sign, single words, that same child, or one who is partially or profoundly deaf, can learn to read single words. The written words have to be presented as a form of play, linked in the child's interest to the meanings to which they refer, and at moments when the child wants to share meanings. The meanings, in all cases, are found in referenda (persons, objects, or events) that greatly interest the child and that find their place naturally in spontaneous, emotional, playful communication with trusted companions and teachers.

How are we to interpret this? There must be some central drive in the child's mind that organizes ideas and their communication for all these superficially very different forms of language in the same way, and this drive to understand and use symbols must be regulated, by growth of brain tissues and their responses to experience, to elaborate at a particular rate and in a particular direction. Developments of the brain in the second and third year appear to be necessary for the process to start. Thereafter, new developments add proficiency in the production of grammatically correct, unambiguous, and context-free utterances. Neuropsychological investigations confirm that the brain mechanisms for speech and hand-signing, while different, have much in common (Poizner, Klima, and Bellugi 1987).

It is striking that the three very different forms of language are learned through a similar cooperative, emotional, and interpersonal exercise of consciousness and volition, at the early preschool age. It is also the case that, as in infancy, the form and content of communication by language in the second and third years depend on the child's motivation for interaction and joint enterprises. What appears to be a cognitive and rational advance, when one focuses attention only on the information and structural conventions the child takes in, recognizes, and remembers, looks more like a change in motives for seeking cooperation with other minds when the whole of the system, child and companions in their joint enterprises with respect to the shared and emotionally colored reality, is taken in view.

Sharpening the specification of the natural course of development, and finding its endogenous "constraints" or "motives," will certainly help in conceiving possible brain mechanisms for language development (Trevarthen 1987b). Conversely, we can hope to clear up some of the differences of interpretation about language learning, both before and after the child starts to make phonemic and graphemic analysis of words, by observing correlated changes that can be identified with structures or processes in the brain.

In the early stage of language, from 18 to 36 months, there is evidence for strengthening of cortical systems of the left half of the brain. Individual children may differ considerably in this period in their speech, consistency of handedness, and general motor coordination. They also give different results in dichotic tests for laterality in perception of verbal and nonverbal sounds and in visuospatial cognitive tasks (Kraft 1984). The majority, however, are clearly right-handed, the males being more varied in the rate of development of handedness and more of them are left-handed than among females. Nearly all toddlers are left-brained for hearing speech and have been so since infancy. A small minority of females shows very early strong left-handedness associated with precocious development of speech (Annett 1970; Trevarthen 1986a). It is important to emphasize that hand preference is shown in performance of imitated conventional forms of behavior, which automatically have communicative or "role-playing" significance, before the child has clear speech (Trevarthen 1986a). Handedness has behind it, therefore, components of motivation for expression of ideas to others independently of language, though clearly linked to forthcoming language. We came to the same conclusion from the asymmetries of gesture observed in early infancy (Trevarthen 1986a). Hand preferences and associated cognitive developments show, besides sex differences, familial consistency; children from dextral families are distinguishable from those with familial sinistrality (Kraft 1984).

After midpreschool, at about the age of four, a child can move into a social world that extends outside the family. Becoming increasingly dependent on an ability to speak like everyone else in the community, he or she needs to perform cultural activities with an acceptable level of some skill and understanding (Trevarthen and Logotheti 1989). The development appears to result from a freeing of the symbolic processes that were practiced in communication with the mother and other family members and tied to that intimate context. The child simultaneously gains an independence and confidence in cooperative fantasy play with peers. All these advances invite interpretation in terms of brain development.

Brain growth after birth: New evidence

After a maximum rate of growth from the midfetal stage, the human brain continues a rapid size increase for one and one-half years after birth. Between birth and one year, it more than doubles in weight (400 to 900 gm); by three, it reaches 80% of the adult brain size (1,100 gm compared to 1,350 gm), and it grows more and more slowly through the years that the body grows to maturity, leveling off about puberty (Lemire et al. 1975; Lecours 1982). Continuing the fetal trend, postnatal size increase takes place mainly in the cerebral hemispheres and neocerebellar cortex, and in the former, more growth occurs in the frontal, temporal, and parietal association cortex than in the primary sensory and motor zones, which are fully functional by two years.

At first sight, the obvious correlate of cultural learning in childhood is the relative expansion of inferoparietal, temporal, and frontal cortex, regions surrounding the Sylvian sulcus that have anatomical asymmetries from late fetal stages. In infants, cortical neurones in all areas develop their dendrites and a complement of synapses somewhat in excess of the final adult number. Cortical synaptogenesis appears to be a "catastrophic" process, the main population, for life, being formed in a synchronous wave throughout the neocortex at about the middle of the first year (Huttenlocher 1979; Huttenlocher et al. 1982; Rakic et al. 1986). Subsequent developments, resulting in major functional changes, appear to involve selective reinforcement of some synapses and loss of others, so the total number decreases, and these crucial advances in patterning for function occur with little change in brain mass.

Histological and histochemical studies confirm that, despite the synchronicity of synaptogenesis, agranular "association" cortices differentiate more slowly than granular "primary" areas. Myelin deposition on axons gives a measure of neurone maturity. The pioneering myelin studies of Flechsig (1901) and the Vogts (Vogt 1900) led to the conclusion that intracortical connections mature first in primary areas and last in perisylvian zones. Cycles of myelin formation in axons ascending and descending between the brainstem and cortex, and in the vast number of axons interconnecting near or distant cortical loci, including the interhemispheric connections, indicate that brain circuits undergo developmental transformation for decades, even though the brain changes little in size and surface appearance (Yakovlev and Lecours 1967; Lemire et al. 1975; Lecours 1982). The same conclusion is reached from observations on dendritic growth and the development of opiate and muscarinic receptor sites for cholinergic neurotransmitters that gate cortical cell function (Bachevalier et al. 1986). The neocortex continues to develop long after birth, in contrast to subcortical, limbic, and allocortical areas, and the primary receptor cortex matures before associative cortex. In monkeys, temporal association cortex maturing after birth contributes to changes in both visual recognition memory and habit formation (Bachevalier and Mishkin 1984). Maturation of the temporal cortex involved in habit formation is retarded by high levels of testosterone that appear in newborn male monkeys (Hagger et al. 1986).

By the myelin density criterion, late-maturing axons include both the long intrahemispheric association fibers inside each hemisphere and their functional equivalents, the interhemispheric fibers of the corpus callosum. Short associative links in the nonspecific "association" cortices (intracortical neuropil) of humans myelinate slowest of all the neocortical systems. Interestingly, axons of the reticular formation of the human brain core also myelinate for decades (Yakovlev and Lecours 1967).

Histological and physiological studies confirm that callosal neurones are equivalent in form, distribution, and function to the neurons that make interconnections between loci within a hemisphere (Innocenti 1986). Indeed, callosal and intracortical links develop from the one type of cell. In some regions of the cortex, these "stem association cells" of the developing cortex lose collaterals within the hemisphere and keep axons that cross in the commissures. In other regions, the reverse selection takes place. Intrahemispheric and commissural connections begin to segregate in this way in late fetal stages (Goldman-Rakic 1981, 1987), but the process continues long after birth. The number of axons in the corpus callosum (and presumably within a hemisphere, too) is at a maximum about birth. Innocenti (1983, 1986) has shown that a considerable proportion of these, perhaps as many as 9/10, are eliminated in the first half year, immediately after the wave of synapse formation on cortical cells. The current estimate of the number remaining is 800×10^6. Myelinization of callosal axons begins shortly after this, but continues for years (Yakovlev and Lecours 1967; Lecours 1982). Developments in intrahemispheric associative links, reflected in the changes in cohesion of electrical activity in the cortex that have recently been shown to continue through adolescence (Thatcher, Walker, and Giudice 1987), will be further discussed.

Functions of the developing commissures should be considered in terms of the mutual regulation of cortical systems, and their anatomicofunctional integration. Neocortical commissures serve not only in the transfer of perceptual information, or in facilitation or inhibition of cortical neuronal activity, but also in the differential activation and patterning of areas of one cortex in relation to areas on the other side to which they are attached through the corpus callosum. This is shown by the developmental effects of callosal agenesis and by comparing effects of early and late hemispherectomy, early and late unilateral lesions, and commissurotomy performed in adolescence or adulthood (Levy 1985).

The first formed interhemispheric commissure is the more primitive anterior commissure that carries allocortical (limbic) connections (see Chapter 11, this volume). In the corpus callosum, fibers of the corpus callosum grow in the anterior portion (genu) before those of the posterior part (splenium). The genu and central body of the corpus callosum increase in size more rapidly before birth, but the splenium grows quickly immediately after birth (Rakic and Yakovlev 1968). This may be connected with the rapid postnatal maturation of the visual cortices that waits on a patterned light environment. Psychologists have concluded that the postnatal maturation of the corpus callosum may increase interhemispheric communication, sharpen interhemispheric inhibition, or favor independence of hemispheric functions in childhood. Most of this thinking now seems too simplistic (Best 1985; Levy 1985).

Schonen and Bry (1987) present evidence that interhemispheric transfer of visual category discrimination learning (between normal and scrambled drawings of faces) develops five to six months after birth, that is, about the time the visual cortex is completing functional differentiation. This may be a consequence of maturation in the splenium of the corpus callosum, but a much slower development of the function of the corpus callosum in transmission of somesthetic information (vibratory stimulation) from the tip of the index finger to the ipsilateral parietal cortex has been demonstrated with the aid of evoked potentials (Salamy 1978). The latter study showed a decrease in callosal conduction time from 25 ms at four years to 5 ms from 10 years to adulthood, that is, over the period in which the body of the corpus callosum becomes increasingly myelinated. Tests for intermanual transfer of touch localization of the fingers also indicate that interhemispheric communication of hand awareness increases between five and seven years (Galin, Diamon, and Herron 1977). O'Leary (1980) demonstrated improvement in hand-to-hand kinesthetic transfer between seven and nine years. Liederman, Merola, and Hoffman (1986) used visual perception tests to show that hemispheric independence (resistance to perceptual interference) increases after 12 years, and they attribute this to maturation of the corpus callosum. Obviously, both contact and separation between the hemispheres can increase with callosal development.

It should not be forgotten that the corpus callosum is not the only system of fibers reaching the neocortex to undergo late myelinization. Nonspecific thalamic afferents, including the pulvinar input from brainstem coordinative systems important in governing orientation, behavior, and attention, also myelinate slowly after birth. Changes in connections of the cortex to and from the brainstem are just as likely to influence the balance of hemispheric activity and the coordination or separation of function in cortical systems as are connections across the corpus callosum, with which they certainly collaborate (Lecours 1982).

Thatcher et al. (1987) used measures of phase relations and coherence in EEG activity to infer development of intrahemispheric connectedness. Their data chart regional developments from birth to adolescence, which correlate well with the myelin studies and add the first reliable evidence of asymmetries in regional postnatal maturation of the cortex (Figure 20.5). Phases of development in long association systems (parietofrontal and temporofrontal) alternate between left and right hemisphere. Furthermore, development of short distance associations in cortical networks, which give increased coherence to their electrical activity, show up regional "hot spots" of growth in different lobes, and these, too, show significant asymmetries. These findings offer many intriguing correspondences with psychological developments, both socioemotional and cognitive. The authors confine themselves, however, to the observation that the important transitional periods seem to coincide with stage shifts in cognitive processes described by Piaget. Particularly interesting in relation to the development of language is a highly significant growth spurt in connections of the left hemisphere between two and four years of age.

We may confidently expect new findings on regional developments of the cortex and new distinctions between the growth patterns in left and right cortices. These may well include differences that relate to gender, handedness, educational level, deafness, or blindness, and other differences between individuals (Neville 1980). It will be increasingly clear that intrinsic regulations of postnatal brain growth, and in hemispheric plasticity of function (Witelson 1985), have relationship to the education of children in skills that they are expected to master to become intelligent members of the society. Underlying all such transformations of the cortex are change in motivation for social engagement and learning mediated by communication, and these will be regulated in subcortical systems of the brain. Very little is known about age-related changes in the functions of these parts.

Evidence from psychological developments to adolescence

With children over five, tests of perceptual discrimination and categorization reveal increasing awareness of significant features. This learning to perceive is correlated with differentiation of many cortical mechanisms, and, to judge from effects of sensory deprivation and brain lesions, competitive growth of complementary systems is involved. Tests with subjects who have had hemispherectomy or hemidecortication in infancy show that the hemispheres have considerable plasticity, in the sense that they can develop compensation for loss of systems that are normally lateralized to the side that has been taken away (Trevarthen 1984a, Goodman and Whitaker 1985). They also have an inborn commitment to different kinds of cognitive activity and memory, which limits this plasticity. Language tests show that an isolated right hemisphere can attain essentially normal phonemic and semantic abilities,

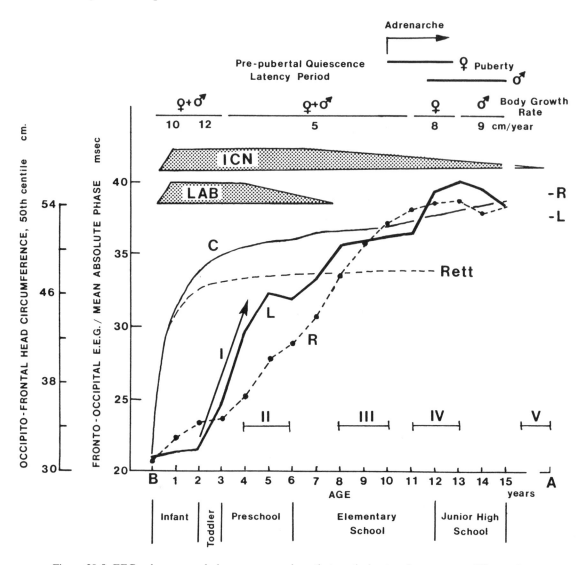

Figure 20.5. EEG coherence and phase measures show that cortical networks mature at different times in the left and right hemispheres (Thatcher et al. 1987). The periods of accelerated development in the cortex relate to histological changes and to phases of psychosocial and sexual development. EEG phase shows the right hemisphere (R) ahead from birth (B) to two and one-half years, and the left hemisphere (L) making a highly significant development from two to four years (I). EEG coherence increases rapidly in the frontal cortex, indicating a significant growth spurt of short-distance fibers about five years in the right frontal lobe (II). At the same time (four to six yrs) there is a pronounced increment in EEG phase for left temporal-frontal electrode pairs. The right temporal-frontal electrodes show a growth spurt from 8 to 10 years (III). Two growth spurts occur in both hemispheres, particularly in frontal cortex, at 11 to 13 years and between 15 and adulthood (A) (IV and V). Myelin deposition studies indicate that most of the long-association bundles (LAB), including the corpus callosum, mature between birth and five years, but short intracortical neuropil (ICN), making associations within each hemisphere, continue to develop through adolescence (from Lecours 1982). Increase in head circumference (C) does not correlate well with later stages of psychological growth. Rett's Syndrome girls show arrest of brain growth after midinfancy (Kerr and Stephenson 1985).

understanding descriptions of reality, and describing experiences and memories, but that a right brain on its own will fail in more complex sentence constructions such as passive negatives (Dennis 1980). Children with the left cortex removed, whom Dennis tested, fell back in grasp of rules for identifying purposeful responsibility of agents. In reading tests, they were deficient in extracting meaning from text and in recognizing correspondences between speech sounds and letters (Dennis, Lovett, and Weigel-Crump 1981). They also found difficulty with rhyming, which shows that awareness of word sounds, or their retrieval from short-term phonological memory, was weak.

The evidence from auditory evoked potentials in infants, mentioned before, indicates that prosodic features and affective content of vocalizations are detected at an earlier age than articulatory and verbal or referential aspects. This fits the evidence for a difference in contribution to communication by right and left hemispheres, respectively, in adults. Left-hemisphere lesions interfere with language expression and more elaborate aspects of word and sentence comprehension, leaving prosody and simple word understanding intact. Right-hemisphere lesions interfere with prosody, melodic expression, and poetic or metaphoric awareness, as well as perception of emotion in the expression of others (see Chapters 13, 18, and 19, this volume). Left hemispherectomy may leave a person with capacity to sing lyrics of well-practiced songs, but little capacity for ordinary speech. In a child, it may reduce the expressive vocabulary, leaving intonation and facial and gestural expression largely intact. This is evidence for an underlying asymmetry of motivation for engagement between the subject and other persons, with left-hemisphere language being organized within a context of nonverbal expression of feeling and understanding of purpose, such as is mastered by a toddler before speech. When a child has a dominant left hemisphere removed later in life, after the age of five, the effects on expressive language are more marked, indicating that developments after infancy lead to lateralization of motive systems governing initiation and patterning of articulation in speech or hand movements of writing.

From tests of visuospatial ability, children appear to move, possibly with enhancement of the effect by education, away from a wholistic intuitive grasp of the solution toward a more systematic rational approach that works out logical rules from critical features and their conjunctions (Trevarthen 1984a). Tests that tend to be solved by the left hemisphere in adults may be strongly affected by a right hemispherectomy in early childhood. That is, tasks that young children perform holistically may become recast in adolescence as verbally or analytically mediated, with a shift in lateralization to the left brain. This recalls the difference Bever and Chairello (1974) reported in cerebral dominance for perceiving music, between skilled musicians, trained to read music, who were left-hemisphere dominant, and untrained listeners, who were right-hemisphere dominant. A lesion in the right hemisphere before the shift may prevent development of the left-hemisphere style of processing. In a very few remarkable cases, supernormal verbal intelligence may occur with only the left-dominant hemisphere remaining, but most infantile hemiplegics have a general loss of intellect.

Skills of speech perception and speaking appear to be established at about adult levels only after about 11 to 13 years. Thus, tests of word perception with dichotic conflict of stimuli (different simultaneous inputs to the two ears), which show changes throughout childhood, test different brain processes at different ages. A right-ear superiority for accurate analytical perception of syllables, independent of short-term memory limitations characteristic of young children, does not appear until 8 to 12 years (Bryden and Allard 1978). This development depends upon support from a responsive human environment. Deprivation, from infancy, of speech and social isolation by pathological parents can lead a teenage child to suffer language retardation, as well as personality change, with atrophy of left-hemisphere language systems (Curtis 1977).

Visual perception of faces is another skill with an innate hemispheric basis that undergoes development through childhood, and it has received extensive study. Carey and Diamond (1980) found that around nine years, children change the way they see faces of unfamiliar people. They become more confused by inversion of pictures of faces, more attentive to defining features or additions (such as hat, glasses, or beard), and more distractable by the absence of such things. Carey and Diamond (1980) made the furthermost interesting observation that comparable developmental curves are seen for face recognition, voice recognition, and tonal memory, all functions served by the posterior-temporal sectors of the right hemisphere in adults. For all these abilities, there is a steep rise in performance level between 6 and 10 years, and then a plateau or dip between 10 and 16 years. Levine and Levy (1986) found a similar development of lateral asymmetries in perception of face expressions viewed as chimeric pictures in a free-field photobook test.

Levine (1985) has observed changes in the way faces are perceived with development of feature-detecting strategies that can show marked differences from subject to subject. Familiar faces, of people who are very well known, are most readily recognized when they are presented in the left visual field (right hemisphere) for all ages (cf. Schonen et al. 1986), but for unfamiliar faces, of strangers, the recognition strategy changes to the adult one, using more features, after age 9 or 10. Before that, strangers are recognized equally well when presented in the right field or the left field. Individual differences in face recognition by children and adults are related to habitual hemispheric activations, presumably of subcortical origin (Gur and Reivitch 1980; Levy et al. 1983; Levine, Banich, and Kim 1987). It is important to note that children change greatly in social autonomy and responsibility over this period in which their ability to recognize strangers is growing (Rogoff et al. 1975, 1980). They are becoming participant members of society.

Childrens' attempts to draw, and to reproduce the layout and detail of a model, change from the toddler stage through school age, and this can be explained by development of collaboration between strategies that are inherently different in the two hemispheres (Kirk 1985). This development will be related to the learning of writing, and reading, skills. Although even infants can, as we have described, begin to read printed words and know them as signs for objects of special interest for them, most children gain literacy as a result of formal instruction beginning at five or six years. Learning to read and write continues to advance for many years after that. Even with the best encouragement for early reading, no child will "crack the code" of grapheme-to-phoneme correspondence before the third year. The advantages of text for organizing narrative thoughts are not utilized until the child is at least five or six years older than this, about 8. It is, therefore, not surprising that an inherent deficit in cortical systems important for advanced reading does not show itself until a child is of school age.

Heritable specific dyslexia is a rare condition (Pennington et al. 1984) that appears to be associated with abnormalities of perisylvian cortex, particularly the angular gyrus, that first came about in prenatal stages (Galaburda et al. 1985). However, the affected child may have normal visual memory, mathematical ability, and general knowledge, and will appear to have normal, even superior, communication until past five or six years (Pennington et al. 1984). Experiments on effects of cortical lesions in monkeys demonstrate how late effects in psychological functioning can arise through maturation of new systems (Goldman-Rakic 1981, 1987). Moscovitch (1987) has reported that, with visual half-field tests, bilingual readers in Israel, who learn Hebrew first and show a left-hemisphere preference for this language at about eight years, do not develop left-hemisphere reading for English, which they start to learn at 10, until they are 16. Clearly, the lateralization depends upon experience in reading. Dyslexic children show their faults after grade 3, when they fail at this learning. They have the same lateral asymmetry as normal children, but are defective in left-hemisphere processes that have specific importance for reading.

Conclusions

I have considered findings in lines of psychological and neurological research that advance separately. They begin now to support one another. Inevitably, bringing them together is difficult. Nevertheless, certain clear and interesting prospects open before us.

The time seems ripe for psychology to

take deliberate interest in deep inherent motivating processes that underly the cognitive and volitional programs for not only language, but the whole of human cooperative intelligence and the way it allows for sharing of consciousness of meaning (knowledge) in the daily life of a society. Much more than a general learning ability or a general-purpose cognitive strategy underlies mutual awareness between humans and their intelligent cooperation. There is a highly organized system of motives and emotional evaluations that, moreover, are adapted to pass knowledge, of what to notice and how to act, on to the young. For their part, infants and children have brains with elaborate psychological adaptations to learn language and other skills of culture by communicating with parents, peers, and teachers.

Brain science, independently, is becoming increasingly concerned with intrinsic determinants or "constraints" on functional systems that learn. These systems have definite anatomical localization in the adult brain and refined microstructure and chemistry. Approaching this developmentally, we find that the associative systems of the neocortex, though genetically prewired to a degree, grow in response to stimulation, but in interaction and under protracted regulation from reticular and limbic structures that have formative primacy in both evolution and ontogeny. Perceptions, cognitions and the forming of memories and habits themselves are gated by these subcortical systems (see Chapter 13, this volume).

Psychology and brain science come together in the scientific analysis of cerebral localization of function. Asymmetries of function, correlated with the deeply separated left and right cerebral hemispheres, have particular value in the opening up of an approach to mental activities at the highest level. Cognitive and voluntary processes that attain maturity only after many years and that have special importance in cultural life tend to be asymmetric in the brain. The basis for this asymmetry seems to be set down very early, probably in fetal stages. It becomes elaborated in the subsequent development of the brain. Throughout childhood, as the brain takes up the lessons of experiences, and even in the moment-to-moment adjustments of adult consciousness, structures beneath the cortex continue to exercise their regulations. They assist in the development of a bihemispheric system in which the two sides have complementary roles.

Finally, completing the picture, we find evidence that the intrinsic regulators of human brain growth in a child are specially adapted to be coupled, by emotional communication, to the regulators of adult brains of people who know more. This seems to be the key generic brain strategy for cultural learning, learning that takes place not in single brains, but in communities of them. Developmental brain science will have great importance in future efforts to understand the growing human mind, and the life of ideas and beliefs in human communities.

No one scientist matches Roger Sperry's breadth of interest in all these basic matters of brain growth and their relation to the psychology of perception and coordinated action or the components of consciousness in a human mind. I could not, and would not, have begun to make the kind of analysis presented here without the inspiration of his work. I have also been greatly impressed by the conclusion he has come to that inherent values govern the patterning and flow of consciousness in the human world.

His ideas on these matters, and on the importance of emotional factors in the formation of human thought patterns, in the individual and socially, are given significant clarification in the Nobel Prize Conversations held at the Dallas Isthmus Institute in 1982 (Nobel Prize Conversations 1985).

References

Annett, M. 1970. The growth of manual preference and speed. *Brit. J. Psychol.* 61: 545–58.

Armstrong, E. 1985. Allometric considerations of the adult mammalian brain, with special emphasis on primates. *In* W. Jungers (ed.) *Size and Scaling in Primate Biology.* Academic Press, New York.

Bachevalier, J., and M. Mishkin. 1984. An early and a late developing system for learning and retention in infant monkeys. *Behav. Neurosci.* 98: 770–8.

Bachevalier, J., L. G. Ungerleider, J. B. O'Neill, and D. P. Friedman. 1986. Regional distribution of [³H]naloxone binding in the brain of a newborn rhesus monkey. *Devel. Brain Res.* 25: 302–8.

Baker, R. S. 1985. Horseradish peroxidase tracing of dorsal root ganglion afferents within fetal mouse spinal cord explants chronically exposed to tetrodotoxin *Brain Res.* 334: 357–60.

Bauman, M. L., and T. L. Kemper. 1985. Histoanatomic observations of the brain in early infantile autism. *Neurol.* 35: 866–74.

Bellugi, U., K. van Hoek, D. Lillo-Martin, and L. O'Grady. 1988. The acquisition of syntax and space in young deaf singers. *In* D. Bishop and K. Mogford (eds.) *Language Development in Exceptional Circumstances*. Churchill Livingstone, London.

Best, C. T. 1985. Introduction. *In* C. T. Best (ed.) *Hemispheric Function and Collaboration in the Child*. Academic Press, Orlando (FL).

Bever, T. G., and R. J. Chiarello. 1974. Cerebral dominance in musicians and non-musicians. *Science* 185: 537–9.

Björklund, A., and U. Stenevi. 1979. Regeneration of monoaminergic and cholinergic neurons in the mammalian central nervous system. *Physiol. Rev.* 59: 62–100.

Bradshaw, J. L., and N. C. Nettleton. 1983. *Human Cerebral Asymmetry*. Prentice-Hall, Englewood Cliffs (NJ).

Bresson, F., L. Maury, G. Pieraut Le Bonniec, and S. de Schonen. 1977. Organization and lateralization of reaching in infants: An instance of dissymmetric functions in hands collaboration. *Neuropsychol.* 15: 311–20.

Brown, W. T., E. C. Jenkins, I. L. Cohen, G. S. Fisch, E. G. Wolf-Schen, A. Gross, L. Waterhouse, D. Fein, A. Mason-Brothers, E. Ritvo, B. A. Ruttenberg, W. Bentley, and S. Castells. 1986. Fragile-X and autism: A multicenter survey. *Am. J. Med. Gen.* 23: 341–52.

Bryden, M. P., and F. Allard. 1978. Dichotic listening and the development of linguistic processes. *In* M. Kinsbourne (ed.) *Hemispheric Asymmetries of Function*. Cambridge University Press, New York.

Carey, S., and R. Diamond. 1980. Maturational determination of the developmental course of face encoding. *In* D. Caplan (ed.) *Biological Studies of Mental Processes*. MIT Press, Cambridge.

Changeux, J.-P. 1985. *Neuronal Man: The Biology of Mind*. Pantheon, New York.

Changeux, J.-P., T. Heidmann, and P. Patter. 1984. Learning by selection. *In* P. Marler and H. S. Terrace (eds.) *The Biology of Learning*. Springer-Verlag, Berlin, Heidelberg, New York, Tokyo.

Chaurasia, B. D., and H. K. Goswami. 1975. Functional asymmetry of the face. *Acta Anat.* 91: 154–60.

Comings, D. E. 1986. The genetics of Rett Syndrome: The consequences of a disorder where every case is a new mutation. *Am. J. Med. Gen.* 24: 383–8.

Conel, J. LeRoy. 1939–1963. *The Postnatal Development of the Human Cerebral Cortex,* Vols. I–VI. Harvard University Press, Cambridge.

Corballis, M. 1983. *Human Laterality*. Academic Press, New York.

Corballis, M., and I. L. Beale. 1976. *The Psychology of Left and Right*. Lawrence Erlbaum, Hillsdale (NJ).

Curtis, S. 1977. *Genie: A Linguistic Study of a Modern Day "Wild Child."* Academic Press, New York.

Damasio, A. R., and R. G. Maurer. 1978. A neurological model for childhood autism. *Arch. Neurol.* 35: 777–86.

Davidson, R. J., and N. A. Fox. 1982. Asymmetric brain activity discriminates between positive and negative affective stimuli in human infants. *Science* 218: 1235–6.

Dawson, G., S. Phillips, L. Galpert, and C. Finley. 1986. Hemispheric specialization and the language abilities of autistic children. *Child Dev.* 57: 1440–53.

Dennis, M. 1980. Language acquisition in a single hemisphere: Semantic organization. *In* D. Caplan (ed.) *Biological Studies of Mental Processes*. The MIT Press, Cambridge.

Dennis, M., M. Lovett, and C. A. Weigel-Crump. 1981. Written language acquisition after left or right hemidecortication in infancy. *Brain and Lang.* 12: 54–91.

Diamond, M. C. 1987. Asymmetry in the cerebral cortex: Development, estrogen receptors, neuron/glial ratios, immune deficiency and enrichment/overcrowding. *In* D. Ottoson (ed.) *Duality and Unity of the Brain,* Wenner-Gren International Symposium Series, No. 47. Macmillan, London.

Dimond, S. 1972. *The Double Brain*. Churchill Livingstone, Edinburgh and London.

Dobbing, J. 1981. The later development of the brain and its vulnerability. *In* J. A. Davis and J. Dobbing (eds.) *Scientific Foundations of Paediatrics,* 2nd Ed. Heinemann, London.

Dunnett, S. B., A. Björklund, and U. Stenevi. 1983. Dopamine-rich transplants in experimental parkinsonism. *Trends in Neurosci.* 6: 266–75.

Fisch, G. S., I. L. Cohen, E. G. Wolf, W. T. Brown, and E. C. Jenkins. 1986. Autism and fragile-X syndrome. *Am. J. Psychiat.* 143: 71–3.

Flechsig, P. 1901. Developmental (myelogenetic) localization of the cerebral cortex in the human subject. *Lancet* 2: 1027–9.

Fox, N. A., and R. J. Davidson (eds). 1984. *The Psychology of Affective Development*. Lawrence Erlbaum, Hillsdale (NJ).

Gainotti, G. 1987. Disorders of emotional behavior and of automatic arousal resulting from unilateral brain damage. *In* D. Ottoson (ed.) *Duality and Unity of the Brain,* Wenner-Gren International Symposium Series, No. 47. Macmillan, London.

Galaburda, A. M., G. F. Sherman, G. D. Rosen, F. Aboitiz, and N. Geschwind. 1985. Developmental dyslexia: Four consecutive cases with cortical anomalies. *Ann. Neurol.* 18: 222–33.

Galin, D., R. Diamon, and J. Herron. 1977. Development of crossed and uncrossed tactile localization in the fingers. *Brain and Lang.* 4: 588–90.

Geffen, G. 1978. The development of right ear advantage in dichotic listening with focussed attention. *Cortex* 14: 169–77.

Gerendai, I. 1987. Laterality and the neuroendocrine system. *In* D. Ottoson (ed.) *Duality and Unity of the Brain,* Wenner-Gren International Symposium Series, No. 47. Macmillan, London.

Geschwind, N., and A. M. Galaburda. 1985. Cerebral lateralization. Biological mechanisms, associations and pathology. I. An hypothesis and a program for research. *Arch. Neurol.* 42: 428–59.

Gesell, A., and L. B. Ames. 1947. The development of handedness. *J. Genet. Psychol.* 70: 155–75.

Glick, S. D., J. N. Carlson, K. L. Drew, and R. M. Shapiro. 1987. Functional and neurochemical asymmetry in the corpus striatum. *In* D. Ottoson (ed.) *Duality and Unity of the Brain,* Wenner-Gren International Symposium Series, No. 47. Macmillan, London.

Goldman-Rakic, P. S. 1981. Development and plasticity of primate association cortex. *In* F. O. Schmitt (ed.) *The Organization of the Cerebral Cortex.* The MIT Press, Cambridge.

–1987. Development of cortical circuitry and cognitive function. *Child Dev.* 58: 601–22.

Goodman, R. A., and H. A. Whitaker. 1985. Hemispherectomy: A review (1928–1981) with special reference to the linguistic abilities and disabilities of the residual right hemisphere. *In* C. T. Best (ed.) *Hemispheric Function and Collaboration in the Child.* Academic Press, Orlando (FL).

Graves, R., H. Goodglass, and T. Landis. 1982. Mouth asymmetry during spontaneous speech. *Neuropsychol.* 20: 371–81.

Grigsby, J. P., M. B. Kemper, and R. J. Hagerman. 1987. Developmental Gerstmann syndrome without aphasia in fragile-X syndrome *Neuropsychol.* 25: 881–91.

Gur, R. C., and M. Reivitch. 1980. Cognitive task effects on hemispheric blood flow in humans: Evidence for individual differences in hemispheric activation. *Brain and Lang.* 9: 78–92.

Hagberg, B., J. Aicardi, K. Dias, and O. Ramos. 1983. A progressive syndrome of autism, dementia, ataxia and loss of purposeful hand use in girls. Rett Syndrome: Report of 35 cases. *Ann. Neurol.* 14: 471–9.

Hagerman, R. J., A. W. Jackson III, M. Braden, B. Rimland, and A. Levitas. 1986a. An analysis of autism in fifty males with fragile-X syndrome. *Am. J. Med. Gen.* 23: 353–8.

Hagerman, R. J., A. W. Jackson III, M. Kemper, R. Ahmad, A. E. Chudley, and J. H. Knoll. 1986b. Autism in fragile-X females. *Am. J. Med. Gen.* 23: 375–80.

Hagger, C., J. Bachevalier, and B. B. Bercu. 1986. The effects of perinatal testosterone on the development of habit formation in infant monkeys. *Soc. Neurosci. Abst.* 12: 23.

Halliday, M. A. K. 1975. *Learning How to Mean,* Arnold, London.

Hamburger, V. 1973. Anatomical and physiological basis of embryonic motility in birds and mammals. *In* G. Gottlieb (ed.) *Studies on the Development of Behavior and the Nervous System.* Academic Press, New York.

Harshman, R. A., and E. Hampson. 1987. Normal variation in human brain organization: Relation to handedness, sex and cognitive abilities. *In* D. Ottoson (ed.) *Duality and Unity of the Brain,* Wenner-Gren International Symposium Series, No. 47. Macmillan, London.

Hebb, D. O. 1949. *The Organization of Behavior.* Wiley, New York.

Hein, A., F. Vital-Durand, W. Salinger, and R. Diamond. 1979. Eye movements initiate visual-motor development in the cat. *Science* 204: 1321–2.

Held, R. 1985. Binocular vision – behavioral and neuronal development. *In* J. Mehler and R. Fox (eds.) *Neonate Cognition: Beyond the Blooming Buzzing Confusion.* Lawrence Erlbaum, Hillsdale (NJ).

Held, R., S. Shimojo and J. Gwiazda. 1984. Gender differences in the early development of human visual resolution. (Proceedings of the ARVO Meeting, April–May 1984, Abstract No. 90.) *Inv. Ophthalmol. Vis. Sci.* 25: 220.

Herrick, C. J. 1948. *The Brain of the Tiger Salamander.* University of Chicago Press, Chicago.

Hofsten, C. von. 1983. Catching skills in infancy. *J. Exp. Psychol.: Human Percep. Perf.* 9: 75–85.

–1984. Developmental changes in the organization of prereaching movements. *Dev. Psychol.* 20: 378–88.

Hofsten, C. von, and K. Lindhagen. 1979. Observations on the development of reaching for moving objects. *J. Exp. Child Psychol.* 28: 158–73.

Hökfelt, T. 1987. Neuronal mapping by transmitter histochemistry with special reference to coexistence of multiple synaptic messengers. *In* G. Adelman (ed.) *Encyclopedia of Neuroscience,* Vol. II. Birkhäuser Boston, Cambridge.

Hubley, P., and C. Trevarthen. 1979. Sharing a task in infancy. *In* I. Uzgiris (ed.) *Social Interaction During Infancy. Vol. 4: New Directions for Child Development.* Jossey-Bass, San Francisco, pp. 57–80.

Humphrey, D. E., and G. K. Humphrey. 1987. Sex differences in infant reaching. *Neuropsychol.* 25: 971–5.

Huttenlocher, P. R. 1979. Synaptic density in human frontal cortex – developmental changes and effects of ageing. *Brain Res.* 163: 195–205.

Huttenlocher, P. R., C. de Courten, L. J. Garey, and H. Van der Loos. 1982. Synaptogenesis in human visual cortex – evidence for synapse elimination during normal development. *Neurosci. Lett.* 33: 247–52.

Imbert, M. 1985. Physiological underpinnings of perceptual development. *In* J. Mehler and R. Fox (eds.) *Neonate Cognition.* Lawrence Erlbaum, Hillsdale (NJ).

Innocenti, G. M. 1983. Exuberant callosal projections between the developing hemispheres. *In* R. Villani, I. Papo, M. Giovanelli, S. M. Gaini, and G. Tomei (eds.) *Advances in Neurotraumatology.* Excerpta Medica, Amsterdam.

–1986. General organization of the callosal connections in the cerebral cortex. *In* E. G. Jones and A. Peters (eds.) *Cerebral Cortex,* Vol. 5. Plenum, New York.

Iverson, L. L. 1987. Neurotransmitters. *In* G. Adelman (ed.) *Encyclopedia of Neuroscience.* Birkhaüser Boston, Cambridge.

Kanner, L. 1943. Autistic disturbances of affective contact. *Nervous Child* 2: 217–50.

Kerr, A. M. 1987. Report on the Rett Syndrome Workshop: Glasgow, Scotland, 24–25 May 1986. *J. Ment. Def. Res.* 31: 93–113.

Kerr, A. M., and J. B. P. Stephenson. 1985. Rett's syndrome in the west of Scotland. *Brit. Med. J.* 291: 579–82.

Kimura, D. 1982. Left-hemisphere control of oral and brachial movements and their relation to communication. *Phil. Trans. Roy. Soc. London, Ser. B* 298: 135–49.

Kinsbourne, M., and M. Hiscock. 1983. Functional lateralization of the brain: Implications for normal and deviant development. *In* M. M. Haith and J. J. Campos (eds.) *Handbook of Child Psychology, Volume 2: Infancy and Developmental Psychobiology.* Wiley, New York.

Kirk, U. 1985. Hemispheric contributions to the development of graphic skill. *In* C. T. Best (ed.) *Hemispheric Function and Collaboration in the Child.* Academic Press, Orlando (FL).

Kraft, R. H. 1984. Lateral specializations and verbal/spatial ability in preschool children: Age, sex and familial handedness differences. *Neuropsychol.* 22: 319–35.

Lancaster, J. 1986. Human adolescence and reproduction. *In* J. Lancaster and B. Hamburg (eds.) *School-Age Pregnancy and Parenthood: Biosocial Dimensions.* Aldine-DeGruyter, New York.

Lecours, A. R., 1982. Correlates of developmental behavior in brain maturation. *In* T. G. Bever (ed.) *Regressions in Mental Development: Basic Phenomena and Theories.* Lawrence Erlbaum, Hillsdale (NJ).

Lemire, R. J., J. D. Loeser, R. W. Leech, and E. C. Alvord. 1975. *Normal and Abnormal Development of the Human Nervous System.* Harper and Row, New York.

Levine, S. C. 1985. Developmental changes in right-hemisphere involvement in face recognition. *In* C. Best (ed.) *Hemispheric Function and Collaboration in the Child.* Academic Press, New York.

Levine, S. C., M. T. Banich, and H. Kim. 1987. Variations in arousal asymmetry: Implications for face processing. *In* D. Ottoson (ed.) *Duality and Unity of the Brain,* Wenner-Gren International Symposium Series, No. 47. Macmillan, London.

Levine, S. C., and J. Levy. 1986. Perceptual asymmetry for chimeric faces across the life span. *Brain and Cog.* 5: 291–306.

Levy, J. 1985. Interhemispheric collaboration: Single-mindedness in the asymmetric brain. *In* C. T. Best (ed.) *Hemispheric Function and Collaboration in the Child.* Academic Press, Orlando (FL).

Levy, J., W. Heller, M. T. Banich, and L. A. Burton. 1983. Are variations in right-handed individuals in perceptual asymmetries caused by characteristic arousal differences between hemispheres? *J. Exp. Psychol.: Human Percep. Perf.* 9: 329–59.

Leiderman, J., J. L. Merola, and C. Hoffman. 1986. Longitudinal data indicate that hemispheric independence increases during early adolescence. *Dev. Neuropsychol.* 2(3): 183–201.

Loehlin, J. C., L. Willerman, and J. M. Horn. 1988. Human behavior genetics. *Ann. Rev. Psychol.* 39: 101–33.

MacKinnon, P. C. B., and B. Greenstein. 1985. Sexual differentiation of the brain. *In* F. Falkner and J. M. Tanner (eds.) *Human Growth: A Comprehensive Treatise. Vol. 2: Postnatal Growth; Neurobiology.* Plenum, New York.

MacNeilage, P. F., M. G. Studdert-Kennedy, and B. Lindblom. 1987. Primate handedness reconsidered. *Behav. Brain Sci.* 10: 247–303.

Marin-Padilla, M. 1970. Prenatal and early post-natal ontogenesis of the cerebral neocortex of the cat (*Felis domestica*): A Golgi study. I. The primordial neocortical organization. *Z. Anat. Entwichlungsgesch.* 134: 117–45.

Mark, R. F. 1974. *Memory and Nerve-Cell Connections.* Oxford University Press, London.

Malsburg, C. von der, and W. Singer. 1988. Principles of cortical network organisation. *In* P. Rakic and W. Singer (eds.) *Neurobiology of the Neocortex,* Dahlem Conference, Life Sciences Research Report No. 42. Wiley, Chichester and New York.

McGeer, P. L., J. C. Eccles, and E. G. McGeer. 1978. *Molecular Neurobiology of the Mammalian Brain.* Plenum, New York.

McNeill, D. 1987. *Psycholinguistics: A New Approach.* New York, Harper and Row.

Mehler, J. 1985. Language related dispositions in early infancy. *In* J. Mehler and R. Fox (eds.) *Neonate Cognition.* Lawrence Erlbaum, Hillsdale (NJ).

Merjanian, P. M., J. Bachevalier, H. Crawford. and M. Mishkin. 1986. Socioemotional disturbances in the developing rhesus monkey following neonatal limbic lesions. *Soc. Neurosci. Abst.* 12: 23.

Michel, G. F. 1981. Right-handedness: A consequence of infant supine head-orientation preference? *Science* 212: 685–7.

Mishkin, M. 1982. A memory system in the monkey. *Phil. Trans. Roy. Soc. London, Ser. B* 298: 85–95.

Morest, D. K. 1970. A study of neurogenesis in the forebrain of the opposum pouch young. *Z. Anat. Entwichlungsgesch.* 130: 265–305.

Moscovitch, M. 1987. Lateralization of language in children with developmental dyslexia: A critical review of visual half-field studies. *In* D. Ottoson (ed.) *Duality and Unity of the Brain,* Wenner-Gren International Symposium Series, No. 47. Macmillan, London.

Moscovitch, M., and J. Olds. 1982. Asymmetries in spontaneous facial expressions and their possible relation to hemispheric specialization. *Neuropsychol.* 20: 71–81.

Murray, E. A., and M. Mishkin. 1985. Amygdalectomy impairs cross-modal association in monkeys. *Science* 228: 604–6.

Murray, L., and C. Trevarthen. 1985. Emotional regulation of interactions between two-month-olds and their mothers. *In* T. Field and N. Fox (eds.) *Social Perception in Infants.* Ablex, Norwood (NJ).

Nauta, W. J. H., and M. Fiertag. 1986. *Fundamental Neuroanatomy.* W. H. Freeman, San Francisco.

Neville, H. J. 1980. Event-related potentials in neuropsychological studies of language. *Brain and Lang.* 11: 300–18.

Newport, E. L., and R. P. Meier. 1985. The acquisition of American Sign Language. *In* D. E. Slobin (ed.) *The Crosslinguistic Study of Language Acquisition. Vol. I: The Data.* Lawrence Erlbaum, Hillsdale (NJ).

Nobel Prize Conversations, 1985. *Nobel Prize Conversations with Sir John Eccles, Roger Sperry, Ilya Prigogine and Brian Josephson.* at the Dallas Isthmus Institute (with a commentary by Normal Cousins). Saybrook, Dallas.

Nomura, Y., M. Segawa, and M. Hasegawa. 1984. Rett's syndrome – clinical studies and pathophysiological consideration. *Brain and Dev.* 6: 475–86.

Nordeen, D. J. and P. Yahr. 1982. Hemispheric asymmetries in the behavioral and sexual differentiation in the mammal brain. *Science* 218: 391–4.

Oke, A., R. Keller, I. Mefford, and R. N. Adams. 1978. Lateralization of norepinephrine in human thalamus. *Science* 200: 1411–13.

O'Leary, D. 1980. A developmental study of interhemispheric transfer in children aged five to ten. *Child Dev.* 51: 743–50.

Oppenheim, R. W. 1984. Cellular interactions and the survival and maintenance of neurons during development. *In* S. C. Sharma (ed.) *Organizing Principles of Neural Development.* Plenum, New York.

Oppenheim, R. W., and J. Reitzel, 1975. Ontogeny of behavioral sensitivity to strychnine in the chick embryo: Evidence for the early onset of CNS inhibition. *Brain, Behav. Evol.* 11: 130–59.

Pennington, B. F., S. D. Smith, L. L. McCabe, W. J. Kimberling, and H. A. Lubs. 1984. Developmental continuities and discontinuities in a form of familial dyslexia. *In* R. N. Emde and R. J. Harmon (eds.) *Continuities and Discontinuities in Development.* Plenum, New York.

Piaget, J. 1962. *Play, Dreams and Imitation in Early Childhood.* Routledge and Kegan Paul, London.

–1970. Piaget's theory. *In* P. H. Mussen (ed.) *Carmichel's Manual of Child Psychology*, Vol. I. Wiley, New York.

Piaget, J., and B. Inhelder. 1969. *The Psychology of the Child.* Routledge and Kegan Paul, London.

Poizner, H. R., E. S. Klima, and U. Bellugi. 1987. *What the Hands Reveal About the Brain.* The MIT Press, Cambridge.

Rakic, P., J.-P. Bourgeois, M. F. Eckenhoff, N. Zecevic, and P. S. Goldman-Rakic. 1986. Concurrent overproduction of synapses in diverse regions of the primate cerebral cortex. *Science* 232: 232–5.

Rakic, P., and P. I. Yakovlev. 1968. Development of the corpus callosum and cavum septi in man. *J. Comp. Neurol.* 132: 45–72.

Ramsay, D. S. 1980. Onset of unimanual handedness in infants. *Infant Behav. Dev.* 3: 377–85.

–1984. Onset of duplicated syllabic babbling and unimanual handedness in infancy: Evidence for developmental change in hemispheric specialization. *Dev. Psychol.* 20: 64–71.

Ramsay, D. S., J. J. Campos, and L. Fenson. 1979. Onset of bimanual handedness in infants. *Infant Behav. Dev.* 2: 69–75.

Rett, A. 1966. Uber ein eigenartiges hirnatrophisches Syndrom bei Hyperammonamie im Kindesalter. *Wien Med. Wochensch.* 116: 723–6.

Richer, J. M. 1978. The partial non-communication of culture to autistic children. *In* M. Rutter and E. Schopler (eds.) *Autism: A Reappraisal of Concept and Treatment.* Plenum, New York.

Rogoff, B., N. Newcombe, N. Fox, and S. Ellis. 1980. Transitions in children's roles and capabilities. *Int. J. Psychol.* 15: 181–200.

Rogoff, B., M. J. Sellers, S. Pirrotta, N. Fox, and S. H. White. 1975. Age assignment of roles and responsibilities to children: A cross-cultural survey. *Human Dev.* 18: 353–69.

Rogoff, B., and J. V. Wertsch (eds.). 1984. *Children's Learning in the "Zone of Proximal Development" (New Directions for Child Development, No. 23).* Jossey-Bass, San Francisco.

Sackeim, H. A., and R. C. Gur. 1978. Lateral asymmetry in intensity of emotional expression. *Neuropsychol.* 16: 473–81.

Salamy, A. 1978. Commissural transmission: Maturational changes in humans. *Science* 200: 1409–11.

Scheibel, A. B. 1984. The brain stem reticular core and sensory function. *In* I. Darian-Smith (ed.) *Handbook of Physiology: The Nervous System III, Part 1.* American Physiological Society, Washington (DC).

Schonen, S. de, and I. Bry. 1987. Interhemispheric communication of visual learning: A developmental study in 3–6 month old infants. *Neuropsychol* 25: 601–12.

Schonen, S. de, M. Gild de Diaz, and E. Mathivet. 1986. Hemispheric asymmetry in face processing in infancy. *In* H. D. Ellis, M. A. Jeeves, F. Newcombe, and A. W. Young (eds.) *Aspects of Face Processing.* Martinus Nijhoff, Dordrecht.

Seth, G. 1973. Eye-hand co-ordination and "handedness": A development study of visuo-motor behaviour in infancy. *Brit. J. Educ. Psychol.* 43: 34–49.

Sherman, G. F., A. M. Galaburda, and N. Geschwind. 1982. Neuroanatomical asymmetyries in non-human species. *Trends in Neurosci.* 2: 429–31.

Shucard, D. W., J. L. Shucard, and D. G. Thomas. 1984. The development of cerebral specialization in infants: Electrophysiological and behavioral studies. *In* R. N. Emde and R. J. Harmon (eds.) *Continuities and Discontinuities in Development.* Plenum, New York.

Sidman, R. L., and P. Rakic. 1973. Neuronal migration, with special reference to the developing human brain: A review. *Brain Res.* 62: 1–35.

Singer, W. 1987. Activity-dependent self-organization of synaptic connections as a substrate of learning. *In* J.-P. Changeux and M. Konishi (eds.) *The Neural and Molecular Bases of Learning.* Wiley, New York.

Singer, W., and J. P. Rauschecker. 1982. Central core

control of developmental plasticity in the kitten visual cortex. II. Electrical activation of mesencephalic and diencephalic projections. *Exp. Brain Res.* 41: 199–215.

Singer, W., F. Tretter, and W. Yinon. 1982. Central gating of developmental plasticity in kitten visual cortex. *J. Physiol.* 324: 221–37.

Söderbergh, R. 1981. Early reading as language acquisition. *System* 9(3): 207–13.

Sperry, R. W. 1940. The functional results of muscle transposition in the hind limb of the rat. *J. Comp. Neurol.* 73: 379–404.

–1963. Chemoaffinity in the orderly growth of nerve fiber patterns and connections *Proc. Nat. Acad. Sci. USA* 50: 703–10.

–1965. Embryogenesis of behavioral nerve nets. *In* R. L. Dehaan and H. Ursprung (eds.) *Organogenesis.* Holt, Rinehart and Winston, New York, pp. 161–85.

–1967. Split-brain approach to learning problems. *In* G. C. Quarton, T. Melnechuk and F. O. Schmitt (eds.) *The Neurosciences: A Study Program.* Rockefeller University Press, New York, pp. 714–22.

–1974. Lateral specialization in the surgically separated hemispheres. *In* F. Schmitt and F. Worden (eds.) *The Neurosciences: Third Study Program.* The MIT Press, Cambridge, pp. 5–19.

–1982. Some effects of disconnecting the cerebral hemispheres (Nobel lecture). *Science* 217 (4566): 1223–6.

–1983. *Science and Moral Priority.* Columbia University Press, New York.

Sperry, R. W., M. S. Gazzaniga, and J. E. Bogen. 1969. Interhemispheric relationships: The neocortical commissures; syndromes of hemisphere disconnection. *In* P. J. Vinken and G. W. Bruyn (eds.) *Handbook of Clinical Neurology,* Vol. 4. North-Holland, Amsterdam, pp. 273–90.

Stern, D. 1985. *The Interpersonal World of the Infant: A View from Psychoanalysis and Developmental Psychology.* Basic Books, New York.

Strauss, E., B. Kosaka, and J. Wada. 1983. The neurobiological basis of lateralized cerebral function: A review. *Human Neurobiol.* 2: 115–27.

Studdert-Kennedy, M. 1983. On learning to speak. *Human Neurobiol.* 2: 191–5.

–1987. Speech development. *In* G. Adelman (ed.) *Encyclopedia of Neuroscience,* Vol II. Birkhäuser Boston, Cambridge.

Thatcher, R. W., R. A. Walker, and S. Giudice. 1987. Human cerebral hemispheres develop at different rates and ages. *Science* 236: 1110–13.

Trevarthen, C. 1974. Cerebral embryology and the split-brain. *In* M. Kinsbourne and W. L. Smith (eds.) *Hemispheric Disconnection and Cerebral Function.* Thomas, Springfield (IL).

–1979. Communication and cooperation in early infancy. A description of primary intersubjectivity. *In* M. Bullowa (ed.) *Before Speech. The Beginnings of Human Communication.* Cambridge University Press, Cambridge (UK).

–1980. The foundations of intersubjectivity: Development of interpersonal and cooperative understanding

in infants. *In* D. Olson (ed.) *The Social Foundations of Language and Thought: Essays in Honor of J. S. Bruner.* Norton, New York.

–1982. The primary motives for cooperative understanding. *In* G. Butterworth and P. Light (eds.) *Social Cognition: Studies of the Development of Understanding.* Harvester Press, Brighton.

–1983. Interpersonal abilities of infants as generators for transmission of language and culture. *In* A. Oliverio and M. Zapella (eds.) *The Behavior of Human Infants.* Plenum, London and New York.

–1984a. Hemispheric specialization. *In* I. Darian-Smith (ed.) *Handbook of Physiology: The Nervous System, III, Part 2.* American Physiological Society, Washington (DC).

–1984b. How control of movements develops. *In* H. T. A. Whiting (ed.) *Human Motor Actions: Bernstein Reassessed.* Elsevier/North-Holland, Amsterdam.

–1984c. Emotions in infancy: Regulators of contacts and relationships with persons. *In* K. Scherer and P. Ekman (eds.) *Approaches to Emotion.* Lawrence Erlbaum, Hillsdale (NJ).

–1985a. Neuroembryology and the development of perceptual mechanisms. *In* F. Falkner and J. M. Tanner (eds.) *Human Growth, A Comprehensive Treatise. Volume 2: Postnatal Growth, Neurobiology,* 2nd Ed. Plenum, New York.

–1985b Facial expressions of emotion in mother–infant interaction. *Human Neurobiol.* 4: 21–32.

–1986a. Form, significance and psychological potential of hand gestures of infants. *In* J. L. Nespoulous, P. Perron, and A. Roch Lecours (eds.) *The Biological Foundation of Gestures: Motor and Semiotic Aspects.* Lawrence Erlbaum, Hillsdale, (NJ).

–1986b. Development of intersubjective motor control in infants. *In* M. G. Wade and H. T. A. Whiting (eds.) *Motor Development in Children: Aspects of Coordination and Control.* Martinus Nijhof, Dordrecht.

–1987a. Brain development. *In* R. Gregory (ed.) *Oxford Companion to the Mind.* Oxford University Press, Oxford.

–1987b. Development of language mechanisms in the brain. *In* G. Adelman (ed.) *Encyclopedia of Neuroscience.* Birkhäuser Boston, Cambridge.

–1987c. Sharing makes sense: Intersubjectivity and the making of an infant's meaning. *In* R. Steele and T. Threadgold (eds.) *Language Topics: Essays in Honour of Michael Halliday.* John Benjamins, Amsterdam and Philadelphia.

–1987d. Sub-cortical influences on cortical processing in "split" brains. *In* D. Ottoson (ed.) *Dual Brain: Unified Functioning and Specialization of the Hemispheres,* Wenner-Gren International Symposium Series, No. 47. Macmillan, London; Stockton Press, New York.

Trevarthen, C., and P. Hubley, 1978. Secondary intersubjectivity: Confidence, confiding and acts of meaning in the first year. *In* A. Lock (ed.) *Action, Gesture and Symbol.* Academic Press, London.

Trevarthen, C., and K. Logotheti. 1987. First symbols

and the nature of human knowledge. *In* J. Montangero, A. Tryphon, and S. Dionnet (eds.) *Symbolism and Knowledge,* Cahier No. 8. Jean Piaget Archives Foundation, Geneva.

–1989. Child and culture: Genesis of cooperative knowing. *In* A. Gellatly, D. Rogers, and J. Sloboda (eds.) *Cognition and Social World.* Oxford University Press, Oxford.

Trevarthen, C., and H. Marwick. 1986. Signs of motivation for speech in infants, and the nature of a mother's support for development of language. *In* B. Lindblom and R. Zetterstrom (eds.) *Precursors of Early Speech.* Macmillan, London; Stockton Press, New York.

Tucker, D. M. 1986. Neural control of emotional communication. *In* P. Blanck, R. Buck, and R. Rosenthal (eds.) *Nonverbal Communication in the Clinical Context.* Cambridge University Press, Cambridge (UK).

Tucker, D. M., and S. L. Frederick. 1987. Emotion and brain lateralization. *In* H. Wagner and T. Manstead (eds.) *Handbook of Psychophysiology: Emotion and Social Behavior.* Wiley, New York.

Tucker, D. M., and P. A. Williamson. 1984. Asymmetric neural control systems in human self-regulation. *Psychol. Rev.* 91: 185–215.

Turkewitz, G. 1977. The development of lateral differences in the human infant. *In* S. Harnad, R. W. Doty, L. Goldstein, J. Jaynes, and G. Krathamer (eds.) *Lateralization in the Nervous System.* Academic Press, New York.

Vogt, C. 1900. *Etude sur la Myelinisation des Hemispheres Cerebraux.* Paris.

Volterra, V. 1981. Gestures, signs and words at two years: When does communication become language? *Sign Lang. Stud.* 33: 351–62.

Volterra, V. 1986. What sign language research can teach us about language acquisition. *In* B. T. Tervoort (ed.) *Signs of Life.* The Dutch Foundation for the Deaf and Hearing Impaired Child, The Institute of General Linguistics of the University of Amsterdam, The Dutch Council for the Deaf, Amsterdam.

Wied, D. de, 1987. Neuropeptides and behavior. *In* G. Adelman (ed.) *Encylopedia of Neuroscience,* Vol. II. Birkhäuser Boston, Cambridge.

Wierman, M. E., and W. F. Crowley. 1985. Neuroendocrine control of the onset of puberty. *In* F. Falkner and J. M. Tanner (eds.) *Human Growth: A Comprehensive Treatise. Vol 2: Postnatal Growth; Neurobiology.* Plenum, New York.

Wilson, A. C. 1985. The molecular basis of evolution. *Sci. Am.* 253(4): 164–73.

Windle, W. F. 1970. Development of neural elements in human embryos of four to seven weeks gestation. *Exp. Neurol. (Supplement)* 5: 44–83.

Witelson, S. F. 1985. On hemispheric specialization and cerebral plasticity from birth. Mark III. *In* C. Best (ed.) *Hemispheric Function and Collaboration in the Child.* Academic Press, New York.

–1987. Brain asymmetry, functional aspects. *In* G. Adleman (ed.) *Encyclopedia of Neuroscience.* Birkhäuser Boston, Cambridge.

Witelson, S. F., and D. L. Kigar. 1987. Neuroanatomical aspects of hemisphere specialization in humans. *In* D. Ottoson (ed.) *Duality and Unity of the Brain,* Wenner-Gren International Symposium Series, No. 47. Macmillan, London; Stockton Press, New York.

Wolf, M. E., and M. A. Goodale. 1987. Oral asymmetries during verbal and non-verbal movements of the mouth. *Neuropsychol.* 25: 375–96.

Yakovlev, P. I., and A. R. Lecours. 1967. The myelogenetic cycles of regional maturation of the brain. *In* A. Minkowski (ed.) *Regional Development of the Brain in Early Life.* Blackwell, Oxford.

Young, G. 1977. Manual specialization in infancy: Implications for lateralization of brain function. *In* S. J. Segalowitz and F. A. Gruber (eds.) *Language Development and Neurological Theory.* Academic Press, New York.

21 Hemispheric specialization in the aged brain

Robert D. Nebes
Geriatric Psychiatry Program
Western Psychiatric Institute and Clinic
University of Pittsburgh

The contributions of the majority of experimental scientists are restricted to the new empirical observations they add to the literature. A very few, however, go far beyond this and stimulate a change in the actual conceptual framework of their field. The work of these individuals generates excitement throughout the field and produces a widespread reevaluation of established facts and concepts. Certainly, Roger Sperry has had this effect in the neurobehavioral sciences. The explosive growth of research on the differing psychological functions of the right and left hemispheres is, in many ways, directly attributable to Sperry's dramatic demonstration of hemispheric specialization in commissurotomized patients. These commissurotomy results have not only revolutionized research in neuropsychology, but they have had a major impact in other fields as well. The theoretical constructs of many different fields have had to be reexamined within the context of Sperry's work. Educators have questioned whether our school systems overemphasize left-hemisphere types of processes to the detriment of right-hemisphere processes (Wittrock 1977). Philosophers have been forced to deal with the issue of whether cerebral commissurotomy produces a "state of separate coconscious awareness" in the two hemispheres (Sperry 1977). The concepts of hemispheric specialization have even penetrated sociology and anthropology, with the suggestion (Bogen et. al. 1972) that cultures may vary in the degree to which their members rely on the information-processing approaches of the right or left

hemispheres (hemisphericity). It has also become common to attribute neurobehavioral disorders (e.g., schizophrenia, depression, autism, dyslexia, stuttering) to a dysfunction in one or the other hemisphere or in their interaction. The data and logic used to justify application of this left brain–right brain dichotomy are often tenuous, at best. However, so strong is the appeal of the commissurotomy syndrome that it has become a popular explanatory mechanism.

How cognitive processes change in old age

Recently, the concept of hemispheric specialization has been used to explain the cognitive dysfunction seen in normal aging. An impairment of central nervous system function is thought to underlie much of the cognitive decline that so often accompanies advancing age. Histological changes, though not uniform, are widespread in the aged brain (Scheibel and Scheibel 1975), and it has been commonly held that the psychological effects of age are due to a progressive diffuse loss of cerebral tissue (Birren, Woods, and Williams 1979). However, when normal elderly individuals are actually compared to patients with documented diffuse brain disease, their psychological test profiles are actually very different (Overall and Gorham 1972, Goldstein and Shelly 1975). Recently, some researchers have suggested that, whatever the anatomical distribution of the underlying structural and physiological changes that occur in old age, certain major regions of the brain may be more affected by aging than are others. In particular, the right hemisphere has been singled out as being particularly sensitive to the deleterious effects of aging (Klisz 1978, Johnson et al. 1979, Goldstein and Shelly 1981).

This interest in the right hemisphere springs from a reinterpretation of the "classic" pattern of cognitive change with age. One of the most consistent findings in the psychology of aging has been that on standardized intelligence tests, such as the Wechsler Adult Intelligence Scale (WAIS), scores on certain subtests remain fairly steady across the adult life span, whereas others show a substantial decline. Typically, subtests making up the performance scale show an age-related decline, but those making up the verbal scale do not (Botwinick 1977). Until recently, most theoretical interpretations of this difference focused on task variables that differentiate verbal from the performance subtests (e.g., the timed nature of the performance subtests, which disadvantages older, slower subjects, or the reliance of the verbal subtests on retrieval of overlearned information, which old people retain well). Over ten years ago, however, a number of investigators (e.g., Elias and Kinsbourne 1974) suggested that the crucial distinction between the two subscales of the WAIS might be that the verbal subtests make heavy demands upon verbal-processing skills, whereas the performance subtests are more dependent upon visuospatial skills. Seen from this perspective, the verbal/performance discrepancy in the WAIS would reflect a greater decrement in the spatial abilities of the elderly than in their verbal abilities.

This new interpretation occurred within the context of a burst of studies from Sperry's group that dramatically demonstrated the differing competencies of the left and right hemispheres for verbal and spatial operations (Bogen 1969; Levy, Trevarthen, and Sperry 1972; Nebes 1974; Sperry 1974). Given the interest in hemispheric specialization generated by this work, it is not surprising that a number of investigators came to the conclusion that the apparently greater decline in spatial abilities in the elderly was a consequence of age having a disproportionately greater effect on right-

hemispheric function than it does on left-hemispheric function.

Several lines of evidence were advanced to support this hypothesis. First, the profile of scores seen in normal elderly individuals on the 11 subtests of the WAIS is almost identical to that seen in patients with damage restricted to the right hemisphere (Schaie and Schaie 1977). Second, on a standardized neuropsychological test battery (Halstead–Reitan) designed to diagnose lateralized brain injury, it is the tasks that are sensitive to right-hemispheric damage that are most difficult for normal elderly subjects (Klisz 1978).

However, just because right-brain-damaged patients and elderly individuals find the same types of psychometric tasks difficult, it does not necessarily follow that the aged have a dysfunctional right hemisphere. Psychometric tests are generally complex, making demands upon a number of cognitive functions; the performance of different populations of subjects may be determined by very different factors. Right-brain-injured patients might, for example, do poorly in the block-design test because they lack the specific spatial skills required, whereas the elderly might do poorly on the same test for a totally different reason, such as a generalized slowing in all cognitive operations, producing low scores on timed tasks. Thus, a mere similarity in the pattern of deficits shown by two types of individuals on such tests is not a sufficient basis for concluding that they share a common underlying cognitive decrement.

Perceptual asymmetries in the elderly

In order to determine whether the functional efficiency of the two hemispheres actually does decline differentially with age, a more direct measure of relative hemispheric performance is needed. One such measure involves comparing the relative speed and/or accuracy with which subjects process stimuli that are selectively presented to one or the other hemisphere. With visual stimuli, this requires the items to be tachistoscopically flashed to the right or left of fixation, whereas with auditory stimuli, a dichotic listening paradigm is necessary to demonstrate lateralized abilities. Typically, normal young people process verbal information faster and more accurately if it is presented in the right visual half-field or right ear, and thus projected first to the left hemisphere. Similarly, the same subjects are faster in processing spatial or nonverbal information presented in the left half-field or ear (see Madden and Nebes 1980).

If, with advancing age, the right hemisphere undergoes a greater decline in processing efficiency than does the left, then in comparison to the young, the old should demonstrate a *larger* visual half-field and ear difference in processing verbal information and a *smaller* difference in processing spatial information. This pattern would be expected because, in the young, the left hemisphere already surpasses the right in verbal processing; therefore, any loss of right-hemisphere ability in the old would augment an already existing lateral performance asymmetry. With spatial information, however, the right-hemisphere processing superiority present in the young would be diminished or eliminated by a right-hemisphere decline in the old.

In a first experiment (Nebes, Madden, and Berg 1983), we measured subjects' response times for naming verbal and pictorial stimuli in their right and left half visual fields. The verbal stimuli were the printed names of the numbers between "one" and "twelve," and the pictorial stimuli were clocks with their hands set at the various hours. Thus, for each number between 1 and 12, there were two representations, one verbal and one spatial, to which the subjects made the same vocal response. Although the numbers represented by the clock faces do have readily available verbal labels, actual identification of the time requires a visuospatial discrimination of the angle formed by the two hands of the clock.

Our use of a vocal response might be expected to confound interpretation of field differences, since expressive language appears to be primarily a function of the left hemisphere. However, the majority of the studies in the literature (e.g., Gross 1972) does not find the pattern of visual-field asymmetries in speed of response to be altered by the nature of the response (vocal versus manual). Thus, the left-field-response time advantage for a spatial discrimination task like the one used here is evident even when a vocal response is used (Berlucchi et al. 1979).

On the basis of previous results, then, we would expect the young to show a right-field superiority in naming words and a left-field superiority in naming clocks (Bradshaw and Gates 1978; Berlucchi et al. 1979). If increasing age does cause a differential decrement in right-hemispheric abilities, then this right-field superiority for words should be increased in the elderly, whereas the left-field superiority for clocks should be decreased.

Forty right-handed subjects were used, half of whom were between 20 and 30 years of age, the other half between 60 and 70. On testing with the WAIS, the classic age pattern was found: on the vocabulary subtest, the two groups did equally well (young, M = 65.7; elderly, M = 64.6), whereas on the object assembly subtest (this task requires subjects to assemble a drawing of a common object that has been cut up and the pieces disarranged), there was a significant age difference (young, M = 34.9; elderly, M = 25.5, t = 3.7, p < 0.01).

The verbal stimuli were vertically printed words (the numbers "one" through "twelve"), and the spatial stimuli were clock faces set on the hour (one o'clock, two o'clock, etc.). The actual clock faces consisted of a circle 1½° in diameter with twelve markings at the usual five-minute intervals (Figure 21.1A). The markings were not numbered. The large hand of the clock always rested on the top mark. The position of the small hand varied randomly across trials, falling on each of the twelve markings equally often.

The stimuli were flashed in a tachistoscope, and fell 1½° to the right or left of the central fixation point. Each of the twelve printed numbers and twelve clock faces appeared eight times in each visual field in a predetermined random order. The presentation of a stimulus started a millisecond timer that was stopped by a voice key triggered by the subject's speech. The subject's response to either a printed number or a clock face was the same – the name of the number between one and twelve represented by that stimulus.

Analysis of the response-time data

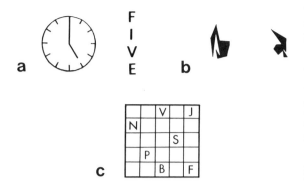

Figure 21.1. Stimuli used in experiments to test spatial abilities, memory for shapes, and memory for letters or for their spatial position in a grid. For further explanation, see the text.

showed that subjects identified the spatial stimuli (i.e., the clock faces) approximately 50 ms faster in the left visual field than in the right (p < 0.001). By contrast, they identified the verbal stimuli (i.e., the words) approximately 15 ms faster in the right field than in the left (p < 0.003). Although the elderly subjects were generally slower than the young by some 140 ms (p < 0.001), the size and direction of their visual-field differences were the same as those of the young (i.e., there was no interaction between age and visual field).

A second study (Nebes et al. 1983) used a dichotic listening approach to examine further the effect of age on hemispheric function. In dichotic listening, two different stimuli are presented simultaneously, one to each ear. When verbal stimuli are presented dichotically, younger subjects generally report those items heard in the right ear more accurately than those heard in the left (Shankweiler and Studdert-Kennedy 1975). This, presumably, reflects the left hemisphere's superior verbal-processing abilities. Any disproportionate decline with age in right-hemispheric function would produce a larger right-ear dichotic advantage in the elderly than in the young.

Twenty-four young (18 to 25 years of age) and twenty-four older (65 to 75 years of age) right-handed individuals were tested. On audiometric examination, all had normal hearing in both ears in the frequency range covered by the human voice. The stimuli, six natural-voice syllables (ba, da, ga, ka, pa, ta), were tape recorded and presented over headphones. On the dichotic trials, two different syllables were presented simultaneously, one to each ear, and the subject was asked to identify both.

The data showed both young and old to be more accurate in reporting syllables from the right ear than from the left (p < 0.001 and p < 0.01, respectively). There was, however, *no* significant age difference in the size of this right-ear advantage.

The results of these two studies thus do not show any evidence of a disproportionate loss in right-hemispheric function with increasing age. We did not see the increase in right visual-field and right-ear superiority for the identification of verbal stimuli, nor the decrease in the left-sided superiority for identification of spatial stimuli that would be expected if older individuals had a greater loss in right- than in left-hemispheric function.

These two studies, however, examined only a few of the many cognitive operations for which lateral performance asymmetries have been demonstrated in young adults. It may well be that the differential effects of age on the two hemispheres are detectable only on tasks that tap more complex forms of information processing and especially those cognitive operations in which the elderly are deficient. In this respect, memory would appear to be an especially appropriate area to investigate, since memory difficulties are a hallmark of aging (Craik 1977), and there is good evidence that certain components of memory function are lateralized to different hemispheres (Milner and Taylor 1972; Milner 1974). There is also a recent study showing an apparent decrease with age in the right hemisphere's ability to carry out a tactual memory task (Riege, Metter and Williams 1980). We, therefore, ran two studies that examined the effect of age upon right- and left-hemisphere memory abilities for verbal and nonverbal material.

Age and lateral asymmetry of memory abilities

In the first study, 24 young and 24 older right-handed individuals served as subjects. On each trial, a single letter was tachistoscopically flashed in either the right or left visual field. In one condition, the subjects had only to identify the letter, saying its name aloud. In the other condition, they had to say the name of a *word* they had learned to associate with that letter prior to beginning the actual task (e.g., S – STAR). In both cases, the sound of the subject's voice stopped a timer started by the presentation of the letter. The letter-naming condition was thus similar to the previous tasks in that it required only that the subject identify the stimulus. In the associated-word condition, by contrast, after identifying the letter, the subject had also to conduct a memory search in order to retrieve the associated word.

The elderly were generally slower in responding than were the young, especially when they had to recall the associated word ($p < 0.004$). In both conditions, subjects responded faster when the stimulus fell in the right field than when it fell in the left ($p < 0.001$). In the letter-identification condition, however, this right-field superiority was only weakly significant ($p < 0.05$), and both young and older subjects showed approximately a 12-ms difference in response time between the two fields. In the condition requiring recall of the associated word, there was a substantially stronger field difference ($p < 0.0001$), with responses to right-field presentations being approximately 40 ms faster in the elderly ($p < 0.0001$) and 22 ms faster in the young ($p < 0.001$). There was, however, no age-by-field interaction in either condition – the size of the right-field advantage in reaction time was *not* significantly larger for the elderly than it was for the young.

The second memory task examined subjects' memory for complex random shapes (Vanderplas and Garvin 1959). On the basis of previous work (e.g., Dee and Fontenot 1973), we expected that such stimuli would be more efficiently processed when they fell in the subjects' left visual field and thus were projected to the right hemisphere.

The subjects first memorized six shapes (see Figure 21.1B for examples). Three of these shapes were designated as targets to which the subjects were to respond in the upcoming task; the other three shapes were nontargets to which they were to withhold their response. This was, therefore, a go/no-go response-time task in which the subjects had to match the presented stimulus against their memory of the six shapes in order to determine whether or not to respond. On each trial, a single shape was tachistoscopically presented in either the right or left visual field. The subjects (16 young, 16 older) responded to the target shapes by saying a single syllable ("po") chosen to trigger reliably the voice key and thus stop the clock.

Analysis of the results showed that subjects responded faster to the shapes when they fell in the left visual field than when they fell in the right ($p < 0.004$). Although the elderly were generally slower than the young in responding ($p < 0.03$), there was no interaction between the effects of the subjects' age and the visual field of presentation; the left-field latency advantage (46 ms in the young, 31 ms in the old) was significant in both the elderly ($p < 0.05$) and the young ($p < 0.02$).

Overall, the results of these two memory studies, and indeed of all four studies, did not yield any evidence suggestive of a disproportionate decline in right-hemispheric abilities with advancing age. Even on the more demanding memory tasks, there was no indication that the right hemisphere suffers any greater age-related decline in processing efficiency than does the left.

Selective spatial disability in the elderly – An artifact?

If the two hemispheres of human beings are not differentially affected by age, why then is there apparently a greater impairment of visuospatial than of verbal skills in the elderly? One possibility is that the verbal/performance subtest discrepancy in the WAIS described earlier may actually have nothing at all to do with age changes in verbal- and spatial-processing abilities. There are many other confounding differences between the verbal and performance subtests (e.g., modality of stimulus presentation, nature of the required response, presence of time limits, amount of sustained attention required). In order to make a valid comparison of the effect of age on verbal and spatial skills, it is essential to equate tasks for such confounding factors. We attempted to do just such a comparison in the context of a short-term memory task (Schear and Nebes 1980).

The subjects in this study (24 young and 24 elderly individuals) were shown a series of 5 × 5 grids. Seven of the cells in each grid contained a letter (see Figure 21.1C for an example). Prior to seeing a given grid, the subject was told to remember *either* the identity of the letters *or* their spatial position within the grid. After a ten-second delay, the subject either wrote down the letters or marked on a blank grid the cells in which the letters appeared. Thus, in this task, the stimuli and the general task demands were constant and only the verbal or spatial nature of the information to be remembered was varied. If spatial processes are truly more sensitive than verbal processes to the detrimental effects of aging, then in comparison to the young, the older subjects should have greater difficulty recalling the spatial locations of the letters than they should their identities.

The data showed that while the older subjects were less accurate than the young in recalling both letter identity ($p < 0.001$) and letter position ($p < 0.001$), there was no indication that they were any less able to encode and recall one type of information than they were the other. Thus, there was no evidence for a greater effect of age on spatial than on verbal processes, once confounding task factors were eliminated.

Conclusion

Where does this leave us? We started with a train of logic in which a discrepancy in the effect of aging on the verbal and performance subtests of the WAIS was taken to reflect a greater decline with age in spatial than in verbal skills. This, in turn, was hypothesized to result from a more severe loss of right- than of left-hemispheric functioning in the elderly. However, on closer investigation, not only is right-hemispheric function found not to be disproportionately affected by normal aging, but even the selective decline in spatial abilities said to occur in the elderly appears questionable. The results of these particular experiments are, instead, more consistent with the presence of a "uniform deterioration of cerebral function"

(Elias and Kinsbourne 1974). Alternatively, these results might also reflect a decline in a part of the cerebral system that is equally implicated in the functioning of both the right and left hemispheres, or that mediates between them.

The actual source of the differential effect that age has upon WAIS verbal and performance scores is still not clear. At present, the most commonly accepted view is that the two scales require different types of intelligence (Horn 1978). The verbal scale is seen to require the retrieval and use of overlearned information and cognitive skills (crystallized intelligence), whereas the performance scale is thought to involve the creative application of problem-solving strategies to novel situations (fluid intelligence). While crystallized intelligence is postulated to increase with age and experience, fluid intelligence is seen to decrease.

The enthusiasm of the scientific community for the research that Sperry initiated in commissurotomized patients has undoubtedly been enormous, especially for the studies that have so dramatically characterized the differing cognitive specializations of the right and left hemispheres in these patients. This enthusiasm has led other researchers to explain a wide variety of behavioral phenomena in terms of possible changes in the specialized functions of the two hemispheres. In many cases, the rationale for using hemispheric specialization as an explanatory mechanism has been based on what turn out to be superficial behavioral similarities. This appears to be the case for the hypothesis that a relative right-hemisphere decline is the explanation for the psychological effects of aging. What started out an attractive neurologically based explanation for the "classic" pattern of psychological change with age now appears to be an instance of the "great tragedy of Science – the slaying of a beautiful hypothesis by an ugly fact" (Huxley 1897). We can console ourselves with the reflection that it is only by ruling out mistaken interpretations of superficially similar phenomena that we can hope to successfully apply the new perspectives on hemispheric specialization generated by Sperry's research and concepts. In this context, the demonstration of an invariance in functional hemispheric lateralization existing over the adult life-span does contribute to our understanding of human brain-behavior relationships.

References

Berlucchi, G., D. Brizzolara, C. A. Marzi, G. Rizzolatti, and C. Umilta. 1979. The role of stimulus discriminability and verbal codability in hemispheric specialization for visuospatial tasks. *Neuropsychol.* 17: 195–202.

Birren, J. E., A. M. Woods, and M. V. Williams. 1979. Speed of behavior as an indicator of age changes and the integrity of the nervous system. *In* F. Hoffmeister and C. Muller (eds.) *Brain Function in Old Age.* Springer-Verlag, Berlin.

Bogen, J. E. 1969. The other side of the brain. II: An appositional mind. *Bull. L.A. Neurol. Soc.* 34: 135–162.

Bogen, J. E., R. DeZure, W. D. Tenhouten, and J. F. Marsh. 1972. The other side of the brain. IV: The A/P ratio. *Bull. L.A. Neurol. Soc.* 37: 49–61.

Botwinick, J. 1977. Intellectual abilities. *In* J. E. Birren and K. W. Schaie (eds.) *Handbook of the Psychology of Aging.* Van Nostrand Reinhold, New York.

Bradshaw, J. L., and E. A. Gates. 1978. Visual field differences in verbal tasks: Effects of task familiarity and sex of subject. *Brain and Lang.* 5: 166–87.

Craik, F. I. M. 1977. Age differences in human memory. *In* J. E. Birren and K. W. Schaie (eds.) *Handbook of the Psychology of Aging.* Van Nostrand Reinhold, New York.

Dee, H., and H. Fontenot. 1973. Cerebral dominance and lateral differences in perception and memory. *Neuropsychol.* 11: 167–73.

Elias, M. F., and M. Kinsbourne. 1974. Age and sex differences in the processing of verbal and non-verbal stimuli. *J. Gerontol.* 29: 162–71.

Goldstein, G., and C. H. Shelly. 1975. Similarities and differences between psychological deficit in aging and brain damage. *J. Gerontol.* 30: 448–55.

–1981. Does the right hemisphere age more rapidly than the left? *J. Clin. Neuropsychol.* 3: 65–78.

Gross, M. M. 1972. Hemispheric specialization for processing of visually presented verbal and spatial stimuli. *Perception and Psychophysics* 12: 357–363.

Horn, J. L. 1978. Human ability systems. *In* P. B. Baltes (ed.) *Life-Span Development and Behavior,* Vol. 1. Academic Press, New York.

Huxley, T. 1897. Biogenesis and abiogenesis. *In Collected Essays, Discourses, Vol. 8: Biological and Geological.* Appleton, New York.

Johnson, R. C., R. E. Cole, J. K. Bowers, S. V. Foiles, A. M. Nikaido, J. W. Patrick, and R. E. Woliver. 1979. Hemispheric efficiency in middle and later adulthood. *Cortex* 15: 109–19.

Klisz, D. 1978. Neuropsychological evaluation in older persons. *In* M. Storandt, I. C. Siegler, M. F. Elias (eds.) *The Clinical Psychology of Aging.* Plenum, New York.

Levy, J., C. B. Trevarthen, and R. W. Sperry. 1972. Perception of bilateral chimeric figures following hemispheric deconnection. *Brain* 95: 61–78.

Madden, D. J., and R. D. Nebes. 1980. Visual perception and memory. *In* M. Wittrock (ed.) *The Brain and Psychology.* Academic Press, New York.

Milner, B. 1974. Hemispheric specialization: Scope and limits. *In* F. G. Worden and F. O. Schmitt (eds.) *The Neurosciences: Third Study Program.* The MIT Press, Cambridge.

Milner, B., and L. Taylor. 1972. Right hemisphere superiority in tactile pattern recognition after cerebral commissurotomy: Evidence for nonverbal memory. *Neuropsychol.* 10: 1–16.

Nebes, R. D. 1974. Hemispheric specialization in commissurotomized man. *Psychol. Bull.* 81: 1–14.

Nebes, R. D., D. J. Madden, and W. D. Berg. 1983. The effect of age on hemispheric asymmetry in visual and auditory identification. *Exp. Aging Res.* 9: 87–91.

Overall, J. E., and D. R. Gorham. 1972. Organicity versus old age in objective and projective test performance. *J. Consult. Clin. Psychol.* 39: 98–105.

Riege, W. H., E. J. Metter, and M. V. Williams. 1980. Age and hemispheric asymmetry in nonverbal tactual memory. *Neuropsychol.* 18: 707–10.

Schaie, K. W., and J. P. Schaie. 1977. Clinical assessment and aging. *In* J. E. Birren and K. W. Schaie (eds.) *Handbook of the Psychology of Aging.* Van Nostrand Reinhold, New York.

Schear, J. M., and R. D. Nebes. 1980. Memory for verbal and spatial information as a function of age. *Exp. Aging Res.* 6: 271–81.

Scheibel, M. D., and A. B. Scheibel. 1975. Structural changes in the aging brain. *In* H. Brody, D. Harman, and J. M. Ordy (eds.) *Aging,* Vol. 1. Raven, New York.

Shankweiler, D., and M. Studdert-Kennedy. 1975. A continuum of lateralization for speech perception? *Brain and Lang.* 2: 212–25.

Sperry, R. W. 1974. Lateral specialization in the surgically separated hemispheres. *In* F. O. Schmitt and F. G. Worden (eds.) *The Neurosciences: Third Study Program.* The MIT Press, Cambridge, pp. 5–19.

–1977. Forebrain commissurotomy and conscious awareness. *J. Med. Phil.* 2(2): 101–26.

Vanderplas, J. M., and E. A. Garvin. 1959. The association value of random shapes. *J. Exp. Psychol.* 57: 147–54.

Wittrock, M. C. 1977. The generative processes of memory. *In* M. C. Wittrock (ed.) *The Human Brain.* Prentice-Hall, Englewood Cliffs (NJ).

22 Forebrain commissurotomy and conscious awareness*

Roger W. Sperry
Division of Biology
California Institute of Technology

The left and right cerebral lobes of the mammalian brain in the natural state are largely separate anatomically except for cables of cross-connecting fibers, the cerebral commissures, most prominent of which is the enormous corpus callosum, the largest fiber system of the brain, estimated to contain in man over 200 million fibers. Experimental investigation of the functional role of the cerebral commissures was stimulated during the early 1940s by a series of clinical reports in which complete surgical section as well as congenital absence of the corpus callosum had seemingly failed to produce any consistent or distinct behavioral symptoms detectable in extensive neurological and psychological testing (Akelaitis 1943; Bremer, Brihaye, and André Balisaux 1956; Bremer 1958). Animal studies started in the early 1950s, mostly on cats and primates (Myers and Sperry 1953; Stamm, Miner, and Sperry 1956; Sperry 1961; Downer 1962; Myers 1962), showed consistently, however, that each hemisphere after surgical separation functions independently to a very large extent in most higher activities, including perception, learning, and memory. In objective behavioral tests involving sensory-discrimination learning, each surgically disconnected hemisphere was found to sense, perceive, learn, and remember independently of the other.

Although deep surgical bisections are possible experimentally that include the roof of the midbrain, the supramammillary commissure, and even the cerebellum (Sperry 1964), it was sufficient merely to cut the forebrain commissures that mediate cross communication between the hemispheres proper to prevent interhemispheric transfer of perceptual learning and memory. The collected animal evidence (Sperry 1961) supported the conclusion that each of the disconnected hemispheres develops its own private chain of learning and memory experiences that are cut off from, and inaccessible to, recall through the opposite hemisphere.

Not only did learning remain lateralized to the one hemisphere receiving the critical sensory input, but also the two hemispheres could be trained concurrently to perform mutually contradictory tasks (Myers 1962). It was shown further by Trevarthen (1962) that with an optical system of light-polarizing filters, the separated hemispheres could be made to perceive two different things occupying the same position in space at the same time. Under these conditions (see Figure 22.1), in which one or the other of two stimulus panels is selectively activated in a series of trial-and-error responses, one hemisphere perceives itself to be receiving rewards for selecting, for example, circles and avoiding crosses, while at the same time with the same responses, the other hemisphere sees itself being rewarded conversely for avoiding circles and selecting crosses. The animals tend to work with one hand in this situation, and the hemisphere controlling the working

Reprinted with permission, from *The Journal of Medicine and Philosophy*, 1977, Vol. 2, No. 2.

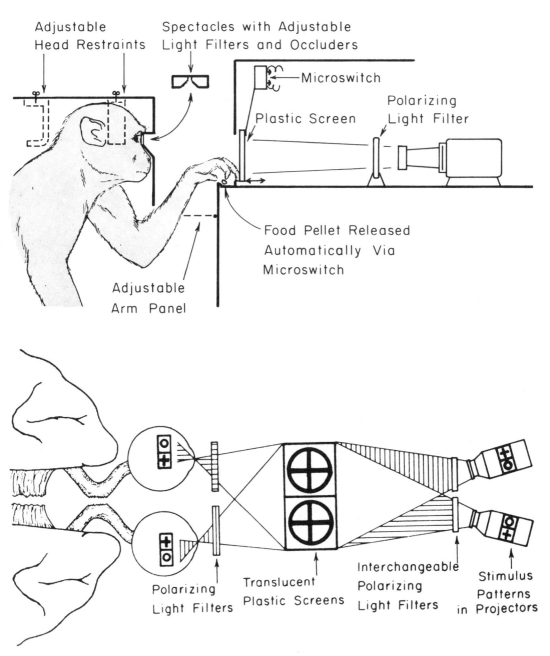

Figure 22.1. Technique of Trevarthen (1962) for showing that a split-brain monkey can perceive two different things occupying the same position in space at the same time. Left and right hemispheres trained under these conditions learn mutually contradictory discrimination habits from the same set of trial-and-error responses.

hand tends to learn more rapidly than does the more passive hemisphere. By forcing use of the inactive hand after learning is established, and by restricting vision to the more passive hemisphere, the cerebral dominance can be shifted, and the animal can be shown to have been learning with the second hemisphere the reverse of what was being learned with the first hemisphere.

Thus, the objective animal evidence suggests that in each disconnected hemisphere, conscious experience (assuming cats and subhuman primates have consciousness) is cut off from conscious experience in the other. Lack of cross communication of awareness between the two hemispheres is further evident in the inability of the split-brain animal to cross compare or integrate sensory information projected simultaneously partly to one and partly to the other hemisphere (Sperry and Green 1964). However, the same kinds of perceptual cross integration that fail with complete surgical deconnection are readily achieved if the anterior commissure or a small one-centimeter strand of the posterior corpus callosum is left intact (Tieman and Hamilton 1974; Doty 1975). The interhemispheric mediation of higher activities can thus be forcibly narrowed down by surgical and other experimental procedures to a small band of roughly several hundred thousand fibers. Such studies hold promising possibilities for the further dissection and analysis of the anatomical substrate of awareness. Whether the impulse traffic crossing such a minimal remnant of the cross-communication system should be regarded as an intrinsic part of the conscious process per se will be considered in what follows in more detail.

Although there is no way to prove firmly that the surgically disconnected hemispheres in the bisected brain of subhuman mammals are separately conscious, this conclusion would seem to follow if one is willing to accept a starting assumption that cats, monkeys, and other mammals normally possess consciousness. The position taken here is that consciousness may be inferred to be present in animals by much the same logic that we infer it to be present in other persons (compare aphasics who have been rendered temporarily mute by brain damage, drugs, or hypnosis, and who may then after recovery be able to recount their conscious experience during the mute period).

Split-brain man

In human patients who have undergone cerebral commissurotomy (see Figure 22.2), carried out for control of intractable epilepsy (Akelaitis 1943; Bogen and Vogel 1976), there similarly are no direct empirical data that can be advanced as firm proof that the surgically separated hemispheres are independently conscious. Human subjects, however, furnish more direct evidence for this conclusion, since the vocal hemisphere of the human brain readily transmits a verbal report of what it introspectively does or does not experience. At the same time, it conversely disclaims any direct awareness of stimulus input that has been restricted to the opposite hemisphere. Meantime, the nonvocal, mute, or "minor" right hemisphere can show by the use of manual signs, nonverbal pointing, or tactual retrieval that it perceives and comprehends correctly the same stimulus input for which the speaking hemisphere disclaims any awareness. Further, the mute hemisphere displays a corresponding lack of ability to respond to stimulus input restricted to the vocal hemisphere. The foregoing applies in general to all sensory modalities thus far tested that can be lateralized, including visual, somaesthetic, olfactory, and auditory. In the case of auditory stimulation, the natural bilateralized projection to the cerebral cortex from each ear necessitates the use of competitive dichotic stimulus input in order to obtain lateralization of conscious effects. This apparently works through suppression of conscious perception of the weaker input from the ipsilateral side (Milner, Taylor, and Sperry 1968).

Studies along the above line have repeatedly confirmed over many years of testing the oblivious unawareness of one hemisphere for conscious experience in the other. This applies not only to perception of the sensory input itself, but also to more central phases of cognitive processing. It is standard procedure in our human testing to ask the vocal hemisphere, following completion of a task performance by the mute hemisphere, to describe what was in the test performed by its silent partner, the contents of the test material, or what had been done or selected by the silent hemisphere. Where the sensory input has been properly controlled and lateralized, the responses of the speaking hemisphere show that it has no direct awareness of the cerebral processing of the partner hemisphere.

Although commissurotomy subjects show a definite tendency to direct attention selec-

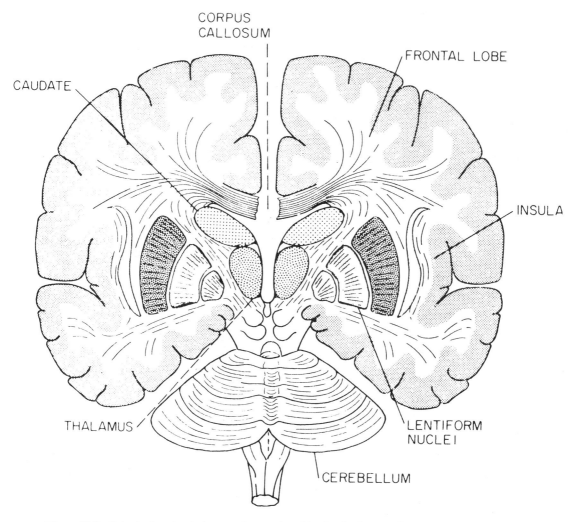

CORPUS
CALLOSUM

FRONTAL LOBE

CAUDATE

INSULA

THALAMUS

LENTIFORM
NUCLEI

CEREBELLUM

Figure 22.2. Extent of anatomical separation produced by forebrain commissurotomy, schematic. (Sperry 1974a.)

tively either to left or right input at the expense of the other, conscious attention to a task confined to one hemisphere does not necessarily switch off conscious awareness in the other. As described before for the split-brain monkey, it is possible to show also that both hemispheres can commonly be coconscious concurrently in split-brain humans and can perform, in parallel, different and even mutually antagonistic cognitive tasks. For example, in tests involving right-hemisphere performance, the vocal hemisphere often tends to offer throughout a running commentary based on those aspects of the situation not restricted to the mute hemisphere.

Because this parallel activity of the second hemisphere may often interfere with the performance of the test hemisphere, the subject is usually instructed to remain silent. Occasionally the commissurotomy subject may become so absorbed in a right-hemisphere task that speech and other left-hemisphere functions are temporarily depressed to the extent that one questions whether consciousness may not have been shifted entirely to the one working hemisphere. This state of affairs occurs more frequently in the reverse direction, that is, where the vocal hemisphere is dominantly active. Parallel cognitive processing is greatly facilitated when left and right tasks involve a common central background of postural and mental sets and is correspondingly disrupted when the background of cerebral and postural sets are in conflict.

Like the split-brain monkey, the human commissurotomy subject also can be made to perceive two quite different things occupying the same position in space at the same time, something rejected, of course, by the normal brain. The method (Levy, Trevarthen, and Sperry 1972) involves the use of compound left–right stimuli composed of the left and right halves of different pairs of stimulus items joined at the vertical midline (see Figure 22.3) and projected half to one hemisphere and half to the other. By the laws of perceptual completion and closure each hemisphere automatically tends to fill in its half stimulus across the midline to form a whole bisymmetric percept on each side (Trevarthen 1976).

Other kinds of evidence further confirm that, while one hemisphere is performing, the nondominant less-active hemisphere, though overtly passive in not exerting control over the motor system, may nevertheless be alert and consciously cognizant of what is going on externally. This is indicated, for example, in disgusted shaking of the head or irked facial expressions triggered from the minor hemisphere after it has heard its speaking partner making what it knows to be an incorrect answer. Also, it is not uncommon, while the informed right hemisphere is performing, for the vocal hemisphere to make remarks like, "Now, why did I do that?" "What's the matter with me anyway?"

In sum, cerebral commissurotomy appears to divide not only the brain but also the mind. Two separate realms of subjective awareness are apparent: one in each disconnected hemisphere, and each in itself seems to be remarkably whole, unified, and capable of supporting behavior comparable in many respects to that of the combined intact system. This latter is most impressive with respect to the dominant left vocal hemisphere, the high-level linguistic and related logistic capacities of which seem largely responsible for earlier impressions that cerebral commissurotomy fails to produce

any definite behavioral symptoms. It may be remembered in this connection that brain bisymmetry provides each hemisphere with a full complement of basic cerebral mechanisms.

Emotional tone appears to be an exception to the rule that each disconnected hemisphere during lateralized testing remains oblivious of the conscious experience of the partner hemisphere. Emotions are rather promptly transferred from one hemisphere to the other, presumably through intact brainstem mechanisms. Similarly, some sensory, attentional, and alertness aspects of awareness are also projected bilaterally via the intact brainstem to both hemispheres, as will be discussed more fully. For the present, it is important to note that each hemisphere thus contains in functional terms much more than the half mind one might predict at first thought without taking into account the extensive bilateral redundancy in brain organization. With the foregoing in mind, and with some further qualifications to be mentioned, we can accept the general conclusion that brain bisection yields two conscious minds or selves within the one cranium.

Functional asymmetry

The two disconnected hemispheres of man not only function as if each is independently conscious, but also as if each possesses distinctive qualitative properties not equally shared with the other. Linguistic, perceptual, cognitive, motor, attentional, and mnemonic asymmetries have been found (Bogen 1969; Gazzaniga 1970; Levy 1972; Levy et al. 1972; Milner and Taylor 1972; Zaidel 1973; Zaidel and Sperry 1973; Milner 1974; Nebes 1974; Sperry 1974a; Dimond 1976; Franco and Sperry 1977), most of which presumably reflect corresponding differences in the content and quality of subjective experience. Most conspicuous among these functional asymmetries is the presence of speech, writing, reading, and calculation in the left hemisphere and the relative absence of these same functions in the right hemisphere.

Prior controversy and uncertainties of the early 1960s as to whether the nonvocal hemisphere has simply lagged behind in human evolution or alternatively has evolved advanced

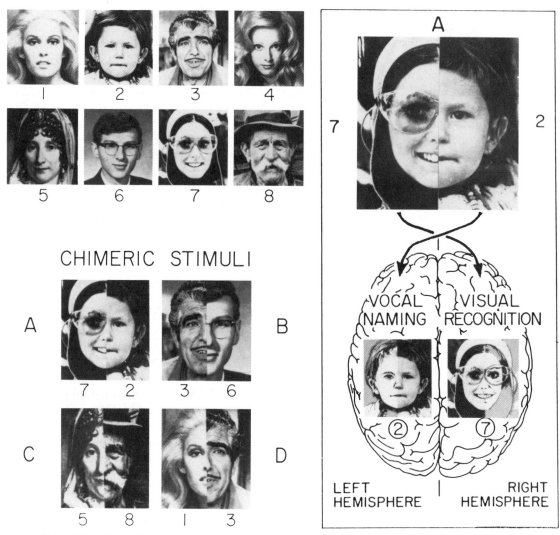

Figure 22.3. Method by which two hemispheres of split-brain human subjects may be shown to perceive two different and mutually exclusive things at the same point in space at the same time. With gaze centered on the nose of the composite stimulus figure, each hemisphere sees a different half stimulus, the missing half of which is automatically completed in each hemisphere to form a bisymmetric whole. (Levy et al. 1972.)

nonverbal specialties of its own (Denny-Brown 1962; Hécaen 1962) seem now to be effectively settled in numerous studies involving direct left–right comparisons within individuals, where many otherwise complicating variables cancel out, and in which the so-called subordinate and relatively passive hemisphere has proven to be the superior and dominant hemisphere. It has been possible further to extend the concept of hemispheric specialization to basic modes in cerebral information processing.

Led by Levy (Levy-Agresti and Sperry 1968; Levy 1972), one may interpret hemispheric specialization in man to be a result of the evolutionary differentiation of two mutually conflicting modes of cerebral processing, holistic-spatial and analytic-sequential in nature. In ordinary mental testing of any series of brain-damaged patients, one tends to take for granted that they will show individual differences in cognitive style and in the kinds of mental strategies employed in approaching test tasks. However, when one sees the same individual consistently approaching and solving a set of problems in two distinct ways, like two different persons, depending on whether the left or the right hemisphere is in use, even subtle left–right cognitive differences become meaningful. Prior doubts and uncertainties resolve and the way is clear to further delineate the nature, extent, and functional role of the left–right differences in cerebral processing.

The demonstrated specialties of the minor hemisphere are, first, nonverbal and nonmathematical and mostly involve spatial and visualizing abilities in which a single mental image is more effective than a long series of words. Geometrical discriminations of topological forms, for example, are performed at a high level by the right hemisphere, but seem to be extremely difficult or impossible for the left hemisphere (Franco and Sperry 1977). The prevailing neurological doctrine of the early 1960s, based mainly on symptoms of unilateral brain lesions, had depicted the minor hemisphere as being typically mute, agraphic, word blind, and word deaf, and correspondingly agnostic in language-related faculties (Geschwind and Kaplan 1962; Geschwind 1976). This older view has now receded before mounting evidence of positive language performance of the minor hemisphere after commissurotomy. The capacity of the disconnected minor hemisphere to comprehend spoken instructions and even read words flashed to the left field of vision (Gazzaniga and Sperry 1967; Sperry and Gazzaniga 1967; Sperry, Gazzaniga, and Bogen 1969) was found from the start to be much more developed after commissurotomy than anticipated in view of the severe receptive aphasias that have been reported to follow unilateral lesions of the language centers in the dominant hemisphere. Initial inclinations to interpret these right-hemisphere language abilities in our commissurotomy cases as an exception to the rule, caused perhaps by diffusing effects of long-term epilepsy or just by individual differences, have now given way to a revised view in which the minor hemisphere of the typical right-hander is credited with substantial, though limited and selective, language functions.

The linguistic faculties of the minor hemisphere have been measured more thoroughly and precisely in recent years by Zaidel (1973) using our two best commissurotomy cases and also three hemispherectomy patients, one of the dominant hemisphere. Zaidel (1975) uses a "stabilized image" technique in which a half-field occluder is mounted on the eye on a scleral contact lens (Figure 22.4). The system allows prolonged exposure of visual material with ocular scanning up to one-half hour. A high-level vocabulary for the comprehension of single spoken words is confirmed, showing in two patients a mental age for the minor hemisphere of eleven and sixteen years, respectively, only two years below that for the vocal hemisphere in these same subjects on the same Peabody Picture Vocabulary Test. In contrast to our earlier results, no specialization was found for nouns as opposed to verbs. The minor hemisphere lexicon appears to follow instead the frequency of word usage. Zaidel finds the right hemisphere to be capable of syntactic and phonetic as well as semantic discriminations.

With respect to reading, writing, and speaking, the results have not much changed our earlier impressions based on tachistoscopic tests. We anticipated that the long exposure and examination of whole sentences instead of single words might reveal a higher level of reading ability, but this is not the case. In general, the ability of the minor hemisphere to process single words stands in marked contrast to its inability to deal with words in series, at least in prose. These limitations do not apply in the same way when words are strung together in singing a familiar melody or in emotional exclamations. In any case, with regard to issues concerning the presence and quality of consciousness in the minor hemisphere, one should keep in mind that the cerebral processing of this hemisphere, though it does not support much speech, is in the current view not at all devoid of linguistic dimensions.

Minor-hemisphere consciousness

The conclusion that cerebral commissurotomy results in the presence of two largely independent conscious entities, one based in each hemisphere, has not gone unchallenged. Some authorities have preferred to think that the unity of the conscious self is preserved in these subjects with its center in the vocal left hemisphere or in a metasystem in the intact brainstem (MacKay 1966; Penfield 1966; Eccles

1973). These and other theoretically possible ways of interpreting the commissurotomy and related findings have been reviewed in a comprehensive philosophical perspective by Nagel (1971).

Our own impression that both hemispheres, the minor as well as the major, are separately conscious after commissurotomy and that the two disconnected hemispheres may commonly be coconscious in parallel, even in mutually conflicting experiences, is based mainly on the kinds of things that the minor hemisphere has been shown to be capable of doing in the course of a long series of tests over many years. The subjective experience of the minor hemisphere has to be inferred almost entirely, of course, from nonverbal manual performance, although facial, linguistic, and emotional expression generated in the minor hemisphere are also involved. Mute test performances of the minor hemisphere show that it can sense, perceive, learn, and remember all at a characteristically human level. The disconnected mute hemisphere can center and hold a focus of attention, perform high-level spatial reasoning and spatial transformation, generate concepts, make cognitive decisions, and carry out volitional actions. It displays goal preferences and can act on value priorities, and it shows typical human emotional responses in reactions to affect-laden stimuli and situations. It further comprehends spoken single words at a moderately high level and to a lesser extent can also read and comprehend single printed words.

In the face of accumulating evidence along these lines, earlier claims that the speechless hemisphere is not conscious are now giving way to intermediate positions contending that we must remain agnostic about consciousness in the minor hemisphere or that the minor hemisphere possesses only an elemental form of consciousness not sufficiently advanced to be the basis of a conscious human person or self. Specifically, the nonvocal hemisphere has been interpreted to be lacking in self-awareness (DeWitt 1975). Self-awareness rates as a comparatively advanced and characteristically human form of consciousness appearing relatively late phylogenetically in primate evolution and also late ontogenetically in childhood.

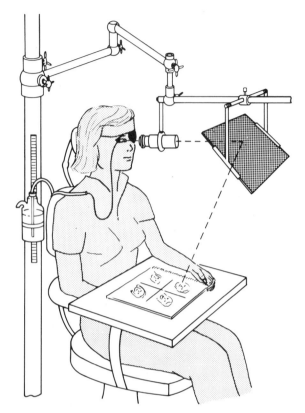

Figure 22.4. Setup employing contact lens technique of Zaidel that continuously blanks out visual input to one hemisphere, used here to test for upper levels of awareness in the minor hemisphere.

In recent efforts to explore further the upper levels of conscious awareness in the disconnected mute hemisphere (Sperry and Zaidel 1973), we have used the stabilized occluder technique developed by Zaidel to test for a sense of self-consciousness and for general social awareness. If these higher peculiarly human levels of conscious awareness can be shown to be present, one may infer that the lower levels of awareness must be there as well. The subject in these tests wears a scleral contact lens on which is mounted a small optical system with an opaque screen that moves with the eye and blocks out the selected half field of vision wherever the gaze is directed. The procedure is to present to the subject for examination a choice array of pictures or photographs, usually four (see Figure 22.4), including items for which the subject might have some familiarity, preference, or an emotional response, such as pictures of the subject, of family, relatives, pets and belongings, political, historical and religious figures, and well-known figures from the entertainment world. After leading questions and remarks by the examiner to establish desired mental sets and associations, the subject is asked to point to the item in the choice array he or she would select for a given situation or reason, the one that he or she most likes or dislikes, or might recognize, and to differentiate by "thumbs-up" or "thumbs-down" his or her feelings about selected individuals, etc.

The kinds of reactions obtained from the mute hemisphere in the two patients thus far fitted with the required corneal contact lens (LB and NG) strongly indicate a characteristic self- and social awareness that is generally normal and roughly comparable to that of the language-dominant hemisphere. If anything, the emotional responses generated in the right hemisphere in these two subjects were more intense and less inhibited than those from the left. Minor-hemisphere reactions included appropriate emotional outbursts when pictures of the subject's self were introduced by surprise among the test items in an unexpected or unseemly context. The emotional tone of these responses promptly crossed to the other hemisphere, presumably by brainstem mechanisms, and affected the vocalization of the blinded hemisphere, changing the tone of voice, evoking exclamations, etc. From the content of the speech, however, which included comments like "what are they?" "something nice," "whatever it was," it was clear that the speaking hemisphere remained unaware of the particular visual material that had triggered (via the mute hemisphere) its emotional reaction. When the speaking hemisphere was allowed a series of follow-up guesses, however, and eventually came to ask, "Was it me?" "Myself?" the minor-hemisphere recognition of the audible stimulus as correct had some kind of a central effect that was registered across and recognized in the speaking hemisphere, which thereon settled with satisfaction on this as the answer.

When the subjects were asked directly if they could find a portrait photo of themselves inserted among similar photos in the choice array, they had no trouble doing so, working with either hemisphere. Pictures of pets, other belongings, and of scenes in and outside the home were readily recognized by either hemisphere and evoked appropriate responses. Pictures of well-known public or historical figures, relatives, and acquaintances also were readily pointed out by the minor as well as the major hemisphere. Evaluative judgments from the right hemisphere expressed by preferential pointing and by "thumbs-up"/"thumbs-down" gestures were consistent with those obtained verbally from the other hemisphere of the same subject and also in free vision. For example, in a series of trials with LB, a 21-year-old male subject, the response from the right hemisphere was "thumbs-up" for Churchill, pretty girls, Johnny Carson, and a ballet scene, and "thumbs-down" for Hitler, Castro, and a war scene. A photo of Nixon (the date of testing was pre-Watergate) evoked some indecision, ending in an intentional and definite horizontal neutral. A photo of the subject himself inserted at the end of this same series evoked a definite "thumbs-down" response, but in this case, unlike the others, the response was accompanied by a distinct, wide, sheepish, and (we think) self-conscious grin generated in the mute hemisphere.

Again, follow-up verbal questioning by the examiner, as well as spontaneous remarks of the subject during testing, indicated that the vocal hemisphere had remained quite unaware of the contents of the test material presented to the minor hemisphere. However, if such verbal questioning were pursued, the subject's left hemisphere was commonly able, with the combined cues from himself and the examiner, to narrow in, after a few exchanges, on the correct category and sometimes on the specific test item. It was concluded that the mute disconnected minor hemisphere does indeed possess self-and social awareness at levels quite comparable to those of the left hemisphere and of the intact brain as a whole.

Incompleteness of psychological division

Although the foregoing and many similar lateralized tests indicate that each surgically disconnected hemisphere has a conscious domain of its own and that the bulk of the content of mental experience in each hemisphere remains cut off from any direct awareness through the other hemisphere, there are important qualifications to be kept in mind in thinking about the degree and nature of this mental separation. This applies especially to behavior under natural nonlateralized conditions. Many unifying factors can be enumerated (Sperry 1968, 1974b) that tend to make at least components of the inner experience of the two disconnected hemispheres similar or identical in orientation and content especially during ordinary unrestricted behavior. The bilateral sensory projection systems of the brain, like those for cutaneous sensibility of the face, ensure a bilateral reduplication of symmetric sensations in both hemispheres. Thus, with conscious attention focused on facial, auditory, or other stimuli that get bilateral representation, both hemispheres presumably develop a full bilateral percept with no vertical split between right and left aspects. Scanning movements of the eyes yield a similar duplication with respect to vision (Sperry 1970a, 1974a). The overall effect in some respects is thus more like a twinning or doubling of the conscious domain of the self rather than midline division. This bisymmetric reduplication of sensory input from proprioception and from some external sources provides a considerable background of left–right unification in the functional organization in both hemispheres and has been an important factor in the concept of two separate minds or selves in the bisected brain. Insofar as mental activities are identical in the two hemispheres, there is no way to prove behaviorally that the two are separate; this can only be extrapolated from analogous conditions where the functions differ.

Unity in conscious experience after hemisphere deconnection tends to be preserved also by cross-integration systems of the intact brainstem like those referred to before that mediate a prompt bilateralization of emotion generated unilaterally. This brainstem cross-integration we presume involves also mood, alertness, and perhaps subtle shades of these as in the more elemental dimensions of mental sets and attention. This latter is inferred from the ability of the vocal hemisphere in tests for social awareness to sense orientational, categorical, or attitudinal cues generated in the mute hemisphere, which then enable the vocal member to center in on the correct general category of a mute hemisphere experience. Cross transmission of some components of auditory verbal images at brainstem levels remains a possibility. At any rate, some affective, cognitive, and attentional aspects of consciousness seem to be effectively transmitted from one side to the other to further help the two disconnected hemispheres to function together in harmony and in some respects as a unit.

Whether the neural cross integration involved in the foregoing as, for example, that mediating emotional tone, constitutes an extension of a single conscious process or is better interpreted as just a transmission of neural activity that triggers a second and separate bisymmetric conscious effect in the opposite hemisphere remains open at this stage. In any case, it is pertinent to remember that the bilateralizing and unifying mechanisms are largely of the nonfocal general background category, whereas conscious awareness tends on the other hand to be correlated predominantly with attentional and focal aspects of cerebral function.

When all unifying factors like the above are taken into account in combination with the evidence for functional deconnection, one is led to conclude with respect to ordinary behavior that the bulk of conscious experience after cerebral commissurotomy is separated into two distinct hemispheric domains, but that these are usually similar in their attentional focus and have a large common overlap in general content. Differences contributed by the lateral specialization of the hemispheres will, of course, be accentuated whenever the cerebral processing becomes centered exclusively around specialties of either hemisphere like speech, calculation, or topological reasoning.

During lateralized testing, prolonged use of a single hemisphere with deprivation of focal input to the other not uncommonly leads to a state in which there is a suppression of functional alertness in the nonworking hemisphere to the point where several trials may be required with input to this hemisphere to restore a state of proper function. In ordinary unrestricted behavior, on the other hand, it is rare that conditions would thus selectively restrict sensory input or central processing to one hemisphere for an extended period. Thus, typically, the two disconnected hemispheres appear to be actively, but separately, conscious in parallel, each working and contributing in its own way to the performance on which attention is focused.

The inference that the disconnected hemispheres are commonly in a state of simultaneous separate coconscious awareness receives additional support from many bilateral tests that involve concurrent but different sensory input and different motor response from each hemisphere. The conclusion is reinforced as well by numerous incidental observations like those involving cross-cueing, which variously require that the second hemisphere be actively alert while the other is performing. Coconscious involvement is indicated also in Zaidel's recent evidence (personal communication 1976) that scores for commissurotomy subjects with free vision are superior to those of either hemisphere working alone on the visual reception subtest of the Illinois Test of Psycholinguistic Abilities. Coconsciousness is further inferred from tests involving competitive double performances, like reading aloud or whistling while counting or sorting blocks with left and right hand. When the two tasks involve the same hemisphere, there is severe interference, whereas tasks performed in separate hemispheres can be carried through in parallel.

Implications for consciousness in the normal intact brain

It has been argued by Anderson (1974) that, if one can have two coconscious entities occupying the same cranium concurrently, as in commissurotomy subjects, and if two or more different persons can occupy the same body successively, as in multiple-personality or fugue states, it follows logically that it is no longer correct to identify a "person" or "self" as being correlated one-to-one with a body. The concepts and definitions of "person," "self," and related terms need accordingly to be more precisely refined in terms of the critical brain states involved. Such definitions become important for medicolegal issues concerning, for example, comatose, anencephalic, or severely deranged mental conditions, in evaluating donors for vital organ transplants, in dealing with different stages in fetal development, etc.

An interesting position in regard to the concept of "personal identity" has been taken by Puccetti (1973, 1976) and Bogen (1969) who infer that each hemisphere must have a mind of its own – not only after brain bisection, but in the normal intact state as well, a conclusion apparently accepted also by DeWitt (1975) with the qualification that only the left cerebral member has self-awareness and is therefore qualified as a person. The argument goes like this: if cutting the cross connections between the hemispheres leaves two coconscious minds, and if surgical removal of a whole hemisphere, that is, hemispherectomy, leaves one conscious person or self, regardless of which hemisphere is removed, then there must have been two present to start with. Puccetti contends that we are, therefore, all of us, really a compound of two conscious persons that coexist in the normal brain, one based in each hemisphere, and that this goes undetected when the commissures are intact and the normally conjoined hemispheres work in perfect synchrony. Because a similar proposal regarding the inherent duality of mind was made back in 1844 by Wigan (see Zangwill 1974), modern dual-mind proponents are known as "latter-day Wiganites." Again, one is impressed with the need for sharpening definitions of mind, person, self, and related concepts. Regardless of terminology, however, the question of whether the normal intact brain contains only one unified realm of conscious awareness or alternatively maintains two separate conscious systems, or minds, one centered in each hemisphere, poses a rather clear dichotomy that should be subject eventually to a definite empirical answer.

My own position on this question has been a relatively conventional one. I see consciousness and the conscious self as being normally single and unified, mediated by brain processes that typically involve and span both hemispheres through the commissures. This interpretation implies: first, that the fiber systems of the brain mediate the stuff of conscious awareness as well as the switching mechanisms, synaptic interfaces, or other interaction sites of the gray matter; and, second, that the fiber cross connections between the hemispheres are not different in this respect from fiber systems within each hemisphere. Third, this interpretation is based on a theory of consciousness that goes back to the early 1950s (Sperry 1952) in which the subjective unity in conscious experience, along with other subjective effects, is ascribed not so much to corresponding spatiotemporal unity in neural activity or to other isomorphic or topological correspondence, but rather to the operational or functional effects in brain dynamics. What counts in determining subjective meaning on these terms is the way a given brain process works in the context of cerebral organization. Subjective unity is accordingly conceived in terms of organizational and functional relations which in turn leads to the idea of a functional (thus causal) impact.

When I tried to put some of these threads together back in the mid-1960s, I found to my initial consternation (as well as that of immediate colleagues) that what seemed to be emerging was a conceptual formula for the way that conscious mind could move matter in the brain and exert causal influence in the direction and control of behavior – in direct contradiction, of course, to the central founding precepts of behaviorism and of twentieth-century scientific materialism generally, and contrary to everything that we had always been taught and believed. When this "unthinkable thought" nevertheless continued to hold up under repeated reexamination, I decided to risk a trial-run publication in a humanist lecture (Sperry 1965, 1966) that might allow me to save face should it promptly be shot down. When, instead, it held up in the marketplace with favorable feedback, it was presented more seriously four years later to the National Academy of Sciences (Sperry 1969a), since when it has had a fairly wide exposure in the literature (Sperry 1969b, 1970a, 1970b, 1972, 1974b, 1976a, 1976b, 1976c, 1976d, 1977). The longer it survives, of course, the less casually it is taken.

Since the main concepts have been presented recently in some detail elsewhere, they are reviewed in rather brief outline to permit added regard for some of the broader implications and humanistic impact. In essence, consciousness was conceived to be a dynamic emergent of brain activity, neither identical with, nor reducible to, the neural events of which it is mainly composed. Further, consciousness was not conceived as an epiphenomenon, inner aspect, or other passive correlate of brain processing, but rather to be an active integral part of the cerebral process itself, exerting potent causal effects in the interplay of cerebral operations. In a position of top command at the highest levels in the hierarchy of brain organization, the subjective properties were seen to exert control over the biophysical and chemical activities at subordinate levels. It was described initially as a brain model that puts "conscious mind back into the brain of objective science in a position of top command . . . a brain model in which conscious, mental, psychic forces are recognized to be the crowning achievement . . . of evolution" (Sperry 1965, 1966). It must be emphasized at the outset that no direct empirical proof is available, any more than proof is available for the opposing behaviorist position. At this stage, we have only a balance in credibility, all things considered, and the most that can be said is that many of us have now come to regard these psychophysical-interaction concepts as being a little more credible in several respects than the older behaviorist-materialist stance.

Broadly speaking, one of the more important revisions brought by the current concepts is a shift in the scientific status of consciousness. In the past, consciousness has been variously dispensed within science as some kind of parallelistic epiphenomenon, aspect, or correlate of brain processing, and has been considered to be entirely passive in cerebral operations without influence on the stream of physical causation in brain activity, and therefore something that objective science could safely ignore. On our new terms, consciousness, as a holistic systemic property and an active dynamic part of high-order brain processing, is now put within the province of science and is something that cannot be ignored where science wants an explanation of higher brain activities. In effect this change means that the whole value-rich qualitative world of innerconscious, subjective experience, the world of the humanities, that has long been explicitly excluded from the domain of science on materialist principles, is now reinstated. In the revised scheme, subjective phenomena have a place and a use in brain function and a reason for having been evolved in a physical system.

An overall consequence of this change is that many of the more objectionable materialistic, mechanistic, deterministic, and reductionistic aspects of science that the humanities have always found difficult to accept and relate to, and which have consistently drawn the fire of antiscience, no longer apply in the new framework. Science, behavioral science in particular, acquires a new look in this perspective to become much more mentalistic, subjectivistic, and humanistic. The swing we have witnessed in recent years toward an increased recognition of conscious subjective experience and referred to variously as the "humanist" or "third resolution" in psychology, the "cognitive revolution" or just the "new psychology," can be seen to be more than just a matter of changing attitudes in science or a reflection of general trends of the time. The new subjectivism in psychology has authentic support and grounding in basic theoretical changes in fundamental mind/brain concepts.

The past strength of the materialist-behaviorist movement has rested in no small measure on the seeming inconceivability that the causal march of neuromechanisms could be influenced by the contents of subjective experience. The present undermining of prior convictions in this area has resulted in a floodgate release of all the pent-up subjectivist pressures held back for decades by behaviorist doctrine. All those disciplines in behavioral science that by preference or by necessity work with subjective experience directly, such as the clinical, cognitive, and humanist schools, also acquire in the new framework a corresponding shift in scientific status. Parallel changes have occurred also in philosophy dealing with mind/brain relations. Today one finds mentalists, dualists, and psychophysical interactionists surfacing again in numbers after having been essentially silent and invisible for decades.

It is important to caution that there is nothing in the current theoretical change that makes subjective experience any easier to work with by scientific methodology and that therefore many of the old arguments against the use of introspection in experimentation still apply. One must caution further that the above legitimate changes toward an increased recognition of subjective mental experience supported by theory have been accompanied in recent years by a series of corollary developments not similarly supported by theory, but which have opportunistically ridden along on the same upsurge of new interest in mental phenomena. Things like mysticism, occultism, astrology, faith healing, and parapsychology also have enjoyed a new vigor and popular acceptance in the past eight or nine years. The current view of consciousness as an emergent property of the living brain in action with all its anatomical and physiological constraints hardly increases the likelihood of things like mental telepathy, precognition, psychokinesis, or the existence of mental domains of experience separate from brain activity.

Formula for psychophysical interaction

Perhaps the simplest and quickest way to approach and explain our current mind/brain concept is to compare it with better-known preexistent theories and thus, largely by elimination, to state what the present view is by describing what it is not. First, consciousness in the current view is not an acausal epiphenomenon as widely held in materialist theory. Second, consciousness is not just an "internal aspect" of brain activity as in "dual-aspect theory." An internal aspect is conceivable for all neural processing, but consciousness is special. Third, conscious experience is not conceived to be identical to neural events as in "psychophysical-identity theory." In the present view, conscious phenomena are different from, more than, and not reducible to, neural events, though it is correct to say that conscious phenomena are built of neural events as elements and perhaps also of glial and other cerebral events. Fourth, consciousness is not a pseudoproblem conjured into our thinking by semantic gymnastics, or something that will disappear with a proper linguistic approach. In brief, we can thus bypass previous interpretations of the epiphenomenal, parallelistic, passive correlate, dual aspect, psychophysical identity, and semantic pseudoproblem types in order to focus on consciousness as an emergent property of brain activity, as upheld especially by the Gestalt school of psychology in ideas that peaked during the 1930s and early 1940s under Kohler (1929), Koffka (1935), Kohler and Held (1949), and others (see Boring 1942).

It then remains to distinguish our present model from these earlier emergent Gestalt concepts. First, the emergent properties of the present view are not conceived to be correlated with, nor derived from, electrical field or volume current conduction effects in the cortex. They are conceived rather in terms of traditional nerve-circuit and nerve-integration theory. Second, the brain processes of consciousness are not conceived to depend on isomorphic or topological correspondence with the mental event. Conscious meaning is a functional derivative conceived in terms of functional impact and potential. Third, while the current view agrees with Gestalt theory that the conscious phenomena are not reducible to the neural elements, it does not take the extreme Gestalt position that categorically rejects analysis and explanation in terms of the parts. Fourth, and most important, the emergent properties in the present view are not interpreted to be mere passive, parallel correlates, or passive aspects or by-products of cortical events, but as active causal determinants essential to the normal cerebral control.

A conceptual explanatory model for psychoneural interaction is provided, stated in terms acceptable to neuroscience without violating the monistic principles of scientific explanation. The main focus is on the feature of causality. By all prior theories of consciousness, at all recognized by science, consciousness was interpreted to be acausal in brain function, and brain research could accordingly confine itself to the neurophysiology, chemistry, and biophysics of brain processing, totally ignoring consciousness, and expect this approach to lead, in principle, to a complete explanation of brain function. This, of course, is not the case with the present view in which consciousness (to repeat) plays a causal role and is neither identical to, nor reducible to, the neural events.

Given our present perspectives, it is not difficult now to stretch the meaning of terms such as "neural events," "brain events," "brain processes," etc., to include their emergent (i.e., holistic, configurational, organizational, gestalt, pattern) conscious properties and to thus bring psychophysical identity theory into line with the current emergent interpretation. On these terms identity theory tends to fuse with emergentism and is then forced to espouse reductionist philosophy to retain identity. Either way we come around to much the same concept. It has been pointed out (Sperry 1970b, 1976c) that the theoretical and semantic distinctions that prevailed in philosophy prior to 1965 no longer hold in the same way in the context of current perspectives.

Even after the meaning of neural events is stretched to include the holistic conscious properties, our current model still differs from identity theory in that it identifies consciousness only with the holistic properties of *select* brain processes and then not with their neurophysiological, biophysical, and chemical infrastructure. The holistic conscious properties are recognized to be distinctive "real" phenomena in their own right with their own distinctive causal properties. Though mainly composed of neural events, conscious phenomena are not conceived to be "nothing but" neural events.

The causal power attributed to the subjective properties is nothing mystical. It is seen to reside in the hierarchical organization of the nervous system combined with the universal power of any whole over its parts. Any system that coheres as a whole, acting, reacting, and interacting as a unit, has systemic organizational properties of the system as a whole that determine its behavior as an entity, and control thereby at the same time the course and fate of its components. The whole has properties as a system that are not reducible to the properties of the parts, and the properties at higher levels exert causal control over those at lower levels. In the case of brain function, the conscious properties of high-order brain activity determine the course of the neural events at lower levels (Sperry 1966). The term "interaction" for the psychophysical relation is perhaps not the best descriptively, but is used for its historical connotations that still apply in the sense that mental phenomena are conceived to exert causal control influence on neural events.

Emergent properties are generally assumed to have causal potency elsewhere at all levels, and one need merely insist that no exception should be made in the case of the yet-to-be-described aspects of cerebral processing responsible for consciousness. On the foregoing terms, psychology and psychiatry are best interpreted as distinct disciplines in their own right, not reducible or identical to neuroscience or behavioral biology. In other words, "The meaning of the message will not be found in the chemistry of the ink." This exaggeration, however, should not be taken to the extreme of depreciating the tremendous explanatory value of analysis and of subdisciplines in science generally, at least those close to the level of the causal unknowns under investigation. Our concepts of the emergent subjective properties and their causality are still, of course, at a general, abstract level. It remains by this and by any other theory thus far available to explain those critical organizational differences that distinguish brain processes with subjective properties from those without, and to define in exact operational and neural terms the essential functional role played by subjective awareness.

From the standpoint of functional control, one may ask what benefits precisely are conferred by the introduction in evolution of subjective conscious effects? Thinking concerning this question is still preliminary and speculative along lines like the following: consider the tactical difference between responding to the world directly and responding to inner conscious representations of the outside world. Wherever displacements in time or in space are advantageous, as, for example, in mental recall, in thinking, and in the formation of anticipatory sets, the use of inner representations has indispensable organizational advantages. The real world can hardly be manipulated as can inner images. Responses involving perceptual constancies in shape, size, position, etc. would seem also to be more effectively managed through the use of inner representations. Further, the employment of implicit trial-and-error responses to inner mental models, and the avoidance thereby of overt response commitments, with possible errors in the real world, is a central rationale in the evolution of thinking.

The development of an inner subjective world may thus be viewed broadly as part of the evolutionary process of freeing behavior from its initial primitive stimulus-bound condition, providing increasing degrees of freedom of choice and of originative central processing. The subjective effects have additional advantages in the driving and directing of behavior as motivational elements and as positive and negative reinforcers. It is difficult to conceive an efficacious motivational system without subjective properties like pain, pleasure, hunger, etc. These subjective effects evolve into controlling ends in themselves in much of human behavior.

Conscious experience may be conceived as a rather distinct entity built into brain organization and expressly designed for specific functional effects, as opposed to viewing it as a general pervasive property of complex neural integration. There is reason to believe it is present in the higher brain centers but not in the spinal cord, for example, or lower brainstem, and probably not in the cerebellum either. The commissurotomy evidence indicates that the system for inner conscious representations in primates and cats, at least, is confined mainly to the cerebral hemispheres proper and the upper brainstem. We assume it to be rather diffusely represented within the forebrain, but by no means extending throughout all neural activity at forebrain levels. On the input side of the conscious system, a great deal of the sensory processing is completed automatically and unconsciously. The integrations required for constancy effects like those for perceived position in space during head, eye, and body movements, or for the union of monocular two-dimensional patterns into novel three-dimensional percepts, or the processing of elemental auditory sounds into perceived speech, etc., are extremely complex neural functions but appear to be processed without conscious mediation. Similarly, on the output side, most or all of the complicated processing required to translate conscious aims, percepts, and volitional intent into appropriate motor-behavior patterns also takes place automatically and unconsciously. The intricate arrays of requisite muscle-contraction patterns involve a complexity that goes far beyond the ability of the conscious mind to understand and direct. This is another reason to identify the conscious properties with the relatively simple holistic features rather than with the whole intricate inframechanism of brain processing.

Though representing a rather small fraction of the total brain activity in physiological terms, the conscious properties are of prime importance from the organizational standpoint. For example, the laying down, storage cataloging, and retrieval of memories seems to proceed very largely on the basis of their holistic conscious properties rather than those of the neuronal inframechanisms. Most higher brain processing in many can be viewed as being designed for, and directed toward, the generation, maintenance, or expression of aspects of conscious awareness. Older stimulus-response and central-switchboard concepts of brain organization that arose out of spinal-cord physiology and were congenial to behaviorist interpretation may be replaced by a model in which the brain is seen to be organized as a decision-making control system monitored with value priorities, and in which conscious phenomena confer certain operational advantages over and above those obtainable in systems that lack consciousness.

Acknowledgments

Portions of this chapter draw substantially on prior presentations for the 9th International Symposium on Brain Research, Netherlands Central Institute for Brain Research, Amsterdam, July 1975, and a symposium on The Psychology of Consciousness, The Institute for the study of Human Knowledge, San Francisco, May 8, 1976. Work of the author is supported by grant no. MH 03372 of the National Institutes of Mental Health and the F. P. Hixon Fund of the California Institute of Technology.

References

Akelaitis, A. J. 1943. Studies on the corpus callosum. VII. Study of language functions (tactile and visual lexia and graphia) unilaterally following section of corpus callosum. *J. Neuropathol. Exp. Neurol.* 2: 226–62.

Anderson, S. L. 1974. *On the Problem of Personal Identity.* PhD dissertation, University of California, Los Angeles.

Bogen, J. E. 1969. The other side of the brain. II. An appositional mind. *Bull. L.A. Neurol. Soc.* 34: 135–62.

Bogen, J. E., and P. J. Vogel. 1976. Neurological status in the long term following complete cerebral commissurotomy. *In* F. Michel and B. Schott (eds.) *Les Syndromes de disconnexion calleuse chez l'homme.* Hôpital Neurologique, Lyon.

Boring, E. G. 1942. *Sensation and Perception in the History of Psychology.* Appleton-Century-Crofts. New York.

Bremer, F. 1958. Physiology of the corpus callosum. *Brain and Human Behav.: Res. Proc. Assoc. Nerv. Ment. Dis.* 36: 424–48.

Bremer, F., J. Brihaye, and G. André-Balisaux. 1956. Physiologie et pathologie du corps calleux. *Schweizer Arch. Neurol. Neuroch. Psychiat.* 78: 31–87.

Denny-Brown, D. 1962. Discussion. *In* V. B. Mountcastle (ed.) *Interhemispheric Relations and Cerebral Dominance.* The Johns Hopkins Press, Baltimore.

DeWitt, L. 1975. Consciousness, mind and self: The implications of the split-brain studies. *Brit. J. Phil. Sci.* 26: 41–7.

Dimond, S. J. 1976. Depletion of attention capacity after total commissurotomy in man. *Brain* 99: 347–56.

Doty, R. 1975. Consciousness from neurons. *Acta Neurobiol. Exp.* 35: 791–804.

Downer, J. L. 1962. Interhemispheric integration in the visual system. *In* V. B. Mountcastle (ed.) *Interhemispheric Relations and Cerebral Dominance.* The Johns Hopkins Press, Baltimore.

Eccles, John C. 1973. *The Understanding of the Brain.* McGraw-Hill, New York.

Franco, L., and R. W. Sperry. 1977. Hemispheric lateralization for cognitive processing and geometry. *Neuropsychol.* 15: 107–14.

Gazzaniga, M. S. 1970. *The Bisected Brain.* Appleton-Century-Crofts, New York.

Gazzaniga, M. S., and R. W. Sperry. 1967. Language after section of the cerebral commissures. *Brain* 90: 131–48.

Geschwind, N. 1976. Discussion. *In* F. Michel and B. Schott (eds.) *Les Syndromes de disconnexion calleuse chez l'homme.* Hôpital Neurologique, Lyon.

Geschwind, N., and E. Kaplan. 1962. A human cerebral deconnection syndrome. *Neurol.* 12: 675–85.

Hécaen, H. 1962. Clinical symptomatology in right and left hemispheric lesions. *In* V. B. Mountcastle (ed.) *Interhemispheric Relations and Cerebral Dominance.* The Johns Hopkins Press, Baltimore.

Koffka, K. 1935. *Principles of Gestalt Psychology.* Harcourt Brace, New York.

Kohler, W. 1929. *Gestalt Psychology.* Liveright, New York.

Kohler, W., and R. Held. 1949. The cortical correlate of pattern vision. *Science* 110: 414–19.

Levy, J. 1972. Lateral specialization of the brain. *In* J. A. Kiger, Jr. (ed.) *Annual Colloquium on Biology of Behavior.* Oregon State University Press, Corvallis.

Levy, J., C. Trevarthen, and R. W. Sperry. 1972. Perception of bilateral chimeric figures following hemisphere deconnection. *Brain* 95: 61–78.

Levy-Agresti, J., and R. W. Sperry. 1968. Differential perceptual capacities in major and minor hemispheres. *Proc. Natl. Acad. Sci. USA* 61: 1151.

MacKay, D. 1966. Discussion. *In* J. C. Eccles (ed.) *Brain and Conscious Experience*. Springer-Verlag, New York.

Milner, B. 1974. Hemispheric specialization: Scope and limits. *In* F. O. Schmitt and F. G. Worden (eds.) *The Neurosciences: Third Study Program*. The MIT Press, Cambridge.

Milner, B., and L. Taylor. 1972. Right hemisphere superiority in tactile pattern-recognition after cerebral commissurotomy: Evidence for non-verbal memory. *Neuropsychol.* 10: 1–15.

Milner, B., L. Taylor, and R. W. Sperry. 1968. Lateralized suppression of dichotically presented digits after commissural section in man. *Science* 161: 184–5.

Myers, R. E. 1962. Transmission of visual information within and between the hemispheres. *In* V. B. Mountcastle (ed.) *Interhemispheric Relations and Cerebral Dominance*. The Johns Hopkins Press, Baltimore.

Myers, R. E., and R. W. Sperry. 1953. Interocular transfer of a visual form discrimination habit in cats after section of the optic chiasm and corpus callosum. *Anat. Rec.* 115: 351.

Nagel, T. 1971. Brain bisection and the unity of consciousness. *Synthese* 22: 396–413.

Nebes, R. 1974. Hemispheric specialization in commissurotomized man. *Psychol. Bull.* 18: 1–14.

Penfield, W. 1966. Speech, perception and the cortex. *In* J. C. Eccles (ed.) *Brain and Conscious Experience*. Springer-Verlag, New York.

Puccetti, R. 1973. Brain bisection and personal identity. *Brit. J. Phil. Sci.* 24: 339–55.

–1976. The mute self. A reaction to DeWitt's alternative account of the split-brain data. *Brit. J. Phil. Sci.* 27: 65–73.

Sperry, R. W. 1952. Neurology and the mind-brain problem. *Am. Scientist* 40: 291–312.

–1961. Cerebral organization and behavior. *Science* 133: 1749–57.

–1964. Problems outstanding in the evolution of the brain function: James Arthur Lecture on the evolution of the human brain. *In* R. Duncan and M. Weston-Smith (eds.) *American Museum of Natural History & The Encyclopedia of Ignorance*. Pergamon Press, Oxford and New York, pp. 423–33.

–1965. Mind, brain, and humanist values. *In* J. R. Platt (ed.) *New Views on the Nature of Man*. University of Chicago Press, Chicago. Reprinted in *Bull. Atom. Scientists* 22 (1966): 2–6.

–1966. Brain bisection and mechanisms of consciousness. *In* J. C. Eccles (ed.) *Brain and Conscious Experience*. Springer-Verlag, New York, pp. 298–313.

–1968. Mental unity following surgical disconnection of the cerebral hemispheres. *The Harvey Lectures, 1966–1967*. Series 62. Academic Press, New York, pp. 293–323.

–1969a. Toward theory of mind. *Proc. Natl. Acad. Sci. USA* 63: 230–1.

–1969b. A modified concept of consciousness. *Psychol. Rev.* 76: 532–6.

–1970a. Perception in the absence of the neocortical commissures. *Res. Publ. Assoc. Res. Nerv. Ment. Dis.* 48: 123–38.

–1970b. An objective approach to subjective experience: Further explanation of a hypothesis. *Psychol. Rev.* 77: 585–90.

–1972. Science and the problem of values. *Persp. Biol. and Med.* 16: 115–30. Reprinted in *Zygon* 9: 7–21, 1974.

–1974a. Lateral specialization in the surgically separated hemisphere. *In* F. O. Schmitt and F. G. Worden (eds.) *The Neurosciences: Third Study Program*. The MIT Press, Cambridge, pp. 5–19.

–1974b. Messages from the laboratory. *Eng. Sci. Caltech* 37: 29–32.

–1976a. Left-brain, right-brain. *Sat. Rev.* (August 9): 30–3.

–1976b. Mental phenomena as causal determinants in brain function. *In* G. G. Globus, G. Maxwell, and I. Savodnik (eds.) *Consciousness and the Brain*. Plenum, New York. Reprinted in *Process Studies* 5: 247–56.

–1976c. A unifying approach to mind and brain: Ten year perspective. *In* M. A. Corner and D. F. Swaab (eds.) *Progress in Brain Research*. Vol. 45: *Perspectives in Brain Research*. Elsevier, Amsterdam, pp. 463–9.

–1976d. Changing concepts of consciousness and free will. *Persp. Biol. Med.* 20(1): 9–19.

–1977. Bridging science and values – A unifying view of mind and brain. *Am. Psychologist* 32(4): 237–45. Reprinted in *Zygon* 14: 7–21, 1979.

Sperry, R. W., and M. S. Gazzaniga. 1967. Language following surgical disconnection of the hemispheres. *In* F. L. Darley (ed.) *Brain Mechanisms Underlying Speech and Language*. Grune and Stratton, New York, pp. 108–21.

Sperry, R. W., M. S. Gazzaniga, and J. E. Bogen. 1969. Interhemispheric relationships: The neocortical commissures; syndromes of hemisphere disconnection. *In* P. J. Vinken and G. W. Bruyn (eds.) *Handbook of Clinical Neurology*, Vol. 4. North-Holland, Amsterdam, pp. 273–90.

Sperry, R. W., and S. M. Green. 1964. Corpus callosum and perceptual integration of visual half-fields. *Anat. Rec.* 148: 339 (abstract).

Sperry, R. W., and E. Zaidel. 1973. Level of the consciousness in the surgically disconnected minor hemisphere. *In Proceedings of the 14th Annual Meeting of the Psychonomic Society* (abstract).

Stamm, J., N. Miner, and R. W. Sperry. 1956. Relearning tests for interocular transfer following division of optic chiasma and corpus callosum in cats. *J. Comp. Physiol. Psychol.* 49: 529–33.

Tieman, S., and C. Hamilton. 1974. Interhemispheric communication between extraoccipital visual areas in the monkey. *Brain Res.* 67: 279–87.

Trevarthen, C. 1962. Double visual learning in split brain monkeys. *Science* 136: 258–9.

–1976. Psychological activities after forebrain commissurotomy in man. *In* F. Michel and B. Schott (eds.) *Les Syndromes de disconnexion calleuse chez l'homme.* Hôpital Neurologique, Lyon.

Wigan, A. L. 1844. *The Duality of the Mind.* Longman, London.

Zaidel, D., and R. W. Sperry. 1973. Performance on Raven's colored progressive matrices tests by subjects with cerebral commissurotomy. *Cortex* 9: 34–9.

Zaidel, E. 1973. *Linguistic Competence and Related Functions in the Right Cerebral Hemisphere following Commissurotomy and Hemispherectomy.* Doctoral dissertation, California Institute of Technology, Pasadena. *Diss. Abst. Intl.* 34: 2350B. University Microfilms no. 73–26, 481.

–1975. A technique for presenting lateralized visual input with prolonged exposure. *Vis. Res.* 15: 283–9.

Zangwill, O. L. 1974. Consciousness and the cerebral hemispheres. *In* S. Dimond and J. Beaumont (eds.) *Hemisphere Function in the Human Brain.* Paul Elek, London.

APPENDIX A   Publications of Roger W. Sperry

1939

R. W. Sperry. Action current study in movement coordination. *J. Gen. Psychol.* 20: 295–313.

R. W. Sperry. The functional results of muscle transplantation in the hind limb of the Albino rat. *Anat. Rec.* 75 (Suppl.): 51 (abstract).

1940

R. W. Sperry. The functional results of muscle transposition in the hind limb of the rat. *J. Comp. Neurol.* 73: 379–404.

P. Weiss and R. W. Sperry. Unmodifiability of muscular coordination in the rat, demonstrated by muscle transposition and nerve crossing. *Am. J. Physiol.* 129: 492 (abstract).

1941

J. M. Snodgrass and R. W. Sperry. Mammalian muscle action potentials of less than a millisecond. *Am. J. Physiol.* 133: 455 (abstract).

R. W. Sperry. The effect of crossing nerves to antagonistic muscles in the hind limb of the rat. *J. Comp. Neurol.* 75: 1–19.

R. W. Sperry. *Functional Results of Crossing Nerves and Transposing Muscles in the Fore and Hind Limb of the Rat.* Unpublished doctoral dissertation, University of Chicago.

1942

R. W. Sperry. Fixed persistence in the rat of spinal reflex patterns rendered extremely maladaptive by cross union of sensory nerves. *Anat. Rec.* 84: 483 (abstract).

R. W. Sperry. Reestablishment of visuomotor coordinations by optic nerve regeneration. *Anat. Rec.* 84: 470 (abstract).

R. W. Sperry. Transplantation of motor nerves and muscles in the forelimb of the rat. *J. Comp. Neurol.* 76: 283–321.

1943

R. W. Sperry. Effect of 180 degree rotation of the retinal field on visuomotor coordination. *J. Exp. Zool.* 92: 263–79.

R. W. Sperry. Functional results of crossing sensory nerves in the rat. *J. Comp. Neurol.* 78: 59–90.

K. S. Lashley and R. W. Sperry. Olfactory discrimination after destruction of the anterior thalamic nuclei. *Am. J. Physiol.* 139: 446–50.

R. W. Sperry. Visuomotor coordination in the newt (*Triturus viridescens*) after regeneration of the optic nerve. *J. Comp. Neurol.* 79: 33–55.

1944

R. W. Sperry. Optic nerve regeneration with return of vision in anurans. *J. Neurophysiol.* 7: 57–69.

1945

R. W. Sperry. Centripetal regeneration of the 8th cranial nerve root with systematic restoration of vestibular reflexes. *Am. J. Physiol.* 144: 735–41.

R. W. Sperry. Fixed persistence in the rat of spinal reflex patterns rendered extremely maladaptive by cross union of sensory nerves. *Fed. Proc.* 4: 67 (film abstract).

R. W. Sperry. Horizontal intracortical organization in the cerebral control of limb movement. *Proc. Soc. Exp. Biol. Med.* 60: 78–9.

R. W. Sperry. Restoration of vision after crossing of optic nerves and after contralateral transplantation of the eye. *J. Neurophysiol.* 8: 15–28.

R. W. Sperry. The problem of central nervous reorganization after nerve regeneration and muscle transposition. *Quart. Rev. Biol.* 20: 311–69.

1946

R. W. Sperry. Ontogenetic development and maintenance of compensatory eye movements in complete absence of the optic nerve. *J. Comp. Psychol.* 39: 321–30.

1947

R. W. Sperry. Cerebral regulation of motor coordination in monkeys following multiple transection of sensorimotor cortex. *J. Neurophysiol.* 10: 275–94.

R. W. Sperry. Effect of crossing nerves to antagonistic limb muscles in the monkey. *Arch. Neurol. Psychol.* 58: 452–73.

R. W. Sperry. Nature of functional recovery following regeneration of the oculomotor nerve in amphibians. *Anat. Rec.* 97: 293–316.

1948

R. W. Sperry. Orderly patterning of synaptic associations in regeneration of intracentral fiber tracts mediating visuomotor coordination. *Anat. Rec.* 102: 63–75.

R. W. Sperry. Patterning of central synapses in regeneration of the optic nerve in teleosts. *Physiol. Zool.* 21: 351–61.

1949

R. W. Sperry and N. Miner. Formation within sensory nucleus V of synaptic associations mediating cutaneous localization. *J. Comp. Neurol.* 90: 403–23.

R. W. Sperry and E. Clark. Interocular transfer of visual discrimination habits in a teleost fish. *Physiol. Zool.* 22: 372–78.

R. W. Sperry. Reimplantation of eyes in fishes (*Bathygobius soporator*) with recovery of vision. *Proc. Soc. Exp. Biol. Med.* 71: 80–1.

1950

R. W. Sperry. Myotypic specificity in teleost motoneurons. *J. Comp. Neurol.* 93: 277–87.

R. W. Sperry. Neural basis of the spontaneous optokinetic response produced by visual inversion. *J. Comp. Physiol. Psychol.* 43: 482–9.

R. W. Sperry. Neuronal specificity. *In* P. Weiss (ed.) *Genetic Neurology*. University of Chicago Press, Chicago, pp. 232–9.

N. Miner and R. W. Sperry. Observations on the genesis of cutaneous local sign. *Anat. Rec.* 106: 317 (film abstract).

1951

R. W. Sperry. Developmental patterning of neural circuits. *Chicago Med. School Quart.* 12: 66–73.

R. W. Sperry. Mechanisms of neural maturation. *In* S. S. Stevens (ed.) *Handbook of Experimental Psychology*. Wiley, New York, pp. 236–80.

R. W. Sperry. Regulative factors in the orderly growth of neural circuits. *Growth Symp.* 10: 63–87.

1952

R. W. Sperry. Neurology and the mind-brain problem. *Am. Scientist* 40: 291–312.

N. Miner, R. E. Myers, H. Zartman, and R. W. Sperry. On brain field forces in visual pattern perception. *Anat. Rec.* 112: 433 (abstract).

1953

R. W. Sperry. Regeneration studies and learning. *In Proceedings of the XIX International Congress of Physiology*, Montreal, pp. 101–5.

R. E. Myers and R. W. Sperry. Interocular transfer of a visual form discrimination habit in cats after section of the optic chiasm and corpus callosum. *Anat. Rec.* 115: 351–2 (abstract).

1954

N. Miner and R. W. Sperry. Pattern perception after implantation of dielectric plates in the visual cortex. *Anat. Rec.* 118: 330 (abstract).

1955

R. W. Sperry. Functional regeneration in the optic system. *In* W. F. Windle (ed.) *Regeneration in the Central Nervous System*. Thomas, Springfield (IL), pp. 66–76.

R. W. Sperry. On the neural basis of the conditioned response. *Brit. J. Animal Behav.* 3: 41–4.

R. W. Sperry. Problems in the biochemical specification of neurons. *In* H. Waelsch (ed.) *Biochemistry of the Developing Nervous System*. Academic Press, New York, pp. 74–84.

R. W. Sperry, N. Miner, and R. E. Myers. Visual pattern perception following subpial slicing and tantalum wire implantations in the visual cortex. *J. Comp. Physiol. Psychol.* 48: 50–8.

R. W. Sperry and N. Miner. Pattern perception following insertion of mica plates into visual cortex. *J. Comp. Physiol. Psychol.* 48: 463–9.

R. E. Myers and R. W. Sperry. Contralateral mnemonic efforts with ipsilateral sensory inflow. *Fed. Proc.* 15: 134 (abstract).

R. W. Sperry. Experiments on perceptual integration in animals. *Psychol. Res. Rep.* 6: 151–60.

R. W. Sperry. The eye and the brain. *Sci. Am.* 194(5): 48–52.

N. Deupree and R. W. Sperry. Functional recovery following alterations in nerve-muscle connections of fishes. *J. Comp. Neurol.* 106: 143–61.

J. S. Stamm, N. Miner, and R. W. Sperry. Relearning tests for interocular transfer following division of optic chiasm and corpus callosum in cats. *J. Comp. Physiol. Psychol.* 49: 529–33.

1957

H. L. Arora and R. W. Sperry. Myotypic respecification of regenerated nerve fibres in cichlid fishes. *J. Embryol. Exper. Morphol.* 5: 256–63.

R. W. Sperry. Brain mechanisms in behavior. *Eng. Sci.* 20: 24–9.

R. W. Sperry. High order integrative functions in surgically isolated somatic cortex in cat. *Anat. Rec.* 127: 371 (abstract).

R. W. Sperry. Review of C. Judson Herrick: The evolution of human nature. *Eng. Sci.* 20: 6–10.

J. S. Stamm and R. W. Sperry. Function of corpus callosum in contralateral transfer of somesthetic discrimination of cats. *J. Comp. Physiol. Psychol.* 50: 138–43.

1958

H. L. Arora and R. W. Sperry. Studies on color discrimination following optic nerve regeneration in the cichlid fish, *Astronotus ocellatus*. *Anat. Rec.* 131: 529 (abstract).

R. E. Myers and R. W. Sperry. Interhemispheric communication through the corpus callosum. *Arch Neurol. Psychol.* 80: 298–303.

R. W. Sperry. Brain mechanisms in behavior. *In* E. Hutchings, Jr. (ed.) *Frontiers in Science*. Basic Books, New York, p. 48.

R. W. Sperry. Concepts re a concept: A review of D. B. Harris (ed.) The concept of development: An issue in the study of human behavior. *Contemp. Psychol.* 3: 76.

R. W. Sperry. Corpus callosum and interhemispheric transfer in the monkey, *Macaca mulatta*. *Anat. Rec.* 131: 297 (abstract).

R. W. Sperry. Developmental basis of behavior. *In* A.

Roe and G. G. Simpson (eds.) *Behavior and Evolution*. Yale University Press, New Haven, pp. 128–39.

R. W. Sperry. Physiological plasticity and brain circuit theory. *In* H. F. Harlow and C. N. Woolsey (eds.) *Biological and Biochemical Bases of Behavior*. University of Wisconsin Press, Madison, pp. 401–21.

1959

M. Glickstein and R. W. Sperry. Contralateral transfer of somesthetic discriminations in monkeys after section of major hemispheric commissures. *Am. Psychol.* 14: 385 (abstract).

M. Glickstein and R. W. Sperry. Intermanual transfer of somesthetic discriminations in split-brain Rhesus monkeys. *Physiologist* 2: 45–6 (abstract).

A. M. Schrier and R. W. Sperry. Visuomotor integration in split-brain cats. *Science* 129: 1275–6.

R. W. Sperry. Preservation of high-order function in isolated somatic cortex in callosum-sectioned cat. *J. Neurophysiol.* 22: 78–87.

R. W. Sperry. The growth of nerve circuits. *Sci. Am.* 201(5): 68–75.

R. W. Sperry. Discussion. *In* M. A. B. Brazier (ed.) *The Central Nervous System and Behavior* (Transactions of the First Macy Conference). Josiah Macy Foundation, New York.

1960

D. G. Attardi and R. W. Sperry. Central routes taken by regenerating optic fibers. *Physiologist* 3: 12 (abstract).

M. Glickstein and R. W. Sperry. Intermanual somesthetic transfer in split-brain Rhesus monkeys. *J. Comp. Physiol. Psychol.* 53: 322–7.

M. Glickstein, H. L. Arora, and R. W. Sperry. Delayed response performance of split-brain monkeys with unilateral prefrontal ablation and optic tract section. *Physiologist* 3: 66 (abstract).

R. E. Myers, A. M. Schrier, and R. W. Sperry. Perceptual capacity of the isolated visual cortex in the cat. *Quart. J. Exper. Psychol.* 12: 65–71.

M. Glickstein and R. W. Sperry. Intermanual transfer in split-brain monkeys after somatic cortical ablation. *Amer. Psychol.* 15: 485 (abstract).

1961

R. W. Sperry. Cerebral organization and behavior. *Science* 133: 1749–57.

R. W. Sperry. Some developments in brain lesion studies of learning. *Fed. Proc.* 20: 609–16.

T. S. Voneida and R. W. Sperry. Central nervous pathways involved in conditioning. *Anat. Rec.* 139: 283 (abstract).

1962

H. L. Arora and R. W. Sperry. Optic nerve regeneration after surgical crossunion of medial and lateral optic tracts. *Am. Zool.* 2: 389 (abstract).

M. S. Gazzaniga, J. E. Bogen, and R. W. Sperry. Some functional effects of sectioning the cerebral commissures in man. *Proc. Natl. Acad. Sci. USA* 48: 1765–9.

R. E. Myers, R. W. Sperry, & N. M. McCurdy. Neural mechanisms in visual guidance of limb movement. *Arch. Neurol.* 7: 195–202.

R. W. Sperry. Some general aspects of interhemispheric integration. *In* V. B. Mountcastle (ed.) *Interhemispheric Relations and Cerebral Dominance*. The Johns Hopkins Press, Baltimore, pp. 43–9.

R. W. Sperry. Problems of molecular coding. *In* E. O. Schmitt (ed.) *Macro-molecular Specificity and Biological Memory*. The MIT Press, Cambridge, pp. 70–2.

R. W. Sperry. Orderly function with disordered structure. *In* H. von Foerster and G. W. Zopf, Jr. (eds.) *Principles of Self-Organization*. Pergamon Press, New York, pp. 279–90.

1963

H. L. Arora and R. W. Sperry. Color discrimination after optic nerve regeneration in the fish (*Astronotus ocellatus*). *Dev. Biol.* 7: 234–43.

D. G. Attardi and R. W. Sperry. Preferential selection of central pathways by regenerating optic fibers. *Exp. Neurol.* 7: 46–64.

M. S. Gazzaniga, J. E. Bogen, and R. W. Sperry. Laterality effects in somesthesis following cerebral commissurotomy in man. *Neuropsychol.* 1: 209–15.

M. Glickstein, H. L. Arora, and R. W. Sperry. Delayed response performance following optic tract section, unilateral frontal lesion, and commissurotomy. *J. Comp. Physiol. Psychol.* 56: 11–18.

M. Glickstein and R. W. Sperry. Visual-motor coordination in monkeys after optic tract section and commissurotomy. *Fed. Proc.* 22: 456 (abstract).

R. W. Sperry. Chemoaffinity in the orderly growth of nerve fiber patterns and connections. *Proc. Natl. Acad. Sci. USA* 50: 703–10.

R. W. Sperry. Evidence behind chemoaffinity theory of synaptic patterning. *Anat. Rec.* 145: 288 (abstract).

R. W. Sperry. Recovery of sight after transplantation of eyes and regeneration of retina and optic nerve. *In* L. L. Clark (ed.) *Proceedings of the International Congress on Technology and Blindness*, Vol. 2. William Byrd Press, New York, pp. 87–97.

1964

H. L. Arora and R. W. Sperry. Selectivity in regeneration and reconnection of the oculomotor nerve in cichlid fishes. *Anat. Rec.* 148: 357 (abstract).

M. S. Gazzaniga and R. W. Sperry. Some comparative effects of disconnecting the cerebral hemispheres. *Fed. Proc.* 23: 359 (Part 1, abstract).

R. F. Mark and R. W. Sperry. Bimanual coordination in monkeys. *Proc. Australian Physiol. Soc.*, May (abstract).

R. W. Sperry. The great cerebral commissure. *Sci. Am.* 210: 42–52.

R. W. Sperry and S. M. Green. Corpus callosum and perceptual integration of visual half-fields. *Anat. Rec.* 148: 339 (abstract).

R. W. Sperry. Problems outstanding in the evolution of brain function: James Arthur lecture on the evolution of the human brain. *In* R. Duncan and M. Weston-Smith (eds.) *American Museum of National History & The Encyclopedia of Ignorance*. Pergamon Press, Oxford and New York, pp. 423–33.

1965

M. S. Gazzaniga and R. W. Sperry. Language in human patients after brain bisection. *Fed. Proc.* 24(2): 522 (abstract).

R. W. Sperry. Corpus callosum and intermodal visuotactile integration in the monkey. *Anat. Rec.* 151(3): 476 (abstract).

M. S. Gazzaniga, J. E. Bogen, and R. W. Sperry. Observations on visual perception after disconnexion of the cerebral hemispheres in man. *Brain* 88(2): 221–36.

R. W. Sperry. Discussion. *In* D. P. Kimble (ed.) *Conference on Learning, Remembering, and Forgetting*, Vol. 1. Science and Behavior Books, Palo Alto (CA) pp. 140–77.

R. W. Sperry. Embryogenesis of behavioral nerve nets. *In* R. L. Dehaan and H. Ursprung (eds.) *Organogenesis*, Vol. 6. Holt, Rinehart and Winston, New York, pp. 161–85.

R. W. Sperry. Selective communication in nerve nets: Impulse specificity vs. connection specificity. *Neurosci. Res. Prog. Bull.* 3(5): 37–43.

R. W. Sperry and H. L. Arora. Selectivity in regeneration of the oculomotor nerve in the cichlid fish, *Astronotus ocellatus. J. Embryol. Exp. Morphol.* 14(3): 307–17.

H. L. Arora and R. W. Sperry. Studies on nerve growth and selective nerve muscle connections in fishes. *Am. Zool.* 5(4): 163.

R. W. Sperry. Mind, brain, and humanist values. *In* J. R. Platt (ed.) *New Views of the Nature of Man.* University of Chicago Press, Chicago, pp. 71–92.

1966

R. W. Sperry. Brain bisection and mechanisms of consciousness. *In* J. C. Eccles (ed.) *Brain and Conscious Experience.* Springer-Verlag, Heidelberg, pp. 298–313.

M. S. Gazzaniga and R. W. Sperry. Simultaneous double discrimination response following brain bisection. *Psychonon. Sci.* 4(7): 262–3.

M. S. Gazzaniga and R. W. Sperry. Visuomotor control in monkeys following brain lesions. *Fed. Proc.* 25: 396 (abstract).

E. Lee-Teng and R. W. Sperry. Intermanual stereognostic size discrimination in split-brain monkeys. *J. Comp. Physiol. Psychol.* 62: 84–9.

R. W. Sperry. Brain research. Some head-splitting implications. *The Voice* 15: 11–16.

R. W. Sperry. Mind, brain, and humanist values. *Bull. Atomic Sci.* 22: 2–6, September (reprint).

1967

R. W. Sperry and M. S. Gazzaniga. Language following surgical disconnection of the hemispheres. *In* F. L. Darley (ed.) *Brain Mechanisms Underlying Speech and Language.* Grune and Stratton, New York, pp. 108–21.

M. S. Gazzaniga and R. W. Sperry. Language after section of the cerebral commissures. *Brain* 90(1): 131–48.

R. W. Sperry. Syndrome of hemisphere deconnection. Second Pan American Congress of Neurology, San Juan, pp. 195–200.

M. S. Gazzaniga, J. E. Bogen, and R. W. Sperry. Dyspraxia following division of the cerebral commissures. *Arch. Neurol.* 16: 606–12.

R. W. Sperry. Split-brain approach to learning problems. *In* G. C. Quarton, T. Melnechuk, and F. O. Schmitt (eds.) *The Neurosciences: A Study Program.* Rockefeller University Press, New York, pp. 714–22.

1968

R. Saul and R. W. Sperry. Absence of commissurotomy symptoms with agenesis of the corpus callosum. *Neurol.* 18: 307.

R. W. Sperry. Psychobiology and vice versa. *Engineer. Sci.* 32(2): 53–61.

R. W. Sperry. Mental unity following surgical disconnection of the cerebral hemispheres. *In The Harvey Lectures, 1966–1967.* Series 62. Academic Press, New York, pp. 293–323.

R. W. Sperry. Hemisphere deconnection and unity in conscious awareness. *Amer. Psychol.* 23: 723–33.

R. W. Sperry. Plasticity of neural maturation. *In* M. Locke (ed.) *Proceedings of the 27th Symposium of the Society of Developmental Biology.* Academic Press, New York, pp. 306–27.

R. W. Sperry and E. Hibbard. Regulative factors in the orderly growth of retino-tectal connexions. *In* G. E. W. Wolstenholme and M. O'Connor (eds.) *Growth of the Nervous System.* Churchill, London, pp. 41–52.

R. F. Mark and R. W. Sperry. Bimanual coordination in monkeys. *Exp. Neurol.* 21: 92–104.

C. R. Hamilton, S. A. Hillyard, and R. W. Sperry. Interhemispheric comparison of color in split-brain monkeys. *Exp. Neurol.* 21: 486–94.

R. W. Sperry. Apposition of visual half-fields after section of neocortical commissures. *Anat. Rec.* 160: 498–9 (abstract).

B. Milner, L. Taylor, and R. W. Sperry. Lateralized suppression of dichotically presented digits after commissural section in man. *Science* 161: 184–6.

J. Levy-Agresti and R. W. Sperry. Differential perceptual capacities in major and minor hemispheres. *Proc. Natl. Acad. Sci. USA* 61: 1151 (abstract).

1969

H. W. Gordon and R. W. Sperry. Lateralization of olfactory perception in the surgically separated hemispheres of man. *Neuropsychol.* 7: 111–20.

R. W. Sperry, M. S. Gazzaniga, and J. E. Bogen. Interhemispheric relationships: The neocortical commissures; syndromes of hemisphere disconnection. *In* P. J. Vinken and G. W. Bruyn (eds.) *Handbook of Clinical Neurology*, Vol. 4. North-Holland, Amsterdam, pp. 273–90.

J. E. Bogen, R. W. Sperry, and P. J. Vogel. Commissural section and propagation of seizures. *In* H. H. Jasper, A. A. Ward, and A. Pope (eds.) *Basic Mechanisms of the Epilepsies.* Little, Brown, Boston, p. 439.

R. W. Sperry. Toward a theory of mind. *Proc. Natl. Acad. Sci. USA* 63: 230–1 (abstract).

R. W. Sperry. A modified concept of consciousness. *Psychol. Rev.* 76: 532–6.

R. W. Sperry and J. Levy. Hemispheric specialization as reflected in the syndrome of the neocortical commissures. *Excerpta Med. Int. Cong.* Series 193: 176 (abstract).

R. D. Nebes, J. E. Bogen, and R. W. Sperry. Variations of the human cerebral commissurotomy syndrome with birth injury in the dominant arm area. *Anat. Rec.* 163: 235 (abstract).

R. Gavalas and R. W. Sperry. Central integration of visual half-fields in split-brain monkeys. *Brain Res.* 15: 97–106.

1970

R. W. Sperry. Cerebral dominance in perception. *In* F. A. Young and D. B. Lindsley (eds.) *Early Experience in Visual Information Processing in Perceptual and Reading Disorders*, National Academy of Sciences, Washington, DC, pp. 167–78.

R. W. Sperry. Perception in the absence of the neocortical commissures. *Res. Publ. Assoc. Res. Nerv. Ment. Dis.* 48: 123–38.

R. W. Sperry. An objective approach to subjective experience: Further explanation of a hypothesis. *Psychol. Rev.* 77: 585–90.

R. W. Sperry, P. J. Vogel, and J. E. Bogen. Syndrome of hemisphere deconnection. *In* P. Bailey and R. E. Fiol (eds.) *Proceedings of the Second Pan-American Congress of Neurology*. Department of Public Education of Puerto Rico, San Juan, pp. 195–200.

H. W. Gordon, J. E. Bogen, and R. W. Sperry. Tests for hemispheric deconnection symptoms following partial section of the corpus callosum in man. *Anat. Rec.* 166: 308 (abstract).

J. Levy and R. W. Sperry. Crossed temperature discrimination following section of fore-brain neocortical commissures. *Cortex* 6: 349–61.

J. Levy and R. W. Sperry. Mental capacities of the disconnected minor hemisphere following commissurotomy. *In Proceedings of the 78th Annual Convention of the American Psychological Association*. American Psychological Association, Washington (DC).

1971

R. W. Sperry. How a developing brain gets itself properly wired for adaptive function. *In* E. Toback, E. Shaw, and L. R. Aaronson (eds.) *The Biopsychology of Development*. Academic Press, New York, pp. 27–44.

R. W. Sperry. Book review of R. M. Gaze: The formation of nerve connections. *Quart. Rev. Biol.* 46: 198.

R. W. Sperry and J. Levy. Minor hemisphere function in the human commissurotomy patient. *Acta Cient Venezuelana* 22: 32.

H. W. Gordon, J. E. Bogen, and R. W. Sperry. Absence of deconnexion syndrome in two patients with partial section of the neocommissures. *Brain* 94: 327–36.

J. Levy, R. D. Nebes, and R. W. Sperry. Expressive language in the surgically separated minor hemisphere. *Cortex* 7: 49–58.

J. Levy and R. W. Sperry. Lateral specialization and cerebral dominance in commissurotomy. *In Proceedings of the 19th International Congress of Psychology*. British Psychological Association, London, p. 244.

R. D. Nebes and R. W. Sperry. Hemispheric deconnection syndrome with cerebral birth injury in the dominant arm area. *Neuropsychol.* 9: 247–59.

1972

J. Levy, C. B. Trevarthen, and R. W. Sperry. Perception of bilateral chimeric figures following hemispheric deconnection. *Brain* 95: 61–78.

R. W. Sperry. Hemispheric specialization of mental faculties in the brain of man. *In* M. P. Douglass (ed.) *The 36th Yearbook Claremont Reading Conference*. Claremont Graduate School, Claremont (CA) pp. 126–36.

R. W. Sperry and B. Preilowski. Die beiden Gehirne des Menschen (The two brains of man). *Bild. Der Wissenschaft* 9: 920–7.

R. W. Sperry. Science and the problem of values. *Persp. Biol. and Med.* 16: 115–30. (Reprinted in *Zygon* 9: 7–21, 1974.)

R. W. Sperry. Cerebral function following surgical separation of the hemispheres in man. *D.S.C. Award Address*, A.P.A. Convention.

1973

E. Lee-Teng and R. W. Sperry. Interhemispheric interaction during simultaneous bilateral presentation of letters or digits in commissurotomized patients. *Neuropsychol.* 11: 131–40.

D. Zaidel and R. W. Sperry. Performance on the Raven's colored progressive matrices by subjects with cerebral commissurotomy. *Cortex* 9: 34–9.

R. W. Sperry. Lateral specialization of cerebral function in the surgically separated hemispheres. *In* J. B. McGuigan and R. A. Schoonover (eds.) *Psychophysiology of Thinking*. Academic Press, New York, pp. 5–19.

R. W. Sperry and E. Zaidel. Level of consciousness in the surgically disconnected hemispheres. *In Proceedings of the 14th Annual Meeting of the Psychonomic Society* (abstract).

C. B. Trevarthen and R. W. Sperry. Perceptual unity of the ambient visual field in human commissurotomy patients. *Brain* 96: 547–70.

L. Benowitz and R. W. Sperry. Amnesic effects of lithium chloride in chicks. *Exp. Neurol.* 40: 540–6.

R. L. Meyer and R. W. Sperry. Tests for neuroplasticity in the anuran retinotectal system. *Exp. Neurol.* 40: 525–39.

1974

R. W. Sperry. Changing concepts of mind and some value implications. Gerstein Lecture Series. *In* R. H. Haynes (ed.) *Man and the Biological Revolution*. Toronto: York University and the University of Toronto Press.

R. W. Sperry. Lateral specializatioin in the surgically separated hemispheres. *In* F. O. Schmitt and F. G. Worden (eds.) *The Neurosciences: Third Study Program*. The MIT Press, Cambridge, pp. 5–19.

R. L. Meyer and R. W. Sperry. Explanatory models for neuroplasticity in retinotectal connections. *In* D. Stein (ed.) *Recovery of Function in the Central Nervous System*. Academic Press, New York, pp. 45–63.

R. W. Sperry. Messages from the laboratory. *Eng. Sci. Caltech* 37: 29–32. (Reprinted in *Academic Therapy* XI(2): 149–55, 1975–6.)

R. W. Sperry. Science and the problem of values. *Zygon* 9: 7–21.

E. Lee-Teng and R. W. Sperry. Interhemispheric rivalry during simultaneous bilateral task presentation in commissurotomized patients. *Cortex* 10: 111–20.

D. Zaidel and R. W. Sperry. Memory impairment after commissurotomy in man. *Brain* 97: 263–72.

E. Zaidel and R. W. Sperry. Dichotic listening to synthetic stop consonants in the disconnected hemispheres of man. *In Proceedings of the 15th Annual Meeting of the Psychonom. Soc.* (abstract).

1975

M. Y. Scott and R. W. Sperry. Tests for left-right che-mospecificity in frog cutaneous nerve. *Brain, Behav. Evol.* 11: 60–72.

R. W. Sperry. Models, new and old, for growth of retinotectal connections. *In* M. Marois (ed.) *From Theoretical Physics to Biology.* North-Holland, Amsterdam, pp. 191–215.

R. W. Sperry. Science looks at human values. *Science of Mind* 48: 18–25 (interview).

R. W. Sperry. In search of psyche. *In* F. G. Worden, J. P. Swzey, and G. Adleman (eds.) *The Neurosciences: Paths of Discovery.* The MIT Press, Cambridge, pp. 425–34.

R. W. Sperry. Mental phenomena as causal determinants in brain function. *Process Studies* 5: 247–56.

R. W. Sperry. Bridging science and values: A unifying view of mind and brain. *In* M. Y. Warder (ed.) *The Centrality of Science and Absolute Values, Proceedings of the Fourth International Conference on the Unity of the Sciences,* Vol. I. The International Cultural Foundation, Inc., New York, pp. 247–59.

1976

R. W. Sperry. Hemispheric specialization of mental faculties in the brain of man. *In* T. X. Barber (ed.) *Advances in Altered States of Consciousness and Human Potentialities* (P.D.I. Research Reference Work), Vol. 1. Psychological Dimensions, New York, pp. 53–63.

R. L. Meyer and R. W. Sperry. Retinotectal specificity: Chemoaffinity theory. *In* G. Gottlieb (ed.) *Neural & Behavioral Specificity, Studies on the Development of Behavior and the Nervous System,* Vol. 3. Academic Press, New York, pp. 111–49.

R. W. Sperry. Changing concepts of consciousness and free will. *Perspect. Biol. Med.* 20(1): 9–19.

R. W. Sperry. A unifying approach to mind and brain: Ten year perspective. *In* M. A. Corner and D. F. Swaab (eds.) *Progress in Brain Research. Vol. 45: Perspectives in Brain Research.* Elsevier, Amsterdam, pp. 463–9.

R. W. Sperry. Mental phenomena as causal determinants in brain function. *In* G. G. Globus, G. Maxwell, and I. Savodnik (eds.) *Consciousness and the Brain.* Plenum Press, New York, pp. 163–77. (Reprinted in *Process Studies* 5: 247–56, 1976.)

R. W. Sperry. Left-brain, right-brain. *Sat. Rev.* (August 9): 30–3.

1977

L. Franco and R. W. Sperry. Hemisphere lateralization for cognitive processing of geometry. *Neuropsychol.* 15: 107–14.

D. Zaidel and R. W. Sperry. Some long-term motor effects of cerebral commissurotomy in man. *Neuropsychol.* 15: 193–204.

R. W. Sperry. Bridging science and values – A unifying view of mind and brain. *Am. Psychol.* 32(4): 237–45. (Reprinted in *Zygon* 14: 7–21, 1979.)

R. W. Sperry. Consciousness from neurons. *Brain Information Service, Conference Report #45.* BRI Publication Office, Society for Neuroscience, Sixth Annual Meeting, University of California, Los Angeles, pp. 34–9.

R. W. Sperry. Forebrain commissurotomy and conscious awareness. *J. Med. Phil.* 2(2): 101–26.

R. W. Sperry. Reply to Professor Puccetti's "Sperry on consciousness." *J. Med. Phil.* 2(2): 145–6.

R. W. Sperry. Absolute values: Problem of the ultimate frame of reference. *In* M. Y. Warder (ed.) *The Search for Absolute Values: Harmony Among the Sciences,* Vol. II, Proceedings of the Fifth International Conference on the Unity of the Sciences, Washington, DC, 1976. International Cultural Foundation Press, New York, pp. 689–94.

1978

R. W. Sperry. Mentalist monism: Consciousness as a causal emergent of brain processes. *Behav. Brain Sci.* 3: 365–7.

1979

R. W. Sperry, E. Zaidel, and D. Zaidel. Self-recognition and social awareness in the deconnected minor hemisphere. *Neuropsychol.* 17: 153–66.

R. W. Sperry. Consciousness, free will and personal identity. *In* D. A. Oakley and H. C. Plotkin (eds.) *Brain Behavior and Evolution.* Methuen, London, pp. 219–28.

L. Ellenberg and R. W. Sperry. Capacity for holding sustained attention following commissurotomy. *Cortex* 15: 421–38.

1980

R. W. Sperry. Mind-brain intereaction: Mentalism, yes; dualism, no. *Neuroscience* 5(2): 195–206. (Reprinted *in* A. D. Smith, R. Llinas, and P. G. Kostyuk (eds.) *Commentaries in the Neurosciences.* Pergamon Press, Oxford, pp. 651–62. (Reprinted in *Mobius* 1(4): 46–65.)

L. Ellenberg and R. W. Sperry. Lateralized division of attention in the commissurotimized and intact brain. *Neuropsychol.* 18: 411–18.

1981

R. W. Sperry. Changing priorities, *Ann. Rev. Neurosci.* 4: 1–15.

E. Zaidel, D. Zaidel, and R. W. Sperry. Left and right intelligence: Case studies of Raven's progressive matrices following brain bisection and hemidecortication. *Cortex* 17(2): 167–86.

1982

J. J. Myers and R. W. Sperry. A simple technique for lateralized visual input that allows prolonged viewing. *Behav. Res. Meth. Instrument.* 14(3): 305–8.

R. W. Sperry. Some effects of disconnecting the cerebral hemispheres (Nobel Lecture). *Biosci. Rep.* 2(5): 265–76. (Reprinted in *Science* 217(4566): 1223–6.)

1983

R. W. Sperry. *Science and Moral Priority.* Columbia University Press, New York.

R. W. Sperry with Y. Baskin. Roger Sperry (interview), *Omni* 5(11): 68–75, 98–100. (Reprinted *in The OMNI Interviews.* Ticknor & Fields, New York, 1983.)

R. W. Sperry. Changed concepts of brain and consciousness: Some value implications (1982–1983 Isthmus Foundation Lecture Series). *Perkins J.* 36(4): 21–32. (Reprinted in *Zygon* 20: 41–57, 1985.)

L. I. Benowitz, D. M. Bear, R. Rosenthal, M. M. Mesulam, E. Zaidel, and R. W. Sperry. Hemispheric specialization in nonverbal communication. *Cortex* 19: 5–11.

1984

L. I. Benowitz, D. M. Bear, M. M. Mesulam, R. Rosenthal, E. Zaidel, and R. W. Sperry. Contributions of the right cerebral hemisphere in perceiving paralinguistic cues of emotion. *In* L. Vaina and J. Hintikka (eds.) *Cognitive Constraints on Communication.* Reidel, pp. 75–95.

G. Plourde and R. W. Sperry. Left hemisphere involvement in left spatial neglect from right-sided lesions: A commissurotomy study. *Brain* 107: 95–106.

R. W. Sperry. Consciousness, personal identity and the divided brain. *Neuropsychol.* 22(6): 661–73. (Reprinted *in* D. F. Benson and E. Zaidel (eds.) *The Dual Brain*, Guilford Press, New York, 1985. (Reprinted *in* F. Leporé, M. Ptito, and H. Jasper (eds.) *Two Hemispheres–One Brain: Functions of the Corpus Callosum*, Alan R. Liss, New York, pp. 3–20, 1986.)

1985

J. J. Myers and R. W. Sperry. Interhemispheric communication after section of the forebrain commissures. *Cortex* 21: 249–60.

R. W. Sperry. The cognitive role of belief: Implications of the new mentalism. *Contemp. Phil.* 10: 2–3.

R. W. Sperry. Response to critique of Howard Slaatte. *Contemp. Phil.* 10: 3–4.

R. W. Sperry. Citation classic. *Curr. Cont.: Life Sci.* 28(6): 21.

R. W. Sperry. *Science and Moral Priority.* Greenwood/Praeger, Westport (CT).

R. W. Sperry with J. Eccles, I. Prigogine, and B. Josephson, and comments by N. Cousins. *Nobel Prize Conversations.* Saybrook, Dallas.

1986

R. W. Sperry. A world security system. *In* D. Paulson (ed.) *Voices of Survival in a Nuclear Age.* Capra Press, Santa Barbara, pp. 219–21.

R. W. Sperry. Discussion: Macro- versus micro-determinism (A response to Klee). *Phil. Sci.* 53(2): 265–70.

R. W. Sperry. Vital holistic phenomena and properties of living things. *The World and I* (May): 264–8.

R. W. Sperry. The new mentalist paradigm and ultimate concern. *Persp. Biol. and Med.* 29(3), Part 1: 413–22.

R. W. Sperry. Science, values and survival. *J. Human. Psychol.* 26(2): 8–23.

R. W. Sperry. The human predicament: A way out? *Contemp. Phil.* 11(6): 2–4.

R. W. Sperry. Toward a higher system of world law and justice (editorial). *Los Angeles Times* (October 5), p. 2.

R. W. Sperry. *Naturwissenschaft und Wertentscheidung.* R. Piper, Munich.

1987

R. W. Sperry. Structure and significance of the consciousness revolution. *J. Mind Behav.* 8: 37–65.

R. W. Sperry. Consciousness and causality. *In* R. L. Gregory (ed.) *Oxford Companion to the Mind.* Oxford University Press, Oxford, pp. 164–6.

R. W. Sperry. The science-values relation: Impact of the consciousness Revolution. *In* D. M. Byers (ed.) *Religion, Science and the Search for Wisdom*, Proceedings of a Conference on Religion and Science, September 1986. United States Catholic Conference, Washington, DC, pp. 110–33.

1988

R. W. Sperry. Psychology's mentalist paradigm and the religion/science tension. *Am. Psychol.* 43(8): 607–13.

APPENDIX B Students and collaborators of Roger W. Sperry

This list was compiled by Chuck Hamilton from records at Caltech. It omits a number of undergraduates who assisted in significant experiments.

GRADUATE STUDENTS

Nancy Miner/McCurdy	Chicago
Ronald E. Myers	Chicago
Ivan Jean Mayfield/Weiler	1956–60
Colwyn B. Trevarthen	1956–62
Charles R. Hamilton	1959–64
Michael S. Gazzaniga	1961–5
Jerre Levy	1965–70
Robert Nebes	1966–71
Larry I. Benowitz	1967–73
Harold W. Gordon	1967–73
Cary Lu	1967–70
Ronald L. Meyer	1968–73
J. Geoffrey Magnus	1968–71
James R. Carl	1970–5
Margaret Y. Scott	1971–6
David S. Isenberg	1972–6
Karen F. Greif	1973–8
Betty A. Vermeire	1974–81
Sheila G. Crewther	1975–8
Larry E. Johnson	1975–80
Karen E. Gaston	1975–81
Alice Cronin-Golomb	1979–84
Jay J. Myers	1979–84

POSTDOCTORAL FELLOWS

Nancy Miner/McCurdy	1953–5
John S. Stamm	1953–6
Ronald E. Myers	1954–6
Frederic G. Worden	1955–7
John T. Eayrs	1956–7
Gilbert M. French	1956–7
Allan M. Schrier	1956–8
Harbans L. Arora	1957–66
Mitchell E. Glickstein	1958–60
Theodore J. Voneida	1959–63
Dominica G. Attardi	1959–60
John Steiner	1959–60
Joseph Bossom	1960–2
John Cronly-Dillon	1960–1
John S. Robinson	1960–2
Douglas B. Webster	1960–3
Herman Teitelbaum	1961–4
Richard F. Mark	1962–7
Colwyn B. Trevarthen	1962–3
Rochelle J. Gavalas	1965–6
Alan I. Maxwell	1965–7
John E. Swisher	1965–9
Robert Biersner	1966–8
Salvatore Giaquinto	1966–8
Stuart R. Butler	1967–9
Linda Fagan	1967–72
Ulf Norrsell	1967–9
Kerstin Norrsell	1968–9
Santosh Kumar	1969–73
Myonggeun Yoon	1969–73
Stanley Jaffee	1969–70
John David Johnson	1970–3
Bruno Preilowski	1970–3
J. Geoffrey Magnus	1971–2
Peggy S. Gott	1971–3
James J. Wright	1971–3
Harold W. Gordon	1972–3
Eran Zaidel	1972–6
Cornelius H. Vanderwolf	1962–4
Rod A. Westerman	1962–3
Emerson Hibbard	1963–6
Evelyn M. Lee-Teng	1963–9
Giovanni Berlucchi	1964–6
Charles R. Hamilton	1964–5
Michael S. Gazzaniga	1965–7

Ronald L. Meyer	1974–7
Laura Franco-Testa	1974–6
Timothy D. Field	1977–8
R. Gilles Plourde	1979–81
Betty A. Vermeire	1982–
Polly Henninger/Pechstedt	1982–7
Alice Cronin-Golomb	1984–5

SENIOR RESEARCH FELLOWS, RESEARCH ASSOCIATES, SENIOR RESEARCH ASSOCIATES

Arthur Cherkin	1964–7
Emerson Hibbard	1967–9
Colwyn B. Trevarthen	1969–71
Evelyn M. Lee-Teng	1970–2
Charles R. Hamilton	1971–
Ronald L. Meyer	1977–9
Eran Zaidel	1977–9

VISITING INVESTIGATORS

R. M. Gaze	1960
Joseph E. Bogen	1960–5
N. S. Sutherland	1962–3
William M. Smith	1964–5
Seymour Benzer	1965–6
Jerzy Majkowski	1965–6
Harbans L. Arora	1969–72
Vachtang Mosidze	1970
Colwyn B. Trevarthen	1976–
Ann Marie Peters	1976–7

Deborah M. Burke	1976–7
Stuart Dimond	1976–7
Carol K. Peck	1976–9
Felicia Huppert	1977–78
Donald M. MacKay	1979–80
Erika M. Erdmann	1983–
Jenny Yates-Hammett	1985
Abu Kamal Abdur Rahman	1986

SHORT-TERM SCIENTIFIC VISITORS (INCOMPLETE LIST)

Brenda Milner
Laughlin Taylor
Marcel Kinsbourne
Oliver L. Zangwill
Gina Geffin
D. I. McClosky
Justine Sergent
Michael Corballis
Morihiro Sugishita

KEY STAFF

Lois E. MacBird	1954–83
Ruth T. Johnson	1960–74
Eef Goedemans	1965–85
Harry Hoepner	1965–69
Dahlia W. Zaidel	1967–77
Peter Jonkhoff	1970–4
Josephine Macenka	1973–9
Edward Ogawa	1974–81
Leah Ellenberg	1976–9
Erika Erdmann	1983–

Index

Italics indicate illustrations

A

Abplanalp, J. M., 184
Abstract words: recall of, 297, 298–301, *299, 300, 301*; right-hemisphere comprehension, 308, 313
Abuladze, K. S., 223
Achievement testing, 261
Activation, hemispheric, 241–5
Acuna, C., 160
Adaptability, 278; to commissurotomy, 147
Adaptive behavior, 37; vestibuloocular reflex changes, 163
Adaptive learning, xvii–xx
Adaptive motives, 340
Adrenergic neurosystem, 255
Affect, 324
Affective disorders, 255
Aged brain, 364–70
Agnosia, for faces, 284–6
Agranoff, B. W., 80
Airplane pilots, 262
Akelaitis, A. J., xxi, xxxiii, 371, 373
Alajouanine, T., 232–4
Albert, M. L., 268, 270, 286, 288, 305, 306
Albino mammals, 134
Albus, K., 133, 161
Alexander, A., 257
Alexander, D., 251, 257
Alexia, 289, 305–6, *305*, 314–17
Allard, F., 355
Allen, R. D., 83
Allman, J. M., 130, 133, 221
Altman, J., 161
Ambient vision, split-brain, 152
Ames, L. B., 346

Amine systems, 255, 256
Amino acids, 79
Amnesia, 285; delayed matching-to-sample, 294–7
Amochaev, A., 241
Amoeboid nerve growth, 82–3
Amphibians, neural studies, xv–xvii, xix–xx, xxiii, xxviii, xxxvii; chemospecificity of retina, 45; eye rotation, 21–3, 47–8; limb grafts, 4–5; nerve connections, 21–3, *22*; peripheral nerves, 62; retinotectal system, 114–15, *114*; somatosensory experiments, 51–4, *51, 54*; vestibular system, 49–50, *49*; visual projection, 104; visuomotor coordination, xvi -embryonic development, 28, *29,* 31, *32, 35,* 114; eye grafts, 76–83; optic nerve, 108–9 -optic-nerve regeneration, xx, xxix, 6, 41–5, *42, 46,* 81, 86, 108, 102, 113; experiments, 21–3, *22, 51, 52–4, 54, 79, 81,* 87
Anatomical basis: of anosagnosia, 233, 270; of auditory attention, 293–4, 373; of autotopagnosia, 283; of bimanual coordination, 169–79; of cognitive differences, 260–2, 270–4, 276–8, 375–6; of conditioning and learning, 161, 163–5, *164,* 177; of consciousness, 373–86, *374*; of emotion, 321; of functional loss, 233; of hand movement control, 158–60, 163, 169–76, *175,* 371–2; of haptic memory, 294, 297, 373; of image-mediated learning, 298, 301–2; of language,

speech, 231–4, 242, 251; of mental illness, 255–6, 323–4; of mental unity, duality, 215–7, 220, 221–4, 227–8; of prosopagnosia, 232, 285–6; of reading, dyslexia, 251, 261, 305–6, 311, 313–5, 316–7, 377; of spatial ability, 232, 242, 250, 282–4, 319; of thinking, story comprehension, 325–7, 329; of visual agnosia, 232, 234, 286–90; of visual memory, 196–209, *197, 199, 200, 204–5, 207,* 270–1, 274, 276–8, 282–3, 329, 371; of visual perception, 129–37, *130, 131,* 140–2, 149–50, 153–4, 234–5, 239, 250–1; of visuomotor coordination, xiii–xxiv, *xx, xxiii,* 41, 44–5, *46,* 55, *56,* 57–9, 86, 101, *104,* 143–5, *143,* 157–65, 169, *170,* 196, *197*; of voluntary movement, apraxia, 269;
Anderson, K. V., 145
Anderson, S. L., 381
André-Balisaux, G., 371
Andrew, R. J., 183
Androgen, 257
Aneurogenic limb innervation, 62
Angelergues, R., 232, 284–5
Angeletti, P. U., 14
Angular gyrus, 305, 356
Animals, hemispheric specialization, 182–4
Annett, M., 350
Anosognosias, 240
Anson, J. M., 183
Anterior commissure, 204–8, *207,* 213
Anterior temporal lobectomy, 274
Antonini, A., 126, 149
Anxiety, 312

Apes: cerebral asymmetries, 183; play of, 343
Aphasia, 234, 297, 315; right-hemisphere reading, 314–16
Apperceptive visual agnosia, 287
Aragao, A. S., 145
Arango, V., 106
ARAS (brainstem ascending reticular activating system), 217
Arcurate fissure, 160
Area TE, 196–209
Armitage, R., 259
Arm movement, xxi
Armstrong, E., 341
Arora, H., xxxii, xxxvi–xxxvii, 24, 40, 55, 58, 60–4, 66, 103, 126
Arousal: asymmetric, 241–4; brain damage and, 325; commissurotomy and, 150
Arriagada, J. R., 145
Arrow model of retinotectal specificity, 93–4, 111
Ashcroft, G., 255
Assal, G., 226
Association neurons, 65
Associative agnosia, 287
Associative cortex, 351
Associative learning, 341
Associative memories, 209
Associative systems, 357
Asymmetric movements, 173
Asymmetries: handedness, 177–9; in infants, 343–7, *344, 345,* 347; in nonhuman primates, 183; hemispheric, 240–6, 334–5, 357; long-term memory, 268; prenatal, 337 -functional, 177, 182, 375–7
Attardi, D. G., xxxii, xxxvii, 7, 22, 24, 55, 57–8, 75, 76, 87, 88, 102–3, 106, 111, 113

Attention: commissurotomy and, 150, 152; and hemispheric regulation, 241; and memory, 302; weight discrimination, 171–2
Audioarticulatory system, 281
Auditory comprehension, 309
Auditory cortex, 294
Auditory systems, 136
Auditory vocabulary, 308
Autism, 348–9
Automaticity premise, 233
Autotopagnosia, 270
Avian retina, 80–1
Awards given to Sperry, xxxv
Awareness, 245, 385–6; right-hemisphere, 378–9, *378*; in split-brain patients, 375
Axelrod, S., 223
Axial gradients of differentiation, 67–8
Axolotls, eye grafts, 76–8
Axons, *25*, 27; erroneous connections, 26–7; growth, 27, 37, 63, 82–3, 102, 108, 337; maturation, 351–2; myelin deposition, 351–2; neuron doctrine, 24; regenerating, 81

B

Baboons, 221–2; split-brain studies, 142. *See also* Apes; Monkeys
Bachevalier, J., 337, 351, 352
Bailey, P., 196
Bakan, P., 241
Baker, J., 161, 162
Baker, R. S., 336
Banich, M. T., 241, 243, 356
Banks, B. E. C., 10
Barbera, A. J., 81
Barrett, J. N., 12, 13, 15, 301
Barry, C., 313
Bartlett, F. C., 268, 329
Basso, A., 234
Bastian, C., 282
Bastiani, M., 103
Bates, J., 160
Bauman, M. L., 348
Baumann, T. P., 149
Beale, I. L., 334
Beazley, L. D., 78
Beecher, M. D., 184, 193
Beers, D., 41
Behan, B., 261
Behavior: asymmetric arousal, 243–4; brain damage and, 320–9; functionalist theory, 37; motivation, 339–40; regulation, 231; visually guided, 142–52, *143*

Behavioral nerve net, 19–20
Behavioral science, 383
Behavior field mapping, 339
Bell, G. A., 222
Bellugi, U., 350
Bender, D. B., 133, 197
Benowitz, L., xxxii, 213, 222, 311
Benson, A. J., 286, 288
Benson, D. A., 183, 286, 287, 289, 306, 323
Bentin, S., 252, 253
Benton, A., 192
Bercu, B. B., 337
Berg, W. D., 366
Beritov, J., 222
Berkley, M. A., 144
Berlucchi, Giovanni, xxxi, 126, 149, 150, 152, 192, 217, 221, 222, 223, 366
Bertelson, P., 241
Bertini, M., 259
Besner, D., 308, 313, 314
Best, C. T., 352
Best fit models, 116
Bever, T. G., 355
Biederman, I., 274
Bihemispheric coordination in perceptions, 140–1
Bilateral lesions, 285–6, 289
Bimanual coordination, 127, 158, 165, 172, 226; split-brain, 163, 169–74
Binocular neurons, 132, *132*, 134–5, 149
Binocular vision, 131, *131*, 134–5
Biorhythms, 259
Bipolar affective disorder, 256
Birds: hemispheric specialization, 182–3; interocular transfer, 177
Birren, J. E., 364
Bixby, J. L., 130, 133
Björklund, A., 336
Blakemore, C., 134–5, 274
Blastophore, dorsal-lip transplants, 28–30
Blood supply, shared by hemispheres, 217
Blood flow, hemispheric asymmetry, 241–2
Bloom, M. 144
Blumstein, S., 323
Bobrow, D. G., 268
Bodamer, J., 284
Body gestures, 321, 322; language and, 349
Body image, 268–71
Bogen, G. M., 221
Bogen, J. E., xxxii–xxxiv, 142, 149, 169, 181, 212, 232, 234, 235, 249, 250, 251, 268, 293, 297, 298, 302, 306, 314, 334, 364, 365, 373, 375, 377, 381; commissurotomy patients, 269–70
Bohn, G., 25, 28, 33
Bohn, R. C., 76
Bok, S. T., 36

Boller, F., 325
Bonin, G., 196
Boring, E. G., 384
Borod, J. C., 323
Bossom, Joe, xxxi
Botwinick, J., 365
Boveri, T., 30
Bower, G. H., 297
Bowers, D., 241
Bradshaw, J. L., 181, 182, 226, 240–1, 334, 366
Brain, R., 319
Brain-core neurones, 336
Brain growth, after birth, 351–7
Brain lesions, 232–4, 239–40, 250, 353–5; auditory effects, 294; compensation and recovery, 224, 232–3; consciousness, 215–6, 228; emotional behavior, 183, 323–4; laterality tests, 252; left hemisphere, 314–5, 330; long–term memory, 274–7; motor coordination, 158, 172, 183; perception, 157–8, 223–4; reading disorders, 305–6, *305*; right-hemisphere, 232, 320–1; tactile pattern matching, 295–7; temporal lobe, 294–5, 297, 301; visual memory, 196–209, *197*, *199*, *200*, *204–5*, *207*, 223, 297, 301. *See also* Commissurotomy patients; Split brain
Brain processes of consciousness, 384, 385–6
Brainstem, 48, 217, 339, 380; human embryo, 336
Brainstem ascending reticular activating system (ARAS), 217; and hemispheric functional asymmetry, 241–5
Brain surgery, xxx
Branch, C., 301
Breger, L., 304
Bremer, F., 371
Bresson, F., 346
Brightness perception, 141
Brihaye, J., 371
Brinkman, C., 172
Brinkman, J., xxxi, 160
Broadbent, D. E., 293
Broca, P., 232, 282
Broca's aphasia, 315
Brodal, A., 161
Brodal, P., 161
Brooks, R. E., 217
Broverman, D. M., 257
Brown, W. T., 348
Brownell, H., 326
Bry, I., 352
Bryant, P. J., 67
Bryant, S. V., 67
Bryden, M. P., 181, 182, 226, 250, 294, 323, 324, 355
Buchbinder, S., 160
Buck, R., 322, 323

Bugelski, B. R., 297
Bundle transplants, optic nerve, 58–9
Bunt, A., 135
Bunt, S. M., 76, 78, 106
Bur, G. E., 257
Bures, J., 223
Buresova, O., 223
Burne, R. A., 161, 162
Burnstock, J., 10
Burton, L., 241, 243
Butler, C. R., 221–2, 223, 226
Butler, S. R., 218, 242

C

Calcium, intracellular, 12
Calderon, M., 226
California Institute of Technology, Hixon Chair of Psychobiology, xxxi
Callosal connections, 312; in cats, 130–1; commissurotomy and, 154; and dichotic listening, 293; in monkeys, 133–6; and visual field, 129–31
Callosal visual input, 131–3
Camarda, R., 149
Caminiti, R., 136
cAMP (cyclic adenosine 3', 5' monophosphate), 12
Campbell, R., 322
Campenot, R. B., 12–13, 14
Campos, J. J., 346
Capranica, R. R., 76, 81
Caramazza, S., 326
Cardiac acceleration, 324
Carey, S., 355–6
Carl, James, xxxi
Carmon, A., 324
Caron, H. S., 323
Carotid amytal test, 224, 301–2
Carpenter, M., 161
Carroll, B. J., 323
Casagrande, V. A., 145
Cats, neural studies, xxii, xxx–xxxi, 161–3, 339; callosal system, 130, 136; crossed-lesions disconnection, 197
-hemispherectomy, 215; interocular transfer, 223; pontine cells, 162; split-brain, 127, 131–5, *132*, 140–55, *143*, 158
CAT scan, 224
Caudal corpus callosum, 141
Caudal parietal lobes, 160
Causality of consciousness, 384
Celesia, G. G., 294
Cell-cell interactions, 67, 80
Cells: retinotectal addition, 114–15, *114*, 118–19, *119*; differentiation, 65, 66–8, 111; spatial relationships, 82; surface factors, 36

Central nervous system, xxviii–xxix, 48, 68, 337–9
Central reflex patterning, 54
Cerebellum, 127, 157–65
Cerebral blood flow, 241
Cerebral cortex, xv–xvi, xix, xxi, 157–8, 353, *354*; and verbal learning, 298–302; growth in utero, 336–7; lesions, 356; rat studies, 4; visual areas, 130, 162
Cerbral duality of function: in split brain, 371–5, 377–9; in intact brain, 215–7, 220–8, 381–2
Cerebral function, 235; aging and, 369–70; hemispheric differences, 376–7; localization, 224
Cerebral peptides, 217
Cetacean hemispheres, 218
Chambers, R., 160
Chamley, J. H., 10
Changeux, J.-P., 338
Charlwood, K. A., 10
Charpentier, A., 171
Chaudhari, N., 16
Chaurasia, B. D., 344
Chavis, D., 160
Chemical mechanisms, 69
Chemical specificity in neurogenesis, 63; amphibian retina, 45
Chemoaffinity theory, 2, 3–16, 39–62, 337–9; alternative hypotheses, 105–10, 112; and developmental biology, 62–8; experimental foundation, 19–39; future of, 120–1; nerve-growth pathways, 81, 82, 106; neuronal specificity, 87; and plasticity, 111–20; retinotectal systems, 75–85, 101–21
Chemotaxis, 8, 39, 59; NGF, 10–14, *13*
Chemotropism, 9, 10–14, *13*, 25–6, 39, 55
Chen, J. S., 9–10, 13
Cherkin, Arthur, xxxii
Chiarello, R. J., 355
Chiasm, split, in cats, 131–3, *132, 134*
Chichinadze, N., 222
Chicks, xxxii; embryos, 8–9, 12, *13*; hemispheric specialization, 183; interhemispheric transfer, 222; retinal studies, 16, 108, 113
Child, C. M., 30, 36
Child: brain of, 225, 335; cultural intelligence, 341–3
Chimeric stimuli, 235–6, *236, 238,* 241
Chlorpromazine, 256
Choo, G., 242
Choudhury, P. B., 149
Christensen, A. L., 257

Chromosomal disorders, 257
Chung, S. H., 69, 104, 108, 109
Cicerone, C. M., 75, 88, 110
Cicone, M., 310, 323, 327, 328
Cima, C., 76
Circulation of blood, 221
Clark, E., 222
Clark, G. A., 165
Clarke, P. G. H., 135
Clarke, R., 183
Classes: of cells, 55; of nerve fibers, 50
Coghill, E. G., 37
Cognitive development, 341
Cognitive function, 251–2, 256–8; left-hemispheric dominance, 193; split-brain, 140–2, 311
Cognitive laterality battery, 252–4, 255–61
Cognitive processes, 231–46, 250–1, 266–8 277, 297, 301–2, 307–10, 313–14, 329, 373–7; in old age, 364–70
Cognitive profiles, *262*
Cognitive styles, 279, 329
Cohen, G., 313
Cohen, J. L., 161
Cohen, L., 173
Cohen, R., 234
Cohen, S., xxxvii, 9, 63
Collaborators with Sperry, 396–7
Collins, A. M., 277
Color recognition, 289, 306
Coltheart, M., 315
Comings, D. E., 347
Commissures, 352, 371, 381–2; and nonverbal cross-cueing, 218–20
Commissurotomy, forebrain, *374*
Commissurotomy patients, xxxiii–xxxiv, 140–55, *143*, 212–13, 249–50, 274, 277, 293; brightness perception, 141; delayed matching-to-sample, 296–7; dichotic listening, 293–4; dual consciousness, 373–5; emotion evaluation, 321–2; hemi-spheric independence, 371; image-related verbal learning, 297–302; laterality, 252; long-term semantic memory, 269–73; nonverbal cross-cueing, 218–20; overlearned skills, 173; perception, 235; right-hemisphere reading, 304–17
Communication, human, 342–7, *342,* 349–51, 357
Complete split-brain, 169–72. *See also* Commissurotomy patients
Compound-eye experiments, 109, 111–12, 113

Compression of retinal projection, 112, *112,* 113–14; system optimization, *117;* vector affinity, 120
Concrete words: recall of, 297, 298–300, *299, 300;* right-hemisphere comprehension, 313–14; right-hemisphere reading, 308, 311
Conditioned reflexes, xxxii, 164–5, 223; neural circuits, 161
Conel, J., 337
Conference on Genetic Neurology, Chicago, 1944, 8–9, *8*
Confusion, right-brain damage, 326
Consciousness, xxv, xxx, 231, 239, 246, 381–6; dual, xxxiii, 140, 168, 212, 380–1; mentalist view, xxxiv–xxxv; regulation of, 231–2, 238–42, 339–40; right hemisphere, 377–9, *378;* unifying mechanisms, 217–20
Constantine-Paton, M., 76, 77, 78, 81, 82, 116
Constructional apraxia, 321, 325–6, 330
Contact lens occluder, 269–70, 306, 309, 310, 378–9, *378*
Context, and detail recognition, 276
Contextual evaluation, right-hemisphere, 330
Contour frame, perceptual dominance, 272–3, *273*
Contralateral auditory pathway dominance, 294
Contralateral transfer of retinal projections, *xxi,* xxii
Conway, K., 69, 114
Cook, J. E., 75, 106, 108, 109, 114
Cooke, J., 69, 104, 108
Cooper, W. E., 323
Coordination: bimanual, 127; visuomotor, 127
Corballis, M. C., 182, 334
Corbin, E. D., 258
Corkin, S., 295, 297
Corollary discharge, xxiv–xxv, xxx, 163, 169–71, 172–3
Corpus callosum, xxxi, 129–39, 158, 178–9, 213, 221, 352–3, 371; and bimanual coordination, 127; commissurotomy, 269; and eye-hand coordination, 158–9; and interhemispheric transfer, 177, 223; and memory, 216; and visual perception, 149, 154; studies, xx–xxii, 157; unifying function, 217
Corpus striatum, 344

Cortex, periarcuate, 160
Cortical neurones, 336, 351
Cortical plate, 336–7
Cortical spreading depression (CSD), 223–5
Corticocortical connections, xxi, xxii, 158, 160, 197
Corticolimbic lesions, 197–201, *199, 200, 204, 205, 207*
Corticolimbic pathways: area TEa, 201–4; visual information, in monkey, *204*
Cortico-midbrain system, 150
Corticopontine cells, 162
Corticopontine fibers, 161–2, 163
Cottee, L. J., 134–5
Cowan, J. D., 116
Cowan, W. M., 2
Cowey, A., 192
Craik, F. I. M., 367
Crandall, P. H., 274
Critchley, M., 284, 286
Cronin-Golomb, A., 220
Cronly-Dillon, J. R., xxxii, 75
Cross-comparison, visual, 223
Cross-cueing, 217–20
Crossed corticolimbic lesions, 197–209, *199, 200, 204, 205, 207*
Crossed-lesion disconnections, 196–209
Crossed morphogenetic gradients, 67
Crossed nerves, 5–6
Crossland, W. J., 108, 111, 113
Cross-midline communication, 141
Cross-modal association, 209
Crowder, R. G., 267
Crowley, W. F., 337
Crystallized intelligence, 369
Cuenod, M., 145
Cultural learning, 334, 357
Culture: genesis theory, 341; and memory schemata, 268; transmission of, 335–6, 341–3
Curtis, A. S. G., 36
Curtis, S., 355
Cutaneous innervation, 23, 51–4
Cutaneous local sign, 49
Cytotropism, 33–6
Czernilas, J., 262

D

Dabbs, J. M., 242
Damasio, A. R., 286, 348
Damasio, H., 286
Davidson, R. J., 242, 324, 341, 344
Davies, I., 242

Davis, R. C., 171
Dawson, G., 348
Dax, M., 232
Day, J., 314
Deaf children, 349–50
de Ajuriaguerra, J., 319, 320
de Beer, G. R., 30
Decision time, 152
Dee, H., 368
Deecke, L., 172
Deficiency syndromes, brain damage, 233, 234
Déjerine, Jules, 305
DeKosky, S. T., 322
Delacour, J., 198
Delayed matching-to-sample tests, 294–7
Delayed nonmatching-to-sample tests, 198–209
Delayed puberty, 257
Dementia, 325
Denenberg, V. H., 182, 183, 223, 225
Denes, G., 327
Dennis, M., 355
Denny-Brown, D., 160, 321, 323, 376
de Olmos, J. S., 145
Depression, 254–6, 323–4
Deprivation, social, 355
De Renzi, E., 192, 213, 234, 250, 284, 325
Desimone, R., 133
Desmedt, John, 227
Detail recognition, 274–6
Detwiler, S. R., 37, 54
Deupree, N., xxix–xxx, xxxii, 24, 40, 60, 63, 64
Development: of brain, 33–4, 335–7, 351–3; of brain asymmetries, 335, 337; of cerebral function, 335–6, 353–6; of corpus callosum, 352–3; of cortex, 339, 351–3; of embryos, 27–36, 29, 32, 35; of face perception, 355–6; of language, 353–5; of nerve connections, 24–7, 25, 36–9, 45–62, 56, 75–83, 87, 101–11, 337–9
Developmental biology, 3; and chemoaffinity, 62–8
Developmental cognitive psychology, 341–2
DeWitt, L., 381
Dewson, J. H., III, 184, 193
Dexamethasone suppression test (DST), 323–4
DeZure, R., 249
Diamon, R., 353
Diamond, I. T., 223
Diamond, M. C., 337
Diamond, R., 355–6
Diamond, S., 334
Diao, Y. G., 134
Dichotic listening, 226, 240–1, 293–4
Differentiation: of cells, 30, 87; of neurons, 48; spatial

control theory, 55; topographical, 96
Dimond, S. J., 325, 375
Direct-access tasks, 312–14; right-hemisphere reading, 316
Disabilities, cognitive, 259–62
Disconnection syndrome, 270, 306
Discrimination learning, 184–5
Distal muscles, visual control, 162
Distance, semantic, 277–8
Di Stefano, M., 134, 223
Diurnal variation, 258–9
Dobbing, J., 336
Doehring, D. G., 260
Dog brain studies, 157
Dolphins, 217
Dopamine systems, 254–5
Dorsal-lip tissue grafts, embryonic, 28–30, 29
Dorsolateral pontine cells, 162
Doty, R. W., 140, 149, 184, 216, 221, 223, 373
Downer, J. L. de C., xxxi, 158, 160, 371
Dreher, B., 134–5, 136
Driesch, H., 30
Dual-aspect theory, 383
Dual consciousness, xxxiii, 140, 168, 212, 215–28, 250; in split brain, 373–5, 380–1
Dual-instruction models, 116, 116
Duffy, R. J., 322
Duration of memory, 267
Durnford, M., 268
Dyslexia, 251, 259–61, 315–16, 356

E

Easter, S. S., 75, 88, 110
Ebendal, T., 10
Eccles, J. C., xxxv, 193, 335, 336, 377
Edds, M. V., 69
Edwards, M. A., 81
Edwards, S. B., 145, 161
EEG desynchronization, 324
Efron, R., 287
Egg cytoplasm, and embryonic development, 30
Egocentricity of child, 342
Ehrhardt, A. A., 257
Ehrlichman, H., 241, 242
Eighmy, B. B., 163
Ekman, P., 321
Ekstron, R. B., 254
Elberger, A. J., 134, 135
Electrical field theory, 37
Electroconvulsive therapy (ECT), 255
Elias, M. F., 365, 369

Ellenberg, L., xxxiv, 302
Elliott, L., 297
Ellis, A. W., 285
Ellis, R. R., 241
Ellsworth, P., 321
Embryonic development, 3, 25, 25, 45, 48–9, 55; eye transplants, 47; limb innervation, 62–3; optic nerves, 105, 108–9; organs, 28–33; tissue affinities, 33–6, 35
Emotional content decoding, 321–2
Emotions: brain damage and, 323–4; human infant, 341–2, 342; neurochemistry of, 341; right-hemisphere, 322, 379; recognition of, 257; split-brain patients, 375
Endocrine system, 337
Endoplasmic reticulum, and nerve regeneration, 79
End-organ induction, 64, 67
End-organ specification, 43–4, 48–50, 54, 63
Entorhinal cortex, 196
Environmental theories of behavior, 37
Epilepsy, 255, 274, 301; commissurotomy for, xxxiii, 212, 269, 293, 373
Episodic memory, 287
Epstein, R., 251, 259
Equipotential systems, 30
Erdmann, A. L., 184
Erlichman, H., 301
Estradiol, 257, 258
Estrogen, absence of, 251
Ettlinger, G., 158, 160, 184
Evaluative judgments, 379
Evoked potential, 227
Evolution: brain motive systems, 340; laterality, 178; thinking, 385
Excitatory receptive visual fields, 135–6
Expansion of retinal projection, 112–14, 112; system optimization model, 117, 118; vector affinity model, 120
Experience, 382–6; values, 319, 339
Experimental memory, 270
Expressive communication of infants, 343–7, 344, 345, 347
Extracallosal unifying mechanisms, 217–18
Extrapyramidal motor system, 220
Extremities, visual control of movement, 160
Eye-field, embryonic, 28
Eye grafts, 76–8
Eye-hand coordination, 158–60

Eyeless axolotls, 76, 77–8
Eye rotation, xvi, xxiii–xxiv, xxx, 21–3, 47–8, 87, 103–4, 105
Eye transplants, 45–7

F

Facial expressions, 321–2; of infants, 344, 345
Facial perception, 257, 355–6; hemispheric differences, 226–7, 232, 270–1; in infants, 346–7; loss of, 284–6; split-brain monkeys, 186–92, 188
Faglioni, P., 192, 234, 284, 324
Falconer, M., 274
Falk, D., 183
Fantz, R. L., 271
Farah, M. J., 301
Farrell, W. S., Jr., 184
Farrington, L., 325
Farthing, T. E., 41
Fasciculation, selective, 55, 65, 76
Faugier-Grimond, S., 160
Fawcett, J. W., 76, 78, 105, 106, 109
Fechner, G. T., 168
Fecock, K., 69, 114
Feinberg, M., 323
Feldman, J. D., 109
Females: cognitive processes, 258; infants, auditory responses, 346; left-hemisphere superiority, 257; monkeys, laterality, 190, 192, 193
Fender, D., 304
Fenson, L., 346
Ferrier, D., 160
Fetal brain growth, 335–7
Fiber interaction, 116; topographic order, 111
Field compression, retinal, 87–8, 96–7, 99
Field concept, in embryonic development, 30–3
Fieldlike differentiation, 45–7, 55, 67
Field positions of neurons, 48–9, 50
Fiertag, M., 339
Filbey, R. A., 312
Finkelstein, S., 323
Finlay, B. L., 107, 109, 111, 113
Fiore, L., 136
Fisch, G. S., 348
Fish, neural studies, xxiii–xxiv, xxiv, xxix, xxx, xxxvii, 24, 86, 92; intraocular transfer, 177, 222; muscle innervation, 24, 59–62, 61, 64; optic-nerve

Fish, (*continued*)
regeneration, 6–7, *22*, 24,
40–1, 47–8, 55–9, *58*, 60–1,
61, 79–80, 81, 87–99, 102–
3, 110–13; retinotectal system, *104*, 114–15, *114*
Fish, S. E., 136
Fisher, C. M., 325
Fisher, E. D., 269, 293, 297
Flanigan, E. F., 217
Flechsig, P., 351
Fleishman, E. A., 169
Flor-Henry, P., 254, 255
Fluid intelligence, 369
Foldi, N. S., 310
Fontenot, H., 368
Force discrimination, 174–7,
175, 176
Ford, M. R., 241
Forebrain, 340, 371, 385;
embryonic eye grafts, 76–
7; tectum transplant, 92–
3, *94*
-commissurotomy, 141,
152–3, 154, *374*; and bi-
manual coordination, 158;
and conditioned response,
161; and eye-hand coordi-
nation, 158–9; and orien-
tation in cats, 144–5; and
response latency, 150–2;
and visual threshold in
cats, 145–50, *148*
Forgays, D. G., 312
Forman, D. S., 79
Form recognition, xxx
Fox, N. A., 341, 344
Fragile X-chromosome dis-
order, 348, 349
Francis, A. C., 221–2, 226
Franco, L., xxxiv, 250, 375,
377
Frank, J. M., 226
Franz, S. I., 312
Fraser, S. E., 69, 108, 111,
116
Frederick, S. L., 341, 344
Freeman, R., 313
French, G., xxxi
French, J. W., 254
French, V., 67
Frenois, C., 160
Frequency of word use, 308
Fries, W., 134, 161
Friesen, W., 321
Fritsch, G. T., 157–8
Frogs. *See* Amphibians
Fromm, C., xxv
Frontal cortex, 173, 324
Frontal lobe, 158, 344
Frooman, B., 259
Frost, D. O., 108, 111, 113,
136
Fujisawa, H., 81
Fukuda, Y., 135
Fuller, J. H., 163
Function, neural, 21–4, 36–
9, 64–5, 103
-asymmetries, 334–5, 357;
and psychopathology, 256;
split-brain studies, 375–7
Functional-association, left-

hemisphere dominance,
238, *238*
Functionalist view of neural
development, 20, 27, 36–
9, 62–5; Sperry and, 39–
41, 69–70
Function words, right-hemisphere reading, 308, 311
Furst, C. G., 242

G

Gaffan, D., 198
Gainotti, G., 322, 323, 341
Galaburda, A. M., 251, 260,
294, 337, 356
Galatzer, A., 251, 257
Gale, A., 242
Galin, D., 225, 241, 353
Ganglion cells of retina,
specificity of, 43
Ganglion innervation, 26
Garcha, H. S., 184, 192
Gardner, H., 310, 321, 323,
326, 327, 328
Garrison, F. H., 221
Garvin, E. A., 368
Gasparrini, W. G., 324
Gaston, K. E., xxxii, 183,
225
Gates, E. A., 366
Gavalas, R., xxxi
Gaze, 324; and cross-cueing,
219; and hemispheric ac-
tivity, 243
Gaze, R. M., 69, 76, 78, 79,
87, 88, 93, 96, 104, 105,
109, 111–15
Gazzaniga, M. S., xxxi,
xxxiii, xxxvii, 129, 142,
149, 160, 169, 181, 193,
212, 217, 223, 225, 234,
235, 249, 269, 293, 302,
306, 310, 312, 334, 375,
377
Gender differences, 257
Genetic disorders, 347–9
Genetic factors: in brain
growth, 334, 335, 349; in
cerebral functions, xxxii,
xxxiv, 2, 257; in hand
preference, 351; in learning disabilities, 260–1; in
motives, 340; in nerve
connections, 6–7, 15, 20,
121; in neural develop-
ment, 251; in neural functions, 3–4, 83
Genetic Neurology Confer-
ence, Chicago, 1944,
8–9, *8*
Genu, 352
Gerard, R. W., 37
Gerendai, I., 337
Germ layers, embryonic, 33
Gerstman, L. J., 324
Gerstmann syndrome, 349
Geschwind, N., xxxiii, 178,
183, 261, 269, 285, 293,
305, 306, 337, 377
Gesell, A., 346

Gestalt psychology, 37, 384
Gibbs, M. E., 222
Gibson, A., 161, 162
Gifted children, 261–2
Gilbert, C., 241
Gild de Diaz, M., 347
Giorgi, P. P., 76, 82
Giudice, S., 352
Glass, A., 242
Gleason, C. A., 172
Glees, P., 172
Glia cells, 336, 339
Glick, S. D., 182, 183, 339,
344
Glickstein, M. E., xxxi,
126–7, 161, 162
Global features, right-hemi-
sphere dominance, 273
Global justice system, xxxv
Goedemans, E., xxxvii
Goldberg, G., 172, 173
Goldberg, M. E., xxv, 133,
160
Goldberg, S., 76
Goldfish. *See* Fish
Goldman-Rakic, P. S., 335,
337, 352, 356
Goldstein, G., 364, 365
Goldstein, K., 37
Goller, I., 10
Gonadal dysgenesis, 251,
256–7
Gonad differentiation, 337
Gonadotropins, 251, 257,
258
Gonshore, A., 163
Goodale, M. A., 145, 222,
344
Goodglass, H., 226–7, 322,
344
Goodman, C. S., 103
Goodman, R. A., 353
Gordon, H. W., xxxiv, 169,
213, 298, 311
Gorham, D. R., 364
Gormezano, I., 163
Gorsuch, R. L., 313
Goswami, H. K., 344
Gowers, W. R., 288
Grafstein, B., 79, 81
Grant, P., 76, 78, 79
Grafts, embryonic, 31–3, *32*
Grapheme-phoneme conver-
sion, 311
Graves, J. A., 222
Graves, R., 226–7, 344
Gray, G. G., 168
Greden, J. F., 324
Green, S. M., 373
Greenberg, J. P., 287
Greenstein, B., 337
Greif, K. F., xxxii, 222
Griffin, C. G., 12, 15
Grigsby, J. P., 349
Grimm, L. M., 38
Gross, C. G., 133, 135, 197
Gross, M. M., 366
Groves, P. W., 36
Growth: of retinotectal sys-
tem, 114–15, *114*, 118–19,
119; selective, 115–16
Growth cones, 25, *25*, 27,

55, 80, 82, 83, 337; che-
motactic behavior, *13*, 14;
optic-nerve fibers, 76, 93
Growth-regulating factors,
xv–xvii, 87
Gruzelier, J. H., 254, 255,
256
Guenther, R. K., 277
Guillemot, J. P., 130, 131
Gulliksen, H., 142
Gundersen, R. W., 12, 13,
15
Gur, R. C., 241, 242, 243,
322, 344, 356
Gur, R. E., 243, 255
Gurwitsch, A., 30
Gwiazda, J., 346

H

Haaxma, R., 160
Haberey, M., 83
Hagberg, B., 347
Hagerman, R. J., 348, 349
Hagger, C., 337
Hahn, W. E., 16
Hall, G. C., 330
Hall, M. M., 330
Halliday, M. A. K., 343
Halstead-Reitan test, 255
Hamburger, V., xxxi,
xxxvii, 2, 5, 9, 10, 14, 15,
37, 63, 336
Hamby, S., 325
Hamilton, C. R., xxxi, 127,
141, 142, 178, 223, 310,
311, 373
Hamm, A., 183
Hammond, B. J., 93, 111
Hammond, N. V., 256
Hampson, E., 334
Hamster, optic nerve, 82,
113, 107–8
Handedness, 177, 241, 350–
1; in infants, *344*, 346; in
monkeys, *159*, 160, 177–8,
184, 191–2
Hands: awareness, 363; bi-
manual control, 127, 158,
163, 165, 169–73
-gestures: evaluation, 321;
of infants, 343–7, *344, 347*
Hannay, H. J., 192
Hardiman, M. J., 165
Harnad, S., 181, 182
Harness, B. Z., 251, 253,
259
Harris. L. J., 226, 243
Harris, W. A., 76, 77–8
Harrison, R. G., 25, 27, 28,
30–3, 37, 45, 46, 62, 66,
82–3
Harshman, R. A., 334
Harting, J. K., 145, 161, 162
Hartje, W., 160
Harvey, William, 221
Hasegawa, M., 347
Heacock, A. M., 80
Head, H., 36, 37, 268, 281,
286
Hearing: commissurotomy

effects, 293; in infants, 346
Hearing-impaired children, 349–50
Heath, C. J., 149
Hebb, D. O., xx, 285, 338
Hécaen, H., 213, 232, 268, 270, 284–5, 319, 321, 326, 376
Heidmann, T., 338
Heifetz, A., 255
Heilman, K. M., 241, 322, 324, 325
Hein, A., 339
Held, R., 346, 384
Heller, W., 241, 242, 322
Hellige, J. R., 182
Hemidecortication, 353–5
Hemispherectomy, 215–16, 224, 353–5
Hemispheres, 252–4, 334–63; differences, 142, 241–2, 266–79, 293–4; independence of, 215–28, 353, 371; single, cognitive capacity, 141; split-brain patients, 141, 234–40; and task parameters, 312 -asymmetry, 142, 335, 340; developmental, 349; in infants, 343–7, *345, 346*; and psychopathology, 245–6 -specialization, 181–4, 213, 216, 232, 240–5, 249–63, 268, 281, 311, 319, 364, 375–7; in animals, 182–93; evolutionary view, 178; in infants, 346
Henry, G. H., 136
Hepp-Reymond, M. C., 173
Heredity. *See* Genetic factors
Heritable specific dyslexia, 356
Herrick, C. J., 36–7, 336
Herring, E., 36
Herron, J., 353
Herron, J. T., 270
Herzog, A. G., 196
Heteroclitic face, 272–3, *273*
Heteropia, "The Rape," *272*
Heteropleural transplants, *32*
Heterotopic callosal connections, 130
Heterotopic transplants, *32*
Hibbard, E., xxxii, 2, 69, 76, 77
Hicks, R. E., 226
Hilgard, E. R., 241
Hillyard, S. A., 234
Hindbrain regions, embryonic eye grafts, 76
Hippocampus, memory, 220
His, W., 24, 37
Hiscock, M., 344
Hitzig, E., 157–8
Hixon Chair of Psychobiology, California Institute of Technology, xxxi

Hodge, R. J., 222
Hoffman, C., 353
Hoffman, K. P., 145
Hofstein, C. von, 346
Hökfelt, T., 335, 336, 339
Holst, E. von, 170
Holtfreter, J., 33–6, 62, 65–6
Homologous response, 4–5, 38–9, 50, 59
Homopleural transplants, *32*
Homotopic callosal connections, 129–31
Hope, R. A., 93, 111
Horder, T. J., 75, 76, 80, 105
Horenstein, S., 321, 324
Hormones, 217, 251, 256–8, *257*, 337, 339
Horn, J. L., 369
Horn, J. M., 334
Howes, D., 324
Hubel, D. H., 77, 129, 133, 134, 149
Hubley, P., 342, 343
Humanist psychology, 383
Humans, brain development, 334, 341; and transmission of culture, 335; cerebral dominance, 193; cross-cueing, 217–20; handedness, 177, 178; hemispheric asymmetry, 142; hemispheric independence, 225–8; hemispheric specialization, 181–2, 240–6; infant communication, 342–7, *342*; massa intermedia, 173; memory, 267; motor-nerve transplants, xxix; neural studies, xxxvii, 62; newborn, 342; split-brain studies, xxxiii–xxxiv, 140, 142, 149, 150, 154–5, 160, 162, 168, 215
Hume, D., 266
Humor, brain damage and, 326, 329
Humphrey, B., 241
Humphrey, D. E., 346
Humphrey, G. K., 346
Hunt, R. K., 2, 104, 108, 111, 114, 115, 116
Huttenlocher, P. R., 337, 351
Huxley, J. S., 30
Huxley, T., 369
Hyden, H., 8
Hypertrophy of regenerating optic cells, 79–82, *81*
Hypothalamus, 258
Hyvarinen, F., 160, 162

I

Iconic store, 267
Ideational praxis in commissurotomy patients, 269
Identity theory, 383, 384
Ideomotor apraxia, 269–71

Ifune, C. K., 184, 193
Image-related learning, 297–302, *298, 299*
Imbert, M., 339
Imming, T. J., 294
Immunofluorescence, 16
Imprinting, 64
Impulse activity-dependent sorting, 116
Impulse specificity, 5
In-vitro NGF experiments, 15
In-vivo nerve-growth experiments, 9–10, *11, 12*, 13–14, 15
Individual differences, 242, 251–2, 334, 356; genetic control, 335; in infants, 346
Individuated behavior, 37
Induction, embryonic, 33–6
Inductive mechanisms, 67
Infants, 346; asymmetrics, 343–7; brain growth, 335–6; cultural intelligence, 341–3; facial recognition, 271, 285
Inferior temporal cortex, 133, 196
Information processing, right-hemisphere, 271
Information-processing psychology, 266–7, *267*
Ingle, D., 177
Ingoglia, N. A., 79, 80
Inhelder, B., 341
Inhibition, 145; of right-hemisphere language, 314–16; of visual fields, 135–6
Innervation: abnormalities, 26–7; of limbs, in rats, 20–1; selectivity, 20–1
Innocenti, G. M., 129, 136, 352
Integumental specification, 50–5
Intelligence tests, 260–1
Interchangeability of neurons, 38–9
Interfiber interactions, *116*
Interhemispheric communication, 137, 141, 154–5, 157, 297; human, 225–7; visual perceptions, 149
Interhemispheric connections, 201–4, 221, 352–3
Interhemispheric interactions, reading, 316
Interhemispheric transfer, xxi–xxii, xxxi, 352–3, 371; and conditioning, 161; incomplete, 221–3; prevention of, 177
Interhemispheric visual projections, 129, 131–5, *131*
International Neurochemical Symposium (1954), 14
Interneurones: prenatal growth, 336; regulatory, 339

Interocular transfer, 177, 222–3
Interpersonal interactions of infants, 342–7, *342*
Interspecies grafting, embryonic, 28–30, *29*
Intracortical connections, xxi, 337, 351
Intrahemispheric connections, 221, 352, 353; corticolimbic, 208
Intrahemispheric visual projections, 130–4, *130*, 136, 149
Ipsilateral projection, 109
Iverson, L. L., 337, 339
Iwai, E., 204
Izard, C. E., 321

J

Jackson, Hughlings, 213, 224, 232, 281–92, 319
Jacobson, C. O., 10
Jacobson, M., 47, 63, 76, 87, 88, 104, 105, 107, 112, 113, 115
James, M., 270
Jargon aphasia, 233
Jason, G. W., 192, 193
Jeffrey, T. E., 254
Jensen, A. R., 152
Jerussi, T. P., 182
Jhaveri, S. R., 82
Johns, P. R., 114
Johanson, G. W., 135
Johnson, M. P., 12
Johnson, N. J., 274
Johnson, N. S., 329
Johnson, R. C., 365
Johnstone, J. C., 313
Jones, E. G., 149
Jones, M. K., 297, 298
Jones-Gotman, M., 213
Josephson, B., xxxv

K

Kaas, J., 223
K-ABC intelligence test, 260
Kalsbeck, F. E., 160
Kandel, E. R., 4
Kanner, L., 348
Kaplan, E., xxxiii, 322, 377
Kappers, C. U. A., 36, 37
Katz, M. J., 76
Kaufman, A. S., 260
Kaufman, N. L., 260
Kawamura, J., 161
Kay, J., 314
Keating, E. G., 160
Keating, M. J., 88, 105, 109
Keller, L. A., 241
Kelter, S., 234
Kemper, M. B., 349
Kemper, T. L., 348
Kerr, A. M., 347, 348, 354
Kertesz, A., 307
Kety, S., xxxi
Kidd, E., 297

Kigar, D. L., 334, 335, 337
Kilduff, S., 312
Kim, H., 356
Kimura, D., 240–1, 268, 274, 293, 294, 349
King, R., 161
Kinsbourne, M., 226, 241, 243, 244, 365, 369
Kirk, U., 356
Klaiber, E. L., 257
Klatzky, R. L., 267, 277
Klein, R., 259
Klima, E. S., 350
Klinefelter's syndrome, 257
Klisz, D., 365
Knapp, M. E., 196
Kobayashi, Y., 257
Koch-Weser, M., 243
Koff, E., 322
Koffka, K., 384
Koh, Y. H., 261
Kohler, G., 16
Kohler, W., xxx, 384
Kolb, B., 322
Komnenich, P., 258
Koriat, A., 314
Kornhuber, H. H., 173
Kosaka, B., 335, 337
Koskoff, Y. D., 216
Kraft, R. H., 350, 351
Krayanek, S., 76
Krieg, W. J. S., 173
Krivanek, J., 223
Kronfol, Z., 255
Krueger, L. E., 313
Kruper, D. C., 216
Kueck, L., 241
Künzle, H., 173
Kushnir, M., 255
Kuypers, H., xxxi, 160

L

Labels, chemoaffinity, 115–16
Ladavas, E., 257
Lamb, A. H., 78
Lamont, D. M., 10
Lamotte, R. H., 160
Lancaster, J., 341
Landis, T., 226–7, 315, 344
Landmesser, L., 103
Langley, J. N., 26, 62, 68
Language, 341, 342–3, 349–51, 353, 355; in autistic children, 348; brain damage and, 324–9; disorders, and schizophrenia, 255; left-hemisphere, xxxiii–xxxiv, 232–3, 249–51, 306, 355; reading, disorders, 305–17; right-hemisphere, 306–11, 377
Lansdell, H., 314
Lasek, R. J., 76
Lashley, K. S., xvii, xx–xxii, xxv, xxix, xxx, 4, 5, 37, 173
Latency responses, 277–8
Lateral eye movements, and

hemispheric activity, 243; in infants, 344
Laterality, 177, 178, 182; in animals, 182–4. *See also* Handedness; Hemispheric specialization
Lateralization: shifts, 355, 356; temporal lobe removal, 273
Lateralized learning hypothesis, 177
Lateral orientation reflex, 241
Lavie, P., 259
Lavoie, P., 329
Law, M. I., 76, 77, 116
Leake, C., 221
Learning, 4, 64, 338–41; adaptive, xv–xx; disabilities, 259–62; genetic factors, xxxii; hemispheric independence, 221–3; lateralization of, 179, 192; perceptual, xxxi, 371; split-brain studies, 142; two-hand coordination, 169; verbal, 207–302
Le Bras, H., 285
Lecours, A. R., 225, 334, 351–54
LeDoux, J. E., 181, 217, 223, 225
Lee, P. A., 258
Lee-Teng, E., xxxi, xxxii
Left-ear suppression, commissurotomy patients, 294
Left-handedness, 241, 350
Left-hand praxis in commissurotomy patients, 269
Left hemisphere, xxxiii–xxxiv, 181, 252, 268, 281, 319, 349, 375–7; and body gestures, 322; cognitive functions, 250–1; damage to, 329, 355; dominance, 193, 232–5, 237–40; and emotional behavior, 321, 323–4; hormones and, 257, 258; infant, 344; inhibition of right hemisphere, 314–16; language abilities, 241, 249–50, 306, 310–11; learning disability, 260; memory impairment, 274; monkey, 184, 192; and prosopagnosia, 289; and reading, 305–6; and schizophrenia, 255–6; semantic memory, 278; visual imagery, 301; and visual-object agnosia, 289
Left-sided neglect, 320, 320, 325
Left temporal lobectomy, and verbal learning, 297
Left visual hemifield testing, 309–10
Lehman, R. A. W., 178
Leicester, J., 135
LeMay, M. J., 178, 183
Lemire, R. J., 351

Lemmo, M. A., 323
Lens of eye, embryonic development, 28, 29
Leohlin, J. C., 334
Lepore, F., 130, 131
Lerner Marine Laboratory, Bimini, xxix
Lesser, R., 302
Letourneau, P. C., 10, 12, 15, 81
LeVay, S., 136
Levi, G., 37
Levi-Montalcini, R., xxix, xxxvii, 8, 63
Levine, R., 75
Levine, R. L., 107, 112
Levine, S. C., 243, 356
Levy, J., xxxiii, xxxiv, 181, 192, 212–13, 219, 250, 251, 268, 286, 293, 308, 313, 323, 352, 356, 365, 375, 376
Levy-Agresti, J., 235, 376
Lewine, J. D., 223
Lewis, M. R., 37
Lewis, W. H., 27–8, 37, 62, 67, 76
Lexical decision, 309–10, 312–14; in deep dyslexia, 316
Ley, R. G., 323, 324
Lhermitte, F., 232–4
Libet, B., 173
Lichtman, J. W., 16
Liederman, J., 353
Lilly, J. C., 217
Limb development, embryonic, 30, 32
Limbic system, 340; and visual memory, 127, 208–9
Limb innervation in rats, 20–1
Limb movement, cerebral control, xxi
Limb position knowledge, 268
Limb transplants, 4–5, 54, 54
Lindblom, B., 178, 346
Lindhagen, K., 346
Lineage markers, 69
Linguistic control mechanisms, 314
Lisberger, S. G., 163
Lissauer, H., 287
Lithium, 256
Local control of neurite growth, 12–14
Local sign, 51–4
Locus-specific differentiation, 66, 67
Logotheti, K., 335, 336, 342, 343, 351
Long association systems, 353
Long-term memory, 267–9; asymmetries, 271–4; in commissurotomy patients, 269–73
Lorente de Nó, R., 163
Lovett, M., 355

Lower vertebrates, visual pathways, 86
Lowery, D. H., 274
Lumley, J. S. P., 160, 173
Lund, J. C., 160
Lund, J. S., 184
Lund, R. D., 136
Lushene, R. E., 312
Luteinizing Releasing Hormone (LRH), 258
Lynch, J. C., 245

M

McAdam, D., 241
MacBird, L., xxxii, xxxvii
McBride, K., 232
Maccabe, J. J., 184
McCasland, J. S., 183
McCloskey, D. I., xxiv
McCormick, D. A., 163
McCurdy, N. M., 158
MacDonald, H., 241
McDonald, P. J., 241
McDonald, W., 67
McFie, J., 232, 319
McGeer, E. G., 335, 336
McGeer, P. L., 335, 336
McGranaghan, K. M., 261
MacKay, D., 377
McKay, R. D. G., 16
McKee, G., 241
McKeever, W. F., 322
MacKinnon, P. C. B., 337
Macko, K. A., 197
MacNeilage, P. F., 178, 346, 349
McNeill, D., 349
MacQuarrie, T. W., 254
Macrodeterminism, xxxiv–xxxv
Macrotopography, in visual projection, 103–10
Madden, D. J., 366
Madigan, S. A., 297, 298
Maer, F., 324
Magalhäes-Castro, B., 145
Magalhäes-Castro, H. H., 145
Magnus, G., xxxii
Magoun, H. W., 217
Magritte, R., "The Rape," 271–2, 272
Mainsell, H. R., 130
Maladaptive nerve connections, 5–6, 20–3, 51–2, 63, 64, 87; experiments, 40–1, 40, 45–6, 46
Males, 257, 258; infants, auditory responses, 346
Malsburg, C. von der, 338
Mammals: brain asymmetries, 337; cortical visual areas, 130
Mandler, G., 267, 274
Mandler, J. M., 329
Mangold, H., 28–30
Manic-depressive psychoses, 255
Manual skill transfer, 226
Marchase, R. B., 81

Marin-Padilla, M., 337
Mark, R. F., xxx, xxxii, xxxvii, 40, 64, 158, 163, 338
Marks, C. E., 216
Marr, D., 163
Marsh, F. J., 249
Marshall, J. C., 315
Marshall, W. H., 150
Martin, K. A. C., 75, 76, 80, 105
Marwick, H., 343
Marzi, C. A., 133, 134, 149, 223
Mascetti, G. G., 145
Massa intermedia, 172–3
Massonnet, J., 319
Matarazzo, J. D., 326
Matelli, M., 153
Materialist theory, 383
Mathivet, E., 347
Matthey, R., xxix, 6, 41, 86
Maturana, H. R., 103, 105
Maturity of brain, 334
Maurer, R. G., 348
May, J., 161
Maze-learning, 285
Meadows, J. C., 285–6
Meaning: achievement of, 267, 268; conscious, 384
Mechanical factors in nerve growth, 37, 63, 75–6, 78–9, 102, 103
Medawar, P. B., 3
Mehler, J., 346
Meier, R. P., 350
Melodic expression, 355
Melville-Jones, G., 163
Memory, 267, 294–302, 340, 357, 386; aging and, 367–8; anatomically specifiable, 220; commissurotomy patients, 297, 301–2; crossed corticolimbic lesions, 197–201; interhemispheric transfer, 371; long-term, 64, 266–79; research, 127; schematic organization, 329; topographical loss, 382–4
Mench, J., 183
Menesini-Chen, M. G., 9–10, 13
Menstrual cycle, 257–8
Mental duality, 215–28, 250. *See also* Dual consciousness
Mental images, 282
Mental structural clusters, 268
Mentalist view of consciousness, xxxiv–xxxv
Merjanian, P. M., 348
Merola, J. L., 353
Mesencephalic tegmentum, 145
Mesial cortex, 289
Mesulam, M. M., 322
Metacontrol of hemispheric function, 237–40
Metamorphopsia, 285
Metania, Y., 259

Metter, E. J., 367
Metzler, J., 253
Meyer, H., 10, 63
Meyer, I. O., 283
Meyer, J. S., 321, 324
Meyers, P. S., 310
Michel, F., 217, 306, 314
Michel, G. F., 344
Midbrain, xxx, 145; embryonic eye grafts, 76–7 -commissurotomy, 141; and bimanual coordination, 158; in cats, 143–54, *148*; and conditioned response, 161
Mihailoff, S. A., 161
Miles, F. A., 163
Milner, B., 213, 224, 274, 285, 314, 367, 373, 375
Milstein, C., 16
Minciacchi, D., 135
Minckler, D. S., 135
Mind: duality of, 215–28, 228; organization of, 268; theory of, xxiv, 381–6
Mind blindness, 286–9
Mind-brain problem, xxv–xxvi, xxx, 383–6
Miner, N., xxx, xxxvii, 23, 50–4, 63, 66, 140, 371
Mingazzini, G., 288
Mishkin, D. B., 133, 135
Mishkin, M., 127, 220, 221, 312, 340, 352
Mismatch of neurons, chemoaffinity and, 115
Mitchell, D. E., 136
Mittelstaedt, H., xxx, 163, 170
Mixed cell aggregates, tissue affinities, 34–6, *35*
Mnemonics, 297, 299–301
Modality specificity, 53
Modulation, 48, 50, 59, 64; of motoneurons, 38–9; systems, 335; of tectal markers, 114
Mohler, C. W., 133
Mohr, J. P., 294
Molecular mechanisms, 69
Molecular model of neuronal differentiation, 66
Money, J., 251, 257
Monkeys: adaptive learning studies, xvii–xx; auditory cortex, 294; autism, 348; callosal connections, 133–4; cerebral cortex studies, xxi; cortical lesions, 356; cortical maturation, 351–2; corticopontine fibers, 161–2; crossed-lesion disconnection, *197*; face perception, 192; handedness, 177–8; hemicerebrectomized, 216; hemispheric specialization, 183–93; intermanual transfer, 173–7, *176*, 221–2, 223; laterality, 178; sex differences, 337; split-brain studies, xxxi–

xxxii, xxxvii, 127, 141, 142, 158–63, 167, 184–93, 235, 371–2, *372*; supplementary motor cortex, 172–3; visual memory, 196–209
Monoclonal antibodies, 16, 80–1
Monocular neurons, 132
Montalcini, Rita, 2
Mood, 323; and brain damage, 323–4
Morais, J., 241
Moran, J., 135
Morest, D. K., 337
Morgan, A. H., 241, 242
Morgan, C. T., xxi, xxii
Morgan, M. J., 182
Morgan, S. C., 222
Morphogenetics, 105
Morphollactic regulation, 113–14
Morton, H. B., 158
Moscona, A., 36
Moscona, H., 36
Moscovitch, M., 182, 185, 322, 344, 356
Mother-child relations, 342–7
Motivation, 340; adaptive, 340; for communication, 350; developmental disorders, 349
Motive systems, 357, 385
Motoneurons, 59–62, *61*; resonance theory, 38–9; selective outgrowth, 67; specificity of, 21, 39–41
Motor asymmetry, 349
Motor axons, prenatal growth, 336
Motor coordination, 165, 169–73
Motor corollary discharge, 169–70, 173–4; weight discrimination, 172–3
Motor cortex, 163; and conditioned response, 161; neural connections, 158
Motor function, xxii–xxiv; overlearned skills, 173; split-brain studies, 234; superior colliculus, 145
Motor learning, 163–5, 169
Motor nerves, regeneration, xxx, 40–1, 59–62, *40*, 61
Movement: central programming, xxii–xxiv; coordination of, xiv–xxvii; response latency, 152; split-brain monkeys, 186–91, *188*; visually guided, 142–50, 158, 160, 162, 165
Moving targets, sensitivity to, 162
Mower, S., 161, 162
Moya, K. L., 325
Mukhametov, L. M., 217

Müller, G. E., 171
Multimodal sensorimotor activity, 145
Munk, H., 157, 286
Murray, D. M., 145
Murray, E. A., 209, 340
Murray, L., 343, 344, 346
Murray, M., 79, 81
Muscle innervation, 64; of fish, 59–62, *61*
Muscle transposition, xiv–xvi, 40, *40*, 59–62, *61*
Muscular activation, resonance theory, 38–9
Musick, F. E., 293
Music perception, 355; infant response, 346
Mutually exclusive perceptions, split-brain, 371–2, 374–5, *376*
Mycek, J., 79
Myelination: of axons, 351–2; of callosal fibers, 225
Myers, J. J., 220, 221, 310
Myers, R. E., xx, xxii, xxx–xxxvi, 2, 69, 126, 129, 140, 157, 158, 167, 196, 197, 371
Myotypic response, 4–5
Myotypic specification, 38–9, 48, 50, 62; respecification, 40

N

Nachshon, I., 323
Nagel, T., 378
Naito, H., 135
Naming, cross-cueing, 219–20
Narrative memory, 329
Natural selection, hemispheric differences, 251
Nauta, W. J. H., 201, 339
Nebes, R. D., xxxiv, 214, 234, 250, 308, 375
Negative emotions, in infants, 346
Negative research findings, 181
Negräo, N., 140, 149, 216, 221
Neisser, U., 329
Neocortex, xxxiii, 336–7, 351, 352, 357; and visual memory, 196–209; visual areas, 129–37
Neonatal rats, NGF experiment, 9–10, *11, 12*, 13–15
Nerve cells, 221
Nerve connections, 101–2; changes, 115, 118 -maladaptive xiv–xix, 5–7, 20–3; amphibian, 21–3, 41–55, *42, 46, 49, 51, 54*, 75–83, 79–80; fish, *22*, 24, 55–62, *56*, 61; rats, 20–21, 40, *40*
Nerve fibers, corticocortical relays, 158; growth path-

Nerve fibers (*continued*) ways, 55–9, *58*, 68, 82–3, 102, 106–10
-abnormal 76–79, *79, 80*; individual specification, 66
Nerve growth, xxiv–xxx, xxxii, 27, 36, active or passive, 82–3, chemoaffinity, 24; cytotropism, 36; pathway-only cueing, 106–10; pathways, 55–9, 68, 102
Nerve-Growth Factor (NGF), 2, 9–15; chemoaffinity theory and, 16; in-vitro effects, 10–14; in-vivo effects, 9–10
Nerve regeneration, 41–4, *42*, 64, 75, 102; in amphibians, xxix–xxx, 45, *46*, 47–8; in fish, 40–1, 55–9, *56*; somatosensory, 51–2; vestibular, 49–50, *49*
Nerve terminals, chemoaffinity, 14. *See also* Chemoaffinity theory, Nerve connections, Nerve growth
Netley, C., 251, 257
Nettleton, N. C., 181, 182, 226, 241, 334
Neural crest removal, 27
Neural development: chemoaffinity theory, 63; functionalist view, 36–9
Neural plate, embryonic transplants, 28–30
Neural specificity, 43–5
Neural tube removal, 27
Neurite growth, 12–14
Neurobehavioral disorders, 364
Neurobiotaxis, 37, 69
Neuroblasts, chemotropism, 26
Neuroembryology, Sperry and, 19
Neuroendocrine, and brain damage, 324–5
Neurogenesis, 15, 63, 65
Neurohumoral systems, 337
Neuron doctrine, 24
Neuronal nets, 15, 338–9; early theories, 19–20
Neurones, 338–40; prenatal growth, 336
Neurons, 14, 27, 63; differentiation, 63; nonspecificity, functionalist theory, 38–9; specificity, xx, 6–7, 48, 66–8, 87
Neuropsychology, 232, 249
Neurosystems, and hemisphericity, 252, 253, 258
Neurotransmitters, 251, 252, 259, 339
-systems: and learning disability, 261; prenatal growth, 336; and psychopathology, 255, 256
Neurotropism, 9–15
Neville, H. J., 353

Newborn humans, voice sensitivity, 346
Newcombe, F., 283, 285, 287, 315
Newport, E. L., 350
Newsome, W. T., 130, 133, 221
Newts. *See* Amphibians
Ng. D. T., 222
NGF. *See* Nerve-Growth Factor
Nicholas, J. S., 31
Nictitating membrane response (NMR), 163–5
Nielsen, J., 257
Nielsen, J. M., 288–9
Niihara, T., 204
Nirenberg, M., 16, 69, 80
Nobel Prize, 215, 262–3
Nobel Prize Conversations, Sperry et al., xxxv
Nomura, Y., 347
Noncallosal hemispheric connections, 217–18
Nonverbal communication, right-hemisphere lesions, 320–3
Nonverbal cross-cueing, 218–20
Nonword pseudohomophone affect, 313
Nordeen, D. J., 337
Normal brain: hemispheric specialization, 311–14; long-term memory, 277–8; right-hemisphere reading, 312–15
Norman, D. A., 267, 268
Norsell, U., 218
Nottebohm, F., 182

O

Object recognition, 196–209, 286–9
Occipital lobe: lesions, 158, 289; and reading, 305
Ochs, S., 177
Oculomotor system development, xix–xx, 59–62, *61*
Ojemann, G., 314, 322
Oke, A., 339, 341
Oldfield, R. C., 283
Olds, J., 322, 344
O'Leary, D., 353
Oppenheim, H., 288
Oppenheim, R. W., 336, 338
Optic-chiasm surgery, xx–xxi, *xxi*, xxii, xxxi
Optic fibers, 66, 86; connections, 75; growth pathways, 76–83, *79, 80*, 87; specificity of, 7, 41–3, 67, 68–9
Optic lobe lesions in amphibians, xvi–xvii, xx, 44–5
Optic nerve, 86; interfiber order, 106
-amphibian, regenerating,

xvi–xvii, xxii, 6–7, 21–3, *22*, 24, 45, *46*, 55–9, *58*, 86, 92–9
-fish, 86, *104*, regenerating, 87–99, 110, 112–15; growth pathways, 102–3
Optic tectum, 86; chemoaffinities, 47–8; of goldfish, *92*, 96; polarization of, 93–9; specificity of connections, 55–7, *58*; surgical experiments, 87–99
Optokinetic response, xxiii–xxiv, xxx, 6, 21–3, *22*
Order, and plasticity, 118
Organ development, embryonic, 28–30; pattern determination, 30–3
Organizer, embryonic, 30
Orientation, 253–4; commissurotomy effects, 142–5, *143*, 152–4, 186–91, *188*
Ornberg, R. L., 77
Ornstein, R., 241
Orthotopic embryo transplants, *32*
Orton, S. T., 259
Oubre, J. L., 196, 198, 203
Overall, J. E., 364
Overlearned motor skills, 173
Overman, W. H., Jr., 184

P

Paivio, A., 297, 298
Palmer, L. A., 131, 149, 161
Palmers, C., 177
Pandya, D. N., 160, 172, 196
Paralimbic region, 172
Parastriate cortex, 223
Parietal lobe, 160, 277
Parker, R., 274
Parkinson, J. K., 209
Parrots, 183
Pasquiline, R. Q., 257
Paterson, A., 283
Pathological inhibition theory, 314
Pathway-only cueing, 105–10
Pathways of nerve growth, 64, 68, 69; optic fibers, 76–83, *79, 80*, 102
Patten, B. M., 297
Pattern, P., 338
Pattern determination, embryonic organs, 30–3
Pattern discrimination, 267, 297; schema concept, 268; split-brain, 141, 186–91, *188*
Patterson, A., 232, 320
Patterson, K., 308, 314, 315
Patton, R. A., 216
Payne, B., 171
Payne, B. R., 134
Penfield, W., 377
Pennington, B. F., 356
Peptides, 337
Perarcuate cortex, 160

Perception, xxx, 231, 245; 266, 357; bihemispheric coordination, 140–1; completion effects, 235; hemispheric specialization, 240–6; in children, 353; split-brain studies, 141, 149, 234–40
Perceptual asymmetries, aging and, 365–7
Perceptual capacity, xviii
Perceptual learning, xxxi
Performance handedness, 177, 178
Peripheral nerves, 62; specificity, xvi
Peripheral visual projection, split-chiasm, 131–3
Perisylvian cortex, 356
Perret, E., 226
Perria, L., 325
Personal identity concept, 381
Persons, recognition of, 284–6
Peters, A. M., 307, 308, 315
Petersen, A. C., 257
Petrinovich, L., 225
Pfenninger, K. H., 12
Phantom limb, 268
Phases of development, theory of, 37
Phenothiazines, 256
Phenotype, cellular, 49
Phillips, R. R., 127, 209, 340
Phoneme-grapheme conversion, 308
Phonetic reading, 308–9, 311
Piaget, J., 341–2
Piatt, J., *8*, 47, 62
Pictorial semantic organization, 274–5, *275*
Piercy, M., 232, 320, 321
Pigeons, interhemispheric transfer, 222
Pioneer-fiber hypothesis, 105–6
Pizzamiglio, L., 257
Place recognition, 282–4
Plasticity, 111–20; in callosal system development, 136; in human brain growth, 353–5
Poetic awareness, 355
Poizner, H. R., 350
Polarity of tectal markers, 111
Polarization of optic field, 46–7, *47*, 86, 93–9
Polyakova, I. G., 217
Pomerat, C. M., 82
Pons, visual information, 161
Pontine nuclei, 161–3
Poranen, A., 160, 162
Porter, R., 172
Positional information, 69, 102; chemoaffinity theory, 67–8; tectal tissue, 93–7
Position-dependent ordering process, 116

Position markers, 66, 67; retinal, 80–1
Position specificity of optic-nerve cells, 55, 102
Positive emotions, left-hemisphere, 324
Posner, M. I., 313
Posterior lobes, 282
Postsynaptic cells, 338
Postural movements, 152
Potzl, O., 288
Precocious puberty, 257
Preconscious information, 236–7
Preference handedness: in humans, 178; in monkeys, 177. *See also* Handedness
Preferential chemoaffinity, 102, 115–20; and best-fit models, 116–17
Preilowski, B., xxxiv, 127, 168–71, 173
Prenatal brain growth, 335–7, 338
Prerepresentational play, 342
Prespeech, 343
Prestige, M. C., 116, 117
Pretectum, 161
Pribram, K. H., 294
Price, L. A., 254
Prigogine, I., xxxv
Primary induction, 30
Primary receptor cortex, 351
Primates: brain development, 341; hemispheric specialization, 183–4; visual system, 133–6. *See also* Apes; Monkeys
Prisko, L.-H., 295
Prismatic visual reversal, VOR and, 163
Procedural learning, in amnesiac patient, 296
Processing, hemispheric specialization, 242–5
Profile face recognition, 270–1
Profile of Nonverbal Sensitivity (PONS), 321, 322–3, *323*
Progesterone, 257, 258
Progressive regional determination, embryonic, 31–3, *32*
Propranolol, 256
Prosody, 355
Prosopagnosia, 236, 284–6, 287, 289
Protein transport, nerve regeneration, 79, 80–1
Protolanguage, infant, 343–4
Protoplasm movement, 82–3
Pseudopodial activity, nerve growth, 83
Psychiatry, 385
Psycholinguistic abilities, 311
Psychological individuality, 334
Psychology, 385; Lashley's theories, 4; subjectivism, 383

Psychometric tests, 365
Psychoneural interaction, 384
Psychopathology, hemispheric asymmetry, 254–6
Psychophysical identity theory, 383, 384
Psychophysical interaction, 382–6
Pu, M. L., 134
Puberty, cognitive asymmetry, 257
Puccetti, R., 217, 381
Purkinje cells, 165
Purves, D., 15, 16
Putnam, W., 277
Pyramidal motor system, 220
Pyramidal tract axons, 163

Q

Qualitative differences in hemispheric function, 251
Quillian, M. R., 277

R

Rabbits: conditioned responses, 163–5; interhemispheric transfer, 222; suppression of interocular transfer, 177
Radant, A., 313, 316
Ratcliff, G., 287
Rainey, C., 183
Rakic, P., 337, 351, 352
Ramon y Cajal, S., 2, 3, 9, 14, 24–7, 36, 37, 55, 62, 68, 82, 163
Ramsay, D. S., 346
Rand, R. W., 274
"The Rape," Magritte, 271, *272*
Raper, J. A., 103
Rasmussen, T., 297, 301
Rats, neural studies, xxviii–xxix, xxxii, 5–6, 20–1, 40, *40*, 51; adaptive learning, xiv–xvi, xxiii–xix; albino, binocular vision, 134; brain asymmetries, 337; cortical lesions, 4; interhemispheric transfer, 177, 223; interocular transfer, 222; laterality, 183; neonatal, NGF experiment, 9–10, *11*, *12*, 13–15
Raushecker, J. P., 339
Reaction time, brain damage and, 324
Reading: comprehension, 309–10; disorders, 305–6; and lateralization, 356; learning of, 350, 356; right hemisphere, 306–17, 377
Reafference principle, xxx
Rebert, C. S., 242
Recall, 282, 329

Receptive fields, visual, 86
Recognition: of objects, 286–91; of persons, 284–6; of place, 282–4; visual memory, 196–209
Recognition molecules on cell surface, 63
Recombinant DNA technology, 16
Red nucleus, 158
Reeves, A., 293
Reflex patterning, 54
Regard, M., 315
Regeneration of nerves, xx, xxix–xxx; abnormal connections, 26–7; axon pathways, 64; pathway-only cueing, 106–10
-optic nerve, 86, 108; in amphibians, xvi–xvii, 21–23, *22*; growth pathways, 76–83, *79*, *80*; retinal connections, 75. *See also* Chemoaffinity theory; Nerve connections; Nerve growth
Regional determination, embryonic, 31–3, *32*
Regulatory neurones, 335, 339–40
Reier, P. J., 76
Reimplantation studies, tectum innervation, 107
Reitzel, J., 336
Reivich, M., 241, 242, 243, 356
Relatedness, semantic, 277–8
Response latency, split-brain, 142–3, 144, 150–4
Response preparation, 245; perception and, 235–9
Response types, chemoaffinity coding, 103
Responses, 266
-cat, experimental variation, 142
Reticular interneurones, 336
Reticular neurones, 335
Retina: fieldlike differentiation, 45; specificity of nerve cells, 16, 43, 55–9
-ganglion cells: differentiation, 87; tectal innervation, *106*
Retinal loci, embryogenic constitution, 7, *7*
Retinal projections: contralateral transfer, *xxi*; pattern determination, 87–99; plasticity, 112; after transplants, *91*, *94*, *96*, *97*, *99*
Retinocular system, 282
Retinotectal system, 75–85; chemoaffinity studies,

101–21; of goldfish, *104*
Retinotopography: and growth, 114–15, *114*; matching systems, 116–20
Retrieval strategies of memory, 268
Rett, A., 347
Rett's syndrome, 347–9
Rhesus monkeys. *See* monkeys
Rhoades, R. W., 136
Ribosomes, 79
Ricci-Bitti, P. E., 257
Rich, S., 169
Richer, J. M., 348
Ridgway, S. H., 217
Riege, W. H., 367
Riesen, A., xx
Right-ear suppression, 294
Right-handedness, 349, 350–1; arousal asymmetry, 243–4; hemispheric asymmetries, 242–3; in infants, *344*, 346; and perceptions, 241
Right hemisphere, xxxiii–xxxiv, 181, 213, 227, 250–1, 252, 261–2, 268, 320, 356, 375–7; aging, 365–70; body part recognition, 270–1; cognitive functions, 250–1; consciousness, 377–9; delayed matching-to-sample, 294–7; and depression, 255–6; dichotic-listening, 294; dominance areas, 237–40; and emotional behavior, 323–4; facial recognition, 236, 284–6, 289; information processing, 271; language ability, 232, 234; and learning disability, 260; lesions, 284, 355; long-term memory, 271; memory impairment, 273; in monkeys, 193; object recognition, 286–9; pattern perception, 297; place recognition, 289; reading, 305–18; semantic memory, 278; semantic processing, 267; spatial processing, 241; tactual pattern matching, 296–7; verbal comprehension, 269; visual recognition, 281–91
Right parietal lesions, 285
Right temporal lesions, 285–6, 297
Right temporal lobectomy, 285, 294
Rigid chemoaffinity, 103, 113–15, 120
Ringo, J. L., 223
Rinn, W. E., 241
Rips, L. J., 277
Risberg, J., 241
Risse, G. L., 302
Rivers-Bulkley, N. T., 275

Rizzolatti, G., 129, 130, 131, 149, 152
RNA, nerve regeneration, 80
Robert, F., 145
Robinson, D. L., 133, 160, 162
Robinson, J. S., xxxi, 126, 223
Robinson, R. G., 183, 323
Rocha-Miranda, C. E., 133, 197
Rodents, laterality, 183
Rodnight, R., 255
Roffwarg, H. P., 217
Rogers, L. J., 183
Rogoff, B., 341, 356
Rosadini, G., 324
Rosch, E., 277, 278
Roscharch tests, brain damage and, 329
Rosenblith, W. A., 294
Rosene, D. L., 172
Rosenquist, A. C., 130, 131, 132, 149
Rosenquist, C., 161
Rosenthal, R., 321
Rosetti, F., 63
Rosina, A., 162
Rosner, B. S., 294
Ross, D. A., 182, 183
Ross, E. D., 310, 323, 324, 325
Rossi, G. F., 325
Rotary Two-Hand Coordination Task, 169–71, *170*
Rotated organs, embryonic, 31, *32*
Rotation of tectum, 112
Rotation of eye, xvi, xxiii–xxiv, xxx, 21–3, 47–8, 87, 103–4, *105*
Roth, R. S., 324
Roth, S., 81
Roux, W., 25, 33, 37
Rovet, J., 251, 257
Rubens, A. B., 286, 287, 289
Rugel, R. P., 260
Rumelhart, D. E., 267, 329
Rush, A. J., 323, 324
Russell, I. S., 177, 222
Russell, S. I., 177
Russell, W. R., 285

S

Sackeim, H. A., 322, 324, 344
Salamanders. *See* Amphibians
Salamy, A., 241, 352
Sandman, C. A., 257
Sanides, D., 133, 149, 161
Sanides, F., 294
Sapiro, J., 76
Saraiva, P. E. S., 145
Saron, C., 242
Saucy, M. D., 322
Scalia, R., 106

Scanning habit in reading, 312
Scars, nerve regeneration, 55–6
Scenes, recognition memory, 274–6
Schaie, J. P., 365
Schaie, K. W., 365
Schear, J. M., 369
Scheibel, A. B., 335, 336, 339, 364
Scheibel, M. D., 364
Schema concept, 268, 329, 341–2; disruption, 324–5; right-hemisphere dominance, 272–3, *273*; right-hemisphere processing, 276, 278
Schizophrenia, 254–6
Schlanger, B. B., 324
Schlanger, P., 324
Schmidt, J. T., 75, 88, 110, 112, 113, 114
Schneider, G. E., 82, 107, 108, 109, 111, 113
Schneider, M. D., 16, 69, 80
Schneps, S. E., 107
Scholes, J. H., 106
Scholes, R., 323
Schonen, S. de, 347, 352, 356
Schrier, A. M., xxxi, 158, 162
Schultz, D. H., 227
Schumann, F., 171
Schwartz, G. E., 324
Schwartz, H. D., 324
Schweiger, A., 314, 315, 316
Schwenk, G. C., 77
Science, and consciousness, 382–3
Scott, M., xxxii
Scotti, G., 192
Scoville, W. V., 294
Seagraves, M. A., 130, 132
Sechzer, J. A., 141
Segarra, J., 286, 288
Segawa, M., 347
Segmens, J., 297
Séguin, J. J., 172
Selecki, B. R., 270
Selective fasciculation, 39, 55, 65, 76
Selectivity, neuronal, 4, 65, 102–3
Self-awareness, 378–9, 381
Self-determination, 231–2
Self-differentiation of embryonic cells, 30, 34
Self-recognition, 168
Self-touching by infants, 346, 347
Semantic faciliation, 313
Semantic knowledge, 267
Semantic memory, 266–79, 339
Semantic organization, 274–6, *275*, 307
Semmes, J., 221
Sensorimotor effort, preference handedness, 177

Sensorimotor integrative functions, 145
Sensorimotor links, prenatal, 336
Sensorimotor stabilization, 173
Sensory cues, and neural adaptation, xviii
Sensory information, 266; new, 268
Sensory local sign, 51–4
Sensory systems, Sperry's experiments, 64
Sentence alexia, 307
Sequence perception, 250, 257; split-brain monkeys, 186–92, *188*
Sequential processing, 250
Serafetinides, E. A., 217, 256
Serotonergic neurosystem, and depression, 255
Serrat, A., 315
Seth, G., 346
Sex differences, 337, 346
Sex-linked factors in learning disability, 260
Sex steroids, 257, 258
Shaffer, J. W., 257
Shankweiler, D., 242, 367
Sharma, S. C., 76, 77, 80, 82, 87, 88, 96, 112, 113, 114
Shatz, C., 129, 134, 136
Sheer, D. E., 241
Shelly, C. H., 364, 365
Shelpin, Y., 160
Shenkman, A., 255
Shepard, R. N., 253
Sherman, G. F., 337
Sherman, S. M., 135
Sherrington, C. S., 3
Shimojo, S., 346
Shoben, E. J., 277
Shorrey, M. L., 37
Short-term memory, 267, 369
Shucard, D. W., 346
Shucard, J. L., 346
Shurley, J. T., 217
Siamese cats: callosal system, 134, 136; interocular transfer, 223
Sidman, M., 294, 295
Sidman, R. L., 76, 337
Sidtis, J. J., 226
Sign language, 349–50
Silver, J., 76
Silverberg-Shalev, R., 255, 262
Simoni, A., 134, 223
Simulation hypothesis, 312
Singer, W., 335, 336, 338, 339
Single hemisphere, cognitive capacity, 141
Skin-graft experiments, 23, 54, *54*
Sleep, callosal activity, 221
Sleep-wake variation, 258–9
Slow learners, commissurotomy effects, cats, 150, 154

Small, I. F., 256
Smallbone, A., 242
Smith, E. E., 277
Smith, E. L., 135
Smith, M. D., 260
Social awareness, 378–9
Social communication, 319; brain damage and, 329
Social development of children, 351
Social sensitivity, 321–2
Society for Neuroscience, Ralph W. Gerard Prize, xxxi
Soderbergh, R., 350
Sodium amytal, carotid injection, 301–2
Somatoesthesic systems, 136
Somatosensory system, 23, 48–9, 50–5
Somesthetic information transfer, 352–3
Sourbeer, E. B., 76
Sparks, R., 293
Spatial ability, 242–3; aging and, 365–70, *367*; right-hemisphere, 232, 250; tactile tasks, 241
Spatial control of differentiation, 55
Spatial discriminations in monkeys, 192, 221–2
Spatial orientation, failure of, 289
Spatial thought, 241
Speaking skills, 355
Spear, P. D., 149
Specialized processing, and perception, 244–5
Specificity in nerve connections, xvi–xvii, xx, xxix–xxx, 4–5, 6–8, 7, 20–4, 43–5; categories of, 65–6; functionalists and, 39; induction of, 48
Speech, 268, 306, 346; comprehension of, 282; learning of, 350; loss of, 281. *See also* Language
Speidel, C. C., 37, 63
Spemann, H., 27–30, 62, 67, 89
Spencer, W. A., 4
Sperling, G., 236
Sperry, N., xxxvi. *See also* Deupree, N.
Sperry, R. W., *frontis.*, 8; antifunctionalist movement, 63–5; career of, xiv–xxvi, xxviii–xxxviii; cerebral function model, 239; chemoaffinity theory, 14, 19–74, 101–3, 337–9; corollary discharge theory, 170; crossed-lesion disconnection, 196, *197*; dual instruction model, 116; on duality of mind, 216; early work, 2, 5–8; and functionalist theories, 39–41; and mind-brain problem, 137; and nerve

growth pathways, 82;
neural net studies, 20–4;
neuronal specificity theory, 6–8, 86–7; and neuropsychology, 249; Nobel
Prize, 212; optic-nerve
studies, 41–8, 77; and
pathway cueing, 106; and
plasticity, 114, 115; publications list, 389–95; on
resonance principle, 5;
students and collaborators, 396–7; supplemental
complementarity principle, 129–30; and tectal
markers, 111
-publications cited, xiv–
xxvi, xxxi, xxxii, xxxiii–
xxxv, 20, 37, 75, 76, 86,
87, 101–3, 105, 111, 113,
131, 140, 141–2, 149, 152,
154, 161, 170, 192, 234–6,
250, 268, 298, 302, 308,
325, 334, 365
-split-brain studies, 126,
129, 141–2, 149, 154, 158–
9, 165, 168, 169, 173, 217,
219, 222, 234, 235, 250,
269, 270, 286, 293, 297,
301, 306; ambient vision,
152; cats, 167; monkeys,
163, 184, 185
-tributes, 3, 8–9, 65–6, 75,
121, 140, 154, 157, 168–9,
181, 212, 215, 228, 231–2,
245–6, 263, 266, 293, 304–
5, 311, 317, 320, 331, 357,
364
Spiegler, B. J., 209
Spielberger, C. D., 313
Spinal cord, 48, 220; human
embryo, 336
Spinal fluid, 217
Spinal regions, embryonic
eye grafts, 76
Spinnler, H., 234
Splenium, 352
Split-brain, dual consciousness, 372–5, 380–1
-studies, xxxi–xxxii,
xxxiii–xxxiv; 126–7, 140–2,
173, 212, 234–40, 306,
364; corpus callosum, 129;
facial recognition, 286;
hemispheric activation,
245; hemispheric regulation, 234–40; monkeys,
184–93; two minds, 215
Split-chiasm experiments,
cats, 131–3, *132*, 134
Sponge cells, 33
Spontaneous optokinetic responses, xxiii–xxiv, xxx
Sprague, J. M., 133, 145,
149, 150, 152, 153
Springer, S. P., 241
Spydell, J. D., 241
Squire, L. R., 196, 220
Stability of tectal markers,
110–11
Stamm, J. M., xxxi, 140,
371

Stanton, G. B., 133, 160
Stein, D., 160
Stein, J., 161
Steinberg, M., 36
Steiner, J., xxxi
Stem association cells, 352
Stenevi, U., 336
Stenslie, C. E., 324
Stephenson, J. B. P., 347,
348, 354
Stereomicroscope, for brain
surgery, xxx
Stereoscopic vision, 135
Stereotype storage, 271–3
Stereotypical arrays, 277
Sterling, P., 162
Stern, D., 343
Stetson, R. H., xxviii
Stevens, S. S., xx
Stimulus encoding, 244
Stoddard, L. D., 294
Stone, J., 135, 136
Stone, L. S., xvi, xxix, 6,
31, 41, 47, 86
Stone, S. C., 257
Story comprehension, 325–
9, 329
Strabismus, and callosal development, 136
Strangers, recognition of,
356
Straschild, M., 145
*Stratum fibrosum et griseum
superficiale*, 86
Stratum opticum, 86
Strauss, E. B., 344, 335, 337
Straznicky, K., 76, 105, 108,
109, 113
Stroer, W. F., 44
Structural clusters, mental,
268
Structural models of hemispheric specialization, 241
Studdert-Kennedy, M. G.,
178, 242, 343, 344, 346,
367
Students of Sperry, 396
Stultz, W. A., 31
Sturmer, C., 106, 110, 111,
113
Subcallosal communications,
217
Subcortical asymmetries, in
infants, 346
Subcortical communication,
217
Subcortical neurones, 340–1
Subcortical processes, 174
Subcortical systems, 353
Suberi, M., 322
Subjective phenomena, xxiv,
xxxiv, 382–6
Subjective unity, 382
Sugarman, J. H., 323
Suib, M. R., 243
Sullivan, M. V., 310
Superior colliculus, 145,
158; callosal connections,
133; of cats, 162; and orienting behavior, 144–5,
154; and response latency,
150–2; and visual percep-

tion, 145–52, *148*, 149,
161
Supernumerary sex chromosomes, 257
Supin, A. Y., 217
Supplemental complementarity principle, 129–30,
130
Supplementary motor cortex, 172–3
Suprasylvian visual areas,
131–3, 135, 149
Surface affinities, 65
Sutcliffe, J., 16
Swett, F. H., 31
Syllable perception, 355
Sylvain sulcus, 337
Symbolic intelligence, genetic disorders, 347–9
Symmes, D., 145
Sympathetic fibers, 26
Synapse formation, 86, 102,
351; chemoaffinity theory,
14, 23, 87; functionalist
views, 41; patterning, xx;
selectivity, 5; vector affinity, 120
Synthetic activity, nerve regeneration, 79, 81
System optimization model,
117–20, *117, 118*
Systems-matching hypothesis, 88–9
Szekely, G., 47, 105
Szentagothai, J., 163

T

Tachistoscopic stimuli,
240–1
Tactile pattern matching,
294–7, *295, 296*
Tactual memory, 209, 367
Tadpoles, limb grafts, 4–5
Talbot, S. A., 150
Talents, and cognitive asymmetries, 261–2
Tangent screen task, 145–7,
146, 147, 148
Target screen task, 150–1
Task-related hemispheric
asymmetries, 243–4
Task-specific hemispheric
activation, 238–9, *238*,
241–2
Taste aversion, 225
Tay, D., 105
Taylor, A. C., 39
Taylor, A. M., 271
Taylor, J., 232, 281
Taylor, J. L., 215
Taylor, L., 213, 322, 367,
373, 375
Taylor, N., 242
Tectal innervation, *106*
Tectal markers, 110–11
Tectoreticular pathways, 154
Tectum, 87; chemical specificity, 43–5, 47–8, 55–8,
56; field compression, 87–
8, 96–7; fieldlike differen-

tiation, 45–7; forebrain
transplant, 92–3, *94*;
optic-fiber connections,
75–85; optic-fiber regeneration, 77–83, *80*; reimplantation, 89–96, *90, 91,
93, 94, 95*, 97, *97, 98*; retinal ganglion cells, *106*;
rotation, 108; selective innervation, 107, *107*; visual
projection, *105*
Teleost fish. *See* Fish
Temporal cortex, 352
Temporal lobe, 196, 274–7;
and alexia, 306
Tenhouten, W. D., 249
Testosterone, 258, 337, 352
Teuber, H. L., xxiv, 170
Thalamic cells, prenatal, 337
Thatcher, R. W., 352, 353,
354
Thinking, evolution of,
385
Thomas, D. G., 346
Thomas, G., 157
Thompson, D. M., 275
Thompson, F., 304
Thompson, R. F., 163
Thorndyke, P., 329
Thought: brain damage and,
324–9; development of,
341–2; and language, 232;
and movement, xxvi
Thrombotic stroke, 224
Thurstone, L. L., 254
Tieman, S. B., 184, 373
Tissue affinities, embryonic,
33–6, *35*
Tissue asymmetries, prenatal, 337
Tissue culture, axonal outgrowth, 27
Tonal evaluation, 324
Tonal memory, 356
Toncray, J. E., 173
Topographic polarity: of tectal tissue, 93–7; of visual
fields, 86, 87
Topographic regulation of
retinotectal projection,
44, 88–97, 103–10
Topographical amnesia,
282–84, 285, 289
Torczyner, H., 271
Touch localization, 353
Townes, P. L., 36
Transcortical associative
links, 340
Transparency hypothesis,
311
Tretter, F., 339
Trevarthen, C. B., xxxi,
xxxiv, 142, 149, 152, 159,
192, 214, 217, 219, 234,
237, 241, 245, 250, 286,
293, 355, 365, 371, 375
Tricyclic drugs, 256
Trinkaus, J. P., 36
Trisler, G. D., 16, 69, 80
Tropisms between cells, 33
Tschirgi, R. D., 215
Tucker, C., 324

Tucker, D. M., 321, 323, 341, 344
Tucker, G. H., 243
Tulving, E., 267, 274
Tumors, cerebral, 224
Tung, Y. L., 114
Turkewitz, G., 344
Turner, B. H., 196
Tusa, R. J., 131, 149
Tweedy, J. R., 241
Two-choice delayed alteration task, 177–8
Tyler, A., 36, 63
Typicality, and response latency, 278
Tzavaras, A., 285

U

Udin, S. B., 106, 108, 109, 111, 113
Umilta, C., 257
Unconcern, right-brain damage, 321
Unconscious information, 236–7
Understanding, 267, 268
Unicellular organisms, 83
Unilateral brain lesions, 250, 274–7, 290–1
Urodeles. *See* Amphibians
Ussher, N. T., 41

V

Values, Sperry's view, xxxv, 383
Van der Loos, H., 76, 82
Vanderplas, J. M., 368
Van Essen, D. C., 130, 133
Van Hoesen, G. W., 196, 286
Van Hof, M. W., 177, 222
Varney, N. R., 192
Vector affinity, 119–20
Vegetative behavior, 323–4
Venables, P., 255
Ventral lateral geniculate nucleus, 161
Verbal ability, 249–51; aging and, 365–70; hemispheric activation, 242–3; and nonverbal cues, 322; right-brain damage, 327–8
Verbal-cognitive set, 323
Verbal cross-cueing, 217–18
Verbal learning, image-related, 207–302
Verbal memory, 326
Verbal processing, 241
Verbal thought, 241
Verbal-visual images, 305
Vermeire, B. A., xxxi, 184, 185–90, 193
Vertical visual meridian, 129–36, 149
Vestiblo-ocular reflex (VOR), 163–4
Vestibular system, 48–50
Vidal, G., 257
VIIIth nerve, 49–50, *49*

Villa, P., 284
Vision, in infants, 344
Visual area TE, 196
Visual cortex, 158, 161–2; postnatal maturation, 352
Visual cues, response latency, 153–4
Visual discrimination, xxii, 197, *197*
Visual-field advantage, 243–4
Visual imagery, 232; and verbal learning, 297–302
Visual information, 267; interhemispheric transfer, 352
Visual memory, 127, 196–209
Visual object agnosia, 286–91
Visual perception, 140–55, 355–6
Visual projection, 86, 103–10, *105*, 112
Visual receptive fields, 86
Visual simularity, 238, *238*
Visual threshold, split-brain, 142–50, *148*, 153, 154
Visually guided movement, 142–50, 158, 160, 162, 165
Visuomotor coordination, xiv, 86, 127; crossed-lesion disconnection, *197*; optic-nerve regeneration, xvi, 87; split-brain, 158–60, 162
Visuomotor reflexes, 21–3, *22*
Visuospatial ability, 355; right-hemisphere, 253–4, 268, 270–71, 282, 319, 325–30, *327, 329*
Vocal tone evaluation, 323
Vogel, P. J., xxxiii–xxxiv, 212, 227, 293, 297, 373; commissurotomy patients, 269–70
Vogt, C., 172, 351
Vogt, O., 172
Voice recognition, 356
Voice sensitivity in infants, 346
Volitional control, 269
Volterra, V., 350
Voluntary movement ability, xviii–xix
von der Malsburg, C., 116, 136
Voneida, T. J., xxxi, 126, 161, 162, 223
Von Holst, E., xxx, 163
Vygotsky, L., 341

W

Waber, D., 257
Wada, J., 335, 337
Wada, J. A., 183
Waddington, C. H., 30
Wakefulness, 217
Walker, H. T., Jr., 257

Walker, R. A., 352
Walker, S. F., 182
Wall, P. D., 172
Walter, R. D., 274
Wang, Y. K., 134
Wapner, W., 322, 325, 327
War injuries, 224
Ward, M. M., 257
Warren, H. B., 184
Warren, J. M., 178, 182, 183, 184
Warrington, E. K., 270, 271, 285
Watson, R. T., 322, 324, 325
Webster, Doug, xxxi
Wechsler, A. F., 326, 327
Wechsler Adult Intelligence Scale (WAIS), 365, 366
Weigel-Crump, C. A., 355
Weight discrimination, 171–2
Weiler, I.-J., xxxii
Weinstein, S., 327
Weis, P., 79
Weisenberg, T., 232
Weisendanger, M., 173
Weiskrantz, L., 192, 217
Weiss, P. A., xv, xvi, xxviii, 4–5, 8, *8*, 9, 20, 27, 30, 36, 44, 50, 59, 60, 62–3, 338, functionalist theory, 37–9; nerve growth theories, 102; resonance theory, 5, 38–40, 62
Wenzel, B. M., 215
Wernicke, C., 232
Wertsch, J. V., 341
Wesner, C. E., 257
Whitaker, H. A., 314, 353
Whitelaw, V. A., 116
Whiteley, A. M., 285
Whitlock, D. G., 201
Whitteridge, D., 135, 149
Whitty, C. W. M., 283
Wickelgren, B. S., 162
Wied, D. de, 336, 337
Wiener, M. S., 241, 242
Wierman, M. E., 337
Wiersma, C. A. G., 5, 38, 60
Wiesel, T. N., 77, 129, 133, 134, 149
Wiesendanger, M., 172
Wigan, A. L., 215, 381
Willbrandt, H., 284
Willerman, L., 334
Williams, M. V., 364, 367
Williamson, P. A., 341
Willshaw, D. J., 116, 117, 136
Wilson, A. C., 340
Wilson, K. G., 109, 111, 113
Wilson, M. E., 149
Wilson, S. A. K., 269
Windle, W. F., 336
Winner, E., 326, 327
Winograd, E., 274
Wise, S. P., xix
Witelson, S. F., 251, 261, 334, 335, 337, 353
Wittrock, M. C., 364

Wolf, M. E., 344
Wollen, K. A., 274
Wolpert, L., 67, 68, 102
Woods, A. M., 364
Woodward, D. J., 161
Word blindness, 314
Word frequency, reading comprehension, 308
Word perception, 355
Word-superiority effect, 313
Wright, E. W., Jr., 172
Writing, learning of, 356
Wurtz, R., 133
Wurtz, R. H., xxv, xxvi
Wuttke, K., 257
Wyke, M. A., xxxvii, 213

X

Xenopus, compound-eye experiments, 111–12, 113; optic-nerve regeneration, *79, 81,* 105–6, 108, 110, 111; retinal ganglion cells, *106. See also* Amphibians

Y

Yaginuma, S. Y., 204
Yahr, P., 337
Yakovlev, P. I., 225, 334, 351, 352, 352
Yamaga, K., 216
Yehuda, S., 259
Yeni-Komshian, G. H., 183
Yeo, C. H., 165
Yerkes Laboratories of Primate Biology, xvii, xxi, xxv
Yeudall, L. T., 255
Yin, T. C. T., 245
Yinon, W., 339
Yntema, C. L., 31
Yoon, M. G., xxxii, 2, 69, 75, 107, 111, 112
Young, G., 346
Yozawitz, A., 255
Yuille, J. C., 297, 298

Z

Zaidel, D. W., xxxiv, xxxvii, 169, 213, 217, 250, 274, 297, 301, 304, 311, 325, 378
Zaidel, E., xxxiii, xxxiv, 181, 213, 217, 220, 227, 234, 252, 322, 375, 377, 381
Zangwill, O. L., xxxvii, 213, 232, 320, 381
Zaur, I., xvi, 41, 86
Zeier, H., 177
Zeki, S. M., 130, 133, 136, 160, 162, 201, 223
Zeuthen, E., 257
Zimmerberg, B., 182
Zoccolotti, P., 257
Zola-Morgan, S., 196, 220
Zurif, E. B., 324